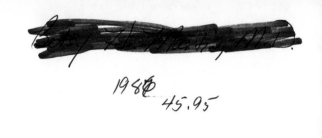

CHEST ROENTGENOLOGY

BENJAMIN FELSON, M.D.

Professor and Director, Department of Radiology,
University of Cincinnati College of Medicine and Medical Center;
Consultant to Cincinnati and Dayton Veterans Administration Hospitals;
National Consultant to the Medical Corps of the United States
Air Force, Army, Navy, and Veterans Administration,
United States Public Health Service,
Armed Forces Institute of Pathology,
and Walter Reed General Hospital

W. B. SAUNDERS COMPANY

Philadelphia   London   Toronto
Mexico City   Rio de Janeiro   Sydney   Tokyo

W. B. Saunders Company: West Washington Square
                           Philadelphia, Pa. 19105

                           1 St. Anne's Road
                           Eastbourne, East Sussex BN21 3UN, England

                           1 Goldthorne Avenue
                           Toronto, Ontario M8Z 5T9, Canada

                           Apartado 26370 – Cedro 512
                           Mexico 4, D.F., Mexico

                           Rua Coronel Cabrita, 8
                           Sao Cristovao Caixa Postal 21176
                           Rio de Janeiro, Brazil

                           9 Waltham Street
                           Artarmon, N.S.W. 2064, Australia

                           Ichibancho, Central Bldg., 22-1 Ichibancho
                           Chiyoda-Ku, Tokyo 102, Japan

Listed here is the latest translated edition of this book together with the language of the translation and the publisher. 1st Ed. 1/12/78. Spanish Editorial Cientifico-Medica, Barcelona, Spain.

Listed here is the latest translated edition of this book together with the language of the translation and the publisher. 1st Ed. 1/31/78. Japanese Hirokawa Publishing Co., Tokyo, Japan.

Chest Roentgenology   ISBN 0-7216-3591-1

Print No.:   19

To my wife Virginia and our children,
for their pride and forbearance.

PROLOGUE

This book started out as a second edition of my previous work, *Fundamentals of Chest Roentgenology*, but in final draft it bore no more resemblance to its predecessor than a hirsute son to his bald-headed father. Although most of the ten chapters from *Fundamentals* have been incorporated, hardly any paragraph remains unchanged and many completely new sections have been inserted. The illustrations, where still pertinent, have been retained but are interspersed with a host of current ones. Further, five additional chapters have been added. So, this is not merely a new lamp for an old, but a modern light that I hope casts a broader, more luminescent beam — if not psychedelic, at least fluorescent.

Why all the changes? For one thing, fresh experiences have bred fresh ideas, and these I was impelled to include. For another, past sins of omission, purposeful and accidental, were too numerous and too obvious to be ignored. Also, newer knowledge had to be incorporated and misconceptions corrected. Finally, though I once believed that fundamental concepts do not change, I have since changed this fundamental concept. A basic principle well conceived and successfully tested should by rights become a fixed, immutable, irrevocable scientific law — but it doesn't. So I've had to take a cue from our professor of psychiatry who solved the problem of hand-me-down medical student examinations by asking the same questions each year — he simply changed the answers.

Chest roentgenography is generally a poor bargain for the patient. The films are quickly obtained and even more quickly interpreted. You can read 20 chest films while your partner is performing one G.I. series, and often do. Important lesions are thereby missed or dismissed with such vague diagnoses as "pneumonitis" or "interstitial infiltrate." I believe we should allot a liberal amount of time to study chest films and spend it scrutinizing them systematically, saving the obvious abnormality, like dessert, for the last. The harm caused by overlooking a lesion needs no emphasis. But just as noxious is the apparent lesion inadequately studied. The two standard views generally suffice if no lesion is visible, but the problem case requires a more detailed and individualized roentgen work-up. Yet, the film jacket may grow fat with monotonously repeated PA and lateral views as the patient is "studied" into oblivion.

All of us have a tendency to make a diagnosis on the basis of past experience with similar shadows. But remember: many dissimilar conditions cast similar shadows. Is there a better way? The drunk is staggering along the street, pulling a chain behind him. The cop stops him and asks, "Why are you pulling that chain?" "Did you ever try to push one?" he replies. Soberly, in radiology there *is* a better way: base your conclusions on solid principles. Obviously, you must know the fundamentals in order to use them; thus, we come to the main purpose of this book—to make you familiar with the rules of chest roentgenology and to show you how to apply them. Specific diseases are considered only as they relate to the principles.

An important feature of this book is personal observation, sometimes called experience. Unfortunately, when I accept the views of others at face value without personal substantiation, I often propagate inaccuracy and false premise. I even have trouble defining such concepts and at times feel as frustrated as a one-armed fisherman trying to describe the size of his catch. What applies to the author applies equally to the reader, who is therefore advised to accept with healthy skepticism what he reads here, and then only until he can test it by his own experience. I trust, then, that you will savor of the repast I have set before you and decide what to swallow and what to spit out.

This book is intended first for cover-to-cover reading and later as an unobtrusive consultant. It reflects mainly my own interests and experience, although I have borrowed freely from others. Whenever my memory and files have not failed me, I have acknowledged my debt. All cases depicted are proved, unless otherwise stated.

Special recognition must be accorded to the pioneering publications and concepts of Dr. Leo G. Rigler and the late Dr. Felix G. Fleischner, who probed the complexities of chest roentgenology and solved many of its riddles. I express my thanks also to the many physicians and editors, most of whom are individually acknowledged in the text, who have given me permission to use their material or have helped me in various other ways. Sections of this book were supported by Grant No. GM-12458-02 of the NIH and by Grant No. TR 170 of the Veterans Administration. Many of the lists and tables were developed for and borrowed from the book-in-process *Gamuts in Radiology—Comprehensive Lists of Roentgen Differential Diagnosis* by Maurice M. Reeder and Benjamin Felson.[970a]

To Miss Claire (Pat) Bittner and to Drs. Henry Felson, Corning Benton, Donald J. Heimbrock, Kenneth Kattan, Harold N. Margolin, Myron Moskowitz, Lee S. Rosenberg, Harold J. Schneider, Frederic N. Silverman, Harold B. Spitz, Aaron S. Weinstein, and Jerome F. Wiot, and all the other members of our staff, past and present, who kept the department afloat when I was submerged, my debt of gratitude is enormous. To Mrs. Margy Himelhoch, who worked long and effectively on a multitude of details, my profound thanks. The same applies to the staff at W. B. Saunders Company, and to Mrs. Sophie Travis and Mrs. Mary Ellen Meyer. Special acknowledgment goes to the late Dr. Leslie Ringel, who helped me understand the nature of the companion shadows of the ribs. Tragically, this brilliant, exciting young resident died in his twenties. Finally, to our many residents and fellows over the years I would like to say that your patience, cooperation, and especially your stimulation helped make this book possible.

BENJAMIN FELSON, M.D.

CONTENTS

CHAPTER 1

THE ROENTGEN WORK-UP

It always irks me to be confronted, in consultation, with a series of PA and lateral chest teleroentgenograms strung along a bank of viewboxes. No obliques, no Buckys, no spots, no tomos, no barium. I look at the films helplessly, thinking "How in the world can I make a diagnosis with so little information? They wouldn't consider a PA and lateral of the stomach an adequate study."

Then I say apologetically, "You ought to fluoroscope him." Everyone seems let down—and I leave, suspecting that the next move will be the surgeon's.

Why the hell am I so defensive? I shouldn't be. A set of PA and lateral teleroentgenograms of the chest serves admirably for *detecting* most lesions and aids in determining what additional studies need to be performed. Unless the clinical or roentgen diagnosis is evident, one should then proceed with further roentgen study of the patient. Depending on the nature of the changes, the roentgen work-up may begin with fluoroscopy or with the exposure of additional films.

FLUOROSCOPY

Fluoroscopy of the chest is becoming somewhat of a lost art. Fear of excessive radiation to the patient is the usual reason given for its omission, although it is generally conceded that, when properly performed, fluoroscopy may provide invaluable information about a chest lesion.[955, 1183, 1340] Complete chest fluoroscopy can be accomplished within a few minutes if the examiner applies a well-organized approach. With modern image amplification equipment, the patient is exposed to little added radiation if certain simple precautions are taken, such as utilizing a small shutter opening, adequate filters, and reasonable speed. It is my firm conviction that the benefits of appropriately indicated fluoroscopy far outweigh the possible hazards.

For purposes of instructing students and residents, I have divided chest fluoroscopy into five phases: *observation, rotation, breathing, ingestion,* and *tilting.* Their first letters spell out the word *ORBIT,* which serves as a mnemonic.

OBSERVATION

After a brief preliminary fluoroscopic scanning of the entire chest, including the larynx and heart, attention is directed to the lesion in question. Its size, shape, homogeneity, and margins are closely studied. Evidence of pulsation should be noted; however, this is of little significance unless much of its circumference is clearly visible. The recognition of intrinsic pulsation depends on the presence of a simultaneous outward thrust of opposite margins of the lesion. Even when this type of pulsation is apparent, an aneurysm cannot be reliably distinguished from a tumor. Aneurysms often contain clot, which dampens the expansile pulsation, and tumors occasionally surround a vessel and may then appear to pulsate expansively.[262] Facetiously stated, if a mass pulsates, I call it a tumor; if it doesn't, it's an aneurysm.

ROTATION

By slightly rotating the patient (10 to 20 degrees) one can quickly establish whether an opacity lies anteriorly or posteriorly.

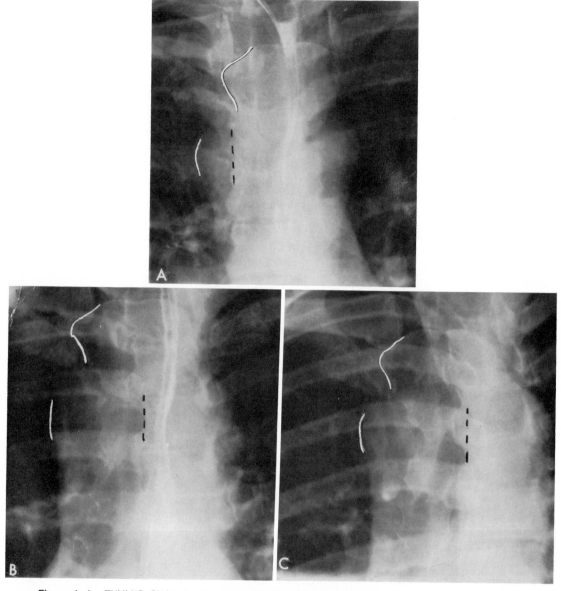

Figure 1–1.   THYMIC CYST OF RIGHT SUPERIOR MEDIASTINUM[673] LOCALIZED BY ROTATION

Spot films: *A,* Frontal view. *B,* 10 degree rotation toward the left anterior oblique. *C,* 20 degree rotation. With increasing rotation, the lateral border of the mass (retouched) shifts away from the right border of the spine (broken line) and moves in the same direction as the manubrium (retouched). This indicates that the mass lies far anteriorly. (From Felson, B.[324]; reproduced with permission of Dis. Chest.)

Storch utilizes the sternum and spine as reference points.[1183] If, on rotation, the lesion appears to move in the same direction as the spine, it is posterior; if it appears to shift with the sternum, it is anterior (Fig. 1–1). The amount of displacement of the lesion with rotation indicates how far it lies from the center of the thorax (the vertical axis on which the patient is rotated). Obviously, a peripheral lesion will shift more with rotation than a central one.

As any lesion is brought closer to the fluoroscopic screen, its image appears smaller and sharper. Thus, if a density is smaller in the PA projection (patient facing the screen) than in the AP, it lies in the anterior portion of the thorax. The patient must be in true frontal position and be in contact with both tabletop and screen for the results of this maneuver to be valid.

Still another method of localization can be utilized. With the patient facing the examiner, the shutters are opened fairly wide and the screen positioned so that the image of the lesion lies along one side of the visible fluoroscopic beam. The screen is slowly shifted transversely in the direction of the lesion, which now seems to move. The greater this apparent movement, the more posterior is the lesion. Localization by this method, called *parallax*, requires considerable practice. However, by taping a coin to the skin over the image of the lesion and then observing the relative displacement of the coin and the lesion as the screen is shifted or the patient rotated, localization is simplified.[1184]

Rotation also serves to separate a lesion from adjacent structures so that a clearer view of it may be obtained. Obviously, if the lesion can be separated entirely from a superimposed structure, there is no likelihood that it is connected with that structure. Rotation is also helpful in differentiating hilar node enlargement from hilar vessels. As the patient is turned, the nodes remain rounded, whereas vascular shadows elongate.

BREATHING

It is important to study the movement of the abnormal shadow during breathing. On inspiration, the spine remains immobile while the ribs move upward, the diaphragm and lower lung fields move downward, and the vascular markings spread apart. By careful observation during respiration, it is often possible to relate a lesion to the thoracic wall, mediastinum, heart, diaphragm, or lung. A point of reference is taken in sequence on each structure in close proximity to the abnormal opacity (rib, vertebra, segment of diaphragm, pulmonary vessel, and so on), and the relative movement between this structure and the density in question is noted. If the two move together synchronously as a unit, a connection between them is postulated, but even the slightest amount of independent motion indicates that they are not intimately associated.

Two cases of mediastinal tumor serve to illustrate the value of this information. The small mass in the left lower posterior thorax adjacent to the spine in Figure 1–2 was observed to move slightly with respiration. This motion appeared to be independent of and less than that of the left hemidiaphragm, the overlying ribs, the heart, the esophagus, and the adjacent lung markings. It was concluded, therefore, that the mass was not connected with any of these struc-

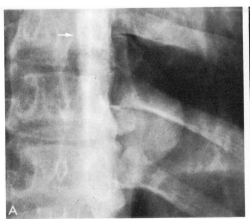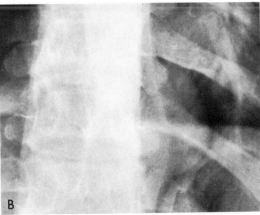

Figure 1–2. RESPIRATORY MOVEMENT IN A MEDIASTINAL BRONCHOGENIC CYST[240, 786]

Inspiration (A) and expiration (B) show a slight respiratory movement which is independent of that of the left hemidiaphragm, lower left ribs, heart, and adjacent lung markings. Note the changing relation of the mass to the transverse processes. The left paraaortic line is elevated, the right (arrow) is difficult to distinguish from the paraesophageal line.

tures or with the immobile spine. By this process of elimination, it was postulated that it lay in the mediastinal soft tissues. At operation a mediastinal bronchogenic cyst was found.[240, 786]

In another patient (Fig. 1–3), a large density was discovered in the left lower posterior thorax adjacent to the spine. Fluoroscopically, the mass appeared to remain fixed while the superimposed posterior ribs, heart, diaphragm, and lung markings showed normal respiratory excursions. It was apparent that we were dealing with a mediastinal mass attached to the spine. At operation, a large neurofibroma arising from multiple spinal nerve roots was found.

The effects of respiration on the heart and mediastinum should also be carefully observed. In obstructive hyperinflation, the heart and other mediastinal structures, even including the esophagus, shift toward the side of the lesion on inspiration and in the opposite direction on expiration. This is attributable to the fact that the trachea and bronchi normally widen on inspiration and narrow on expiration. Air is able to pass the site of bronchial constriction on inspiration, but is partially trapped behind the obstruction on expiration, as the lumen of the diseased bronchus narrows. The pressure in the affected lung remains relatively constant throughout the respiratory cycle, so on expiration the mediastinum swings toward the lower pressured contralateral lung. It returns to its initial position with each inspiration, when there is less discrepancy in pressure between the two lungs[1007] (Figs. 1–4 and 3–67).

In obstructive collapse, the pressure differential between the two lungs is greater on inspiration, since more air enters the normal than the collapsed lung. Again, the swing of the mediastinum is toward the affected lung on inspiration. Thus, regardless of the initial position of the mediastinum—

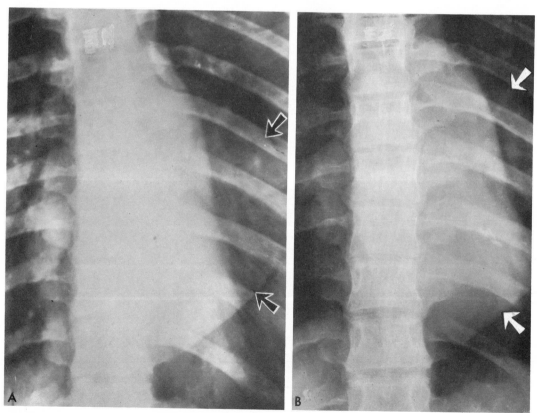

Figure 1–3. LACK OF RESPIRATORY MOVEMENT IN A HUGE POSTERIOR MEDIASTINAL NEUROFIBROMA

On inspiration *(A)* and expiration *(B)* the ribs, heart, and diaphragm are seen to move independently of the mass (arrows), which maintains a constant relationship to the spine.

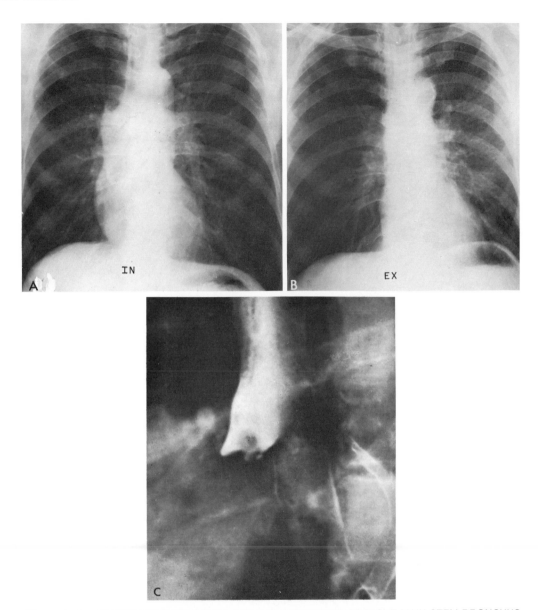

Figure 1–4. OBSTRUCTIVE HYPERINFLATION IN CARCINOMA OF RIGHT MAIN STEM BRONCHUS

On inspiration *(A)*, the heart and mediastinal structures are displaced toward the right. On expiration *(B)*, the right lung retains its radiolucency and, if anything, enlarges. The mediastinal structures swing toward the left. The bronchogram *(C)* shows an irregular occlusion in the right main bronchus, surprisingly complete in the absence of collapse. The lumen is undoubtedly partially patent but the viscosity of the oil prevents it from passing farther into the bronchus.[1053]

often displaced toward the normal side in obstructive overaeration and toward the affected side in collapse—the *direction* of mediastinal swing on inspiration is always toward the side of the lesion. Holinger and Rigby have described a variety of valvelike mechanisms that occur during respiratory exchange in obstructive emphysema and in collapse.[559] Recognition of mediastinal shift is facilitated by placing an index finger or other marker along each border of the heart shadow on the fluoroscopic screen and observing the direction of displacement on deep inspiration and expiration.[1053]

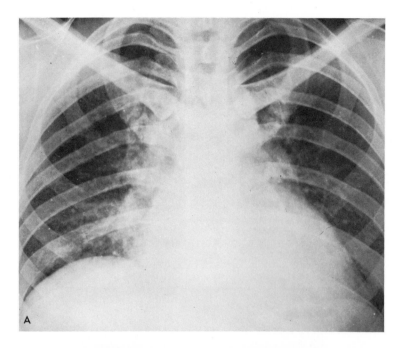

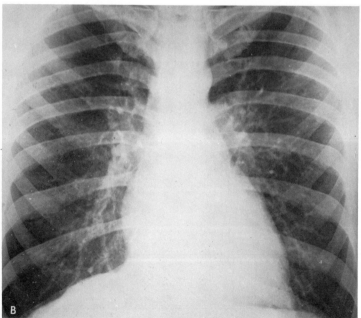

Figure 1–5. NORMAL RESPIRATORY EFFECTS

Expiration *(A)* and inspiration *(B)* films in a healthy young adult. The appearance in *A* simulates congestive fail-ure. The films were exposed a few moments apart.

In normal individuals, the cardiac silhouette usually appears to shrink on inspiration and to enlarge on expiration, the degree of change being more pronounced in children. In a group of 280 normal individuals for whom we had inspiration and expiration films, made without any special coaching, about one fourth showed little change in cardiac size between the two films; the rest showed an obvious alteration in all cardiac dimensions. The lung bases showed striking "clouding" on expiration (Fig. 1–5), resembling pulmonary edema, in 28 per cent, mild to moderate haziness in 46 per cent, and little or no change in 25 per cent.

Paradoxical enlargement on inspiration and diminution on expiration occur in partial tracheal or laryngeal obstruction from a tumor or foreign body, in bilateral chronic emphysema (Fig. 1–6), in acute bronchial asthma, and in diffuse bronchiolitis of infants.[855, 1000] In these conditions, the lungs appear unusually radiolucent on both inspiration and expiration, and the diaphragm excursion is restricted. The intrapulmonary vascular markings may also diminish paradoxically on expiration.[1004]

When dealing with cystic lesions in the lung, breathing maneuvers are extremely valuable. Cystic bronchiectasis will infallibly show a striking enlargement on inspiration and shrinkage on expiration and cough because of the wide-open bronchial com-munication (Fig. 1–7). An emphysematous bulla will not change significantly with respiration. A fluid filled cyst may elongate on inspiration, but a solid mass will not.[1346]

The Valsalva and Müller maneuvers may aid in differentiating between a vascular and nonvascular shadow, since alteration of the intraalveolar pressure often causes vascular structures to change in size.[441, 1004, 1278] These techniques may be of particular help in differentiating mediastinal and hilar lymph node enlargement from vascular shadows. With the Valsalva maneuver, there is an increase in intrathoracic pressure and a reduction in cardiac output. These result from lowering of the effective filling pressure of both ventricles, principally because of obstruction of venous return to the right heart. The heart diminishes in size for a few beats, then enlarges.[1127] Our simple instructions to the patient are, "Take in a deep breath; now hold it; now strain down as if you're moving your bowels—only don't!" Once someone did.

Sniffing (mouth closed, rapid forceful inspiration through nose), snorting (rapid forceful expiration), and coughing provide more dramatic alterations of intrathoracic pressure. Such breathing tactics are of particular value in eliciting diaphragmatic excursion and paradoxical motion in phrenic paralysis or eventration.[1346] The changes are rapidly produced, so that cine or video tape

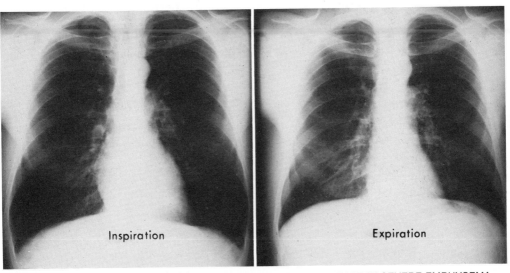

Inspiration   Expiration

Figure 1–6. PARADOXICAL RESPIRATORY EFFECT ON THE HEART IN SEVERE EMPHYSEMA

Fluoroscopy revealed marked limitation of diaphragmatic excursion with increase in heart size during inspiration. *A*, Inspiration. *B*, Expiration.

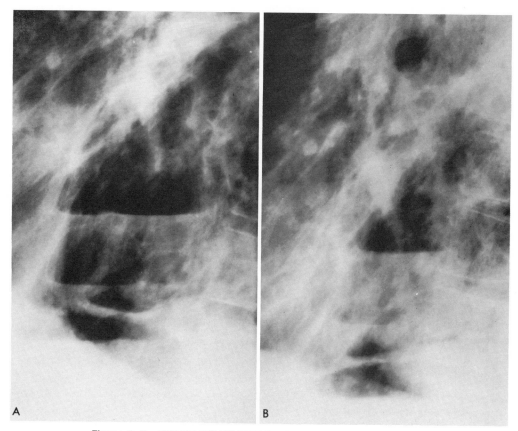

Figure 1–7. RESPIRATORY EFFECT ON CYSTIC BRONCHIECTASIS

Inspiratory enlargement *(A)* and expiratory collapse *(B)* of three air-fluid filled cavities. Lateral projection.

recording with slow playback is helpful. Because the image permitted by the cine screen is small, it is often necessary to use the oblique or lateral projection for comparison of the motion of the two hemidiaphragms.

INGESTION

Barium study is absolutely essential in any instance of an intrathoracic density of unknown nature. The abnormal shadow may actually represent the esophagus or stomach itself, as in the case of a diaphragmatic hernia or cardiospasm; or an unsuspected gastrointestinal abnormality may prove to be the underlying cause of the intrathoracic lesion, as in chronic aspiration pneumonia secondary to esophageal obstruction.[517]

Indentation or displacement of the esophagus often aids in the localization of a mediastinal mass. Esophageal impingement may be the only roentgen sign of enlarged mediastinal lymph nodes.[373, 829] This is especially true of the bifurcation nodes (Figs. 1–8, 2–2 and 6–7), enlargement of

Figure 1–8. CARCINAL NODE ENLARGEMENT (Opposite)

Probable histoplasmosis in a young physician. *A,* Right parahilar pneumonia at the time of an acute respiratory illness. Chest films 2 months earlier and 2 months later were normal. *B* and *C,* AP and left oblique views show carinal node imprint on the esophagus (arrows). The histoplasma complement fixation test showed a rising titer and the skin test became positive. *D,* 6 months later. Contraction of the lymph node has resulted in a traction diverticulum at the site of the previous imprint.

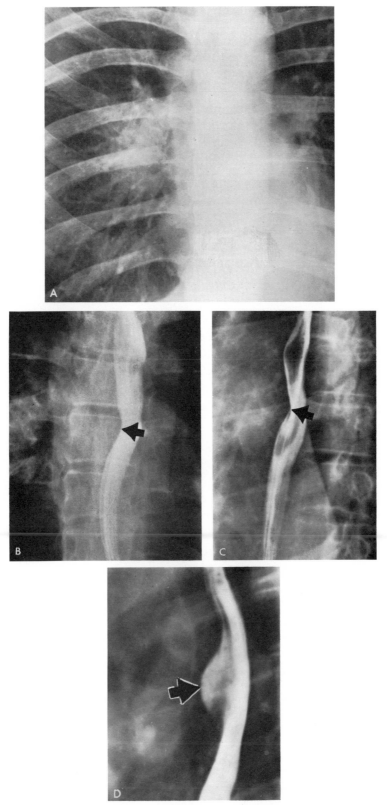

Figure 1–8. See opposite page for legend.

which often produces an extrinsic pressure defect on the esophagus at the level of the carina, usually seen best in the left oblique view (see Chap. 6). The combination of such a defect and a pulmonary lesion usually indicates bronchogenic carcinoma in the older patient and tuberculosis or histoplasmosis in the young (Fig. 1–8).

All of us have difficulty in judging the significance of a prominent hilar shadow. In a number of these cases, an extrinsic imprint on the esophagus at the level of the carina establishes that lymph node enlargement is truly present.

TILTING

Examination of the patient in the prone, supine, Trendelenburg, lordotic, or decubitus position is often rewarding. The decubitus examination can be made by having the patient lie on his side on a stretcher in front of the vertical fluoroscope, but tilting the upright patient to the right and left in the frontal view and having him bend at the waist in the lateral view are more practical methods for obtaining the same information. The lordotic position can be assumed during upright fluoroscopy and may be accomplished through the use of sandbags under the lower ribs in supine fluoroscopy. The recognition of pleural fluid, confirmation of fluid levels, delineation of middle lobe disease, and displacement of pulmonary opacities from overlying structures are facilitated by applying these gravitational methods.

Tilting techniques may also be useful in determining whether a mass is fixed. In Figure 1–9, the upright and right lateral decu-

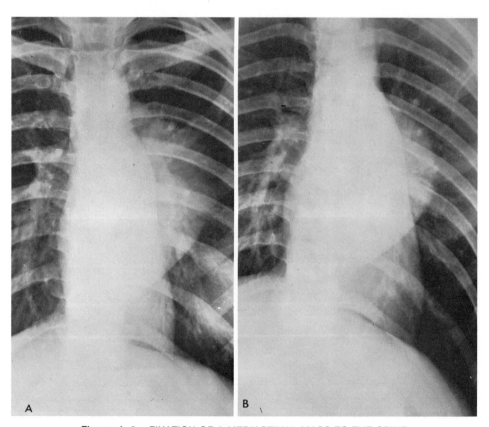

Figure 1–9. FIXATION OF A MEDIASTINAL MASS TO THE SPINE

Same patient as Figure 1–3. *A,* Upright film shows a large left posterior mediastinal mass. *B,* Right lateral decubitus film (reproduced upright for comparison). The large mass does not fall toward the right, indicating its fixation to the bony structures. Neurofibroma arising from multiple spinal nerve roots. Note the high position of the right hemidiaphragm, normal for this decubitus position.

bitus views demonstrate that the large posterior mediastinal mass is fixed to the bony
structures of the left paravertebral gutter. It
proved to be a neurofibroma. By similar
means, we have been able to recognize the
free movement of a fungus ball within a thin
walled cavity[732] (Fig. 8–16).

Spot films or cine obtained during fluoroscopy are an important part of the examination since they provide a permanent record
of the findings and bring out details that are
difficult to see on the screen or on conventional films. Fluoroscopy also facilitates the
selection of the optimal position, centering,
rotation, and angulation for additional
roentgenograms. Cine or television tape recording may provide key information by
permitting slow motion study of a moving or
pulsating lesion. Fluoroscopy and filming
are both important. Like two kids sleeping
together on a wet sheet, it's often impossible to determine which has made the larger
contribution.

Obviously, fluoroscopy is not indicated in
every problem case. It is often immediately
apparent from the initial films that fluoroscopy has little to offer. However, this procedure should be considered in every diagnostic dilemma, for there is no adequate
substitute for it. As one gains experience
with this often neglected method, its value
is soon appreciated.

ROENTGENOGRAPHY

Many of us fall into the habit of attempt-
ing to make a definitive diagnosis from one
or two films, seldom thinking of the advantages of other technical facilities. This attitude is much like that of my little boy who,
when I asked him why he always held his
thumb in his mouth, replied, "Where else
can I put it?" Although the obvious answer
was not supplied in that instance, it should
be emphasized here that one should give
conscious consideration to additional
roentgen studies in every case presenting a
diagnostic problem. A variety of supple-
mental views and procedures is available in
the roentgenologist's repertoire, and each
has its special indications.[199, 955, 1000, 1020, 1342]

THE LATERAL VIEW

This view hardly requires discussion but
several points bear emphasis. Since so
much of the lung and mediastinum are hidden on the frontal view by the shadows of
the heart, diaphragm, and bony structures, it
is not surprising that lesions obscured in
PA projection are often clearly visible on
the lateral film. Mediastinal emphysema
and the small thymoma fall into this category.[455] The value of *routine* lateral views is
therefore apparent.

Customarily, the left lateral view is obtained because more of the left lung is obscured than the right on the frontal view. If
a pathologic process is known to be present,
obviously the lateral view that brings it
closer to the film should be selected. To
delineate the anterior mediastinum, it is
better to obtain the lateral view with the
arms and shoulders drawn back (military
position) rather than extended upward.

The lateral view is of inestimable value in
revealing enlargement or collapse of a diseased lobe or segment and is often the only
projection that will provide this information. The compartment in which a mediastinal lesion is located is of considerable
diagnostic importance and is best determined from the lateral film. This view is
also essential for localizing encapsulated
fluid prior to tapping. These represent but a
few of its many indications.

I do not mean to imply that the lateral
view will *invariably* demonstrate a lesion
that has been visualized in the frontal projection. On the contrary, I have often been
disappointed because the lateral film has
failed to demonstrate a density of considerable proportion that has been clearly shown
in other projections (Fig. 2–27). This will be
discussed in greater detail in the next
chapter.

THE OBLIQUE VIEW[931]

As mentioned earlier, oblique views are
helpful in localizing a lesion, in visualizing
its borders, and in projecting it free of overlying structures. They are preferable to the
lateral view in the case of bilateral disease,
since the likelihood of superimposition of
the images on the two sides is obviated.

The pulmonary vasculature is particularly well shown in oblique projection, especially when made with a grid.

The appropriate degree of obliquity is best determined by fluoroscopy. For lung lesions, a lesser degree is best (e.g., 25 degrees); for cardiac conditions, greater rotation is required (on the order of 60 degrees). An oblique projection in the swimmer's position provides an excellent view of the length of the trachea (Fig. 1–10). Hereafter, I will use *left oblique* to indicate left anterior and right posterior oblique views, and *right oblique* to indicate right anterior and left posterior oblique views.

THE RECUMBENT VIEW

We prefer the supine to the erect view for the very ill patient and the young child. Technical difficulties in obtaining satisfactory upright views in these patients often negate the advantages of the conventional

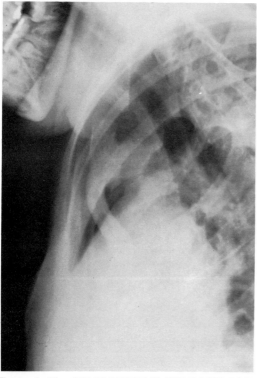

Figure 1–10. OBLIQUE VIEW IN SWIMMER'S POSITION

The film was obtained with patient upright and back to cassette, right arm raised, and left arm lowered.

position. It is possible to obtain a teleroentgenogram of the recumbent patient, but seldom necessary.

The recumbent view is useful in distinguishing between free and encapsulated fluid and between an elevation of a hemidiaphragm and the free fluid trapped below the inferior surface of the lung (Fig. 9–4).

THE LATERAL DECUBITUS VIEW

This cross-table frontal view is actually superior to the recumbent view for demonstrating small amounts of free fluid, since the X-ray beam strikes the fluid surface tangentially rather than vertically. The dependent side should be elevated from the table by a folded sheet or the like so that the lateral portion of the thorax is not obscured by the shadow of the X-ray table. Decubitus (the word merely means *recumbent*) views in lateral, prone, and supine positions with the horizontal beam are also useful in shifting free fluid about so that the portions of the underlying lung obscured by the fluid in other positions are uncovered. The lateral decubitus view may be helpful in determining the confines of a cavity (Fig. 1–11) and in demonstrating a small pneumothorax. It should be noted that in the lateral decubitus position the dependent hemidiaphragm normally rises considerably in the thorax (Fig. 1–9) and its excursion is increased. For years I assumed the "up" side showed the greater respiratory movement; I learned the hard way—from a resident.

THE LORDOTIC VIEW

In this AP view, "invented" by Felix Fleischner,[368] the patient leans backward with his back arched in lordosis so that only the interscapular region touches the plate changer. The shoulders should be rotated forward. Bucky technique enhances the detail.[1341] Someone conceived the brilliant idea that angling the tube upward would be simpler than angling the patient backward, and now this is generally the method of obtaining these views. By a quirk of logic, it is still called the lordotic view.

The clavicles are projected above the lung and the ribs lie more or less parallel to the floor, so that their anterior and posterior

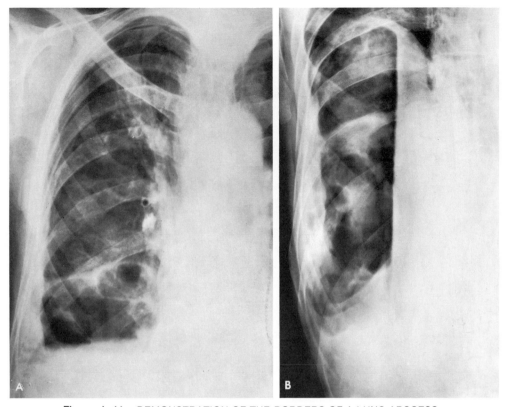

Figure 1–11. DEMONSTRATION OF THE BORDERS OF A LUNG ABSCESS

A, Upright film. *B,* Left decubitus (reproduced upright for comparison). In *B,* the fluid level helps to delineate the thin superior wall of the huge right lower lobe abscess, which extends much higher than is apparent in *A.*

portions are superimposed. In this position, an anterior lesion is projected upward (Fig. 1–12).

The lordotic view gives a relatively bone-free view of the upper lung fields (Fig. 1–13). It is also extremely valuable in confirming the presence of middle lobe[260] and lingular disease, often inconclusively demonstrated on the routine PA and lateral teleroentgenograms. In the lordotic position, the roentgen beam traverses a longer axis of the middle lobe and lingula than in the upright, producing a denser shadow when collapse is present. Furthermore, in this position the lower portion of the major septum sometimes lies perpendicular to the film, resulting in sharp demarcation of the lower margin of the infiltrate (Fig. 1–14). The lordotic view often clearly depicts mediastinal herniation. It is also helpful in determining the anteroposterior location of a lesion by indicating the parallax shift between the lesion and a segment of rib (Fig. 1–13).

A 15 to 30 degree *kyphotic* view has been recommended for the demonstration of upper rib and apical lesions and abnormalities in the posterior costophrenic sinus.[596, 598] I have had little experience with either of these projections.

STEREOSCOPIC VIEWS

Stereoscopy of the chest can be useful in studying apical lesions partially obscured by the bony structures, in detecting cavities, in localizing densities, and so forth. Since it provides two views from slightly different angles, a lesion entirely hidden by a rib or another structure on one film may be projected free and clearly seen on the second. Stereoscopic Bucky films are more successful than conventional films in demonstrating calcification within a pulmonary nodule. Although I was schooled in this

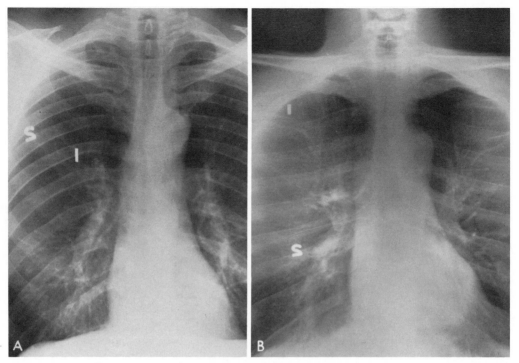

Figure 1–12. EFFECT OF LORDOTIC VIEW ON APICAL LESIONS

A, PA teleroentgenogram. Lead letters are taped to the chest wall, no. 1 anterior and no. 2 posterior. *B,* In the lordotic position, anterior lesions (no. 1) are projected upward and posterior lesions (no. 2) downward.

method—Dunham,[281] its enthusiast, was one of my teachers—I seldom use it now. Other methods, particularly tomography, better provide this type of information.

THE EXPIRATORY FILM

Respiratory techniques have already been discussed, but several additional points should be emphasized. Occasionally a pneumothorax will be demonstrated only on an expiratory film (Figs. 1–15 and 9–22). Vascular lesions can be distinguished from solid or cystic ones if they shrink on inspiration or on Valsalva maneuver. This sign is infallible in the recognition of an enlarged azygos vein (Fig. 5–45). However, a soft or mobile nonvascular mass may *appear* to shrink on inspiration if it changes shape or shifts in the mediastinum.

THE GRID FILM

When dealing with a heavy patient or dense infiltrate, the routine nongrid film does not adequately portray the roentgen details. Increasing the penetration by adding kilovoltage or milliamperage will provide better penetration, but the scatter effect of the secondary radiation is so enhanced that the contrast and detail are still poor. A moving or fixed grid, by blocking out much of the scatter, will provide infinitely better contrast and detail.[1196] The grid film is therefore essential in studying a dense pleural or pulmonary opacity (Fig. 1–16); a condition involving the bony cage (Fig. 1–17); an abnormality obscured by the heart or diaphragm or, in a heavy patient, by the chest wall or breast (Fig. 2–36); and a lesion in which cavitation, calcification, or foreign body is suspected. The grid film shows the trachea and mediastinal structures well; it is superb for the delineation of an air bronchogram and may even show the normal pulmonary vascular markings through a pleural effusion.

Because a small pulmonary infiltrate may be "burned out" by the grid technique, in my opinion the *routine* use of grids for PA teleroentgenography is not warranted.

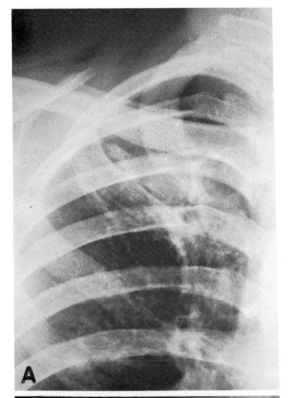

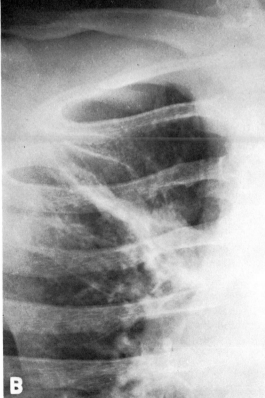

However, a number of my colleagues disagree. I believe a better case can be made for routine grid lateral views.

I have not personally utilized supervoltage technique but, from the films I have seen, this method is capable of beautifully delineating mediastinal and certain intrapulmonary lesions.[626]

TOMOGRAPHY

This procedure is so valuable that it should be available wherever definitive chest roentgen diagnosis is attempted. Its importance in the detailed study of an intrathoracic lesion has long been established and need only be emphasized for those who have had little experience with the method. The demonstration of cavitation (Fig. 1–18), of calcification within a pulmonary nodule (Fig. 14–21), of a tracheobronchial lesion, of fat in a mediastinal mass, of normal and abnormal pulmonary vessels, and of an air bronchogram are but a few of the many advantages of this technique. If tumor cells are discovered on sputum cytology in the absence of a positive roentgenogram, serial tomography through both lungs may show the occult cancer.[722, 819] Tomography often provides key information obtainable by no other means. [67, 622, 753, 891, 899, 1006, 1008, 1268, 1334]

Oblique and lateral tomograms are particularly suited to study of the bronchial and vascular trees and the lymph nodes.[305, 315, 754, 915] The optimal position for showing the bifurcation of the left main bronchus in a single tomographic plane is a left posterior oblique view with the right posterior chest wall elevated 35 degrees from the table. For the right lobar bronchi, a 55 degree right posterior oblique is recommended.

Figure 1–13. VALUE OF LORDOTIC VIEW IN APICAL TUBERCULOSIS

A, Routine PA film. *B,* Lordotic view. Note the improved visibility of the lesion in *B* because of less interference from the ribs and clavicles. The lesion lies posteriorly, since it relates fairly well to the posterior segment of the 4th rib in both projections.

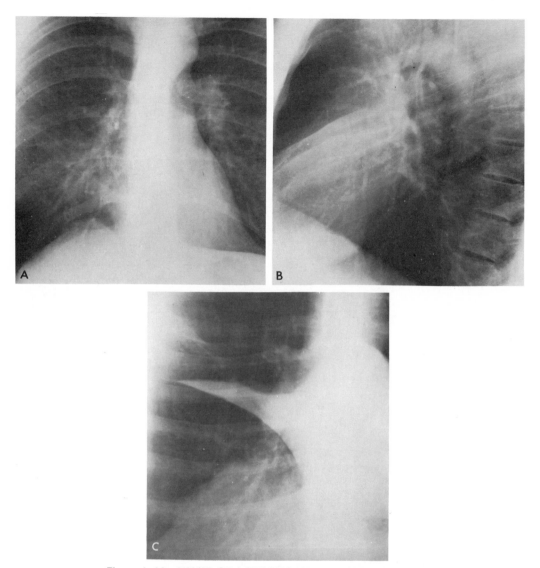

Figure 1–14. VALUE OF LORDOTIC VIEW IN RML COLLAPSE

The involvement is difficult to outline and localize in the routine PA and right lateral teleroentgenograms (*A* and *B*). The lordotic view (*C*) shows the typical triangular appearance of RML collapse. The sharp lower border defines the major fissure.

BRONCHOGRAPHY

I add my own voice to the many who advocate the free use of bronchography for the diagnosis of bronchial carcinoma and other pulmonary lesions (p. 265)[10, 120, 133, 254, 257, 871, 1309] When inhalation bronchography becomes clinically feasible, as it inevitably will, the applications of bronchography will be considerably extended.[363, 548, 610, 862, 1112] In fact, at this writing our new "atomizer" promises to be a great improvement. Even with the earlier

one, however, we had a number of reasonably good double-contrast demonstrations of the larynx, trachea, and central bronchi in both animals and man (Fig. 1–19).

We have found cinebronchography advantageous, especially in the diagnosis of bronchogenic carcinoma. Extensive rigidity of the bronchial tree in the vicinity of a lesion suggests a malignant process. Delineating a bronchus as the patient is rotated may facilitate the detection of a subtle obstructing neoplasm.[1313]

(*Text continued on page 20.*)

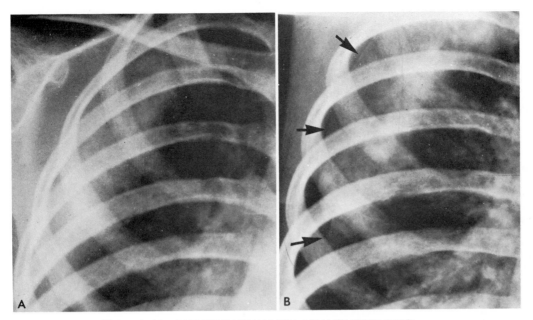

Figure 1–15. PNEUMOTHORAX SEEN ONLY ON EXPIRATION

A, Inspiration. *B*, Expiration.

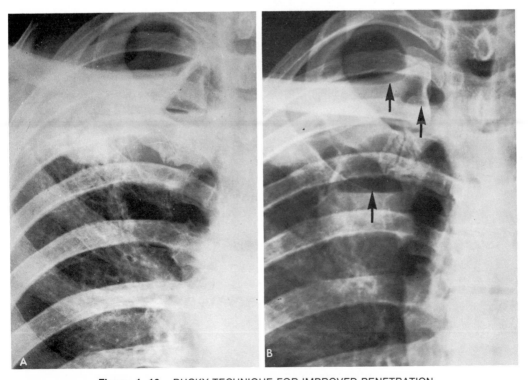

Figure 1–16. BUCKY TECHNIQUE FOR IMPROVED PENETRATION

Infected cysts or bullae in right apex. The true nature of the opacities is not appreciated on the nongrid teleroentgenogram *(A)*. The upright Bucky film *(B)* shows three air-fluid levels (arrows) and a fluid filled cyst.

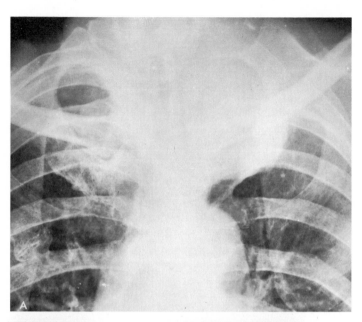

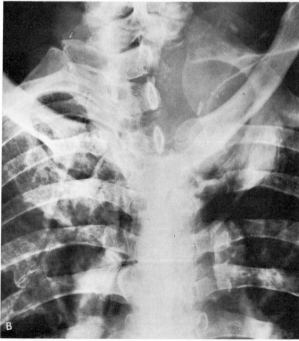

Figure 1–17. VALUE OF BUCKY TECHNIQUE
FOR VISUALIZING A BONE LESION

Superior sulcus carcinoma. *A*, Bone destruction is hardly recognized on the nongrid teleroentgenogram. *B*, The Bucky film shows
striking destruction of the upper ribs and spine.

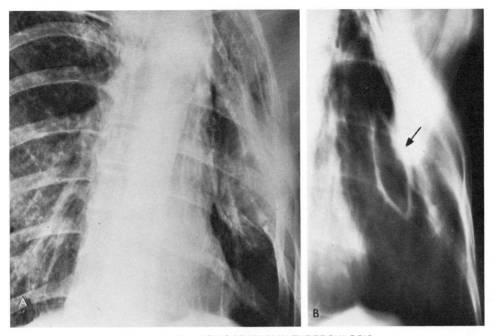

Figure 1–18. TOMOGRAPHY IN TUBERCULOSIS

Positive sputum several years after thoracoplasty. *A*, Teleroentgenogram fails to show a cavity. Various other views and Bucky films were also unrevealing. *B*, The tomogram clearly depicts the compressed cavity (arrow).

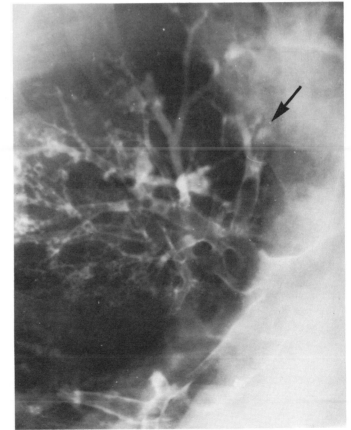

Figure 1–19. INHALATION BARIUM BRONCHOGRAM

The arrow points to the apical bronchus of the RUL, occluded by carcinoma. (From Shook, C. D., and Felson, B.[1112]; reproduced with permission of Chest.)

Our experience with bronchography for the diagnosis of chronic bronchitis is limited (p. 265),[968] but roentgen signs similar to those reported in this condition are often seen incidentally during bronchography for carcinoma. The value of bronchography in the investigation of congenital anomalies of the lung is well established.[133]

The problem of distinguishing between a mediastinal, pleural, or extrapleural lesion and an intrapulmonary one can sometimes be resolved only by bronchography (Fig. 9–

14). Segmental and topographic localization of a lesion for surgical removal also often depends on bronchography. A more detailed discussion of bronchography will be found in Chapter 7.

ANGIOGRAPHY

Pulmonary arteriography affords the only definitive method currently available for the diagnosis of acute pulmonary embo-

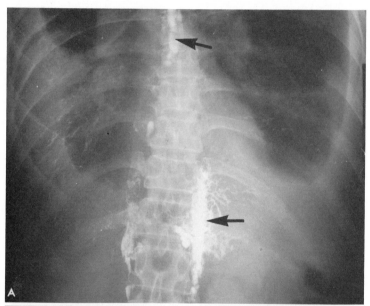

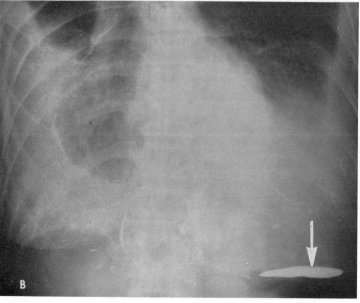

Figure 1–20. LYMPHANGIO-GRAM IN BILATERAL CHYLOTHORAX

A, 3 hours after bilateral lymphatic injection in both feet. The cisterna chyli (lower arrow) and thoracic duct (upper arrow) are shown. Retrograde flow of contrast medium into the pulmonary lymphatics has occurred, especially on the right. *B,* 24 hour upright film. Contrast medium has pooled in the left pleural cavity (arrow; unretouched). Lymphangiomatous transformation of the thoracic lymphatic system was found at autopsy.[1100]

lism.[216, 360, 711] This diagnostic procedure has uncovered the fact that pulmonary embolism with recovery is an amazingly frequent event. Angiography is, of course, also valuable in distinguishing aneurysm from other mediastinal tumors. Its use in depicting pulmonary vascular abnormalities, such as arteriovenous fistula and pulmonary artery coarctation, is essential[496] (Fig. 5–19). On occasion, congenital or acquired intrathoracic extracardiac shunts occur between the mediastinal and the pulmonary vessels. These are recognizable only by angiography.[496, 1146]

Angiography is of little more than academic interest in most other pulmonary conditions.[490, 637, 1087] Pulmonary, intraosseous, or bronchial angiography for diagnosing or assessing the operability of bronchogenic carcinoma[288, 799, 1058, 1078, 1134] has not received wide acceptance.

OTHER TECHNIQUES

There are many other views and diagnostic procedures that are at times useful in the study of chest lesions. It is not my aim to cover this subject completely but merely to discuss those facets which, from personal experience, seem to merit emphasis. Many of these views and techniques will be illustrated in the following pages.

I have occasionally profited from diagnostic pneumoperitoneum in the elucidation of lesions in the vicinity of the diaphragm (Figs. 12–6 and 12–13); from diagnostic pneumothorax in the demonstration of pleural metastases (Fig. 9–12) and the differentiation between pleural lesions and those of the chest wall, lung, or mediastinum; from lymphography in determining the source of chylothorax[180, 702, 1042, 1293] (Fig. 1–20); and even from myelography in the diagnosis of lateral thoracic meningocele. I have had little personal experience with gas mediastinography[37, 70, 1055] or fluorodensitography.[791, 894] Magnification techniques are now feasible and should soon receive wide usage.[480,1144] Of course, we will all have to change the norms in our cerebral computers before we can interpret the enlarged shadows accurately.

CHAPTER 2

LOCALIZATION OF INTRATHORACIC LESIONS

Knowledge of the exact location of an intrathoracic lesion is of great assistance in diagnosis and surgical management. Establishing whether a density is pleural or mediastinal rather than intrapulmonary is of obvious importance. Pinpointing a lesion in a particular pulmonary segment or compartment of the mediastinum is often helpful in differential diagnosis.

GENERAL PRINCIPLES

It would appear axiomatic that AP and lateral views alone should serve to localize any intrathoracic lesion. Unfortunately, this is by no means true. Often the lesion is visible in only one of the two views—and occasionally in neither! There are other reasons for this besides small size or obscuration by overlapping structures, such as the shoulders or ribs. Tuddenham has shown experimentally that a lesion with tapering borders, i.e., shaped like a discus or flying saucer, may not be seen on the roentgenogram, whereas a coin-shaped or round lesion of identical thickness will be clearly delineated.[1233, 1234] The X-ray beam striking the edge of the coin or ball tangentially produces an abrupt sharp shadow on the film, usually readily visible to the eye. A tapering lesion does not provide this sharp border so that optic stimulation is minimal and the lesion more difficult to discern. Retinal stimuli are required in order to see, moreso at lower thresholds of visibility. Any father spying on his children from a doorway knows they won't see him unless he moves.

I read somewhere that this retinal phenomenon accounted for the fact that the Indians had better long distance vision than the cowboys. Their eyes were the same but the Indians had a gimmick: they waggled their heads from side to side stimulating the rods (or is it the cones?) as visual objects flitted across the retina. Unfamiliar objects in the panorama were thus perceived. I had noted this head motion in movies, but I assumed these were nervous Indians. I don't vouch for this quasiscientific fact, but it does make a fine conversation piece. I can already envision vibrating viewboxes for radiologic interpretation! Figures 2–26 and 2–37 illustrate this frequently encountered radiologic paradox: the large invisible lesion.

Obviously, then, we must become versatile and localize chest lesions by other methods. One of these, fluoroscopy, has already been discussed. Stereoscopic and oblique views are also valuable in this regard.

It is often possible to determine the exact position of an intrathoracic density from the posteroanterior film alone. Certain findings have been helpful in this regard. A radiopacity involving the extreme apex of a lung is almost invariably situated in the apical segment of the upper lobe. One that involves the lateral costophrenic angle usually lies in the lateral or anterior basal segment of the lower lobe. An infiltrate in the right upper lung whose lower border is delineated by the minor fissure lies in the RUL, usually in its anterior segment. In like fashion, an opacity in the right midlung field with a sharp horizontal upper border lies in the RML.* At times a lesion may erode a rib,

---

*Exceptions are shown in Figures 3–7 and 3–40.

the sternum, or the spine, thereby indicating its extrapleural location. Displacement of the trachea or the barium filled esophagus will indicate the depth of a mass on the anteroposterior axis.

On the frontal view of the chest, a considerable portion of the lung field is obscured by the heart, great vessels, and diaphragm. Rigler has shown that a disease process in the lower lobe or posterior mediastinum behind the heart shadow may be recognized in the well-penetrated PA view by the increased density of the heart on that side.[997] This is true because the cardiac thickness is approximately the same on both sides of the spine; thus the heart normally casts a uniform roentgen shadow over its entire area. If then the left side of the heart appears more opaque than the right, it may safely be stated that there has been displacement of the air in the left lower lobe, even though the disease process itself is not clearly depicted (Fig. 2–1). Thus, we see through the heart shadow on an adequately penetrated film.[553, 874, 1165] A markedly collapsed LLL will often present as a well-defined triangular opacity framed in the heart shadow[989, 1260] (Fig. 2–27).

The same principle applies to areas obscured by the great vessels (Fig. 2–2) and by the leaves of the diaphragm. For example, a lesion in the posterior costophrenic

angle is often visible through the upper portion of the liver shadow on the frontal projection; similarly, the heart shadow, when shown on an abdominal film, normally appears "burned out." On many occasions, because the heart shadow was seen too clearly on the abdominal film, I have been able to recognize a previously unsuspected intrathoracic abnormality (Fig. 2–3).

Another variation on this theme makes use of the normal density of the shadow of the dome of the liver on a well-penetrated frontal view of the chest. Because of the tapering lappet of lung that occupies the posterior costophrenic sinus, the liver shadow is densely white caudally and gradually appears grayer as the eye travels toward the dome. A uniform liver density on a well-exposed film bespeaks lower lobe consolidation or displacement of the lung from the posterior costophrenic sinus by free pleural fluid (Fig. 9–5). The sign seldom occurs on the left in relation to the spleen because of overlapping of the gas densities of the splenic flexure and stomach.

Hodson has pointed out that if the intervertebral spaces are visible on the AP or PA film, the medial section of the posterior ribs should also be clearly seen.[553] If they are not, pulmonary disease should be suspected. Similarly, in the normal lateral view, the density of the vertebral bodies

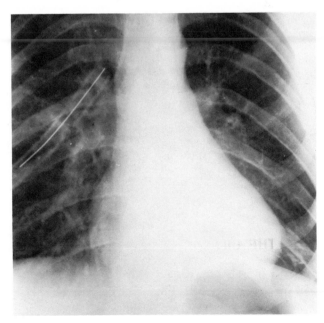

Figure 2–1. UNILATERAL OPACIFICATION OF THE CARDIAC SHADOW

Postoperative collapse of the LLL. A thoracic tube is present on the right.

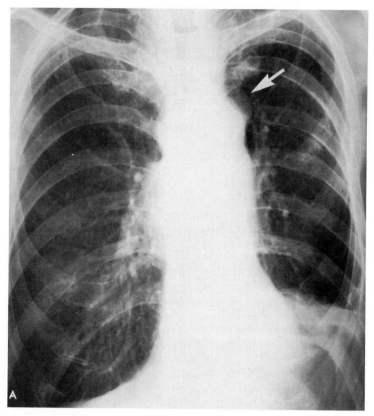

Figure 2–2. EXTENSIVE MEDIASTINAL INVOLVEMENT OBSCURED BY CARDIOVASCULAR STRUCTURES

A, Teleroentgenogram shows a density in the right hilar region. The mediastinal structures on this well-penetrated film appear quite radiopaque except for the aortic knob (arrow).

(Figure continued on opposite page.)

gradually and evenly decreases from above downward. Equal or greater density of the lower vertebral bodies indicates a pathologic process, even though it is otherwise invisible (Figs. 2–26 and 2–27).

Despite the usefulness of the above signs, they are not often applicable. It is the main purpose of this chapter to stress two other important methods of localization, the *silhouette sign* and the *air bronchogram.*

THE SILHOUETTE SIGN

General Remarks

The *silhouette sign* is based on the premise that an intrathoracic radiopacity, if in *anatomic* contact with a border of the heart or aorta, will obscure that border. To my

knowledge, the first reference to this phenomenon was made around 1935 by the late Dr. H. Kennon Dunham of Cincinnati, who often stated that obliteration of the left border of the heart by a contiguous pulmonary density indicated disease of the lingula.[280] Surprisingly, he never mentioned to us that a similar finding occurred on the right. Subsequently, Robbins and Hale, in their classic series of articles on the roentgen signs of lobar and segmental collapse, made numerous references to obliteration of portions of the outline of the heart, aorta, and diaphragm by disease in the lung in contact with these structures.[1019, 1020] They pointed out that the lung in immediate proximity to the right border of the heart consisted almost exclusively of middle lobe, and demonstrated that disease in this location produced loss in definition of the right heart border. They also noted that infiltrate in the lingula obscured the left car-

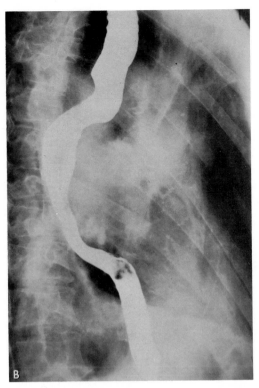

Figure 2–2. *Continued.* Right oblique esophagram (*B*) shows extensive lymph node involvement. A prior left thoracotomy had revealed a nonresectable bronchogenic carcinoma.

diac border. These findings were also mentioned by Walker[1253] and Towsend.[1220] Bachman et al., in discussing pleurisy in primary atypical pneumonia, noted that blurring of the usually sharp left cardiac border was produced by pleural disease involving the lower end of the left major fissure.[26]

The basic tenet of this method of localization may be restated as follows: *An intrathoracic lesion touching a border of the heart, aorta, or diaphragm will obliterate that border on the roentgenogram. An intrathoracic lesion not anatomically contiguous with a border of one of these structures will not obliterate that border.* We have applied the term *silhouette sign* to indicate the *loss* of the silhouette of any of these borders by adjacent disease.[343]

In an effort to reproduce this phenomenon experimentally, the following procedure, suggested to me by the late Dr. Felix Fleischner, was carried out: a small quantity of heated paraffin was poured into an empty X-ray film carton. The carton was

then tilted so that the paraffin, on cooling, solidified as a wedge-shaped mass in the corner of the box. The carton was placed back to back with a second empty film container of identical size. A roentgenogram was made with the central ray traversing the two boxes. Mineral oil was then poured into the box containing the paraffin wedge and a second film was exposed in a manner similar to the first. Finally, the mineral oil was poured from the first into the second carton and another film was exposed (Fig. 2–4).

The first film (*A*) revealed the triangular shadow of the paraffin wedge sharply outlined by air. This represents the normal heart-lung relationship. The second film (*B*) showed obliteration of the border of the paraffin shadow along its zone of contact with the mineral oil (silhouette sign), illustrating that the "heart" border is obscured by "consolidation" in the contiguous portion of the "lung," e.g., the RML. In the third film (*C*), the border of the paraffin shadow was preserved (absent silhouette sign), demonstrating that the "heart" border is not oblit-

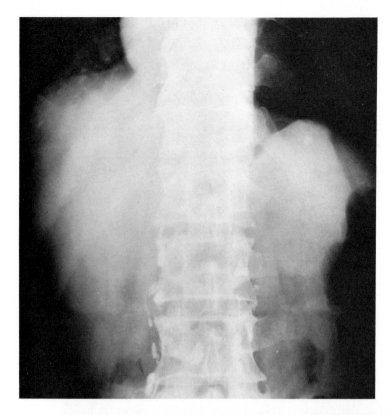

Figure 2–3. RADIOPAQUE RIGHT HEART SHADOW ON AN ABDOMINAL FILM

The RLL, collapsed by an obstructive carcinoma, is overpenetrated except where overlapped by the right side of the heart and upper part of the liver. The lymph nodes are opacified from prior lymphangiography.

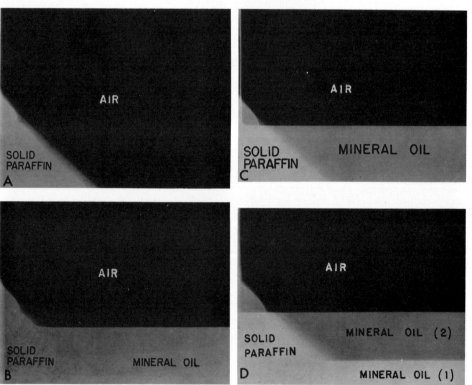

Figure 2–4. EXPERIMENT ILLUSTRATING THE PRINCIPLE OF THE SILHOUETTE SIGN

(From Felson, B., and Felson, H.[343]; reproduced with permission of Radiology.)

erated by "disease" in noncontiguous areas of the "lung," e.g., the RLL. The experiment was repeated using a small quantity of mineral oil in the carton containing the paraffin wedge and a larger quantity in the second carton, with the relative positions of the roentgen tube and film reversed. These changes did not alter the results (D).

The demonstration in Figure 2–5 was devised by Dr. E. Martinez, a radiologist in Prescott, Arizona. A plastic model of a heart with ascending aorta was placed in one empty container and a model of the aortic knob and descending aorta (the banana-shaped structure) was placed in another. The two containers were set front to back and radiographed (A). Water was then added to the container with the heart model and the exposure repeated (B). Below the

water level, the right and left heart borders are obliterated but the descending aorta is still vividly seen. In (C), water is present only in the container with the descending aorta. The findings are reversed: the cardiac outline is now well seen while the descending aorta shadow below the fluid level is obliterated.

The explanation of the silhouette sign rests on the fact that the delineation of any roentgen shadow depends partly on differences in radiographic density.* The ar-

---

*Here are some relative absorption values for 60 kilovolt radiation[1077]:

Water	1.0	Air	.0001
Carbon	0.7	CaPO₄	22.00
Fat	0.5	CaCO₃	15.00
Paraffin	0.4		

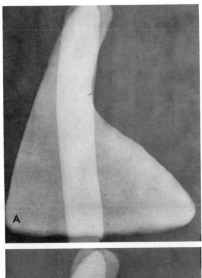

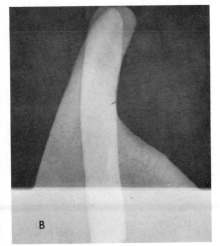

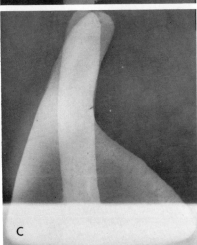

Figure 2–5. SILHOUETTE SIGN ILLUSTRATED BY ROENTGENOGRAMS OF A MODEL

(Courtesy of Dr. E. Martinez.)

rangement in the body of the four basic roentgen densities — gas, fat, water, and metal (or calcium) — determines what we see on the roentgenogram. Thus the cardiac outline is visible in the normal chest because the heart (70 to 80 per cent water) is bordered by the gas density of the lung. We do not visualize the blood within the heart or the heart within the pericardium* because these structures are all of water density. Opacification of the blood with a metal-containing contrast medium enables us to delineate the interior of the heart. Since the pulmonary opacities under consideration are of water density, if they replace the gas shadow abutting a segment of the heart, that segment will no longer be visible roentgenographically.

Tuddenham does not accept this explanation for the silhouette sign, but instead attributes the phenomenon to a summation effect, i.e., to the fact that the absorption pattern of the heart and adjacent consolidation are so complementary that no density gradient between them is recorded on the film.[1234] This presupposes a thickness of the consolidation equal to that of the cardiac surface. He was able to line up two paraffin blocks in different spatial planes so perfectly that the roentgen silhouette between them was lost despite lack of anatomic contact. In other words, the identical thickness of density traversed by the X-ray beam through the two blocks caused loss of their adjoining silhouettes, even though air was present alongside each of the blocks. He further noted that this perfect alignment could hardly occur clinically, so that the silhouette sign was still valid.

In rebuttal, I believe Tuddenham's explanation could hardly apply to the many examples I have seen of a very thin sliver of infiltrate appropriately located, obliterating the cardiac profile as effectively as a large mass (Fig. 4–43). Furthermore, when a wedge-shaped infiltrate abuts the heart the cardiac silhouette is lost equally along the zone of contact. For example, in collapse of the entire LUL, the heart border adjacent to the slender lingula is just as obscure as that over the much thicker anterior segment (Fig. 3–46). Another point: small intrapul-

monary vessels in air containing lung are clearly depicted on a well-penetrated film through a thick pleural effusion (Fig. 2–25) or even through the normal heart shadow. Would you expect the X-ray beam to be able to detect them merely because they have added a few millimeters to a shadow already perhaps 10 cm thick?

I have been unable to reproduce Tuddenham's experimental results and suspect that the loss of the silhouette between his two paraffin blocks was simply the result of roentgen underpenetration. So I still cling stubbornly to my earlier explanation. Whichever is correct, the silhouette sign serves as an extremely effective means of localizing intrathoracic lesions.[986]

Perhaps this is as good a time as any to explain my propensity for naming signs. The name saves time, helps you remember the sign, and advertises it. The sobriquet selected should be appropriate and on target — anal ataxia (circumflatulence) is not permitted. Terms such as rat-tail, eggshell, butterfly, and meniscus conjure an immediate mental hotline — direct, patent, quick. Air bronchogram, fungus ball, and downhill varices are a few that I've invented. They say what I mean.[337]

Heart and Aorta, Frontal View

On the basis of more than 20 years of experience with the silhouette sign on the heart and aorta, the following general applications appear to be justified:*

1. A shadow that causes obliteration of part or all of a heart border (silhouette sign) is anterior in location and lies in the RML, lingula, anterior segment of an upper lobe, anterior mediastinum, lower end of the oblique fissure, or anterior portion of the pleural cavity.

2. A radiopacity that overlaps but does not obliterate the heart border is posterior in location and lies in a lower lobe, the posterior mediastinum, or the posterior portion of the pleural cavity.

3. A lesion that obliterates the right border of the ascending aorta (silhouette sign) is located anteriorly and is situated in the anterior segment of the RUL, the RML,

---

*Occasionally, as Kremens[674] has shown, the heart is outlined within the pericardial cavity by the epicardial fat.

---

*Exceptions are discussed on page 49.

the anterior mediastinum or the anterior portion of the right pleural cavity.

4. A shadow that overlies but does not obliterate the right border of the ascending aorta lies posteriorly and is located in the superior segment of the RLL, the posterior segment of the RUL, the posterior mediastinum, or the posterior portion of the pleural cavity.

5. An opacity that obliterates the left border of the aortic knob (a posterior structure) lies in the apicoposterior segment of the LUL* or in the posterior mediastinum or pleura adjacent to this segment.

6. A shadow that overlaps but does not obliterate the aortic knob is anterior or far posterior and lies in the anterior segment of the LUL, the superior segment of the LLL, or in the anterior or far posterior portion of the mediastinum or pleural cavity.

7. The silhouette sign applied to the right border of the trachea is unreliable because in many *normal* individuals the right tracheal border cannot be seen, even on adequately penetrated films. The same is true of the cephalic aspect of the aortic knob (Chap. 15)

Many years ago, we made a study of the silhouette sign in 84 patients with various types of intrathoracic disease.[343, 352] These included acute and chronic pneumonia,

*Actually, it lies in the posterior subdivision of this segment, which anatomically shows an indentation from the pressure of the aortic knob.

tuberculosis, pulmonary collapse, encapsulated pleural effusion, and tumors of the lung and mediastinum, among others. Roentgenographic evidence of a pulmonary density in contact with or overlapping a cardiovascular border was the only requisite in the selection of case material. Localization of the pulmonary shadows was attempted from the PA roentgenogram alone and the accuracy was then checked by means of the lateral view. When the principles of the silhouette sign were not utilized it was found that accurate placement of the lesion was possible in only 20 of the 84 patients (23 per cent); in several instances incorrect localization resulted. In striking contrast, when the present method was applied we obtained correct results in all but one case (Table 2–1). Here are the salient points indicated by this table:

1. A density in the RML or lingula can produce the silhouette sign on the heart or ascending aorta, but one in a lower lobe cannot (Fig. 2–6).

2. Involvement of the apicoposterior segment of the LUL (really its posterior subsegment) almost always obliterates the aortic knob. The occasional exception is the result of one of two situations: (a) The knob—the posterior portion of the aortic arch—is actually obliterated, but the proximal descending aorta shows through and simulates the knob. (b) LUL collapse has caused so much forward displacement of the upper section of the major fissure that

TABLE 2–1. *Application of the Silhouette Sign to 84 Consecutive Patients*

Location of Density	No. of Cases*	HEART BORDER Silhouette Sign Present	Absent	ASCENDING AORTA Silhouette Sign Present	Absent	AORTIC KNOB Silhouette Sign Present	Absent
RLL	17	0	14	0	5	—	—
LLL	14	0	14	—	—	0	1
RML	13	13	0	2	0	—	—
Lingula	12	12	0	—	—	—	—
LUL, apicoposterior segment	8	—	—	—	—	7	1**
LUL, anterior segment	4	2	0	—	—	0	2
RUL, anterior segment	8	3	0	8	0	—	—
RUL, posterior segment	1	0	1	0	1	—	—
Anterior mediastinum	5	5	0	3	0	1†	2
Posterior mediastinum	2	0	2	0	2	—	—
Posterior encapsulation of fluid	4	0	4	0	2	—	—

*In some, more than one location was involved.
**See text and Fig. 3–47.
†Tumor involved over half of the anteroposterior diameter of the chest.

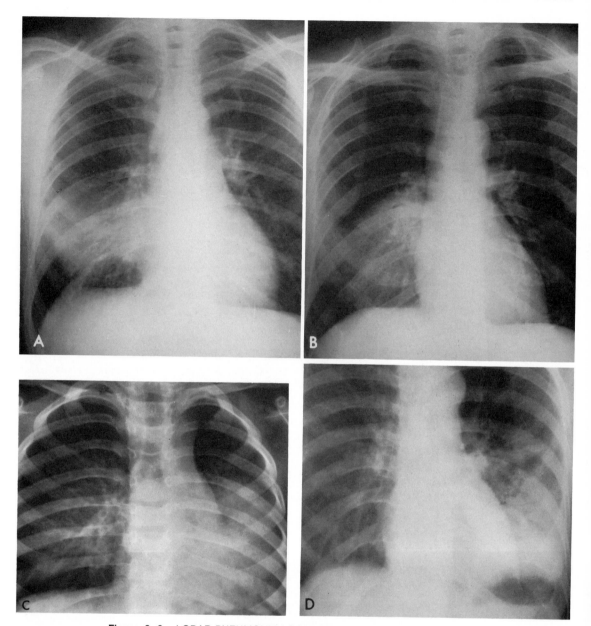

Figure 2–6. LOBAR PNEUMONIA LOCALIZED BY THE SILHOUETTE SIGN

A, RML. *B*, RLL. *C*, Lingula. *D*, LLL. Note the visible right hemidiaphragm in *A* and *B* and the invisible left hemidiaphragm in *C* and *D*. Don't mistake the gastric outline for the diaphragm in *D*.

the superior segment of the air filled LLL now lies in apposition to the aortic knob.

3. An appropriately located lesion in the anterior segment of an upper lobe shows the silhouette sign on the heart or ascending aorta, whereas a posterior segment lesion does not.

4. An anterior mediastinal mass causes a silhouette sign on the heart or ascending

aorta, but a posterior one does not, although it may obliterate the aortic knob.

5. Posterior encapsulation of pleural fluid does not produce the silhouette sign on the heart or ascending aorta, but anteromedial encapsulation or free pleural effusion does.

These points are demonstrated in a series of roentgenograms on the next few pages (Figs. 2–7 to 2–16). I suggest you cover the

(*Text continued on page 37.*)

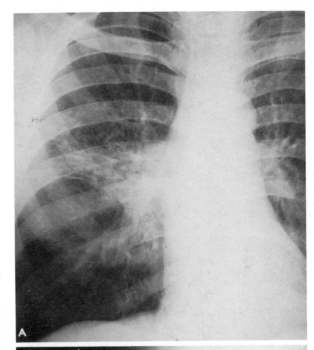

Figure 2–7. SILHOUETTE SIGN IN ANTERIOR SEGMENTAL COLLAPSE OF RUL

A, Obliteration of the right border of the ascending aorta denotes anterior location of the radiopacity. *B,* On the right lateral view, the infiltrate (arrows) is seen to lie in the anterior segment of the RUL. Note on the PA view that the right hilar shadow is also obscured. There is increased density of the right hilar region. Dilated air filled bronchi visible within the infiltrate indicate bronchiectasis.

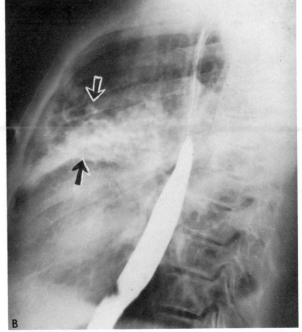

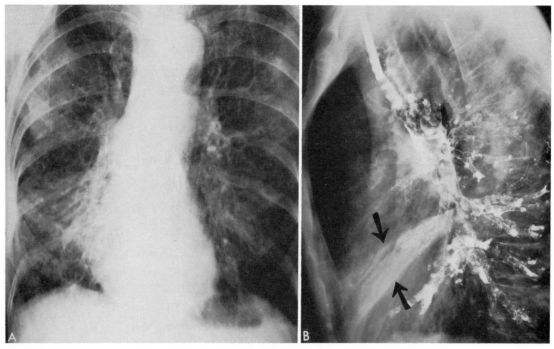

Figure 2–8.   SILHOUETTE SIGN IN COLLAPSE OF RML

A, The right heart border is obliterated. Some of the bronchi contain air and are therefore visible. *B,* The lateral bronchogram reveals widespread bronchiectasis, but only the RML appears collapsed (arrows).

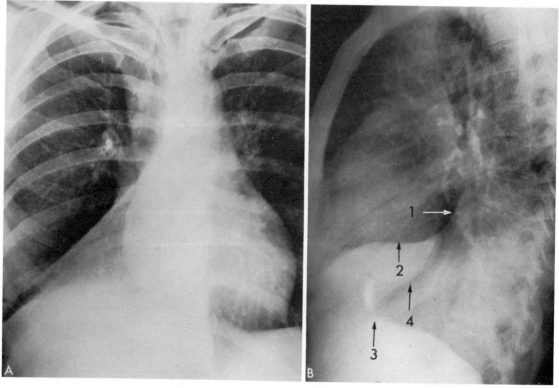

Figure 2–9.   See opposite page for legend.

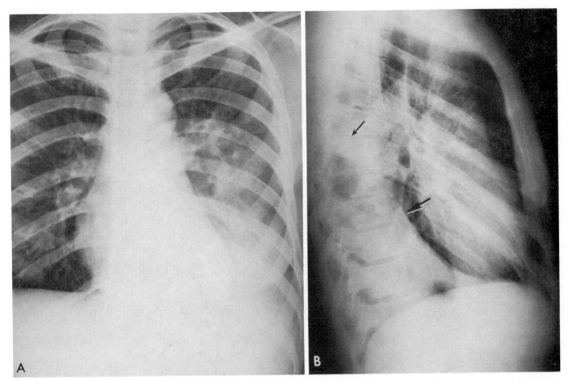

Figure 2–10.   ABSENT SILHOUETTE SIGN IN COLLAPSE OF LLL

Tuberculosis with cavitation and bronchostenosis. *A*, The left heart border is preserved in the frontal view, indicating LLL disease. The left hemidiaphragm is obliterated. *B*, The left lateral view confirms the localization (arrows). Note the obliteration of the posterior half of the hemidiaphragm by the airless LLL and of its anterior half by the heart. The collapsed lobe has pulled away from the back of the heart, which is therefore visible, an unusual finding in extensive LLL disease. There is a "mediastinal wedge" (p. 107) between the arrows. (From Felson, B., and Felson, H.[343]; reproduced with permission of Radiology.)

Figure 2–9.   ABSENCE OF SILHOUETTE SIGN IN RLL COLLAPSE (Opposite)

The right heart border is preserved in *A*, indicating posterior location of the opacity. The right hemidiaphragm is obscured. In the right lateral view *(B)*, RLL involvement is confirmed. The major fissure is displaced posteriorly *(1)* because of the collapse. The elevated right hemidiaphragm *(2)* is obliterated posteriorly by the airless RLL, and the anterior third of the left hemidiaphragm *(3)* is obscured by the bottom of the heart. Note the overlapping shadows of the back of the heart *(4)* (which lies in the left thorax) and the right hemidiaphragm, simulating interlobar effusion. Bronchogenic carcinoma.

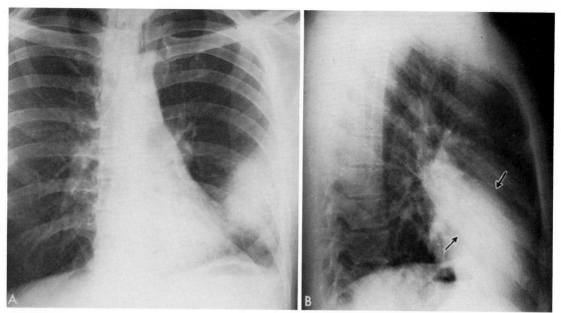

Figure 2–11. SILHOUETTE SIGN IN LINGULAR PNEUMONIA

A, The left lower heart border is obliterated. Pleural reaction is present in the left costophrenic angle. *B*, Most of the lingula is involved (arrows).

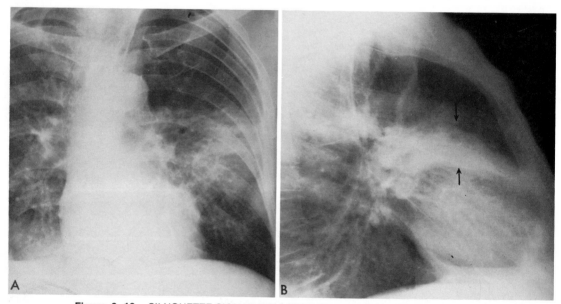

Figure 2–12. SILHOUETTE SIGN IN COLLAPSE OF ANTERIOR SEGMENT OF LUL

In *A*, the obliteration of the left heart border extends above the usual position of the lingula. This indicates involvement of the anterior segment of the LUL. Note loss of the left hilum. In the left lateral view (*B*), the anterior segment shows collapse (arrows). Bronchogenic carcinoma.

Figure 2–14. ABSENCE OF SILHOUETTE SIGN IN POSTERIOR ENCAPSULATED RIGHT PYOPNEUMOTHORAX (Opposite)

A, The right border of the heart and ascending aorta (arrows) is preserved. *B*, Extreme left anterior oblique view verifies the posterior location (arrow). The posterior silhouette of the heart, in the left thorax, overlaps the empyema shadow in the right thorax. (From Felson, B., and Felson, H.[343]; reproduced with permission of Radiology.)

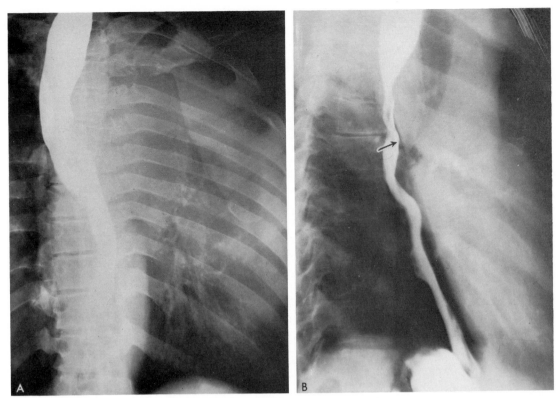

Figure 2–13. WHERE IS THE HEART?

One of the residents made a diagnosis of nocardia! *A,* The shadow parallel to the left border of the dorsal spine represents the lower descending thoracic aorta; the left hemidiaphragm is visible. Preservation of these two shadows indicates that there is little or no involvement of the LLL. The right heart border is displaced toward the left and hidden in the spine shadow. The left heart border is obliterated below by the radiopaque lingula and above by the involved anterior segment. The aortic knob, which lies posteriorly, is obliterated by disease in the apicoposterior segment. The sum of all these segments equals the entire LUL. *B,* Left lateral view shows a diseased LUL (arrow) and a normal LLL. The patient had a carcinoma in the LUL bronchus. (From Felson, B., and Felson, H.[343]; reproduced with permission of Radiology.)

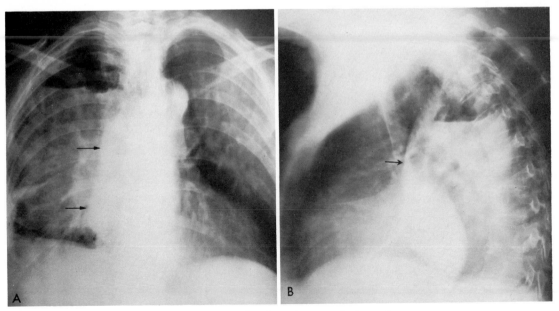

Figure 2–14. See opposite page for legend.

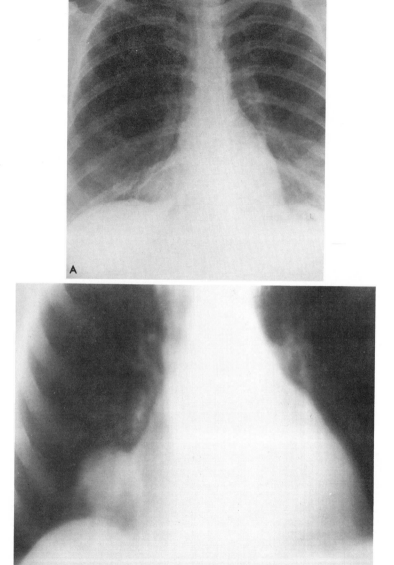

Figure 2–15.   SILHOUETTE SIGN CAUSED BY AN ANTERIOR MEDIASTINAL LESION

A, The lower right heart border is obliterated by a small soft tissue mass which was not present 8 months earlier. Right thoracic pain and tenderness in a 28 year old obese woman. *B,* Tomogram. At operation, necrosis of the pericardial fat pad was found. (Courtesy of Dr. Douglas M. Behrendt and Dr. John G. Scannell.)

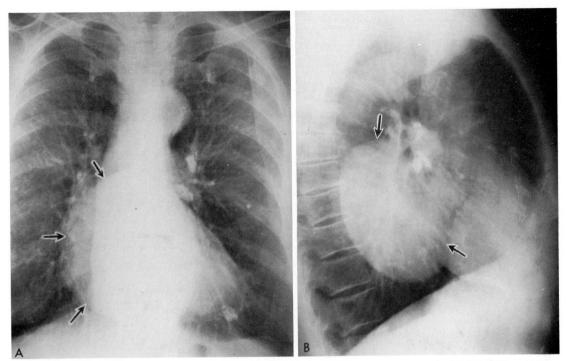

Figure 2-16. ABSENCE OF SILHOUETTE SIGN IN A BRONCHOGENIC CYST OF THE POSTERIOR MEDIASTINUM

A, The PA view shows preservation of the right border of the heart and aorta. The mass (arrows) must then lie posteriorly. *B,* The lateral view shows it to lie behind the heart (arrows). Note that the posterior border of the heart is obliterated, indicating that the mass extends into the left thorax. (From Felson, B., and Felson, H.[343]; reproduced with permission of Radiology.)

bottom half of each page before you look, then try to localize the lesion from the upper illustration alone. If you're a born cheater, have your wife cover it, or your girl friend. Or have them take turns.

DESCENDING THORACIC AORTA

The lateral border of the descending thoracic aorta in its downward course to the diaphragm is usually clearly visible on the adequately exposed frontal view except in infancy. Its medial border is seldom seen, probably because the esophagus is in contact along most of this border and the spine shadow overlies it. The descending aorta indents the superior and posterior basal segments of the LLL and its lateral margin is therefore obliterated by lesions in these segments (Fig. 2–17). The descending aorta may also be obliterated by pleural fluid along the mediastinum, as well as by an ap-

propriately located mediastinal mass. Remember, though, that the most distal segment of the descending thoracic aorta must dip back into the mediastinum before it can traverse the aortic hiatus in the diaphragm so that at this level it may normally disappear from view (Fig. 2–17). In an occasional elderly individual, the distal aortic segment may buckle into the right thorax so that the right aortic border becomes visible as a small posterior mass. Its source is usually easily determined by tracing the descending aorta.

The Diaphragm, Frontal View

The effect of pulmonary densities on the outline of the diaphragm has hardly been mentioned in the literature. Robbins and Hale stated that collapse of a lower lobe often resulted in obliteration of a large segment of the diaphragm in the frontal view,

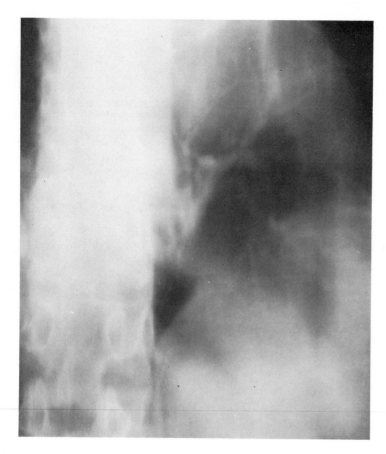

Figure 2–17. OBLITERATION OF LEFT MARGIN OF DESCENDING AORTA

The branching structures on this laminagram represent the arteries feeding an area of sequestration in the posterior basal segment of the LLL. The aorta distal to the lesion is not seen because it has curved back into the mediastinum before entering the abdomen.

whereas collapse of the middle lobe had no such effect.[1020] Our own study is at variance with this.[343] Persistence or loss of the outline of the *right* leaf of the diaphragm is of little value in localizing pulmonary densities to the anterior or posterior thorax. There are several reasons for this:

1. Like noses, the shapes of diaphragms vary from one individual to the next, in health and in disease. The right hemidiaphragm, as seen on the frontal film, represents the highest *plateau* traversed tangentially by the X-ray beam. Usually this is the anterior portion, under the middle lobe, but sometimes it is a more posterior segment under the lower lobe. Thus, the right hemidiaphragm may be obliterated by middle lobe disease in some patients and by lower lobe disease in others (see Figs. 2–6, 2–9, and 2–28).

2. In the frontal projection, when an intrathoracic lesion obliterates the highest portion of the right hemidiaphragm, the next highest plateau may show through, so that the diaphragm does not appear obliterated at all.

Surprisingly, the above rules do not apply to the left hemidiaphragm. The difference lies in the position of the heart, the bottom of which is in broad contact with the anteromedial portion of the left hemidiaphragm and obscures it *normally*. The left hemidiaphragm shadow seen through the heart on the frontal view actually represents only the more posterior phrenic segment. It is often effaced by lower lobe disease but occasionally may normally fail to visualize. On films of average penetration, I was unable to detect any portion of the diaphragm under the heart in 2 per cent of 800 normal individuals; less than half of the lateral portion of the subcardiac segment was visible in another 8 per cent. In the remaining 90 per cent, most of the diaphragm was seen. Lateral to the heart, obliteration usually means a lower lobe lesion (Fig. 2–6D). A rare exception is shown in Figure 2–6C.

Pulmonary Arteries

The silhouette sign is also applicable to the right and left main pulmonary arteries. Although the undivided pulmonary trunk is said to leave the pericardium before bifurcating,[1241] in five of the six adult autopsies I observed with this point in mind, the bifurcation was entirely intrapericardial. To be sure, a short segment of the left pulmonary artery and a longer segment of the right lay in the extrapericardial portion of the mediastinum. The left pulmonary artery quickly entered the left lung through the mediastinal pleura before branching. The right pulmonary artery extended behind the ascending aorta and superior vena cava for some distance before bifurcating into upper and lower divisions.

Thus, only the lateral portion of the right and left main pulmonary arteries is profiled by the lung and is therefore visible on the normal PA chest film. The medial segment lies within the water density of the mediastinum. The visible point of origin of each vessel, then, marks the right and left lateral borders of the mediastinal silhouette at the cardiac waist. At its takeoff, the left pulmonary artery obliterates a small segment of the cardiopericardial border in three of every four individuals. The incidence is much lower on the right side, occurring in about one of six (Chap. 15). In the remainder, the cardiac silhouette shows through the hilum as a continuous line.

HILUM OVERLAY AND HILUM CONVERGENCE SIGNS

The proximal segment of the visible left pulmonary artery (identified by the convergence of its most medial bifurcation) lies lateral to the cardiac shadow or just within its outer edge in over 98 per cent of individuals and lies slightly more than 1 cm within the silhouette in the remainder (Chap. 15). A similar situation occurs on the right. Even with pericardial effusion or cardiac enlargement, this relationship holds, with only an occasional exception. This normal apposition of the main pulmonary arteries to the lateral edges of the cardiopericardial silhouette is the rationale behind the *hilum overlay sign,* a term I have applied to the visibility, on the PA film, of either the right or left pulmonary artery more than a

centimeter within the lateral edge of what appears to be the cardiac silhouette.[338]

The configuration of an anterior mediastinal mass may closely resemble that of an enlarged heart or pericardial sac, but the mass can hardly lie directly medial to the pulmonary artery, since the heart and pericardium preempt this location. Such a tumor will often overlap the main pulmonary arteries which then become well seen within the margins of the mass (Fig. 2–18). On the other hand, if the pulmonary artery derives from the lateral edge of such an anterior mediastinal shadow, enlarged heart or pericardial sac is indicated.

The sign doesn't always work (Figs. 11–2 and 14–12). An AP Bucky film enhances it (Fig. 2–18*B*). Be sure that the film is a true frontal view. Slight obliquity may project a normal pulmonary artery medially.

A corollary of the hilum overlay sign is sometimes useful in distinguishing between a large pulmonary artery and a juxtahilar mediastinal tumor. If the pulmonary artery branches converge toward the mass rather than toward the heart, you are dealing with an enlarged pulmonary artery. The reverse indicates a mediastinal mass. I call it the *hilum convergence sign* (Fig. 2–19).

A less useful variation on the silhouette theme as it relates to the pulmonary arteries is the visibility of the smaller intrapulmonary vessels through pulmonary, pleural, or mediastinal densities. Obviously, vessels will "disappear" when surrounded by pulmonary infiltrate.[1280] If the pulmonary vessels are seen through a large thoracic density, the surrounding lung must be aerated (Fig. 7–11). For example, on a well-penetrated grid film, you may see vessels through a pleural encapsulation[1085] (Fig. 2–20). Similarly, the RLL vessels may show through a RML consolidation, or vice versa. With a little *chutzpah,* you can distinguish between pulmonary consolidation and pleural encapsulation by estimating whether the vessels showing through represent the vasculature of one or two lobes. But go easy, it's risky.

The Silhouette Sign on Thoracic Lesions

A member of our radiology staff, Dr. Kenneth Kattan, called my attention to the fact

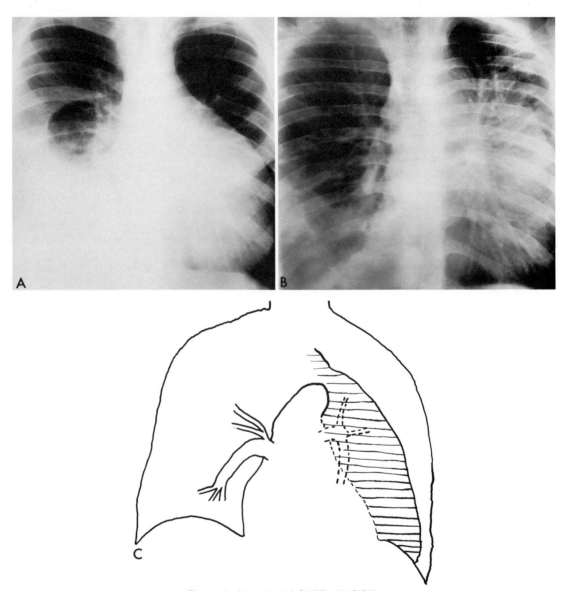

Figure 2–18. HILUM OVERLAY SIGN

    A, The configuration of this anterior mediastinal lymphangioma simulates an enlarged heart. Note that the left hilum is seen well within the "cardiac" border. *B,* The sign is better shown on the AP Bucky film. The anterior tumor is magnified more than the heart behind it, so the discrepant position of the left pulmonary artery is accentuated. *C,* Diagrammatic representation. (Courtesy of Dr. Marvin L. Daves.)

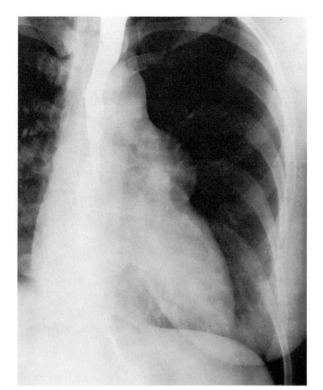

Figure 2–19. HILUM CONVERGENCE SIGN

The left pulmonary vessels converge toward the waist of the heart rather than toward the abnormal shadow at the left cardiac border. A large pulmonary artery can thus be excluded. Thymolipoma of the anterior mediastinum. (Courtesy of Benton, C., and Gerard, P.[57]; reproduced with permission of J. Thorac. Cardiovasc. Surg.)

that the silhouette sign can be applied to sizable thoracic lesions. Like the heart, the borders of such a lesion can be obliterated by adjacent shadows of water density. Coalescence of two large pulmonary alveolar infiltrates is one example; loss of a border of a pulmonary arteriovenous fistula at the site of a feeding vessel is another.

CERVICOTHORACIC AND THORACOABDOMINAL SIGNS

A more important use of this principle, however, is in relation to superior mediastinal lesions. The *cervicothoracic sign* is based on the tenet that if a thoracic lesion is in anatomic contact with the soft tissues of the neck, its contiguous border will be lost.[336] The cephalic border of the anterior mediastinum ends at the level of the clavicles, whereas that of the posterior mediastinum extends much higher (Fig. 2–21). Hence, a lesion clearly visible above the clavicles on the frontal view must lie posteriorly and be entirely within the thorax (Fig. 2–22). If anterior, the cervical soft tis-

sues would have obscured it. Conversely, when the cephalic border of a shadow disappears as it approaches the clavicles, it is cervicothoracic, i.e., it lies partly in the anterior portion of the mediastinum and partly in the neck (Fig. 2–23). The trachea is the dividing line—a mediastinal mass anterior to it loses its superolateral margins as it reaches the lower border of the clavicles; a posterior mass remains visible above the clavicles; a mass alongside the trachea is visible part way above the clavicles (Fig. 2–24).

Similarly, since the abdominal structures are mainly of water density, a sharply marginated mediastinal mass seen through the diaphragm on either a chest or an abdominal film must lie in the thorax. A silhouette sign on its lowermost margin indicates that the mass ends at the diaphragm or extends below it. Convergence of the lower lateral margin toward the spine indicates that the bottom of the lesion is nearby and, therefore, that the lesion is probably entirely intrathoracic. Conversely, lack of convergence or actual divergence of

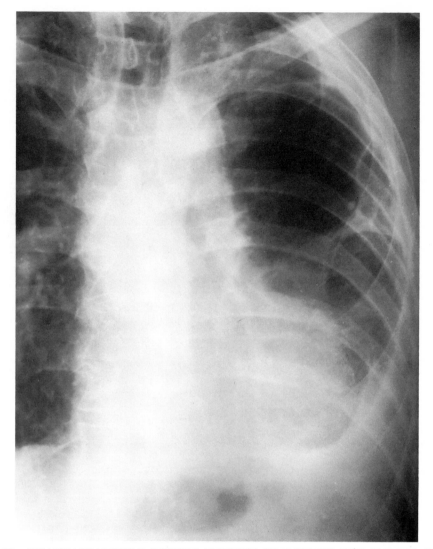

Figure 2–20. PULMONARY VESSELS SHOWING THROUGH AN ENCAPSULATED PLEURAL EFFUSION

the lower border indicates an iceberg configuration, with a segment hidden below in the water density of the abdomen. The *thoracoabdominal sign* is seen in such conditions as aneurysm, neoplasm, and azygos continuation of the inferior vena cava[935] (Fig. 2–25).

The silhouette sign can also be applied to the lateral roentgenogram. This occasionally helps to identify a lesion not visible on the frontal view and is sometimes useful when bilateral lesions require specific localization. Intrathoracic lesions commonly obliterate segments of the contours of the diaphragm, back of the heart, and the aorta (Figs. 2–9B, 2–10B, and 2–16B).

The Diaphragm, Lateral View

Frequently encountered is an opacity clearly seen on the frontal view but not visible at all on the lateral. As explained earlier, a lesion of considerable size, even a completely collapsed lung, is often surprisingly difficult or even impossible to delineate in the lateral view, especially if its margins are beveled, tapered, or unsharp.[767, 1233] In such cases, careful study of the diaphragm, aorta, and posterior border of the heart in the lateral view often indicates the exact site of the opacity (Fig. 2–26). Obliteration of its anterior portion under the heart helps to identify the left hemidiaphragm in the lateral

(*Text continued on page 47.*)

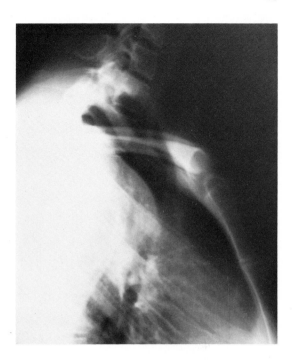

Figure 2–21. LATERAL VIEW OF NORMAL THORACIC INLET

Anteriorly, the thorax ends at the clavicles; posteriorly it extends considerably higher. Therefore, in the frontal view, if a mediastinal lesion is outlined by air above the clavicles it must lie posteriorly and within the thorax. An anterior lesion must either terminate at the clavicular level or enter the water density of the neck.

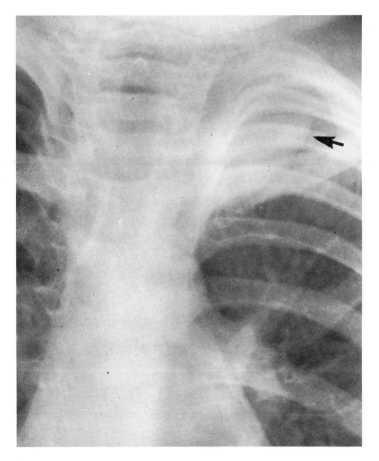

Figure 2–22. NEUROGENIC TUMOR IN THE POSTERIOR THORAX

Note the density above the left clavicle sharply defined by air (arrow). This indicates it is not a cervicothoracic lesion.

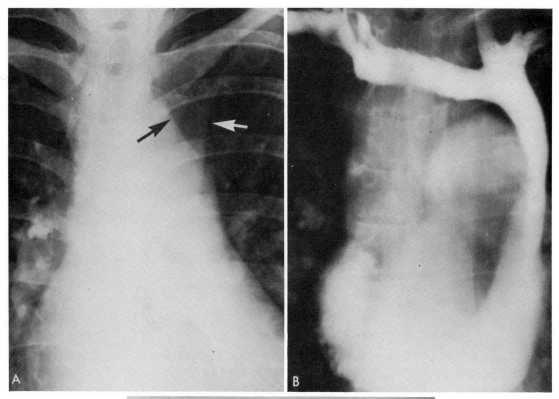

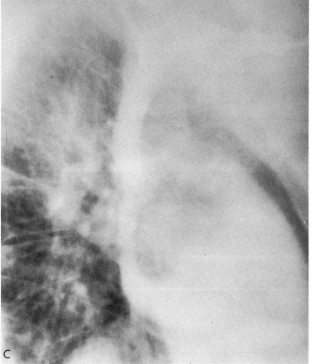

Figure 2–23. CERVICOTHORACIC SIGN

A, The vertical shadow (white arrow) lateral to the aortic knob (black arrow) must lie anteriorly, since it disappears as it approaches the clavicle. (This explains the Hindu rope trick.) *B* and *C,* Venous phase of angiocardiogram in AP and lateral views. A left superior vena cava en route to the coronary sinus is responsible for the abnormal shadow. Note that the anomalous vena cava lies anterior to the trachea in *C.*

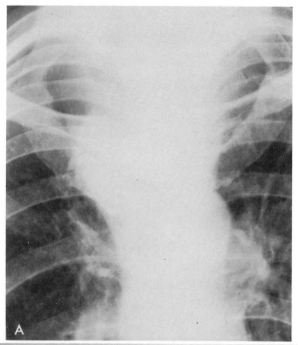

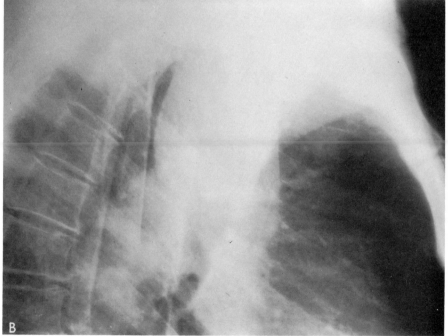

Figure 2–24. CERVICOTHORACIC SIGN IN A THYROID TUMOR

The mass, which is visible slightly above the clavicular level *(A)*, lies alongside the trachea *(B)*.

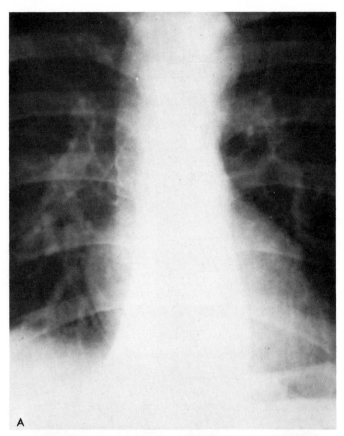

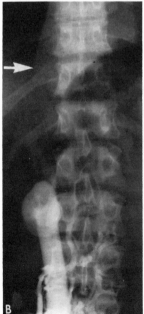

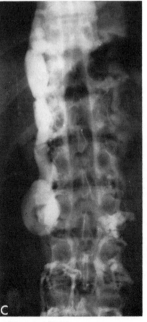

Figure 2–25. THORACOABDOMINAL SIGN

Azygos continuation of the inferior vena cava. *A,* Both right and left lower paravertebral lines are displaced laterally, the right diverging from the spine as it disappears into the abdomen. *B,* Inferior vena cavogram shows abrupt termination of the cava at the level of L1. The right thoracoabdominal sign is again seen (arrow). *C,* Later film in the series shows filling of the enlarged azygos vein, which accounts for the abnormal right paravertebral shadow.

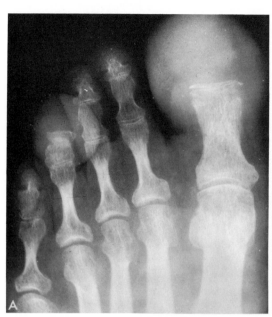

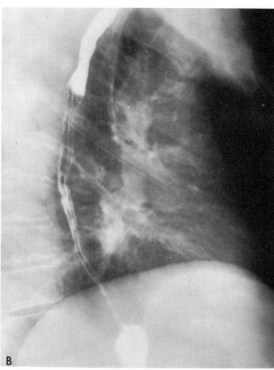

Figure 2-26.   WHY A FOOT FILM IN A CHEST BOOK?

A, Destruction of terminal phalanges sometimes occurs from metastatic bronchogenic carcinoma as a result of tumor embolism secondary to pulmonary vein invasion.[853a] B, Where is the tumor? One hemidiaphragm is visible front-to-back; it must be the right. Loss of the back of the left hemidiaphragm indicates basal segment involvement in the LLL. Loss of the back of the heart shadow indicates disease in the superior and the anterior and medial basal segments of the LLL. The aortic knob is missing, indicating apicoposterior segment opacification in the LUL. Note also that the lower vertebral bodies are equal in density to the upper ones. (See next page for answer.)

view. The remainder of both hemidiaphragms should be clearly outlined. Failure to delineate a normally visible segment of the diaphragm in the lateral view indicates the site of disease (Figs. 2–9, 2–27, and 2–28).

Back of the Heart

The profile of the back of the heart is anatomically located to the left of the midline of the chest. Consequently, unless the heart is displaced into the right thorax, the posterior cardiac silhouette can be obliterated only by left-sided lesions—either pulmonary, mediastinal, or pleural (Figs. 2–16, 2–26, and 2–27). In marked LLL collapse, the posterior surface of the heart may remain visible because the lower lobe is pulled away from it and is replaced by overaerated LUL

(Fig. 2–10). But a word of caution is indicated. On the *normal* lateral film, the posterior border of the heart is not always clearly depicted. This may be attributable to overlying pulmonary vessels or cardiac pulsation. So don't use the silhouette sign here unless you can see a lesion in the vicinity.

The Aorta, Lateral View

The appearance of the aortic arch and descending aorta in the lateral film beautifully portrays the logic of the silhouette sign. In the infant, we seldom see either the arch or descending aorta; in the older child, the knob becomes visible but not the descending aorta. With increasing age, more and more of the distal aorta comes into view, but never all the way down to the dia-

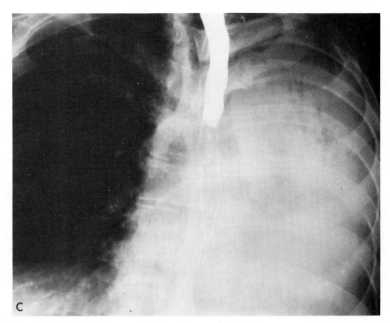

Figure 2–26. *Continued. C,* Here's the proof. Believe it or not, this film was made at the same time as *B.* The patient had bronchogenic carcinoma involving the left main stem bronchus with collapse of the entire left lung. Note the air bronchogram distal to the bronchial obstruction.

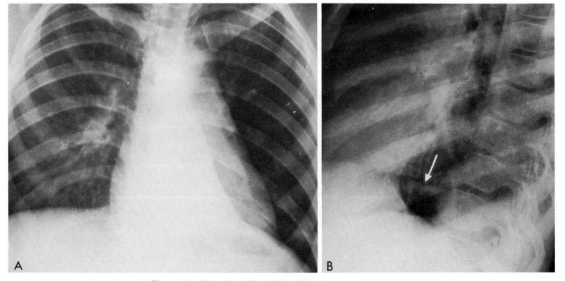

Figure 2–27. SILHOUETTE SIGN IN LATERAL VIEW

    LLL collapse secondary to pneumonia. *A,* The classic triangular opacity of lower lobe collapse is visible through the heart. *B,* Left lateral view. The airless LLL is not visible. Only the middle third of the left hemidiaphragm (arrow) can be seen. Its anterior third is obliterated by the heart and its posterior third by the airless LLL. The lower vertebral bodies are slightly denser than the upper ones. The back of the heart is not visible.

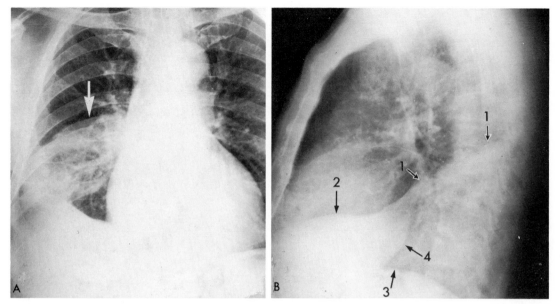

Figure 2–28. THE DIAPHRAGM IN RLL COLLAPSE

A, The frontal view shows loss of the right hemidiaphragm except for a short medial segment. The major fissure is pulled down and parallels the central beam (arrow). The minor fissure is in normal position. The right heart border is visible. *B, 1,* Collapsed RLL. *2,* Elevated right leaf of the diaphragm. The posterior half is obliterated by the collapsed lobe. *3,* Left hemidiaphragm obliterated anteriorly by the bottom of the heart. *4,* Back of the heart.

phragm (Fig. 2–29). The explanation for this is given in Figure 2–29*I,* drawn and sent to me by Dr. Fleischner and reproduced for its unsurpassed clarity and historical interest.[367]

It is purely a matter of aging and silhouettes; the older we get, the bulgier our silhouettes. The more the aorta elongates, the more to the left it extends and the more likely its anterior and posterior walls will come in contact with air bearing lung. Distally, however, the thoracic aorta must return to the water density of the lower mediastinum before entering the abdomen, so it once again disappears from the lateral view. Occasionally, as stated earlier, it may buckle across the midline into the right lower thorax, and so reappear in the lateral view as an ill-defined nodule just above the diaphragm (Fig. 2–30).

The anterior border of the *ascending* aorta is nearly always seen on the lateral view, but its posterior border is not because it is in contact with other structures of water density. Similarly, the top of the arch, except where the great vessels exit, is often seen but the bottom is not.

Admonitions

In utilizing the silhouette sign, mistakes in localization can be avoided if the following points are borne in mind:

1. The technical quality of the roentgenogram must be such that the diseased area is adequately penetrated. Underpenetration may result in spurious obliteration of a cardiovascular border (Fig. 2–31). This is not to say that the film must necessarily be dark. Standard film penetration is usually satisfactory, except for large lesions.

2. Part of the outline of the cardiovascular structure in question must be clearly visible beyond the shadow of the spine. In about 5 per cent of normal individuals, the right border of the heart and of the aorta does not project into the right thorax (Chap. 15). In these patients, the silhouette sign cannot be applied on the right side (Fig. 2–31).

3. The abnormal opacity must either overlap or be contiguous with a segment of the cardiovascular border. Obviously peripheral lung lesions cannot be localized by this method.

4. The lesion must be of water density.

(*Text continued on page 53.*)

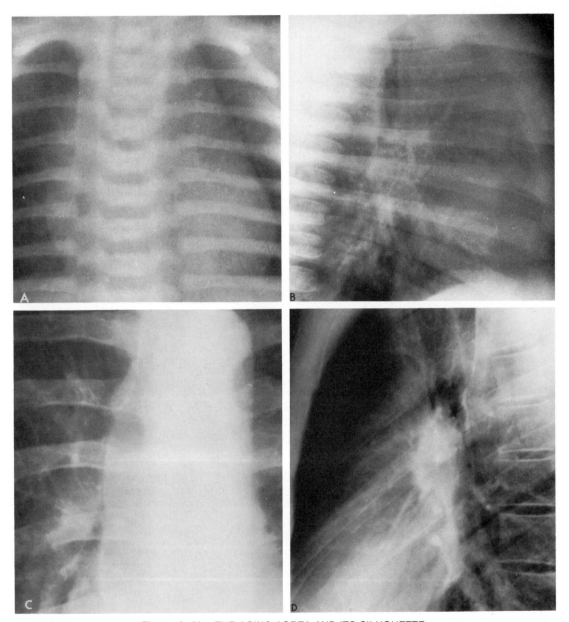

Figure 2–29. THE AGING AORTA AND ITS SILHOUETTE

A and *B*, Infant. The arch and descending aorta are invisible. *C* and *D*, Young adult. Only the aortic arch is seen in the lateral view.

(*Figure continued on opposite page.*)

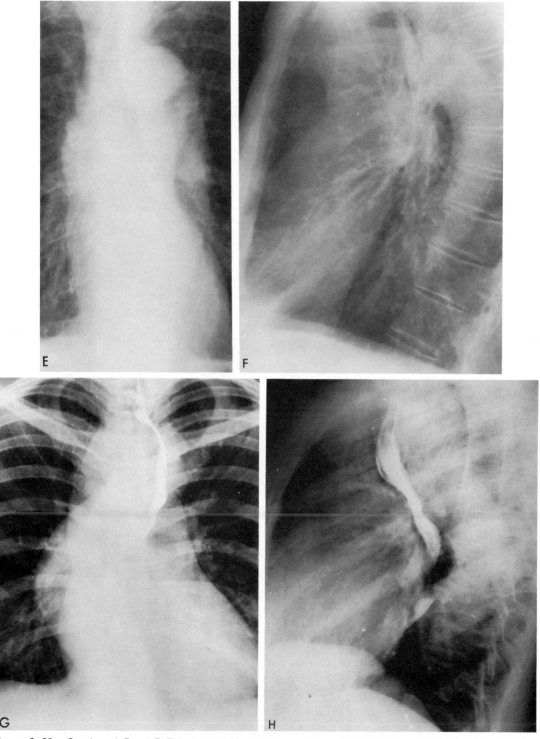

Figure 2–29. *Continued. E* and *F,* Elderly man. Most of the aorta is visible in *F. G* and *H,* Right aortic arch in an elderly man. Note also the absence of a cervicothoracic sign. In this anomaly, the aorta often extends high in the posterior thorax.

(Figure continued on following page.)

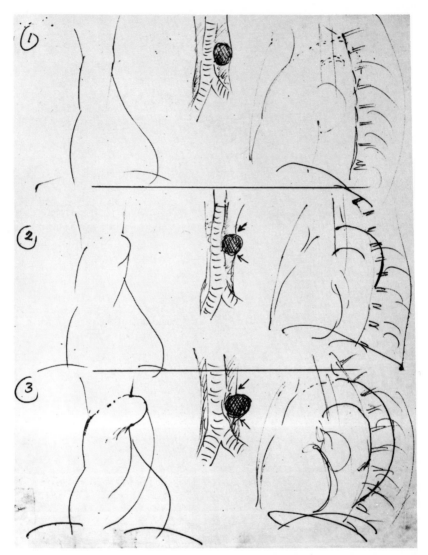

Figure 2–29. *Continued. I,* Felix Fleischner's explanation of these findings. The more the aorta elongates, the more to the left it extends and the more distally we see it on the lateral view.

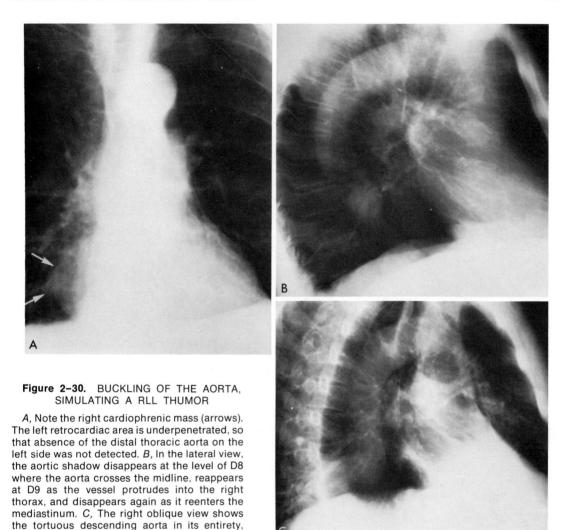

Figure 2–30. BUCKLING OF THE AORTA, SIMULATING A RLL THUMOR

A, Note the right cardiophrenic mass (arrows). The left retrocardiac area is underpenetrated, so that absence of the distal thoracic aorta on the left side was not detected. *B,* In the lateral view, the aortic shadow disappears at the level of D8 where the aorta crosses the midline, reappears at D9 as the vessel protrudes into the right thorax, and disappears again as it reenters the mediastinum. *C,* The right oblique view shows the tortuous descending aorta in its entirety, profiled by the lung.

The sign cannot be applied to air filled cavities or to calcified lesions, but theoretically should hold true in any situation in which like densities come into contact, e.g., fat against fat or calcium against calcium. In fact, I tricked you in Figure 2–4; mineral oil and paraffin are both of *fat* density!

5. When two lesions are superimposed in the PA roentgenogram, only the lesion that obliterates a cardiovascular border can be localized. For example, if the RML and RLL are both involved, the right cardiac border will be obliterated by the RML disease. The presence or absence of RLL involvement cannot then be determined by this method.

6. In patients with funnel breast, the right lower heart border is commonly obliterated[277, 925] (Fig. 2–32). This occurs because the depressed thoracic wall replaces the air bearing lung alongside the cardiac silhouette. Similarly, a chest wall mass outlined by room air may create confusion (Fig. 13–12).

7. Rarely, an anterior lesion in the lung or mediastinum will fail to obliterate the border of the heart or ascending aorta because it is confined to the shallow area in front of the silhouette (Fig. 2–33).

8. In the healthy patient, a segment of the heart border may occasionally be invisible. In at least some instances, this is attributa-

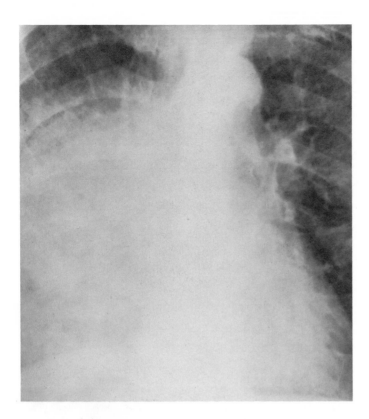

Figure 2–31. SILHOUETTE SIGN MIMICKED ON AN UNDERPENE-TRATED FILM

Lobar pneumonia of the RLL. The right heart border is not visualized because the pneumonic process is inadequately penetrated. Possibly the heart border does not project to the right of the spine in this patient. Localization should not be attempted under these circumstances.

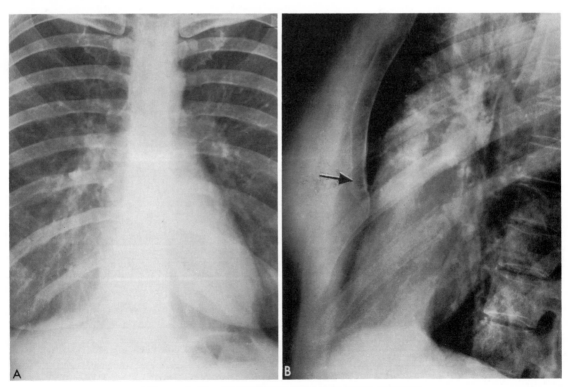

Figure 2–32. SILHOUETTE SIGN IN FUNNEL BREAST

Note the obliteration of the right upper heart border in *A*. The depressed chest wall has replaced the aerated lung alongside the right cardiac border. *B,* The lateral view demonstrates sternal depression (arrow) in this well-endowed young lady.

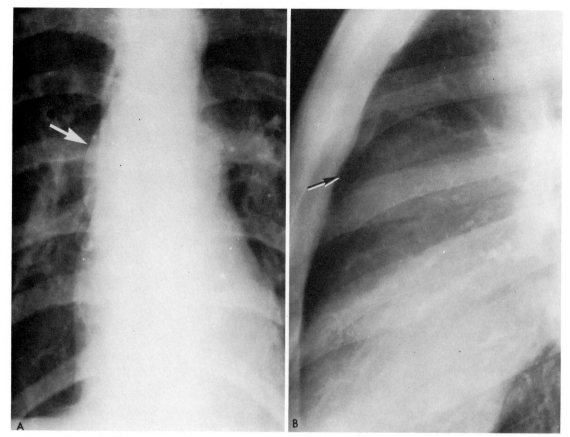

Figure 2–33. FAILURE OF THYMOMA TO OBLITERATE BORDER OF ASCENDING AORTA

The tumor (arrow) lies in the anterior clear space in front of the aorta. A pulmonary lesion anterior to the broadest tangent of the heart (which produces the silhouette) will also fail to obliterate the cardiac border in the frontal view.

ble to a large pulmonary vessel paralleling the cardiac silhouette or to fat on the pericardium. For reasons that escape me, fat in the thorax is often impossible to differentiate from water density. Perhaps the adjacent pulmonary gas density has something to do with this illusion.

I once reviewed over a thousand apparently normal PA teleroentgenograms of asymptomatic patients to determine how often a part of the heart border was normally invisible. In 8 per cent, a very short segment of obliteration clearly attributable to a visible fat pad or overlapping pulmonary vessel was noted on the right side. In about 4 per cent, the obliterated segment was longer and simulated that seen in patients with RML collapse. The left heart border showed very short segment obliteration in

11 per cent, and longer obliteration (somewhat resembling lingular disease) in about 2 per cent (Chap. 15).

An unexplained silhouette sign on one side or the other was thus found in approximately 3 per cent of these presumably normal individuals.* In about one third of these, the resemblance to middle lobe or lingular collapse was close. This surprisingly high figure is embarrassing to me, since I have often expressed the opinion that the silhouette sign is exceedingly rare in the healthy chest. The motto, "My mind's

---

*As my tired eyes began to stare,
  I saw a spot that wasn't there.
  It wasn't there again today.
  I wish that it would go away.
  (Paraphrased from:
      Hughes Mearns' "The Psychoed (Antigonish)."

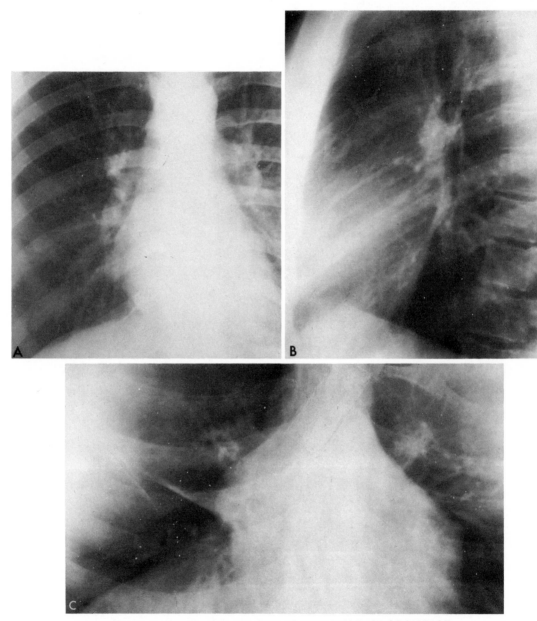

Figure 2–34.   SILHOUETTE SIGN AS MAIN EVIDENCE OF DISEASE

A, Teleroentgenogram. There is obliteration of a short segment of the right heart border without other evidence of pulmonary disease. In the lateral view *(B),* there is a questionable streak in the RML. *C,* Lordotic view shows collapse of the RML. The lung subsequently cleared. RML pneumonia with collapse.

made up—don't confuse me with facts!" certainly applies here.

It is not unusual to encounter patients in whom the silhouette sign represents the *only* roentgen evidence of disease. This occurs most often in RML and lingular collapse (Figs. 2–34 and 3–47) but also under other circumstances (Fig. 2–35). Although, as mentioned earlier, similar findings may on occasion be seen in the normal, the silhouette sign is nonetheless an important indication for additional views and procedures to attempt to explain the loss of the normal aeration (Figs. 2–36 and 2–37).

Attempts to apply the silhouette sign to cutaneous masses (Fig. 2–38) and to abdominal lesions have met with limited success.[821] One of our residents even applied it to a work of art (Fig. 2–39). However, a high degree of accuracy has been maintained when this sign is applied to the thorax. Although occasional mistakes in interpretation do occur, the silhouette sign has af-

forded us an excellent means of localizing intrathoracic lesions.

Shortly after our first article on the silhouette sign appeared, I went to visit a colleague at a hospital in New York City. On my arrival, a film reading session was in progress, so I slipped unobtrusively into a seat in the back row, between two radiology residents. As a new case appeared on the viewbox, one resident leaned across me and whispered to the other, "There's the silhouette sign!"

"What's that?" I asked, and he whispered a brief letter-perfect description of the sign, attributing it to "some fellow out west." He then called out, "Middle lobe disease." It was, and I acted impressed.

At this moment, the Chief saw me in the audience and said, "Oh, Dr. Felson from Cincinnati is visiting us today. Would you come up front, Ben?"

As I edged by the resident he hissed, "You son of a bitch!"

(*Text continued on page 60.*)

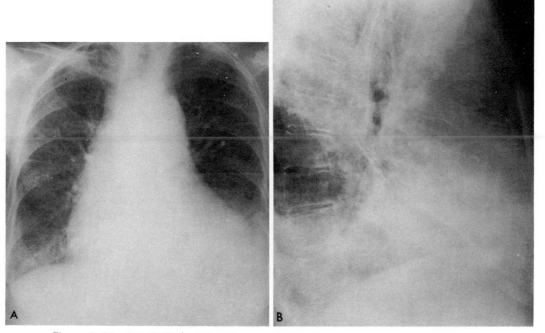

Figure 2–35. SILHOUETTE SIGN AS THE MAIN EVIDENCE OF MEDIASTINAL DISEASE

The clinical and roentgen diagnosis was heart failure. At autopsy, a normal heart was encased in a tremendously thick envelope of mediastinal fibrosis which also extended into the left pleural sac. The diagnostic error could have been avoided. *A,* PA view shows loss of the normal indentations of the heart and aorta. In fact the descending aorta is not visible. The central segment of each main pulmonary artery lies well within its border of the "cardiac" silhouette (hilum overlay sign). *B,* The entire aorta, the back of the heart, and the left hemidiaphragm are obliterated in the lateral film.

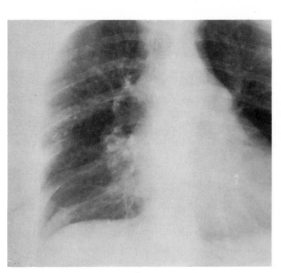

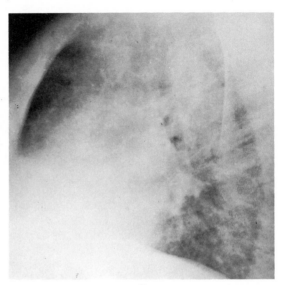

A

B

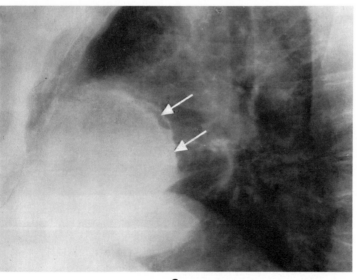

C

Figure 2–36. SILHOUETTE SIGN AS ONLY EVIDENCE OF DISEASE

*A,*Frontal view of the chest of a tremendously obese woman. Note the obliteration of the right cardiac border. *B,* Right lateral teleroentgenogram. No abnormality is recognized. Breast tissue partly obscures the lower anterior thorax. *A* and *B* were at first interpreted as normal. *C,* Bucky right lateral view was obtained because of the right heart border changes. A large anteroinferior mediastinal mass is now visible (arrows). Operative confirmation was not obtained. (From Felson, B.[326]; reproduced with permission of Charles C Thomas, Publisher.)

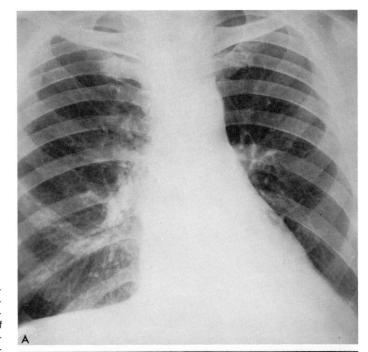

Figure 2–37. SILHOUETTE SIGN AS MAIN EVIDENCE OF DISEASE

A, The left hemidiaphragm is invisible; the left lung is slightly more radiolucent than the right because of compensatory hyperaeration. The left side of the heart shadow is unusually radiopaque. *B,* The lower lobe appears radiolucent. However, only the midportion of the left hemidiaphragm is visible (arrow). Its posterior segment is obliterated by the airless lower lobe and its anterior part by the heart. Carcinoma. (From Felson, B.[325]; reproduced with permission of Amer. J. Med. Sci.)

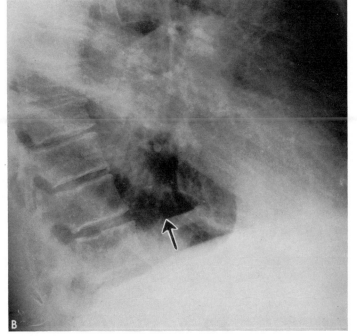

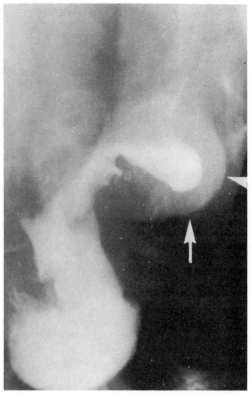

Figure 2–38.   CUTANEOUS SILHOUETTE SIGN

Small postoperative ventral hernia containing the greater curvature of the stomach. Note the sharp lateral and inferior borders (arrows) of the hernia sharply outlined by the room air. The medial and upper margins blend with the abdominal shadows. This has been called the *incomplete border sign.*[822]

THE AIR BRONCHOGRAM

Intrapulmonary bronchi are not visible on the normal chest roentgenogram because they contain air and are surrounded by alveolar air, and their walls are too thin to cast a significant shadow. Parenchymal consolidation may result in the visualization of these bronchi, since the air within their lumens will then stand out in contrast to the surrounding opaque lung.[369] I have called this phenomenon the *air bronchogram.*

Fleischner illustrated this sign in a beautifully simple manner.[371] Figure 2–40 represents a slight modification of his classic demonstration. Paper straws were inserted horizontally through the walls of an upright cylindrical carton and a radiograph was then made with the X-ray beam passing

vertically through the carton *(A)*. Next, water was poured into the carton to a level just below the straws and a second film was exposed *(B)*. Water was then added to *barely* cover the straws and a third film was exposed *(C)*. The straws are barely visible in *A* and *B* because of the lack of contrast between their thin walls and the air within and surrounding them. Their air filled lumens are strikingly visible in *C* because they contrast with the surrounding water density.

In *A*, if the carton is considered to be the lung and the straws the bronchi, it becomes apparent why we do not see the bronchial shadows within the normally aerated lung. In *B*, a pleural effusion is simulated. The "bronchi" are still surrounded by aerated "lung." Thus, an air bronchogram is never seen with pleural effusion per se or, for that matter, with mediastinal or chest wall lesions. Now, let us assume that in *C* the water represents pulmonary consolidation, as in lobar pneumonia, and that the bronchi are patent. The bronchial lumens are clearly

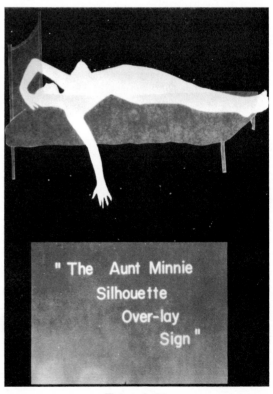

Figure 2–39.

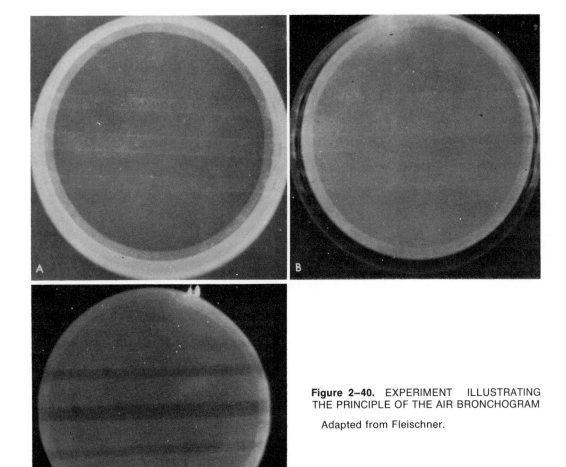

Figure 2–40. EXPERIMENT ILLUSTRATING THE PRINCIPLE OF THE AIR BRONCHOGRAM

Adapted from Fleischner.

seen. Obviously, then, an air bronchogram always indicates infiltrate in the immediately surrounding lung.

Visibility of the bronchi within an intrathoracic density indicates that the lesion is intrapulmonary. The absence of an air bronchogram is of little significance, since it indicates *either* that the lesion is extrapulmonary (e.g., pleural or mediastinal) or that it is intrapulmonary, but the bronchi do not contain air.

An air bronchogram is often seen in pneumonia (Fig. 2–41), and pulmonary edema (Fig. 2–42), and at times in pulmonary infarction (Fig. 2–43), although some disagree.[27] It has been noted many times in hyaline membrane disease.[936] Occasionally, we have seen air filled bronchi in pulmonary lymphoma of the alveolar type (Fig. 7–24) and in alveolar cell carcinoma (Fig. 2–44).

Originally, I theorized that the presence of an air bronchogram in a collapsed lobe or segment could be used to exclude an obstructing bronchial lesion such as carcinoma. I assumed that all the air distal to an obstruction, including that in the bronchi, would be absorbed. However, on reviewing 85 cases of obstructing bronchial carcinoma, we found an air bronchogram in nine (10.5 per cent). Apparently the obstruction from a bronchogenic carcinoma is sometimes in-

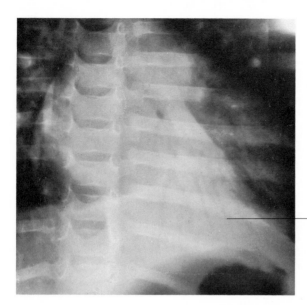

Figure 2–41. AIR BRONCHOGRAM IN PNEUMO-
NIA

The branching air filled bronchi stand out in the otherwise radiopaque LLL. Subsiding lobar pneumonia with collapse (in a child).

Figure 2–42. AIR BRONCHOGRAM IN
PULMONARY EDEMA

The edema in the upper lung fields occurred following a stroke. The lungs cleared in a week. Three months earlier the patient had suffered an episode of congestive failure with pulmonary edema of the more conventional butterfly distribution. Autopsy proof.

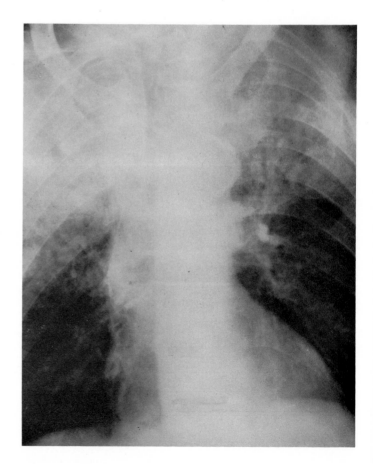

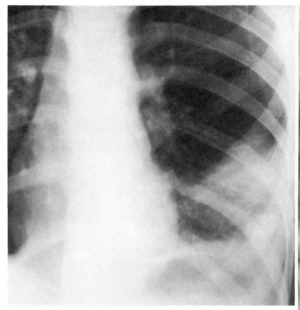

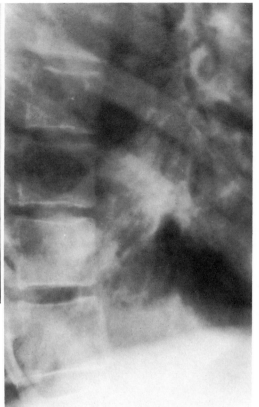

Figure 2–43. AIR BRONCHOGRAM IN PULMONARY
INFARCT

The lateral basal segment of the LLL is involved.

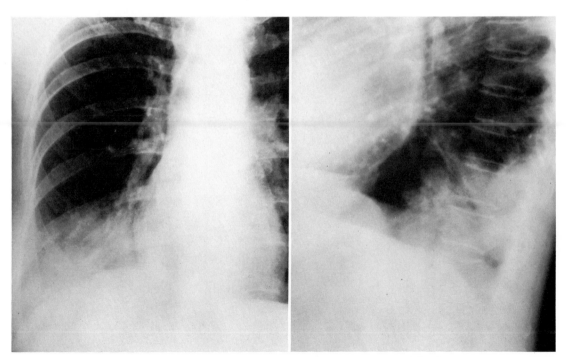

Figure 2–44. AIR BRONCHOGRAM IN ALVEOLAR CELL CARCINOMA

An unusual finding in this neoplasm. The tumor was confined to the RLL and histologically was almost entirely alveolar.

complete, or else the bronchi in the collapsed lung may retain some air (Fig. 2–45). The same applies to bronchial adenoma (Fig. 2–46).

Let's take this air bronchogram concept one step further. What structures in the lung surround the bronchi? The alveoli, of course. So, the air bronchogram is essentially diagnostic of alveolar disease (Chap. 7). The inevitable exceptions are rare: bronchiectasis and chronic bronchitis.[554, 978] The thickened bronchial walls cast a tramline shadow profiled by the surrounding and enclosed air (Fig. 2–47).

An air bronchogram excludes a pleural or mediastinal lesion simply because there are no bronchi traversing these regions (Fig. 2–48). Similarly, an air bronchogram cannot occur within a solid tumor or cyst of the lung, since the bronchi related to such lesions are either engulfed, occluded, or displaced. The same applies to the so-called pulmonary granuloma, in which central destruction is the rule. Conversely, if an air bronchogram is seen within a round pulmonary density you may safely conclude that the lesion is not a tumor but is an alveolar lesion—an inflammatory process, infarct, contusion, alveolar cell carcinoma,[1028a] or lymphoma, in decreasing likelihood (Fig. 2–49).

Tiny areas of radiolucency within an intrathoracic radiopacity often represent normal groups of alveoli within the lesion (Figs. 2–50 and 2–51). Since this pattern has the same genesis and significance as the air bronchogram, I call it an *air alveologram.* However, it isn't as reliable a sign. Nothing else looks quite like an air bronchogram, but pulmonary infiltrate surrounding honeycombing, fine cavitation, or bronchiectasis simulates an air alveologram.

Occasionally the presence of an air bronchogram may provide the only evidence of a pulmonary abnormality. For example, in LLL disease, air filled branching bronchi seen through the cardiac shadow may be the only abnormality detectable on the PA film (Fig. 2–52).

Pulmonary collapse can be postulated if the air filled bronchi appear crowded together. Dilatation of the bronchi can also be recognized and implies the presence of bronchiectasis (Figs. 2–45 and 2–47).

(*Text continued on page 70.*)

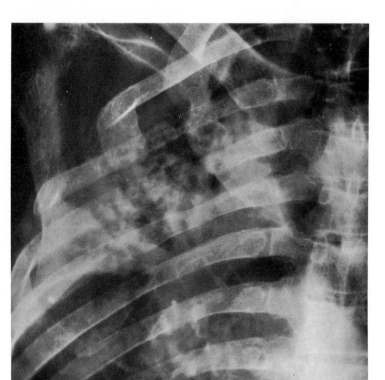

Figure 2–45. AIR BRONCHOGRAM DISTAL TO AN OBSTRUCTING BRONCHOGENIC CARCINOMA

The bronchi are dilated and crowded together, indicating bronchiectasis and collapse.

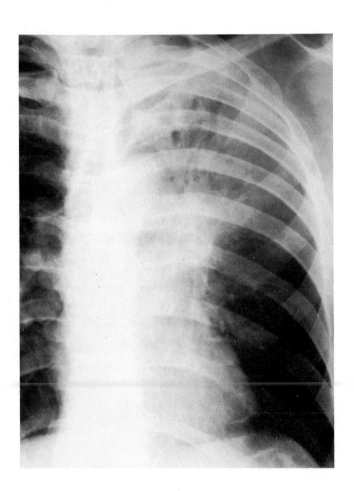

Figure 2–46. AIR BRONCHOGRAM
DISTAL TO A BRONCHIAL ADENOMA

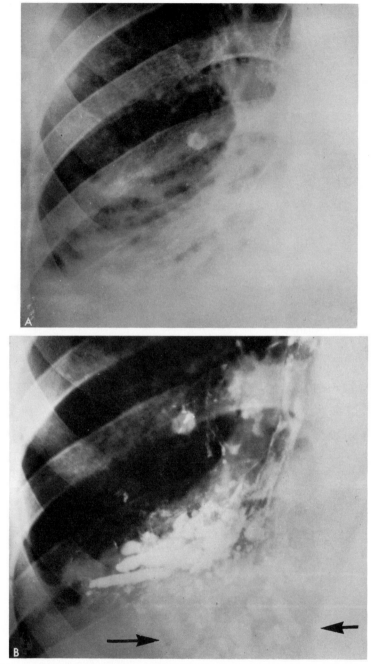

Figure 2–47. AIR BRONCHOGRAM IN BRONCHIECTATIC COLLAPSE OF THE RML AND RLL

A, Plain film shows an air bronchogram. Note the tramline air containing shadows. Crowding of the bronchi indicates collapse and the dilatation denotes bronchiectasis. *B,* Bronchography confirms the diagnosis. The normal patency of the lobar bronchi eliminates tumor as the cause of the collapse. Arrows point to the RLL.

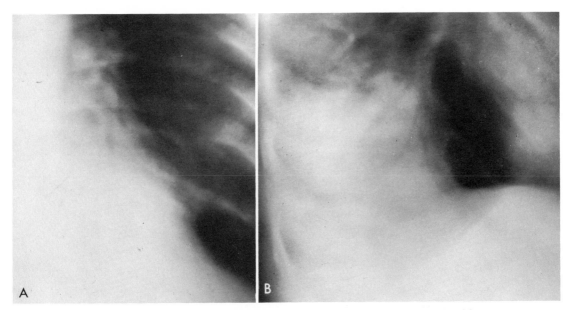

Figure 2–48. AIR BRONCHOGRAM IN A SUSPECTED MEDIASTINAL MASS

AP (*A*) and lateral (*B*) laminagrams of the left lower thorax. The opacity behind the heart was originally thought to be a posterior mediastinal mass, but the air filled bronchi indicated pulmonary infiltrate. Operation revealed a chronic pneumonic process in the LLL.

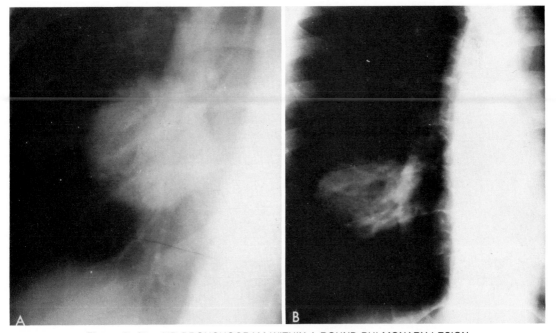

Figure 2–49. AIR BRONCHOGRAM WITHIN A ROUND PULMONARY LESION

This indicates an alveolar lesion and excludes a solid tumor, cyst, or granuloma. The lesion cleared in 2 weeks. Probable pneumonia. *A*, Oblique teleroentgenogram. *B*, Bucky AP film.

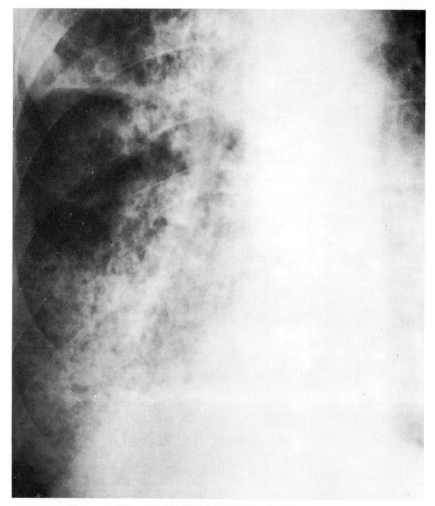

Figure 2–50.   AIR ALVEOLOGRAM IN LOBAR PNEUMONIA

This usually indicates beginning resolution. The lung cleared completely in 8 days.

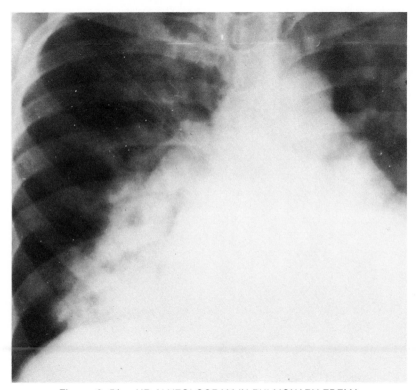

Figure 2–51. AIR ALVEOLOGRAM IN PULMONARY EDEMA

The radiolucencies represent normal aerated lung showing through the water density of the edematous lung.

The normal lung tissue between the almost parallel vascular markings in the medial portions of the lung bases may resemble an air bronchogram (Fig. 2–53). However, on close inspection it will become apparent that the radiopaque lines, rather than the radiolucent ones, show the branching and that the radiolucent areas become wider peripherally. In infants and young children, the proximal ends of the lobar bronchi often lie within the soft tissues of the mediastinum or are surrounded by the hilar blood vessels, especially on the left. Their air filled lumens may then be delineated within the water density.[144] This is a normal finding and should not be mistaken for pulmonary infiltration (Fig. 2–53).

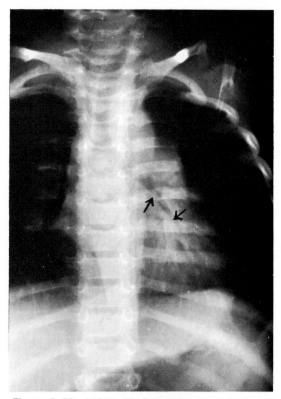

Figure 2–53. VISIBILITY OF LEFT LOBAR BRONCHI (upper arrow) IN A NORMAL CHILD

The radiolucent space between the LLL vessels (below lower arrow) is sometimes mistaken for an air bronchogram.

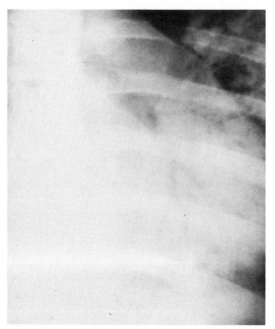

Figure 2–52. AIR BRONCHOGRAM AS THE MAIN IN-DICATION OF DISEASE

The pneumonia in the LLL behind the heart was recognized because of the presence of an air bronchogram within it. The lower portion of the left side of the heart appears more radiopaque than the upper.

The air bronchogram should be specifically searched for in all chest lesions, since it is often quite faint and may not strike the eye. It is generally more readily shown on Bucky films and is particularly difficult to recognize on underexposed teleroentgenograms. To avoid errors in interpretation, one should look for branching of the radiolucent lines. It is again emphasized that *no significance should be attached to the absence of an air bronchogram* within an intrathoracic lesion. However, its presence, properly evaluated, is extremely useful in the elucidation of intrathoracic disease.

CHAPTER 3

THE LOBES

The detection of alterations in lobar size is of paramount importance in the interpretation of chest films. Both lobar collapse and lobar enlargement have significant diagnostic and therapeutic implications, and the roentgenogram provides the best and often the only approach to their recognition. Obviously, a thorough knowledge of the normal size and position of the lobes of the lung is indispensable to roentgen interpretation.[325]

ROENTGEN ANATOMY AND VARIATIONS

The normal septa* which separate the lobes are often seen on chest roentgenograms, but usually not in their entirety.[734] They may be anatomically incomplete[818] or obscured by superimposition of ribs or other structures. Normal and pathologic variations of the lobar contours may also interfere with visibility of the septa. The septa are best demonstrated on Bucky films and are less clearly depicted on improperly centered roentgenograms and those of low contrast. Their average thickness is about 0.2 mm.

The location of the oblique or major septum of each lung in relation to the chest wall is variable. It seldom extends as high as is

*The visceral pleura bordering adjacent surfaces of two lobes forms a double layered interlobar *septum*. The space between is an interlobar fissure. Get the distinction? A fissure is a narrow space, a septum is a divider; e.g., anal fissure, nasal septum. If in doubt, palpate. The two terms, *fissure* and *septum*, are actually used interchangeably. Fleischner preferred *interlobe*, but I can't break my habits.

usually stated in anatomy texts, which are based on postmortem studies. In the lateral view the upper posterior extent of the septum usually lies at the level of the vertebral end of the fifth rib or fifth interspace, often slightly lower on the right than on the left.[128, 751] The oblique fissure usually parallels the sixth rib and reaches the diaphragm several centimeters behind the anterior costophrenic angle. The point of junction with the diaphragm is also variable, but I can recall no instance in which the normal oblique fissure terminated against the anterior thoracic wall.

The oblique septum presents a smooth flat or gently curved surface. In the frontal view it is normally invisible because the roentgen beam does not strike it tangentially. Only when considerable pathologic downward displacement brings it parallel to the beam is it seen in this view (Fig. 2–28). The major fissure is said to be incomplete in about 30 per cent of anatomic dissections.[395, 818]

Portions of the major septa of both lungs are often clearly delineated on the lateral roentgenogram, and the two may be confused. Recognition of septal displacement may depend on their differentiation. The septum on the side nearer the roentgen tube is usually not as distinct as that on the side closer to the film, but the difference, especially on teleroentgenograms, is minimal and should not be relied upon. The right major septum is, of course, readily identified if its junction with the horizontal septum is demonstrable (Fig. 3–1).

If the point where the major fissure touches a leaf of the diaphragm is visible, one need only identify the hemidiaphragm concerned to recognize the side of the fissure. Generally this is not difficult because

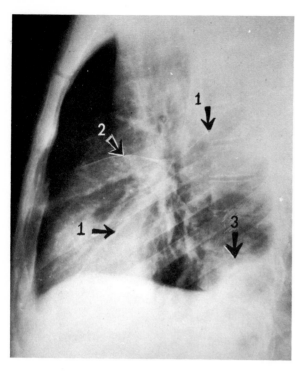

Figure 3–1. RIGHT LATERAL UPRIGHT TELE-ROENTGENOGRAM SHOWING RIGHT INTER-LOBAR SEPTA

The oblique *(1)* and horizontal *(2)* septa are slightly thickened. The right diaphragm is elevated as the result of a pulmonary infarct *(3)*. Note the convexity of the infarct toward the hilum ("Hampton's hump").

the left leaf is obliterated along its line of contact with the undersurface of the heart, and the gastric air bubble can usually be seen below it (Figs. 2–9 and 2–28). In the recumbent lateral view, the hemidiaphragm on the dependent side normally rises a considerable degree above the contralateral one, facilitating differentiation (Fig. 3–2). If necessary, oblique or even stereoscopic lateral views can be obtained for clarification.

As with the major septum, there is considerable variation in the position of the normal right minor or horizontal interlobe. In the lateral roentgenogram, this septum is seen in more than half of normal individuals. It usually meets the oblique septum in the midaxillary line at the level of the fifth rib or interspace. The middle lobe varies in size, depending on the location of this junction, which may lie well above or below the midpoint of the major fissure. The minor septum is usually not truly horizontal but is gently curved, with the convexity upward. It generally extends to the level of the anterior end of the fourth rib.[685, 751]

Sometimes an interlobar septum may present as two lines, more or less parallel, on a single frontal or lateral film. This may occur normally or be associated with collapse and merely means that a step-off or curve in the septum has permitted two parts of its surface to present tangentially to the X-ray beam.

A similar explanation also applies to the *vertical fissure line*, initially described by Davis.[241] This line, a centimeter or two within the lower lateral thoracic wall and paralleling it, extends from the vicinity of the minor fissure to the diaphragm (Fig. 3–3). It represents either a turn or a displacement of the anterolateral portion of the major fissure which presents end-on to the beam. Although encountered normally, it often coexists with cardiac enlargement[241] and with a variety of pulmonary and pleural conditions.[407, 1264] It is more common on the right than on the left. The line may be visible one day and not the next; it may even disappear on expiration because of a change in its relationship to the central beam. A similar line has been reported on the left as a result of LUL collapse in association with cardiomegaly.[322]

The minor fissure is absent or poorly developed in about 20 per cent of anatomic dissections.[639] According to Hilgert,[540] it is visible on PA roentgenograms in 44 per cent of adults and 15.5 per cent of children. In a recent study of 500 normal PA teleroentgenograms in adults, I was able to see the minor septum in 56 per cent. In 24 per cent, the septum was visible for more than half its length; in 32 per cent, a shorter segment was seen. The lateral extent of the septum, when visible, was noted at the level of the fourth anterior interspace in two thirds of the patients, with variations up to two interspaces higher or lower in the remainder. Correlation with the position of the dome of the diaphragm was also poor, but there was a remarkably constant relationship to the right hilum. The medial end of the septal line, or an imaginary continuation of it, generally terminated at the lateral margin of the right inferior pulmonary artery about 0.5 cm distal to its takeoff from the right heart border.

From the preceding discussion, it is apparent that there is so much variation in the position of the minor fissure—and, therefore, in the size of the middle lobe—that abnormal displacement cannot be recognized with certainty unless it is striking or unless other considerations, such as change in contour, are taken into account.

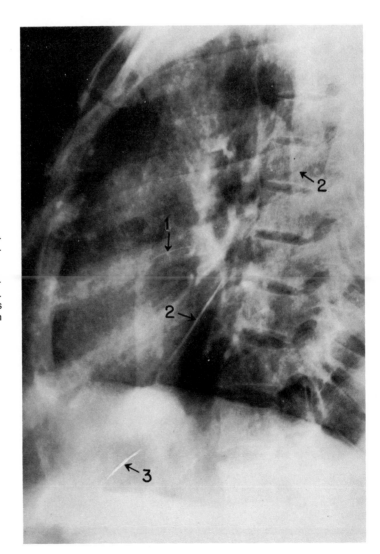

Figure 3–2. NORMAL RIGHT LATERAL BUCKY VIEW SHOWING INTERLOBAR SEPTA

1, Minor septum. *2,* Right major septum. *3,* Left major septum (retouched). The patient was recumbent on his right side, accounting for the elevation of the right leaf of the diaphragm.

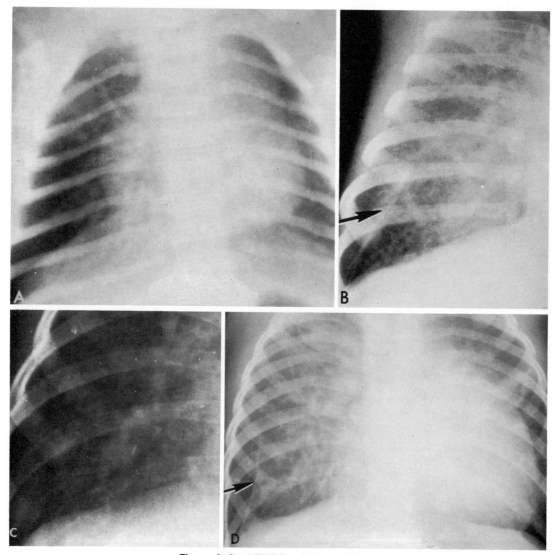

Figure 3–3.   VERTICAL FISSURE LINE

A mongoloid with septum primum cardiac defect. *A,* The line is absent at birth. *B,* It is present at 5 months of age (arrow), during a bout of congestive failure. *C,* At 7 months it is invisible, probably because of rotation, since it reappeared a week later. *D,* At 1 year it is clearly seen (arrow). Congestive failure is again present.

Anomalous Lobes

THE AZYGOS LOBE

Anomalous fissures are not uncommon and often can be recognized roentgenographically. The best known of these is the azygos fissure, which subtends a variable amount of the superomedial portion of the RUL to form the azygos lobe. It is present in 1 per cent of anatomic specimens and is visible in about 0.4 per cent of chest roentgenograms.[11, 560] The site of this fissure bears no constant relationship to the anatomic segments of the lung, a situation contrary to that of other anomalous fissures.[486]

The development of this anomalous fissure is considered by some to be related to the embryologic descent of the heart from its cervical to its thoracic position before the azygos vein has reached its normal medial

A   B

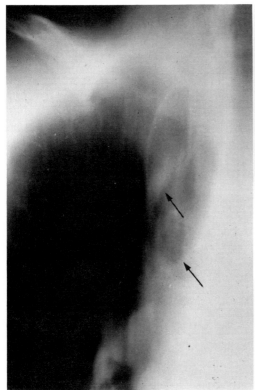

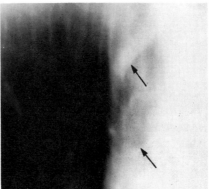

Figure 3–4. TWO EXAMPLES OF AZYGOS LOBE

A and *B*, High position of vein. The tomograms show the azygos vein in profile rather than end-on (upper arrow). Its shadow is missing from its normal site (lower arrow) on these recumbent tomograms. *C*, Upright film in another patient. A lesion in the medial apex was suspected. *D*, Recumbent film shows the vein, now larger, at the lower end of the azygos fissure instead of adjacent to the RUL bronchus. (Courtesy of Tuskegee VA Hospital.)

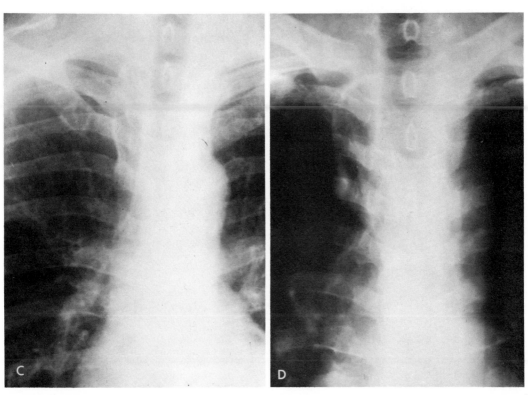

C   D

position. Others have attributed it to too rapid expansion of the pulmonary apex with trapping of the developing azygos vein.[560] In either event, paired folds of parietal and visceral pleura form a mesentery-like structure, the mesoazygos, containing in its hammock the azygos vein.[1124, 1254]

The comma shaped, end-on shadow of the azygos vein, normally positioned in the crotch between the upper lobe bronchus and the trachea, falls short in its migration and lies well within the lung (Figs. 3–4A and B). At the origin of the mesoazygos on the internal thoracic wall, there is a triangular shadow known as the *trigonum parietale* (Fig. 3–5). This represents areolar tissue between the layers of the parietal pleura as it deviates into the lung.

At times it is difficult to be certain that the shadow of the vein is not something more significant. Recumbent films or fluoroscopy will quickly settle the issue. The normal

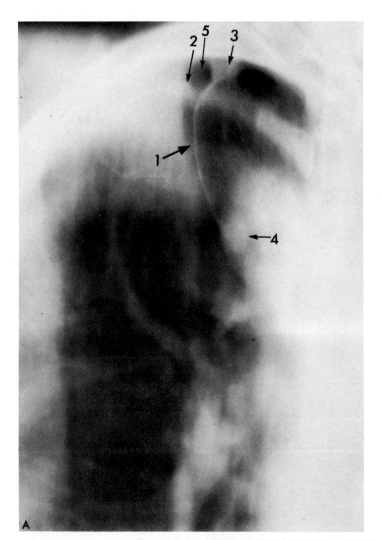

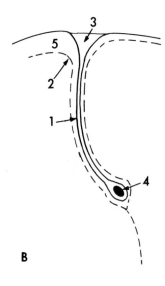

Figure 3–5. AZYGOS LOBE OUTLINED BY PNEUMOTHORAX

A, Tomogram. Air in the pleural sac *(5)* outlines the lateral side of the mesoazygos *(1)* and the visceral pleura of the lung *(2).* The *trigonum parietale (3),* areolar tissue lying along the costal edge of the fissure between the two indented layers of parietal pleura, is clearly depicted. The azygos vein *(4)* lies in the lower end of the fissure between the two layers of parietal pleura. It is slightly superolateral to its normal position. In *B,* solid lines are parietal pleura, broken lines are visceral pleura. (Courtesy of Dr. W. L. Orr.)

azygos vein is invariably visible in recumbency and shrinks notably on Valsalva maneuver and in the erect position (Fig. 5–44). The same applies to the misplaced vein associated with an azygos lobe. Thus, in the supine position, absence of an azygos vein at the usual site and enlargement of the shadow in question identify it as the azygos vein (Figs. 3–4C and D). Azygography has been used to opacify the anomalous vein,[1195] but is hardly necessary.

The azygos lobe is not particularly susceptible to disease.[793] Occasionally a pneumothorax produces a space between the parietal and visceral pleura, nicely demonstrating the various components (Fig. 3–5).

A left azygos lobe is a rare anomaly (Fig. 3–6). The accessory hemiazygos vein which descends on the left side of the upper thoracic vertebral bodies and receives the upper left intercostal veins is probably the vessel responsible (Fig. 5–43). It is not a wrong-sided azygos vein; a left azygos lobe has been found in association with a normal right-sided azygos vein (shown by angiography).[880] The vein is usually visible as a small rounded shadow at the outer edge of the aortic knob.[676, 725, 1084, 1254, 1284]

OTHER ANOMALOUS LOBES

Any bronchopulmonary segment or subsegment may be separated from its neighbors by a fissure, creating an anomalous lobe.[395] The superior segment of either lower lobe may be separated from the remainder of the lobe by a substantial incisura or even a complete septum, thus forming a *superior accessory lobe.* This occurs in about 5 per cent of anatomic specimens and is considerably more common on the right.[128] Not infrequently, the septum can be demonstrated roentgenographically as a horizontal pleural line. In the frontal view, it is seen at the approximate level of the minor septum and is often mistaken for it. In the lateral view, however, it extends *backward* from the major septum to the posterior pleural surface. In this projection it often, but not always, appears to be a posterior continuation of the minor septum, the two forming an X with the major septum.

Consolidation of the superior accessory lobe presents a sharp lower border on the frontal roentgenogram and is usually mistaken for upper lobe disease, especially when it occurs on the right side (Fig. 3–7).

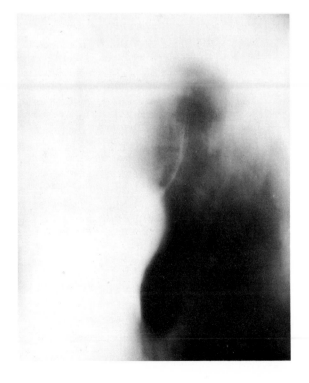

Figure 3–6. LEFT AZYGOS LOBE

Note the small bump on the aortic knob. The trigonum parietale cannot be seen on this tomographic cut.

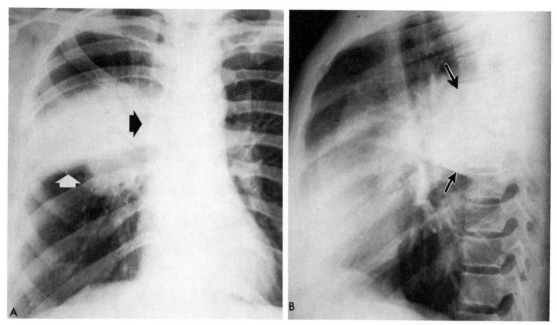

Figure 3–7. PNEUMONIA IN A SUPERIOR ACCESSORY LOBE

A, In the frontal view, the posterior location of the infiltrate is indicated by its failure to obliterate the right border of the ascending aorta (upper arrow). Therefore the sharply defined horizontal lower border (lower arrow) indicates consolidation of a superior accessory lobe rather than of the anterior segment of the RUL. *B,* Right lateral view confirms the localization (arrows). (From Felson, B., and Felson, H.[343]; reproduced with permission of Radiology.)

Similarly, the upper border of the infiltrate in the basal segments of the lower lobe may be sharply demarcated by the anomalous fissure, thus simulating RML disease. Since the superior accessory lobe is not anatomically contiguous with the heart, opacification does not result in obliteration of the right heart border. Localization is readily confirmed on the lateral view.

In about a third of anatomic dissections, an incisura separates the lateral border of the medial basal segment from the other basal segments of the RLL.[395] Not infrequently, a pronounced septum is visible as an oblique line near the right or left cardiophrenic angle on the frontal roentgenogram. The segment thus outlined is called the *inferior accessory lobe* (Fig. 3–8). This septum is not visible in the lateral projection because the roentgen beam strikes perpendicular to its flat surface. Rigler and Ericksen visualized this fissure roentgenographically in 8.2 per cent of 500 patients,

6.6 per cent on the right, 1.0 per cent on the left, and 0.6 per cent bilaterally.[1005] I saw it on the right side in 5 per cent of 500 roentgenograms, but Figure 3–8C is the only time I've ever seen it on the left. Simon believes this line is more often caused by a part of the major fissure.[1125]

As stated earlier, the minor fissure is absent or minimally developed in 25 per cent of anatomic specimens. However, in these cases the segmental anatomy is normal and RML consolidation still presents roentgenographically with a fairly sharp upper border. Rarely, the RML bronchus arises from the RUL bronchus and mirrors the arrangement of the lingula of the left lung so that only two lobes are present.[495] Figure 3–9 illustrates a one-of-a-kind lobar anomaly.

Boyden described a left middle lobe in 8 of 100 anatomic specimens; it represented separation of the lingula from the rest of the LUL by an anomalous minor fissure, often incomplete.[105] Although roentgen visualiza-

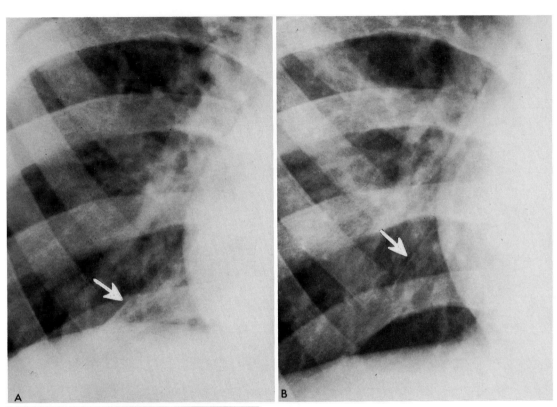

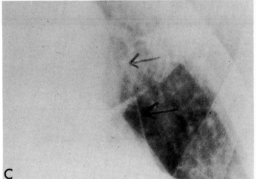

Figure 3–8. INFERIOR ACCESSORY LOBES

A and *B*, Pneumonia in a right inferior accessory lobe. These roentgenograms were made 10 days apart. The inferior accessory fissure (arrow) subtends the right medial basal segment. *C*, Left inferior accessory fissure. It parallels the left heart border to meet the diaphragm. Do not clean the page or your glasses—the spots are in the film. Sorry, but this is my only example.

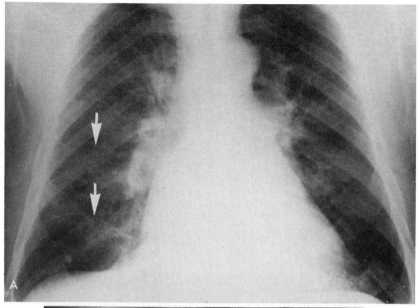

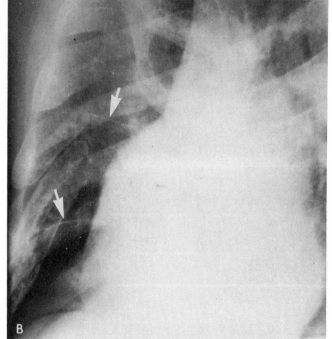

Figure 3–9. TWO MINOR SEPTA

A and *B*, PA and left oblique teleroentgenograms show parallel interlobar septa in the right lung (arrows).

(*Figure continued on opposite page.*)

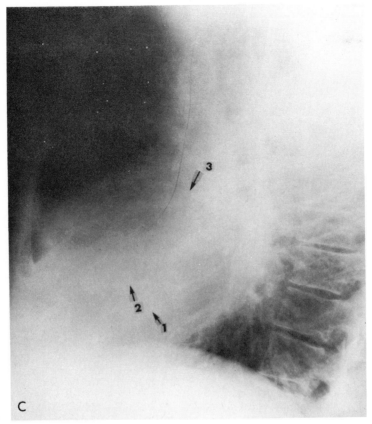

Figure 3–9. *Continued. C,* Lateral view. *(1)* Right major fissure. *(2)* Lower minor fissure. *(3)* Upper minor fissure.

tion of this septum is rare,[1273] I encountered two instances of pneumonia delineating it in one week (Fig. 3–10).

Pulmonary Agenesis and Related Anomalies

Congenital absence or underdevelopment of a lobe is surprisingly common. It is rare in the left lung.[246] Three forms, all usually asymptomatic, have been described: *agenesis,* in which there is complete absence of the lobe as well as of its bronchus (Fig. 3–11); *aplasia,* in which there is no lung tissue but a rudimentary lobar bronchus (Fig. 3–12A); and *hypoplasia* in which bronchi and alveoli are present but the lobe is underdeveloped.[45, 1082, 1157, 1199]

Roentgenologically, there is displacement of the mediastinal structures toward the affected side, more so on inspiration.[361] The involved side shows normal or diminished radiolucency along with diminution in volume. Often there is loss of the silhouette of the right side of the heart and ascending aorta at the site of the absent lobe (Fig. 3–12B). This is difficult to understand, since compensatory overexpansion of the remaining lobes should bring them alongside the heart border. The explanation lies in the failure of the remaining aerated lobes and the parietal pleura encasing them to extend anteriorly all the way to the chest wall. Instead, extrapleural areolar tissue has

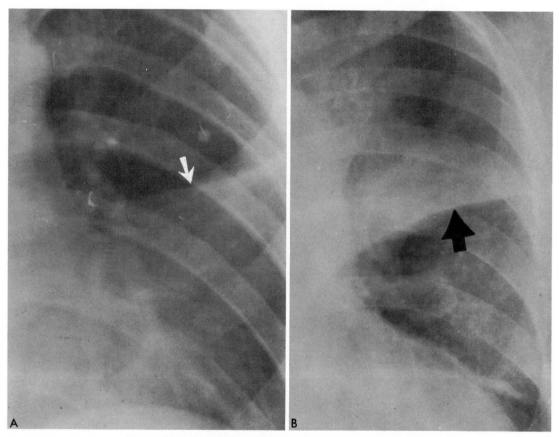

Figure 3–10.   TWO EXAMPLES OF A LEFT MINOR FISSURE

A, Left middle lobe pneumonia. Note the sharp superior border of the infiltrate abutting the anomalous fissure (arrow). The left heart border is obliterated. The lateral view confirmed the localization. *B,* LUL pneumonia outlined against a left minor fissure (arrow). Here too the lateral projection verified the anterior location.

taken the place of the missing lobe and occupies the anteromedial portion of the thoracic cavity alongside the right heart border, between the parietal pleura posteriorly and the thoracic cage anteriorly.[243] This extrapleural tissue is better seen in the lateral view as an anterior opacity paralleling the sternum from diaphragm to clavicle (Figs. 3–12 and 3–20B). In this projection, it simulates LUL collapse except that there is no hilar connection (mediastinal wedge) and of course it's generally on the wrong side. Its sharp posterior border represents the parietal pleura covering the anterior margin of the remaining normal right lung.

The diagnosis of agenesis or aplasia is readily established by bronchography.[576] In agenesis, the bronchus to the missing lobe is simply not there. In aplasia, the blind bronchus often has a distinctive smooth round-bottomed termination, about the shape of September Morn (Fig. 3–13). The only other condition I have seen resembling it is a bronchus severed by trauma (fractured) or by the surgeon (Fig. 3–24).

The bronchial tree supplying the remaining overexpanded pulmonary tissue spreads out to accommodate itself to the increased intrathoracic space. Interestingly, the large bronchi become rearranged to simulate the normal anatomy. In fact, when two lobes remain, the bronchial tree is said to mirror that of a normal left lung.[74, 100, 134, 228, 353] Not to me, however; because they extend over a larger area than they were designed to, the bronchi are smaller in caliber than normal segmental bronchi (Fig. 3–14).

Absence of an *entire* lung is more readily recognized because the thorax is completely opaque and there is striking displacement of the mediastinal structures, diaphragm, and normal lung into the affected hemithorax.[237, 356, 423] Daves and Walsh claim that, unlike acquired gross loss of pulmonary volume, in congenital absence the external diameter of the affected hemithorax is not significantly smaller than the normal side.[235] Either lung may be totally absent (Figs. 3–13 and 3–15). The pulmonary and bronchial arteries are lacking.

(*Text continued on page 87.*)

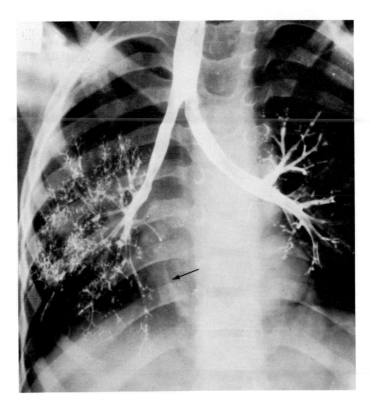

Figure 3–11. LOBAR AGENESIS

There is only one lobar bronchus on the right, probably supplying the RML. An anomalous vessel (arrow) is visible in the right medial lung base. The trachea and heart are deviated to the right but the right hemidiaphragm is in normal position. The right heart border showed partial obliteration on the plain film. The left main stem is unusually long and the anatomy of the left bronchial tree is probably also abnormal.

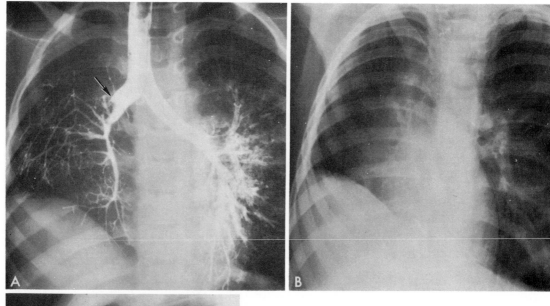

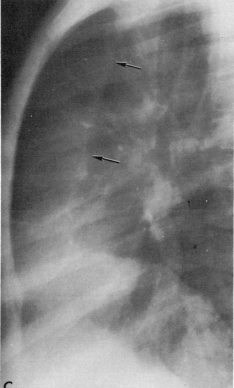

Figure 3–12. APLASIA

A, The rudimentary lobar bronchus (arrow) is the only vestige of the congenitally absent RUL and RML. *B,* PA teleroentgenogram, same patient. The right border of the heart and ascending aorta are obliterated. The right leaf of the diaphragm is elevated, especially laterally. *C,* Lateral view. The arrows point to the anterior border of the right lung separated from the chest wall by a thick layer of extrapleural tissue. Same patient as Figure 3–17.

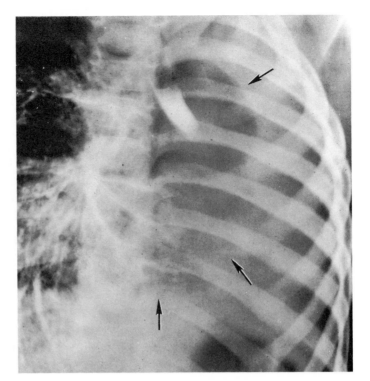

Figure 3–13. APLASIA OF ENTIRE LEFT LUNG

The termination of the left main bronchus is rounded off. A similar appearance is seen in fractured bronchus. Note the herniated right lung (arrows).

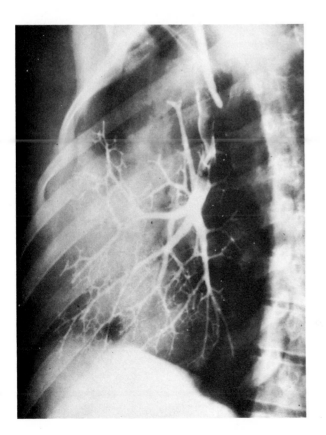

Figure 3–14. BRONCHIAL REARRANGEMENT IN CONGENITAL ABSENCE OF RUL AND RML
Similarity to the bronchial pattern of a normal left lung is noted. However, the bronchi here are smaller in caliber.

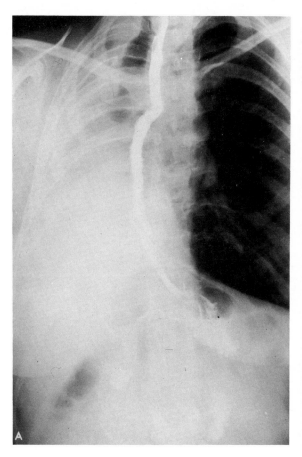

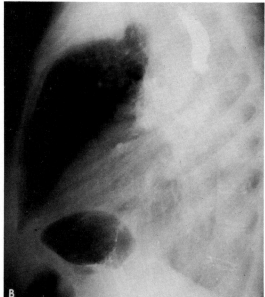

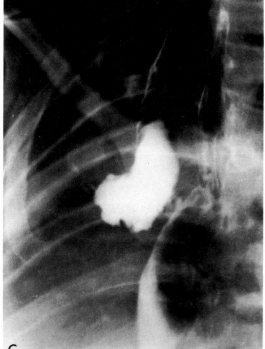

Figure 3–15. APLASIA OF ENTIRE RIGHT LUNG

A, Frontal view. The mediastinal structures, including the heart and esophagus, are shifted far to the right. There is little alteration in the size of the right thoracic cage, as compared to the left. Note the high position of the hepatic flexure, which marks the lower border of the liver. *B,* Lateral view. The heart lies posteriorly, outlined in front by the grossly herniated left lung. The back of the heart, which in this instance lies in the right thorax, is not profiled by air, and so is not visible. *C,* Bronchogram. The right main bronchus terminates blindly except for a few tiny twigs. Contrast medium has also entered the esophagus.

THE CONGENITAL PULMONARY VENOLOBAR SYNDROME

Lobar agenesis or aplasia is frequently associated with other anomalies in the thorax and reported under such interesting titles as the *scimitar syndrome*,[353] the *hypogenetic lung syndrome*, the *epibronchial right pulmonary artery syndrome*,[993] and the *mirror image lung syndrome*,[228] all of which are the same entity. I call it the *congenital pulmonary venolobar syndrome* because one of its major components may be absent in a given case. The term *scimitar syndrome* implies the presence of partial anomalous pulmonary venous return below the diaphragm.[74, 100, 412, 848] This anomalous vessel, occurring much more often on the right side, drains into the inferior vena cava, portal vein, or a hepatic vein. Rarely it enters the lower right atrium directly (Fig. 3–20C). The left to right shunt is hardly ever of clinical magnitude. The roentgen shadow of the anomalous vein has been likened to a Turkish scimitar[228, 812, 1170, 1172] (Fig. 3–16), although it reminds me more of a woman's leg. But then, anything does.

In addition to the lobar agenesis and anomalous pulmonary vein, there are other less constant components of the syndrome. A systemic artery may arise from the lower thoracic or upper abdominal aorta and supply the right lower lung. It occasionally feeds an area of pulmonary sequestration. The right pulmonary artery, which is small to begin with because it serves fewer lobes than normal, provides no branches to the pulmonary tissue supplied by the anomalous systemic artery.[1176, 1199] In fact, the right pulmonary artery may be completely absent and the entire blood supply to the right lung be derived from the aorta (Fig. 3–17).

Anomalies about the right hemidiaphragm are commonly associated with the venolobar syndrome. These include accessory diaphragm (Fig. 3–18), hepatic herniation, phrenic cyst, sequestration, and, rarely, absent inferior vena cava (Fig. 3–19). Accessory diaphragm is a partially duplicated diaphragm that is fused an-

(*Text continued on page 92.*)

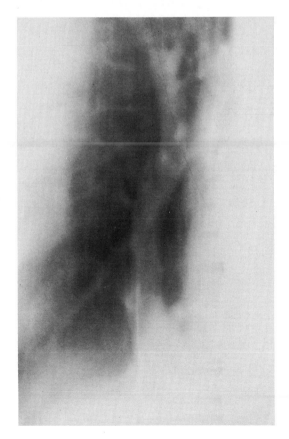

Figure 3–16. ANOMALOUS DRAINAGE OF RIGHT PULMONARY VEIN BELOW THE DIAPHRAGM (SCIMITAR SHADOW)

PA teleroentgenogram. The aberrant vessel receives branches from most or all of the right lung and enlarges as it passes inferiorly toward the cardiophrenic angle where it enters the abdomen, usually via the esophageal hiatus. Drainage is usually to the portal vein or inferior cava. Not proved.

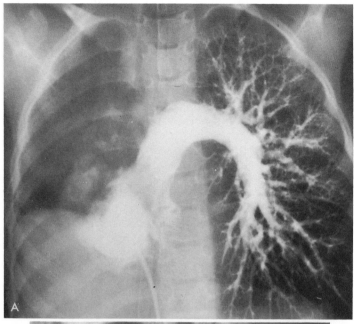

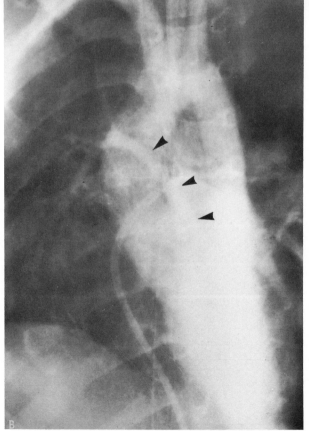

Figure 3–17. PULMONARY APLA-SIA WITH TOTAL ABSENCE OF THE RIGHT PULMONARY ARTERY

Same patient as Figure 3–12. *A,* AP dextroangiocardiogram. The heart is rotated into the right thorax. The right pulmonary trunk is absent. *B,* Levoangiocardiogram. The right lung is supplied from the descending thoracic aorta by a single large vessel (arrowheads). (Courtesy of Dr. Dan R. McFarland.)

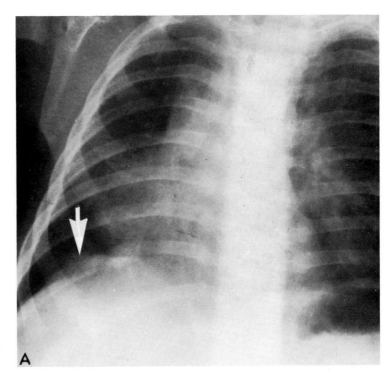

Figure 3–18. ACCESSORY DIA-
PHRAGM

A, There is loss of the right heart
border and a peculiar flat-topped
hump on the right hemidiaphragm
(arrow) in this infant. The heart is
deviated to the right. *B,* AP bronchogram shows a bronchus constricted (arrow) as it passes
through the accessory diaphragm.
It supplies a small section of lung
contained between the two layers
of the right hemidiaphragm. At
operation, an artery and vein accompanied the bronchus through a
small defect in the anomalous diaphragm. (Courtesy of Dr. James W.
Passino.)

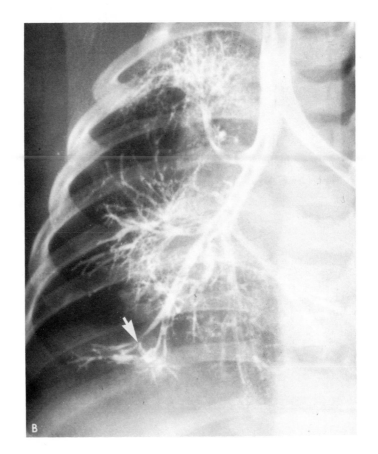

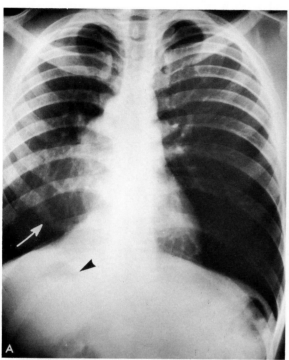

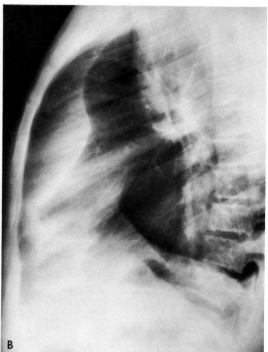

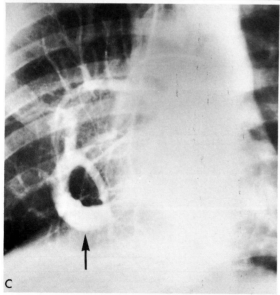

Figure 3–19. VENOLOBAR SYNDROME WITH PROBABLE ABSENCE OF THE INFERIOR CAVA

A, On the PA teleroentgenogram, the gastric bubble is seen under the *right* hemidiaphragm (arrowhead). The end-on azygos vein visualized alongside the upper trachea is enlarged. The right heart border is lost and an anomalous vessel is seen in the right cardiophrenic angle (arrow). *B,* Lateral view. The extrapleural tissue replacing the missing lobe is clearly seen. *C,* Levoangiocardiogram shows entry of an anomalous pulmonary vein into the right atrium. An inferior vena cavagram was not performed. Absence of the hepatic portion of the inferior cava with right-sided stomach is nearly always associated with polysplenia.

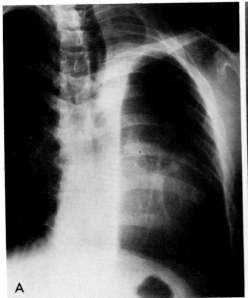

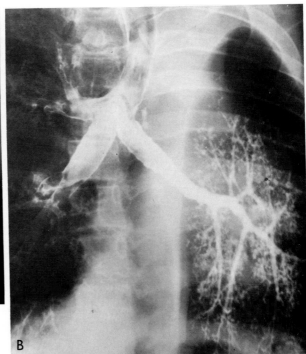

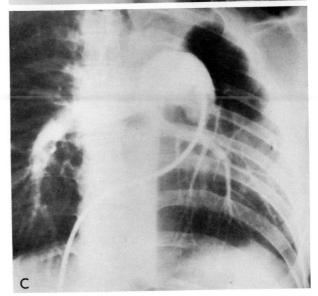

Figure 3–20. LEFT-SIDED VENOLOBAR SYNDROME

A, Plain film. The heart and trachea are shifted to the left. A peculiar branching structure is visible through the heart. *B,* The bronchogram shows absent LUL and trifurcation of the trachea. *C,* Pulmonary arteriogram. The small left pulmonary artery arises medially. The branching structure, probably an anomalous pulmonary vein, is not filled. What's the vertical shadow in the left medial thorax that extends over the pulmonary apex? I believe it's extrapleural areolar tissue. (Courtesy of Dr. Manuel Viamonte, Jr., of Miami, who obtained it from Japan.)

teriorly but separated posteriorly. The cephalic component extends upward and backward to join the posterior thoracic wall. Part or all of the RLL and sometimes the RML is contained between its layers.[243] Figure 3–20 is one of two examples of left-sided venolobar syndrome I have seen.

Tomography, bronchography, or angiography can establish which features of the venolobar syndrome are present. However, they are seldom necessary, since the plain films are generally adequate for diagnosis. There is no need for a detailed demonstration of the specific anomalies, since the condition is usually asymptomatic and seldom requires surgical treatment.

LOBAR COLLAPSE

The term *collapse* is used here to indicate a diminution in volume of a lung, lobe, or

segment from any cause.* Although collapse, by this definition, may result from fibrosis (*contraction collapse*) as in tuberculosis or silicosis, and from extrinsic pressure (*compression collapse*) as in pneumothorax, the discussion that follows is concerned only with the so-called *obstructive* form of collapse.

The volume of a collapsed lobe varies with the cause and rapidity of onset of the obstruction.[550, 888] Pure collapse, as seen with fractured bronchus (Fig. 3–24), results in a mere sliver, since parenchyma comprises so little of the lung volume. At the other extreme, a slowly occluding neoplasm permits secretions and inflammatory products to accumulate distal to it, preventing much reduction in size. In fact, bronchial obstruction does not always result in col-

---

*I prefer *collapse* to *atelectasis* (incomplete distention) because the latter has acquired other meanings, such as *airlessness*.

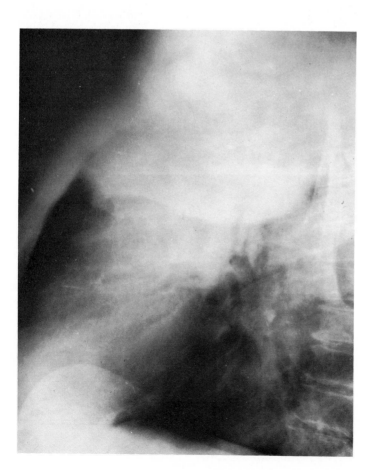

Figure 3–21. "DROWNED LUNG" DISTAL TO BRONCHOGENIC CARCINOMA

The RUL is enlarged posteriorly by accumulated secretions. Confirmed pathologically.

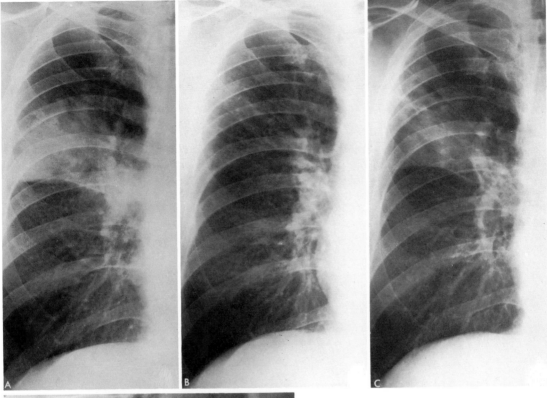

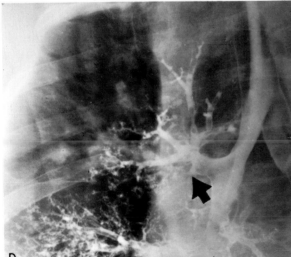

Figure 3–22. COMPLETE CLEARING OF PNEU-
MONIA DISTAL TO A CARCINOMA

A, Consolidation of the anterior segment of the
RUL. The patient was acutely ill but promptly
recovered, both clinically and roentgenologically.
B, 5 months later. Heavy branching markings in
the upper lobe are visible but the patient was still
asymptomatic. The film was interpreted as normal. *C,* 3 months later. Symptoms and roentgen
signs of pneumonia have recurred. There is now
evidence of collapse. *D,* Bronchogram shows a
conical constriction of the anterior segment
bronchus (arrow). Bronchogenic carcinoma was
found at operation.

lapse; distal infection may actually enlarge the affected lung tissue, a condition to which the term *drowned lung* has been applied.[1151] Bulky masses of tumor may also contribute to this enlargement (Fig. 3–21).

The inflammatory changes distal to an ob-structed bronchus may masquerade as pneumonia both clinically and roentgeno-logically. Subsequent disappearance of symptoms accompanied by regression of the roentgen signs may add to the confusion. However, complete clearing of the pulmonary infiltrate hardly ever occurs. Hence, if you adopt the rule that all pneumonias are to be followed to complete roentgen clearing, unduly slow resolution will be detected and necessary studies will be performed. I have seen only two instances in which the pneumonia distal to a tumor *completely* cleared (Fig. 3–22).

Causes and Mechanisms of Collapse

Obstruction of a lobar bronchus with collapse may occur in many dissimilar conditions.[983] These fall into four main categories: (1) intrinsic mass, such as primary or metastatic neoplasm or eroding lymph nodes; (2) intrinsic stenosis, as from tuberculosis; other inflammatory processes; or fracture of a bronchus; (3) extrinsic pressure, as from enlarged lymph nodes, mediastinal tumor, aortic aneurysm, or cardiac enlargement; and (4) bronchial plugging, as by foreign body or mucous accumulation.

Several of these causes of bronchial obstruction deserve further comment. Hypernephroma seems to have a propensity for metastasizing to the wall of a large bronchus and may present as an intrabronchial tumor.[882] I have seen a number of examples[438] (Fig. 3–23). Breast carcinoma,[436] melanoma, and occasionally other neoplasms may do the same. Fracture of a major bronchus, a not-so-rare effect of severe thoracic trauma, results in a marked degree of collapse because it is sudden and complete[550, 888, 897] (Fig. 3–24). Lobar collapse caused by cardiac enlargement is not uncommon.[1017] The types of heart disease include rheumatic mitral stenosis, endocardial fibroelastosis, atrial septal defect, and patent ductus arteriosus (Fig. 3–25). The collapse results from compression of a lobar bronchus by an enlarged left atrium or pulmonary artery. The LLL is generally the one involved, although I have seen collapse of the entire left lung and of the RML from this cause.

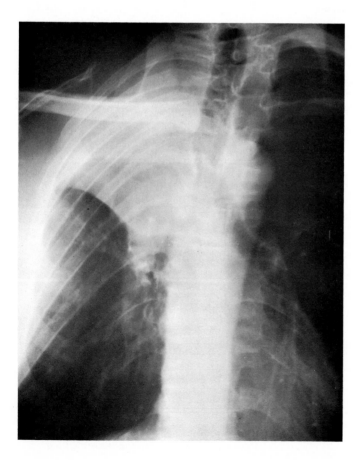

Figure 3–23. BRONCHIAL METASTASIS AS A CAUSE OF PULMONARY COLLAPSE

A hypernephroma had metastasized to the bronchial wall. Note Golden's *S* sign (see p. 121).

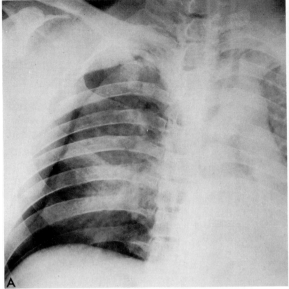

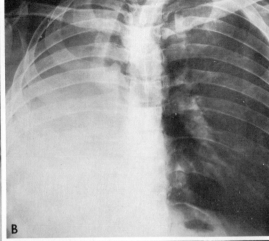

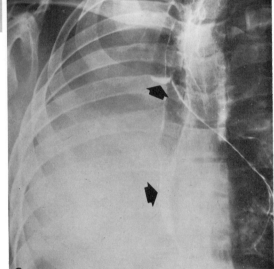

Figure 3–24. COLLAPSE OF RIGHT LUNG SECONDARY TO FRACTURED BRONCHUS

A, Film at the time of injury shows pneumomediastinum and right pneumothorax. B, Several days later. The lung is now completely collapsed. C, Bronchogram shows occlusion of the right stem bronchus (upper arrow). This type of rounded bronchial occlusion is seen only in aplasia, surgical resection, and fracture. The left lung is herniated into the right thorax. The esophagus (lower arrow) is deviated to the right. After operative reconstruction of the right main stem bronchus, the chest appeared essentially normal. (Courtesy of Dr. Hans F. Plaut.)

Chronic non-neoplastic RML collapse has illogically acquired the name *middle lobe syndrome*.[5, 199, 893, 926, 1304] The term is frequently applied to central obstructive collapse of the RML by chronic, usually quiescent granulomatous lymphadenitis caused by histoplasmosis or tuberculosis (Fig. 6–18), but occasionally by silicosis[583] (Fig. 7–13). The term is a poor one, since other lobes or segments are often involved by a similar mechanism and it seems foolish to define them by lengthy anatomic location such as "anterior segment of the RUL syndrome."[104, 767, 783, 786] Furthermore, chronic RML collapse is more commonly the result of multiple peripheral obstruction[222] (Fig.

2–8). This will be discussed later in the chapter.

The lymph node producing the compression often contains calcium and thereby its relationship to the obstructed bronchus can usually be demonstrated on laminagraphy or bronchography (Fig. 14–4). Of course, calcium near a bronchus may be purely coincidental. Before assuming a cause-and-effect relationship, the calcification must be demonstrated at the exact site of an extrinsic compression. Occasionally, a traction diverticulum of the esophagus is produced by retraction of the lymph node causing the collapse.[628]

A foreign body is one of the commonest

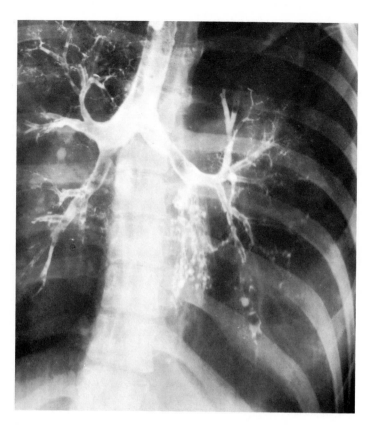

Figure 3–25. COLLAPSE OF LLL FROM CARDIAC ENLARGEMENT

The patient had an atrial septal defect. Compression collapse with bronchiectasis was found at operation.

causes of central obstructive collapse. About two thirds occur in the main stem bronchus and most of the remainder are found in a lobar bronchus. They cause obstructive emphysema about five times as often as collapse.[130] Foreign bodies may shift about from one lobe to another, but rarely, and may fragment, affecting several lobes. Bucky films, tomography, and bronchography are useful in detecting them.

Lobar collapse with a widely patent lobar bronchus, as revealed by bronchoscopy or by bronchography, is frequently encountered.[25, 372] Various theories have been offered to explain this apparent paradox. Reflex bronchospasm with pulmonary vascular dilatation has been implicated,[959] as well as surfactant deficiency.[434] It has been attributed to paralysis of the diaphragm and intercostal muscles.[972] Closure of the pores of Kohn after anesthesia or pulmonary inflammation, preventing collateral ventilation from popping out mucous accumulations, has also been mentioned as a cause.[222, 739] Failure of ciliary action to remove the excessive mucus which accumulates because of pain and splinting has been blamed for postoperative collapse.[539, 1321] Viswanathan[1250] and others[695, 959] have pointed out that air distal to complete central obstruction must be absorbed by the bloodstream and this takes 4 to 24 hours. However, in postoperative and other situations in which secretions accumulate in the lung, the soft plugs move distally on inspiration, entering and completely blocking the smaller bronchi. On expiration, they move proximally, permitting the air to leave and thus accounting for rapid collapse (in a matter of 10 minutes).

My own theory is that during the resolution of pneumonia, after contusion of the lung, or following operation, secretions accumulate centrally. Pain, diminished diaphragmatic motion, and depressed cough reflex prevent expulsion of the exudate, and the air distal to these large plugs is gradually absorbed into the bloodstream. The increasing distal negative pressure pulls the soft semifluid material peripherally and it splits at each of the many bifurcations, moving to the smallest bronchi as the last bit of air is absorbed. The mechanism described by Viswanathan may play a role in the rate of absorption of the air.[1250]

The presence of plugs of mucus, blood, and inflammatory secretion in the small bronchi in collapse is not theoretical. As far back as 1861 Barthel noted them.[186] In a resected collapsed lobe secondary to pneumonia, Simon saw many peripheral plugs protruding from the cut surface.[1121] I have encountered them at the autopsy table in lobar collapse from asthma, pneumonia, and radiation pneumonitis, and so has Rigler.[998] A physician friend, aware of my views, had a bout of pneumonia with RML collapse. Bronchography showed peripheral plugging in this lobe (Fig. 3–26). During recuperation, he expectorated over 100 tiny branching plugs which he brought to me triumphantly as evidence to substantiate my theory!

Fleischner called attention to the absence of bronchographic filling of the finer twigs of the bronchial tree in bronchiectasis ("leafless tree" appearance)[372] (Fig. 7–19). I have consistently noted a similar failure of "alveolar" filling on bronchography in lobar collapse, even when this collapse was not associated with bronchiectasis (Fig. 3–27). To sum up, then, innumerable peripheral obstructions are just as effective in causing lobar collapse as a single central lesion.[372, 1156, 1331]

This peripheral form of obstructive collapse is as frequent as the central type. Although it is seen in a variety of conditions,[983] it is most common in lobar pneumonia,[26] particularly during the period of early resolution.[1111] It also occurs in viral pneumonia as well as in pneumonia complicating pertussis,[710, 878] diphtheria, and measles.

Peripheral obstructive collapse is also seen after operation, chest trauma, administration of respiratory depressants (e.g., morphine), in kerosene aspiration, cystic fibrosis of the pancreas, bronchial asthma, early radiation pneumonitis,[601] and in bronchiectasis.

So-called *reversible* or *pseudo*bronchiectasis provides striking evidence of the nature of peripheral obstructive collapse.[26, 79,

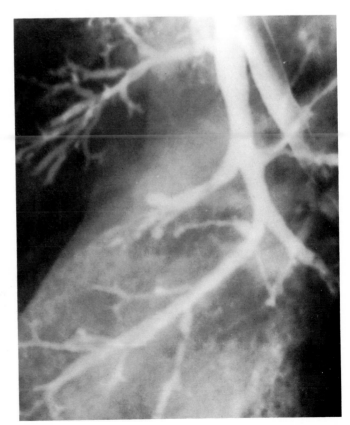

Figure 3–26. PERIPHERAL PLUGS IN RML PNEUMONIA WITH COLLAPSE

Same patient as Figure 1–14. Normal bronchial branching is present in the uninvolved RUL and RLL.

[491, 1138] In this condition, which is probably always the result of pneumonia with pulmonary collapse, bronchography reveals the leafless tree appearance and an associated relatively mild cylindrical or fusiform bronchiectasis confined to the collapsed lobe or segment.[25] Fleischner attributed the bronchial dilatation to the absence of air filled alveoli—the negative pleural pressure then pulls directly upon the bronchi and widens their lumens.[372] My own fanciful theory is that the long slender bronchi of the normal sized lobe become wider as they shorten to conform to the size of the collapsed lobe. Reexpansion of the collapsed lung tissue occurs, often after many months.[601] Bronchography then shows normal sized bronchi and alveolar filling (Fig. 3–28). This phenomenon obviously cannot be explained by fibrosis, which is irreversible, or by central obstruction of a large bronchus, which would be obvious on the bronchogram. It is almost certainly attributable to innumerable peripheral plugs which are subsequently expectorated or absorbed.

Direct Roentgen Signs of Collapse

DISPLACED SEPTA

The most direct and reliable roentgen sign of lobar collapse is displacement of the interlobar septa bounding the affected lobe (Figs. 2–10, 2–28). The degree of displacement varies with the extent of collapse, but decreased volume is always evident if the septa are visible. Occasionally the collapsed lobe retains much of its air, so that septal shift may represent the only sign of collapse (Fig. 3–29). In general, the more rapid the onset of obstruction the more complete is the collapse and the greater the septal displacement.

LOSS OF AERATION

Radiopacity of the affected lobe, reflecting the loss of aeration, is another direct sign of collapse, but, of course, must be accompanied by other signs to be valid.

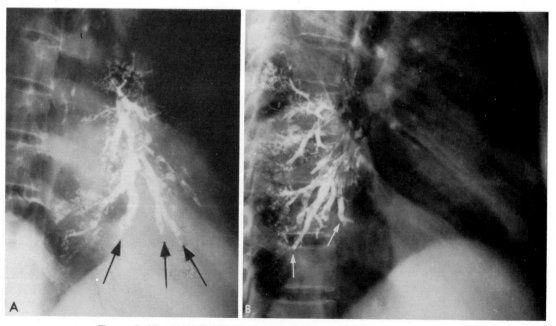

Figure 3–27. "LEAFLESS TREE" APPEARANCE IN LOBAR COLLAPSE

Two different patients with pneumonia of the LLL showing irregular clearing. The bronchogram shows the presence of "alveolar" filling in the aerated portions and its absence in the airless segments (arrows).

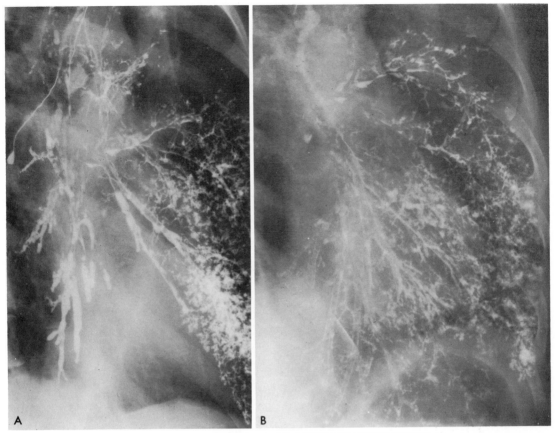

Figure 3–28. REVERSIBLE OR PSEUDOBRONCHIECTASIS

A, Partially collapsed LLL secondary to slowly resolving pneumonia. The lower lobe bronchus and its segmental branches are patent. The bronchi show fusiform dilatation and are crowded together. Alveolar filling is seen only in the normal LUL. *B,* Repeat bronchogram a year later, after reexpansion of the lower lobe, is normal. (Courtesy of Dr. Lee S. Rosenberg.)

Surprisingly, the airlessness may not be apparent on conventional frontal and lateral roentgenograms. In such cases, lordotic or oblique views, especially under fluoroscopic control, are sometimes required for its demonstration. We have found the silhouette sign particularly useful in detecting loss of aeration in lobar collapse. In RML collapse, the frontal and sometimes even the lateral view may show little or no evidence of the airless lobe. However, the right border of the heart is almost invariably obliterated in such cases (Fig. 2–34). Similarly, in lower lobe collapse, the opacity of the affected lobe is sometimes visible in neither or only one view. In this situation, the loss in outline of a segment of diaphragm may help to establish the location of the pathologic process (Figs. 2–37, 3–30).

VASCULAR AND BRONCHIAL SIGNS

In a collapsed lobe that still contains some air, the vascular markings may remain visible and the vessels will lie close together (Fig. 3–29). The same is true of the bronchi if an air bronchogram is visible within the collapsed lobe (Fig. 2–47). Crowding of the bronchial or vascular markings thus also serves as a direct roentgen sign of collapse. Vessels in the adjacent lobes may spread out and curve in an arcade toward the collapsed lobe, indicating compensatory overexpansion.[1122] Bronchographic demonstration of similar rearrangement of the normal bronchi to fill the space abdicated by the collapsed lobe is also a useful sign (Fig. 3–14). I've noted that pulmonary angiography consistently shows ar-

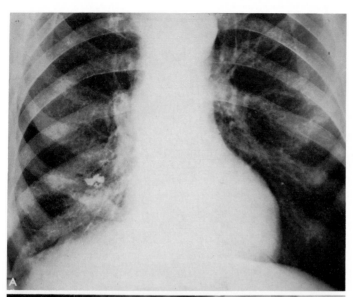

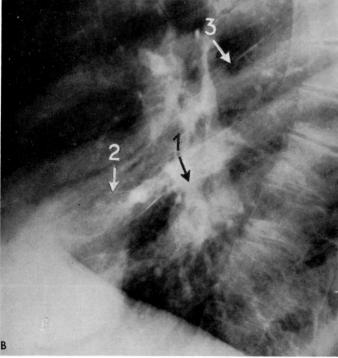

Figure 3–29. COLLAPSE WITHOUT AIRLESSNESS

Note the crowded vascular markings in the right lower lung in *A*. The right hilum is depressed. In the right lateral view *(B)*, the RLL appears radiolucent. The right major septum *(1)*, identified by its junction with the minor septum *(2)*, is displaced posteriorly. The RML is also small. The left major septum *(3)* is visible in normal position. Broncholithiasis[405] in the intermediate bronchus with collapse of the RML and RLL was confirmed at operation. (From Felson, B.[325]; reproduced with permission of Amer. J. Med. Sci.)

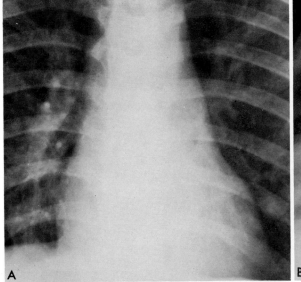

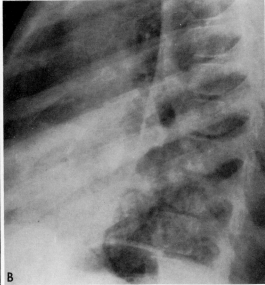

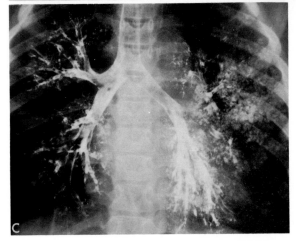

Figure 3–30. LOBAR COLLAPSE POORLY SEEN ON CONVENTIONAL FILMS

A, There is compensatory overaeration of the LUL, the chief sign of collapse in this patient. The left hilum is slightly depressed. *B*, Normal lateral view. *C*, Bronchogram shows crowding and dilatation of the bronchi in the collapsed LLL and overexpansion of the flooded LUL. No operative confirmation. (From Felson, B.[325]; reproduced with permission of Amer. J. Med. Sci.)

terial crowding, vascular "staining," and slow emptying in collapsed lung (Fig. 3–31). Dr. Harold B. Spitz and I have collected about seven such cases associated with lobar or segmental collapse. He has also shown it in experimental pulmonary collapse in dogs.[1154] A similar change has been reported in pulmonary infarction.[96]

Indirect Roentgen Signs of Collapse

The secondary signs of lobar collapse include elevation of a leaf of the diaphragm, shift of the mediastinal structures toward the side of the affected lobe, ipsilateral de-

crease in size of the thoracic cage, compensatory hyperaeration of the uninvolved lobes, and hilar displacement. Of these, the last mentioned is the most reliable and is the only indirect sign which, by itself, is conclusive evidence of collapse.

UNILATERAL ELEVATION OF THE DIAPHRAGM

This is infrequently encountered in collapse of the RUL, RML, or LUL, and is not even a constant finding in lower lobe collapse. Furthermore, diaphragm elevation not only is a common feature of many abdominal and thoracic conditions unas-

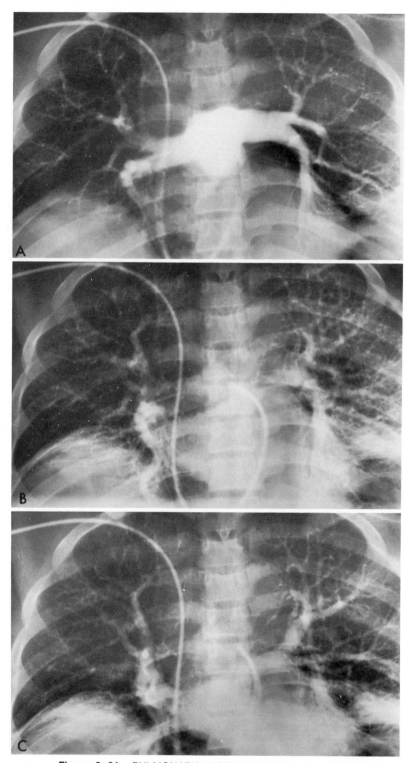

Figure 3–31. PULMONARY ANGIOGRAPHY IN COLLAPSE

A, Early arterial phase. Large segments of collapsed lung at both bases are beginning to fill. *B,* Later arterial phase. The collapsed segments now show "staining." *C,* Venous phase. Drainage from the uninvolved lung is normal but contrast medium remains in the collapsed portion.

(*Figure continued on opposite page.*)

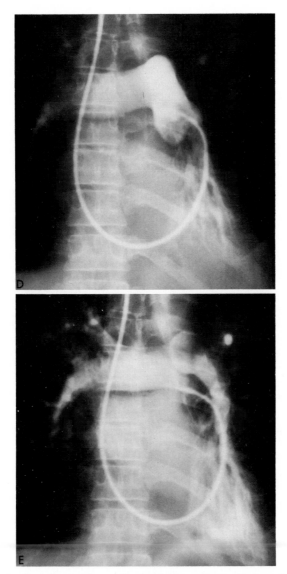

Figure 3–31. *Continued. D* and *E,* Another patient with LLL collapse. Early and late arterial phases, respectively. Note the "blush" in the collapsed lobe. There was a delay in emptying of the lobe.

sociated with collapse, but is also often encountered in the normal patient. I recorded the diaphragm levels in 500 normal PA teleroentgenograms of the chest (army inductees) and found that 11 per cent showed a significant degree of elevation of a leaf of the diaphragm, 2 per cent on the right and 9 per cent on the left. In the latter group, the left hemidiaphragm was either at the same level or actually higher than the right. The degree of diaphragm elevation in collapse varies directly with the amount of collapse

and inversely with the extent of hilar displacement and compensatory overinflation.

DEVIATION OF THE TRACHEA

Tracheal deviation is commonly but not invariably seen in upper lobe collapse (Figs. 3–36 and 3–47). It is infrequent in collapse of the lower or middle lobe or of the lingula. Tracheal deviation is also seen in association with scoliosis, pleural disease, and fibrotic lesions in an upper lobe. Poor positioning of the patient for the frontal roentgenogram is a common cause of *apparent* displacement of the trachea. Among another group of healthy army inductees, 100 PA teleroentgenograms that showed minor degrees of patient rotation were studied. In two thirds of these, the rotation was toward the right anterior oblique position (right shoulder closer to the film) as determined from the fact that the medial end of the left clavicle lay farther from the spine than that of the right. In this group, the trachea was located to the left of the midline of the spine in 39 per cent, in the midline in 57 per cent, and to the right of the midline in 3 per cent. In the last group, no explanation for the deviation, which was in the direction opposite to that expected, was found. In the remaining one third, the rotation was toward the left anterior oblique position, and in these instances, the trachea lay to the right of the midline in 30 per cent, in the midline in 69 per cent, and to the left of the midline in 1 per cent. Of 500 patients in whom no roentgen evidence of rotation could be detected, 2 per cent showed tracheal deviation to either the right or left of the midline, without apparent cause. The tracheal deviation was definite, as much as that seen in many patients with upper lobe collapse.

SHIFT OF THE HEART

Cardiac displacement toward the side of the collapsed lobe occurs relatively infrequently, since it requires considerable negative pressure to move a structure of this bulk. Minor shift is difficult to evaluate. For example, the right side of the heart in normal individuals often fails to clear the spine. Cardiac deviation may also result from pleural or pulmonary fibrosis, thoracic deformity, diaphragmatic eventration or hernia, and intrathoracic mass. Occasionally the heart may lie predominantly in the right thorax without apparent cause. This is thought to represent a developmental variation and has been called *dextroversion of the heart*.[142] Apart from its position, the heart is usually normal or, at most, shows a simple shunt. The term *dextroversion* has also been applied to a group of complex congenital heart conditions,[296] so I now call this abnormality *dextrorotation* to distinguish it. We reported it in 14 asymptomatic patients (Fig. 3–32), including two newborn infants, and have seen many examples since.[1274]

NARROWING OF THE RIB CAGE

This occurs on the side of the collapsed lobe and is a frequent secondary sign of

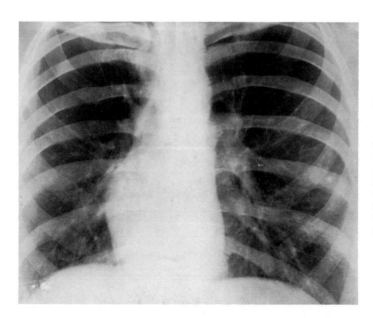

Figure 3–32. DEXTROVERSION OF THE HEART

Asymptomatic woman, age 32. There were no cardiac murmurs and the electrocardiogram was normal. Teleroentgenogram shows the heart predominantly in the right thorax with the aortic knob normally located. The angiocardiogram showed the cardiac chambers in normal relationship to each other.

collapse but is difficult to evaluate unless considerable in degree. It also results from thoracic deformity and pleural or pulmonary fibrosis and is simulated by slight patient rotation. It is said to be minimal or absent in congenital agenesis of a lobe or lung.[235]

COMPENSATORY OVERAERATION

The normal lung tissue adjacent to the diseased lobe becomes overdistended and hyperlucent. This is sometimes a helpful secondary sign of lobar collapse. The overexpansion is recognized in the frontal view by increased radiolucency and spreading of the vascular markings (Figs. 2–37 and 3–30). To recognize this relative oligemia, George Simon actually counts the vessels that cross oblique lines drawn symmetrically in each of the two lung fields. He compares the number of vessels per unit area in one lung with a corresponding area in the other.[1123] Since the changes are seldom striking, it is necessary to make comparison with similar areas in the opposite normal lung. Compensatory overaeration can be distinguished from other forms of pulmonary distention by noting that it clouds up on expiration. Many cases of LLL collapse with LUL overexpansion have been mistakenly diagnosed as idiopathic hyperlucent lung (Swyer-James syndrome) or obstructive emphysema because of failure to appreciate this simple fact.

With marked degrees of collapse, a portion of lung from the normal side may herniate across the midline to fill some of the space evacuated by the collapsed lobe.[*267, 1051] This occurs more often with collapse on the left side.[1019] There are three main locations in the mediastinum through which herniation may occur: (1) anterior to the ascending aorta (Figs. 3–46 and 3–69D); (2) in the lower thorax behind the heart (Fig. 3–51); and (3) under the arch of the aorta. The first mentioned is by far the most frequent,

_____

*Strictly speaking, mere displacement across the midline is not a hernia, since the lung does not necessarily pass through an aperture. True herniation is recognized on the frontal view by displacement of the lung into the contralateral thorax beyond the ascending aorta.

or at least the easiest to identify. Although a herniation here can usually be demonstrated on a well-exposed PA teleroentgenogram, it is usually seen better on a Bucky or lordotic film.[460] The lateral view is confirmatory, demonstrating a distinct widening of the clear space anterior to the ascending aorta.

HILAR DISPLACEMENT

Displacement of a hilum is the most important indirect sign of collapse. Appreciation of the normal position of the hila is therefore essential. The relative levels of the two hila vary somewhat on the normal PA teleroentgenogram. In a survey of 500 roentgenograms of normal adults, I recorded the hilar levels (Table 3–1). In 97 per cent, the left hilum was higher than the right (Fig. 3–33); in 3 per cent the two hila were at the same level. In no instance was the right hilum higher than the left, and in only 0.4 per cent was the left more than 3 cm higher than the right.

Sometimes a hilar shadow is obscured by an abnormal pulmonary density, and its position then becomes difficult to ascertain. In such cases, the hilar level can usually be determined by tracing the arterial markings from the central portion of the lung medially to their confluence.

Elevation of the hilum is the rule in upper lobe collapse (Fig. 3–34) and depression is frequent in lower lobe collapse. However, hilar displacement is usually absent in collapse of the middle lobe or lingula. In lower lobe collapse, there is a reciprocal relationship between hilar displacement and elevation of the diaphragm.

TABLE 3–1. *Relative Hilar Levels in 500 Normal Adults*

RELATIVE LEVELS	NUMBER OF CASES	PER CENT OF CASES
Left Higher Than Right		
Less than 0.75 cm	57	11.4
0.75 to 2.25 cm	402	80.4
2.25 to 3.00 cm	24	4.8
More than 3 cm	2	0.4
Same Level	15	3.0
Right Higher Than Left	0	0

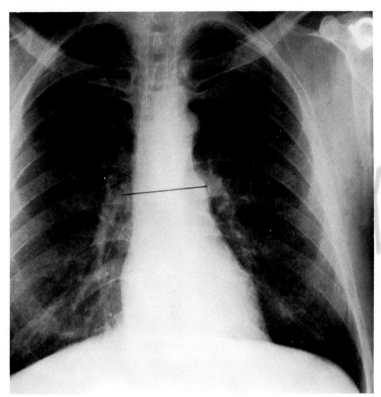

Figure 3–33. NORMAL POSITIONS OF THE TWO HILA

The left hilum is slightly higher than the right in 97 per cent of normal persons.

Figure 3–34. ELEVATION OF HILUM IN RUL COLLAPSE

The right hilum is higher than the left. Phrenic nerve involvement accounts for the elevated right hemidiaphragm. Carcinoma of the apical segment bronchus.

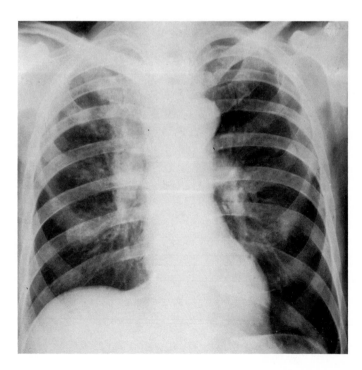

A contracting fibrotic process in the lung or pleura may, of course, also cause hilar displacement. This is often particularly striking in tuberculosis or conglomerate silicosis in an upper lobe, where elevation of a hilum may be so pronounced that the vascular markings emanating from it travel vertically downward to the lower lobe in a manner that has been likened to a waterfall. Severe permanent upper lobe collapse was common (but seldom recognized) in the era of therapeutic pneumothorax for tuberculosis after reexpansion of the lung. Hilar displacement may be the only evidence of collapse if a lobe is so shrunken as to be hidden by the mediastinal structures (Figs. 3–35 and 3–36).

Collapse of the Individual Lobes

Many excellent descriptions of the roentgen findings in collapse of the individual lobes are available, including those by Robbins et al.,[1019, 1020] Lubert and Krause,[766] and Simon.[1127] Lubert and Krause have depicted diagrammatically some of the more common patterns of lobar collapse.[766] The following discussion incorporates some of their material along with my own experiences.

LOWER LOBE COLLAPSE

The lower lobe collapses downward, posteriorly, and medially toward the spine, retaining its connection with the hilum through a tongue of opaque lung tissue that has been called the *mediastinal wedge*[672] (Fig. 3–37). On the *frontal view*, the radiopacity of the affected lobe is usually clearly visible (Fig. 3–38). However, with marked collapse, especially of the LLL, it may be hidden by the heart density. In this situation, a well-penetrated film will usually reveal the airless lung through the heart, the cardiac shadow on the affected side appearing denser than on the normal side[1260] (Figs. 2–1 and 2–37).

The heart border is visible in lower lobe collapse. However, the left border of the descending aorta, the diaphragm, and back of the heart are obliterated by the collapsed LLL (Fig. 3–39). The minor fissure may be displaced downward but more often retains its normal position. Evidently the compensatory hyperaeration and pulmonary rearrangement may spare the region of the minor fissure. Occasionally, the upper part of the major septum may be displaced downward and medially to such a degree that the roentgen beam strikes it tangentially, producing a sharp superior border. On the right side, this appearance closely simulates that of RML disease (Fig. 3–40), except that the heart border is not obliterated.

The hilum is often depressed and small, and there are sparse bowed pulmonary vessels[211, 760] representing only the vessels to the normal lobes; those to the collapsed lobe are incorporated in its radiopacity (Fig. 3–39). The degree of hilar depression and compensatory hyperaeration occurring with lower lobe collapse is variable, depending on the degree of collapse and amount of shift of the mediastinal structures, diaphragm, and thoracic cage. It is not unusual for most of these secondary signs to be absent (Fig. 3–41). Mediastinal herniation is seldom recognized in lower lobe collapse.

On the lateral view, the major septum is displaced posteriorly. This displacement is sometimes detected even before the increased density of the collapsed lobe is apparent (Fig. 3–29). The septum may remain straight or may show an anterior concavity. Often its central segment is invisible because of the mediastinal wedge (Figs. 3–38 and 3–41). The shadow of the diaphragm is lost along the zone of anatomic contact with the airless lobe. In fact, obliteration of a segment of the diaphragm may be the only evidence of loss of aeration apparent in this view (Figs. 2–27 and 3–39).

The right oblique view is sometimes useful in confirming LLL collapse.[367] A well-defined triangular shadow is seen in the angle between the spine and the left hemidiaphragm. Fluoroscopy is helpful in selecting the appropriate degree of obliquity.

COLLAPSE OF MIDDLE LOBE AND LINGULA

The collapsed RML or lingula* may cast only a faint shadow on the frontal roentgen-
(*Text continued on page 112.*)

---

*Since the lingula often behaves as a counterpart of the RML, it is discussed in this section rather than with the LUL.

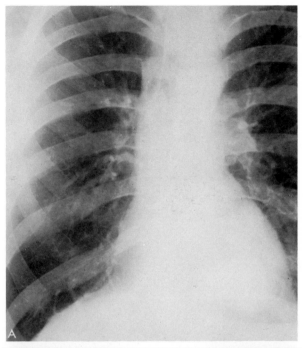

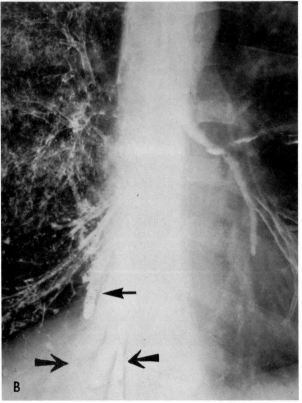

Figure 3–35. DEPRESSED RIGHT HILUM AS
THE SOLE MANIFESTATION OF COLLAPSE

A, The pulmonary arterial branches on the
right converge well below the normal position of
the hilum. The lateral view appeared normal. *B,*
The bronchogram shows marked collapse of the
RLL (between lower arrows) and RML (upper
arrow) with bronchiectasis.

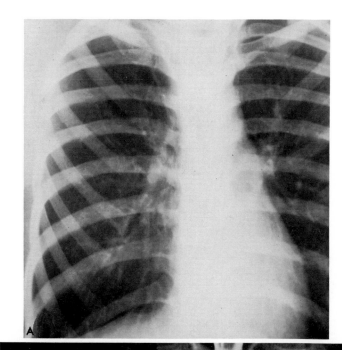

Figure 3–36. ELEVATION OF RIGHT HILUM AS THE CHIEF SIGN OF COLLAPSE

A, The shadow of the collapsed RUL blends with the superior mediastinum and is easily overlooked. However, elevation of the right hilum is apparent. *B,* The bronchogram reveals occlusion of the RUL bronchus (arrowhead) caused by an inflammatory granuloma. Note the midline position of the trachea despite the marked degree of collapse. (From Felson, B.[325]; reproduced with permission of Amer. J. Med. Sci.)

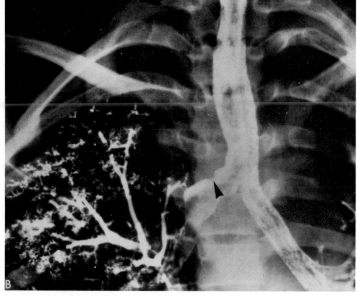

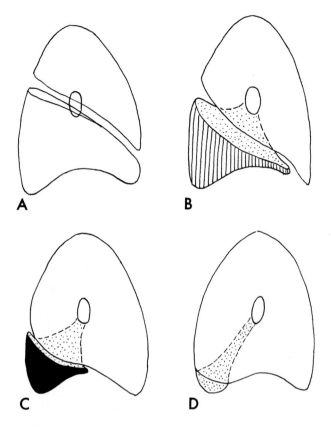

A   B   C   D

Figure 3–37. DIAGRAMMATIC REPRESENT-
ATION OF PROGRESSIVE LLL COLLAPSE

Varying degrees of collapse are illustrated in
lateral projection. The RLL collapses in similar
fashion. (From Lubert and Krause.[766])

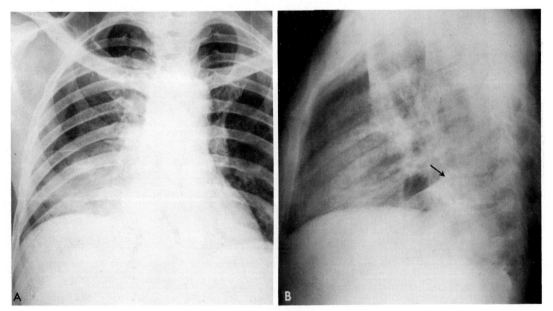

Figure 3–38. POSTOPERATIVE COLLAPSE OF RLL

A, Preservation of outline of the right heart border and of the elevated right hemidiaphragm. *B,* The right lateral
view shows backward displacement of the major septum, the sharp border of which is lost at the level of the
"mediastinal wedge" (arrow).

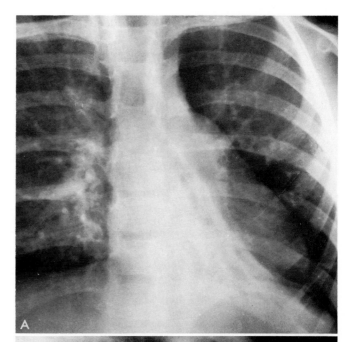

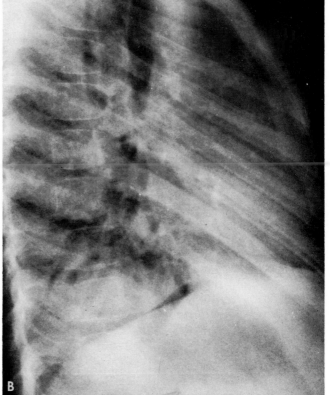

Figure 3–39. LLL COLLAPSE IN BRON-
CHIECTASIS

   A, The left hemidiaphragm and descending aorta are obliterated. The left hilum is
depressed. There is compensatory hyperaeration of the LUL. The air filled
bronchi appear dilated and crowded. *B,*
On the lateral view, the left hemidiaphragm
and posterior cardiac border are obliterated.

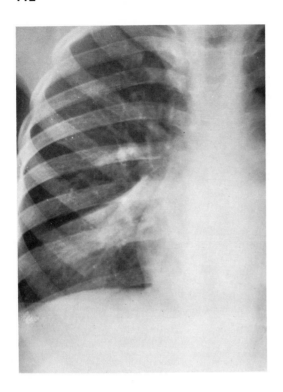

Figure 3–40. COLLAPSE OF SUPERIOR SEG-MENT OF RLL SIMULATING MIDDLE LOBE COLLAPSE

There is downward displacement of the major septum so that it is tangential to the roentgen beam. The heart border is *not* obliterated.

ogram because of its relatively small an-teroposterior diameter.[500, 749] However, al-most invariably the adjacent heart border is obliterated, so that the silhouette sign is often the best and sometimes the only clue of collapse (Fig. 3–42). Secondary signs are usually lacking because of the relatively small potential for shrinkage in volume. Collapse of the RML is often but not always associated with downward displacement of the minor fissure. The lateral portion of the collapsed lobe is frequently so thin that it casts no shadow against the outer segment of the minor fissure on the frontal view. The collapse then appears to be confined to the medial segment. The situation is often clari-fied by the lordotic view (Fig. 1–14).

On the lateral view, the minor and the lower half of the major septa move closer together (Fig. 3–43) and may be bowed toward each other. Occasionally one of the septa is tethered by an adhesion and will re-tain its normal position, the other moving toward it.[1046, 1127] Lingular collapse presents similar findings. There is generally forward displacement of the lower half of the major fissure, but this may be minimal (Fig. 3–46). Sometimes the collapse is poorly shown in lateral projection and an oblique view, pre-ferably controlled by fluoroscopy, is required.

UPPER LOBE COLLAPSE

The roentgen appearance of collapse of the upper lobe varies somewhat on the two sides.[672, 766, 1122] The RUL is displaced su-periorly, resulting in elevation of the minor fissure in the frontal view. There is usually a mild upward bowing of the septum, its lat-eral portion being higher than its medial, so that the opacity is somewhat triangular. With marked collapse, the density of the lobe may blend with that of the right supe-rior mediastinum so that it is easily over-looked (Fig. 3–36). In this event, the sec-ondary signs of collapse, particularly elevation of the right hilum, tracheal shift, and compensatory emphysema, may direct attention to the collapsed lobe. In the lateral view (Figs. 3–44 and 3–45), the superior half of the major septum is displaced for-ward and the minor septum shifts upward, especially anteriorly. The radiopacity of the upper lobe may be completely hidden by the mediastinum or shoulders in this view, but its presence is suggested by obliteration

(*Text continued on page 117.*)

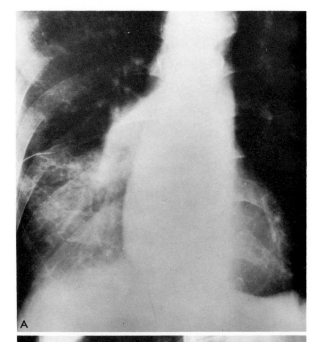

Figure 3–41. RLL COLLAPSE

A, Frontal view. No hilar displacement, compensatory hyperaeration, or other secondary signs of collapse. The right hemidiaphragm is obliterated. *B,* A small mediastinal wedge and an overlap shadow are present. The collapse is of relatively small degree. Bronchogenic carcinoma.

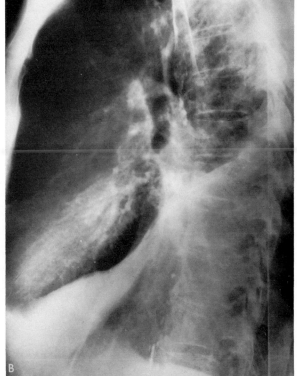

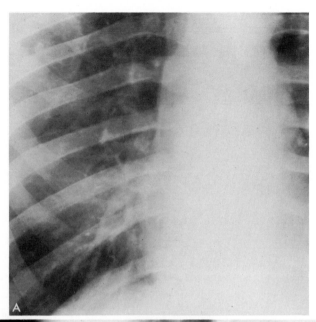

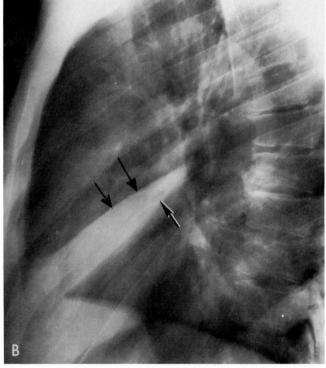

Figure 3–42. RML COLLAPSE

A, The shadow of the collapsed lobe is faint and ill-defined. The right heart border is partly obliterated. *B,* Lateral view. The downward displacement of the minor fissure is evident (upper arrows). The fissural margins are sharp and the borders, unlike those of interlobar effusion, are straight rather than convex. An air bronchogram is present in the collapsed lobe (lower arrow).

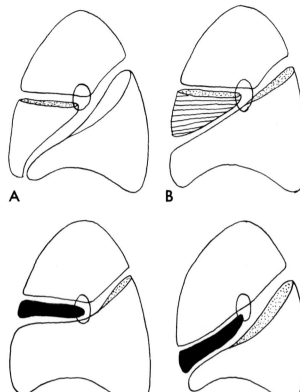

Figure 3–43. DIAGRAM OF PROGRESSIVE RML COLLAPSE

Lateral projection. (From Lubert and Krause.[766])

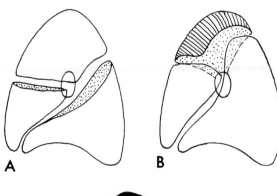

Figure 3–44. DIAGRAM OF PROGRESSIVE RUL COLLAPSE

Lateral view. Note the umbrella shaped shadow in C. (From Lubert and Krause.[766])

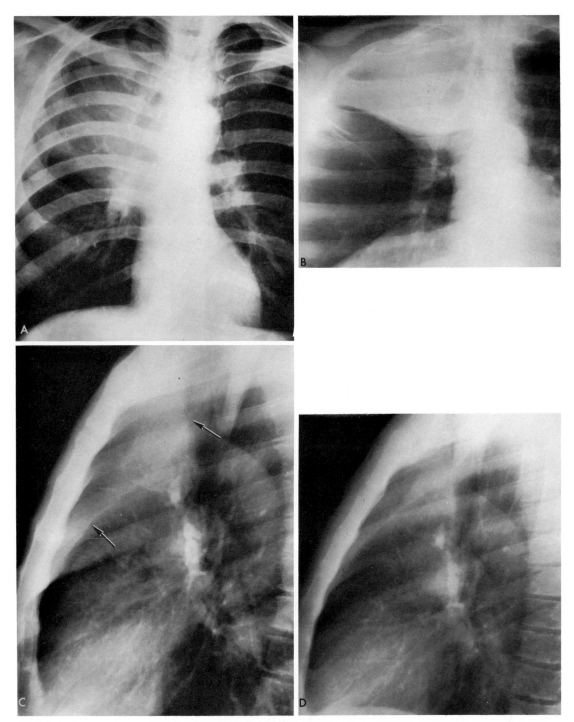

Figure 3–45. RUL COLLAPSE

A, The right upper hilum and ascending aorta are obliterated. The minor fissure is poorly shown. The trachea is sharply deviated to the right. *B,* Lordotic view. The minor fissure is now in profile. *C,* Lateral view. The upper half of the major fissure (upper arrow) and the minor fissure (lower arrow) are shifted anteriorly. There is a mediastinal wedge centrally. *D,* Two weeks later. The collapse has progressed. Again note the "open umbrella" shadow. Bronchogenic carcinoma.

of a segment of the anterior border of the ascending aorta. Rarely, the pattern in combined collapse of the RUL and RML or in collapse of an upper lobe having a long downward extension of its anterior segment (Fig. 4–12) may simulate that of collapse of the LUL.

The LUL collapses anteriorly and upward. On the frontal view, there is a moderate radiopacity of the medial portion of the lung. Unlike its counterpart on the right, the collapsed lobe does not show a sharply defined border. Instead, its lateral margin blends imperceptibly into normal lung density (Fig. 3–46). Sometimes the opacity is so faint that it is practically invisible (Fig. 3–47). In these cases, the silhouette sign saves the day. The aortic knob is usually oblit-

erated by the airless apicoposterior segment adjacent to it, and the upper left cardiac border by the anterior segment. The lingula has already been discussed, but it should also be included here since it is generally a part of LUL collapse. It too shows an ill-defined lateral margin in frontal projection and accounts for downward continuation of the left cardiac border obliteration.

Tracheal deviation and hilar elevation are often evident, and the vascular markings to the lower lobe take a more vertical course than normal. Rarely, the overaerated lower lobe may extend all the way to the apex of the lung and present as a radiolucent area above the collapsed lobe[1216] (Fig. 3–48).

In the lateral view (Figs. 3–46B, 3–47B, and 3–49), the major septum is displaced

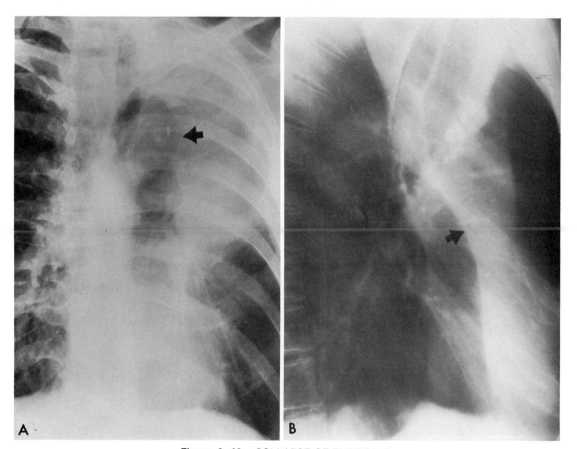

Figure 3–46. COLLAPSE OF ENTIRE LUL

A, The left heart border and aortic knob are obliterated. The right lung is herniated across the midline (arrow). The trachea shows considerable deviation. *B,* The major septum is displaced forward (arrow) and the lower lobe is overexpanded. Herniated right lung occupies the clear space anterior to the ascending aorta. Note the mediastinal wedge behind the arrow.

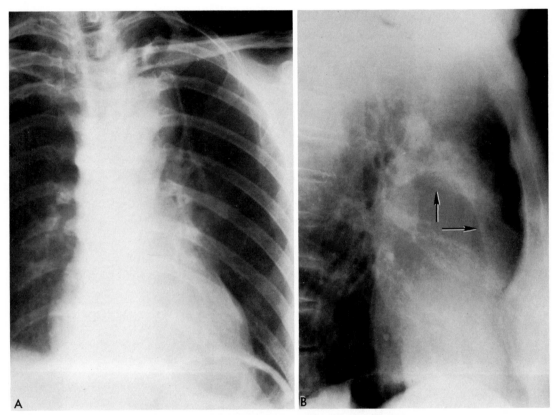

Figure 3–47. MARKED COLLAPSE OF ENTIRE LUL

The roentgen signs are subtle, especially in the PA view *(A)*. Note the obliteration of the upper portion of the heart border (the lingula was pulled cephalad). The aortic knob is preserved. The trachea is not displaced. In the lateral view *(B)*, the major fissure is displaced and bowed anteriorly (horizontal arrow). The mediastinal wedge is visible (vertical arrow). A funnel breast is present.

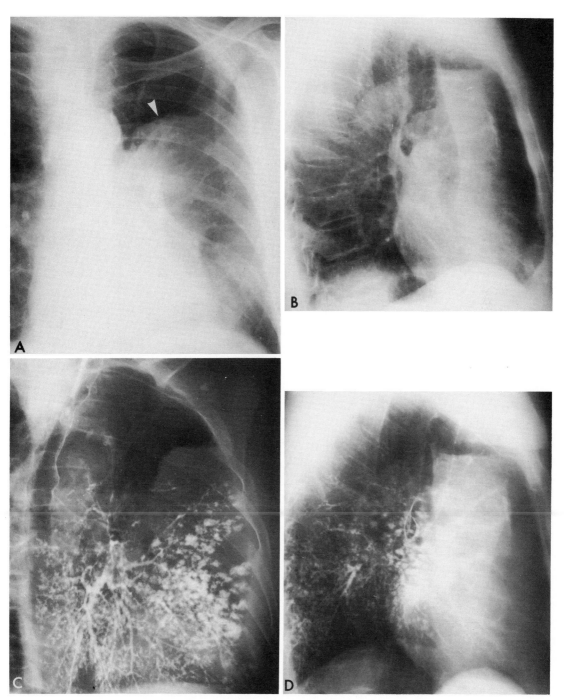

Figure 3–48. LUL COLLAPSE WITH LLL RISING ABOVE IT

A, PA teleroentgenogram. The sharp edge (arrowhead) represents the upper border of the collapsed LUL. Part of the LLL extends above it. *B,* Lateral view. Typical LUL collapse except for the flat top. *C,* Right oblique bronchogram. The flat top is again shown. *D,* Lateral bronchogram. No contrast material has entered the LUL. Spot films showed an occluded LUL bronchus, which was confirmed at operation. Bronchogenic carcinoma.

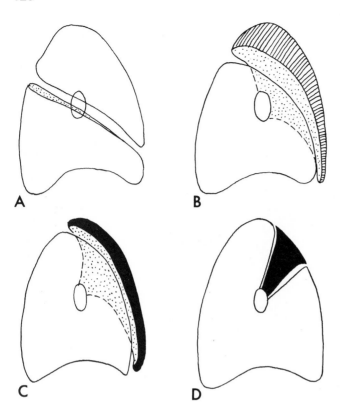

A

B

C

D

Figure 3–49. SCHEMATIC REPRESENT-ATION OF PROGRESSIVE COLLAPSE OF LUL

Lateral view. (From Lubert and Krause.[766])

and bowed anteriorly, paralleling the internal surface of the anterior thoracic wall. The anterior clear space may be obliterated, but herniation of the right lung across the midline often results in a radiolucent strip anterior to the collapsed lobe. When the lingula is also involved, as it often is, the collapsed lobe may follow the sternum down to the diaphragm. A mediastinal wedge of opaque lung tissue may be visible (Fig. 3–47B). A similar shadow is also seen in congenital absence of a lobe (Figs. 3–12 and 3–20) but mostly on the right side. It doesn't represent a collapsed lobe, but rather areolar tissue lying extrapleurally as a result of failure of the remaining lung to grow all the way forward.[243] This shadow does not show a mediastinal wedge.

MULTIPLE LOBAR COLLAPSE

Collapse of multiple lobes reflects the sum of the signs of collapse of the individual lobes (Fig. 3–50) with one notable exception: collapse of an entire lung is often difficult to see in the lateral view because its tapered anterior border often does not cast a sharp shadow[1233] and its density is balanced by the radiolucency of the overexpanded contralateral lung—the uniform filter effect of Lubert and Krause[767] (Fig. 2–26). Collapse of an entire lung is more common on the left side. The collapsed lung shifts dorsally against the posterior thoracic wall. The heart is also displaced backward and its posterior border is usually obliterated. The opposite lung herniates across the midline, sometimes even reaching the lateral thoracic wall on the affected side, and there may be scoliosis of the spine toward the involved side (Fig. 3–51). The site of bronchial occlusion is often visible on the plain PA film, outlined by the water density of the mediastinum and the airless lung.

Differential Diagnosis of Collapse

Roentgenologically, two conditions may simulate lobar collapse: pulmonary consolidation and encapsulated pleural fluid.

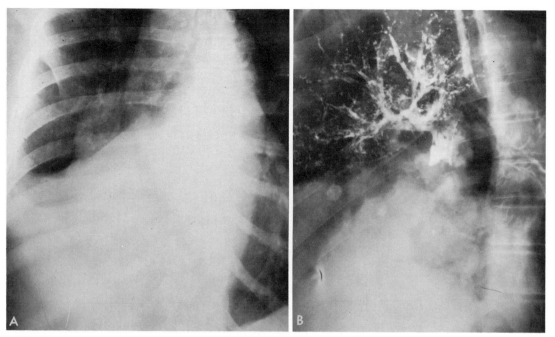

Figure 3–50. RML AND RLL COLLAPSE

A, Frontal view. A right hilar mass is present. The right cardiac border is obliterated and an opacity is seen through the displaced heart. *B,* Left oblique bronchogram shows an abrupt irregular occlusion of the intermediate bronchus by carcinoma.

Lobar consolidation is easy to differentiate, since septal displacement does not occur unless collapse supervenes. The secondary signs of collapse are also lacking. Encapsulated pleural fluid, on the other hand, may closely resemble collapse. This is especially true when the encapsulation is situated in the lower posteromedial portion of the pleural cavity where it can be mistaken for lower lobe collapse; along the anterior upper left thorax where it can resemble LUL collapse; and in the minor or inferior part of the major fissure where it can closely simulate RML or lingular collapse. The presence of pleural thickening elsewhere in the thorax, the absence of an air bronchogram, the demonstration of a nearby interlobar septum separate from the shadow in question, and the presence of rounded contours all favor encapsulation. This subject will be discussed further in Chapter 9.

As mentioned previously, there are many causes of obstructive lobar collapse, and it is seldom possible to distinguish between them on plain roentgenograms. Nevertheless, certain leads obtained from roentgen studies may have important etiologic connotations. For example, enlarged lymph nodes, a foreign body, mediastinal mass, or cardiac enlargement may suggest the cause of the obstruction.

The reverse S shaped curve sometimes seen in the frontal view in collapse of the RUL has been described as a sign of carcinoma.[448, 449] The upper laterally concave segment of the S is formed by the elevated minor fissure; the lower medial convexity is caused by the tumor mass responsible for the collapse (Fig. 3–52A). In lateral or oblique views, a similar S curve may be seen with tumor of other lobes as well (Fig. 3–52B, C, D). Though highly suggestive, the sign is not pathognomonic of bronchogenic carcinoma, since enlarged lymph nodes, a mediastinal tumor, or bronchial metastases associated with lobar collapse may occasionally give an identical appearance (Fig. 3–23).

Collapse accompanied by pleural effusion on the ipsilateral side usually indicates carcinoma (Fig. 3–53). Shift of the mediastinal structures toward the side of an

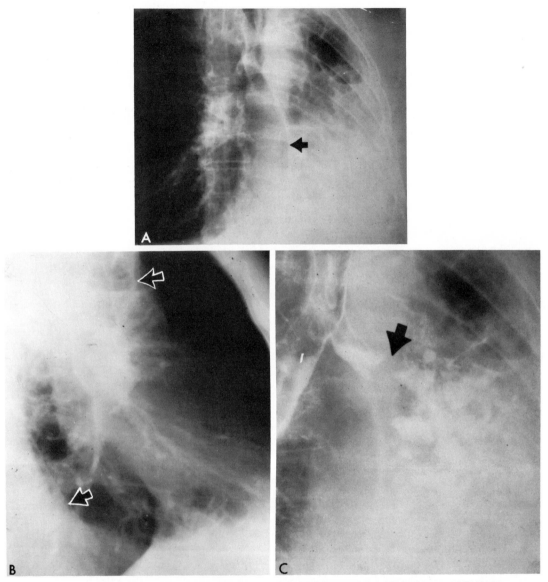

Figure 3-51. COLLAPSE OF ENTIRE LEFT LUNG SECONDARY TO BRONCHIAL ADENOMA

A, PA teleroentgenogram. The heart and aorta are invisible. Mediastinal herniation is striking. The lower herniation (arrow) probably lies behind the heart. *B,* Left lateral view. The lower half of the left lung lies far posterior
(lower arrow), but the upper half shows less collapse and its anterior border is poorly defined (upper arrow). The
clear space behind the heart probably represents herniated right lung. There is also a huge herniation anterior to
the ascending aorta. *C,* Bronchogram showing the tumor (arrow) and marked cystic and saccular bronchiectasis
beyond it. (Courtesy of Dr. Joseph N. Ganim.)

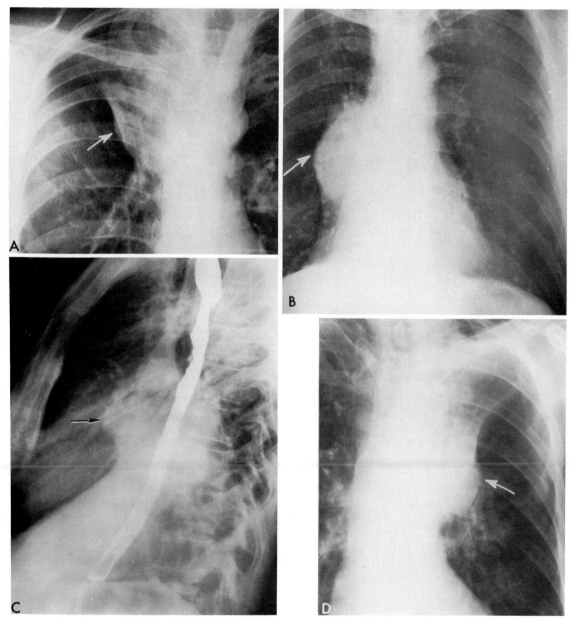

Figure 3–52. FOUR EXAMPLES OF THE *S* SIGN OF GOLDEN

A, RUL. *B,* RLL. *C,* RLL in lateral view (same patient as *B*). *D,* LUL. In each instance, the arrow points to a bronchogenic carcinoma.

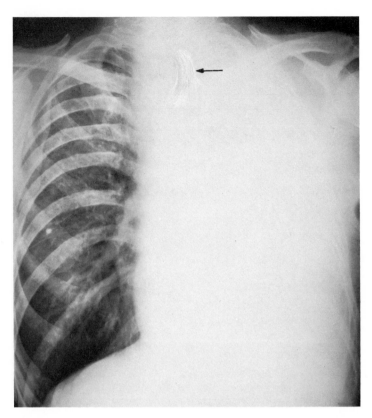

Figure 3–53. COLLAPSE ACCOMPANIED BY PLEURAL EFFUSION

The trachea (retouched, arrow) is deviated toward the same side as the fluid. Bronchogenic carcinoma of the left main stem bronchus.

obvious pleural effusion indicates that the negative pressure in the affected lung is greater than the positive pressure of the pleural fluid. In such cases, bronchial obstruction is implied, since the combination cannot occur from extrinsic compression of the lung alone. There is one exception, though: severe, long-standing pleural fibrosis may by itself draw the mediastinal structures to that side.

Laminagraphy or bronchography commonly reveals an obstructing or stenosing lesion in the lobar bronchus and the cause of the collapse can often be recognized or at least strongly suspected from its configuration. This is discussed in detail under *The Bronchi* in Chapter 7.

Certain signs, although they do not indicate the cause of the collapse, are still extremely useful because they help to eliminate the possibility of bronchogenic carcinoma. I have dubbed them the *open bronchus* and the *double lesion* signs. The following discussion of these signs applies to segmental as well as to lobar collapse.

THE OPEN BRONCHUS SIGN

The *open bronchus sign* applies when the bronchus supplying a collapsed lung, lobe, or segment is normal on bronchography, laminagraphy, or bronchoscopy.[326] It indicates that the collapse is of the peripheral type. When the sign is present, neoplasm can be excluded (Fig. 3–54). So far I have encountered no exception to this rule. In one patient, nearby small bronchi overlapped a large nodule and were mistakenly interpreted as lying within it. Because the mass was undiagnosed, the patient was operated on anyway and carcinoma was found (Fig. 3–55). This error can be avoided by cinebronchography technique with rotation of the patient.

Even the rare case of alveolar cell carcinoma in which peripheral collapse occurs is not an exception. The larger bronchi are abnormally elongated and compressed by the submucous infiltration of the neoplasm and the threadlike appearance is readily recognized (Fig. 3–56). In fact, this

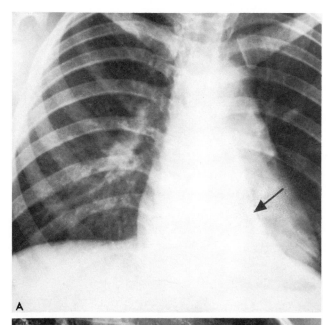

Figure 3–54. THE OPEN BRON-
CHUS SIGN IN CHRONIC LOBAR
COLLAPSE

A, Triangular shadow of LLL collapse is seen through the heart
(arrow). *B,* Bronchogram showing a
normal lobar bronchus leading into
the collapsed lobe.

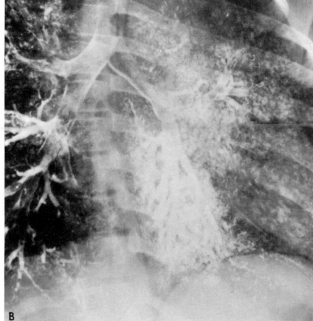

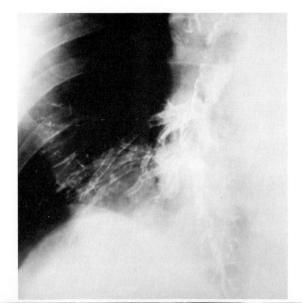

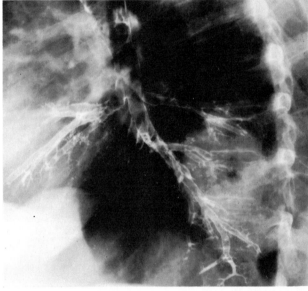

Figure 3–55. MISINTERPRETED OPEN
BRONCHUS SIGN

The contrast filled bronchi appear to enter
the right posterior basal segment mass in both
AP and lateral projections. On careful scrutiny,
it becomes apparent that this is an illusion
caused by superimposition of the lesion on
some bronchi in the AP view and other bronchi in the lateral view. Cinebronchography
would almost surely have prevented this
error.

roentgen appearance has been considered
diagnostic of alveolar cell carcinoma.[1338]

The open bronchus sign is also useful, if
less reliable, in the absence of collapse. In
the differential diagnosis of an infiltrate, if a
normal bronchus can be demonstrated entering it (on bronchography or laminagraphy), carcinoma can be excluded. However, it is important to remember that in the
alveolar form of pulmonary lymphoma (Fig.
3–57) and alveolar cell carcinoma *unasso-
ciated with collapse*, the bronchi may remain normally patent.[1338]

The explanation for the reliability of the
patent bronchus sign is tripartite: (1) To
cause collapse, a malignant tumor must
grossly alter the bronchus supplying the
collapsed tissue. (2) If the pulmonary opacity represents the tumor itself, there
should be no collapse and no open bronchus within it. (3) The peripheral form of
obstruction is not caused by neoplasm.

Bronchography is the most reliable
method of demonstrating the open bronchus sign. One must be certain that the
bronchus definitely extends into the pulmo-

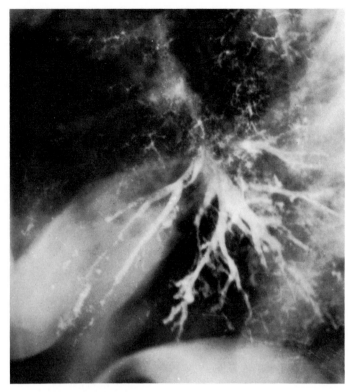

Figure 3–56. COMPRESSED BRON-CHI IN ALVEOLAR CELL CARCINOMA

This lateral bronchogram shows RML collapse without a localized en-dobronchial lesion. However, most of the visible bronchi within the collapsed lobe are elongated and constricted by submucosal extension of the neoplasm.

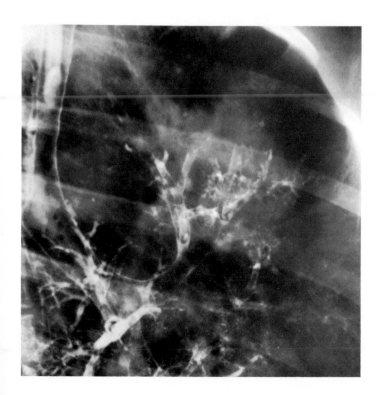

Figure 3–57. OPEN BRONCHUS SIGN IN HODGKIN'S DISEASE

(Courtesy of Dr. Harold N. Margolin.)

nary density in question and that adjacent overlapping bronchi are not misleading on this score (Fig. 3–55). Views in various projections are essential for proper evaluation. Cinebronchography is particularly reliable.

The importance of this simple sign cannot be overemphasized. Many pulmonary lesions of unknown etiology are encountered and the present tendency is to assume that they are malignant and should be operated upon. The open bronchus sign is reliable for excluding neoplasm and thereby unnecessary exploration can often be averted.

THE DOUBLE LESION SIGN

The value of fingertip knowledge of the normal bronchial anatomy in chest roentgenology has already been stressed. One additional by-product of this knowledge bears further emphasis: if collapse of multiple lobes or segments occurs in certain combinations, the likelihood of bronchogenic carcinoma is small. For example,

combined collapse of the RUL and RML is seldom encountered in bronchogenic carcinoma[724] (Fig. 3–58), but simultaneous collapse of the RML and RLL is frequently seen (Fig. 3–50). The reason for this becomes apparent when it is realized that the anatomic takeoff of the RUL bronchus is so situated that a tumor occluding it could hardly extend to involve the RML bronchus without also affecting the orifice to the lower lobe (Fig. 3–59). On the other hand, a single mass in the intermediate bronchus readily obstructs the airway to both the lower and middle lobes.

By the same token, if collapse of two or more pulmonary *segments* cannot be explained by a single bronchial lesion, one has reasonable assurance that a neoplasm is *not* present. Thus, combined collapse of the LLL (or any of its segments) and any one segment of the LUL, sparing the others, is rarely caused by a bronchial neoplasm (Fig. 3–60). Many similar non-neoplastic combinations of collapse may occur: RML and any one of the segments of the RLL (Fig.

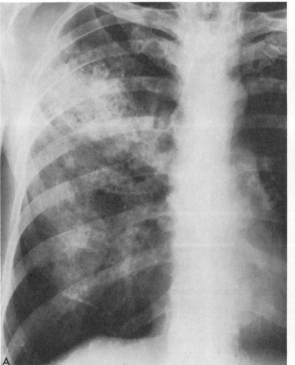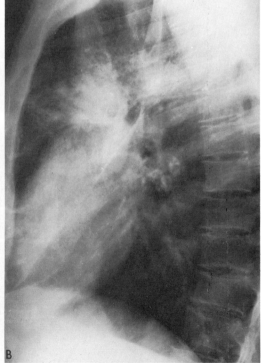

Figure 3–58. DOUBLE LESION SIGN

RUL and RML pneumonia with mild collapse. This lobar combination is rare in bronchogenic carcinoma.

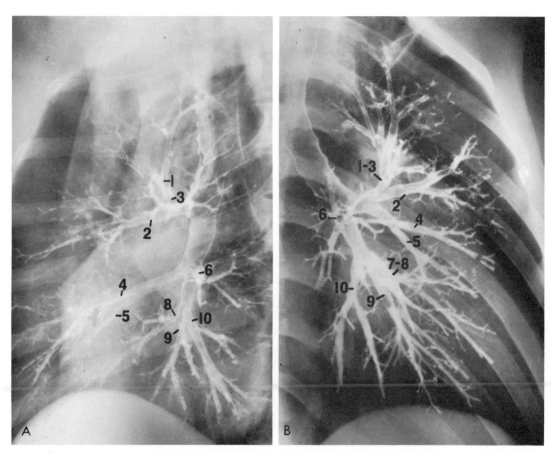

Figure 3–59. NORMAL SEGMENTAL BRONCHIAL ANATOMY

A, Right lung, left oblique projection. *B*, Left lung, right oblique projection. The numbers indicate the segmental bronchi (see Chap. 4).

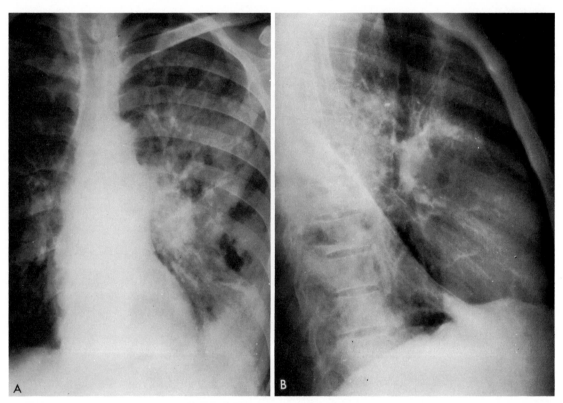

Figure 3–60. DOUBLE LESION SIGN

Collapse of the LLL and posterior subsegment of the LUL. A single bronchial lesion cannot explain this distribution. Staphylococcal pneumonia.

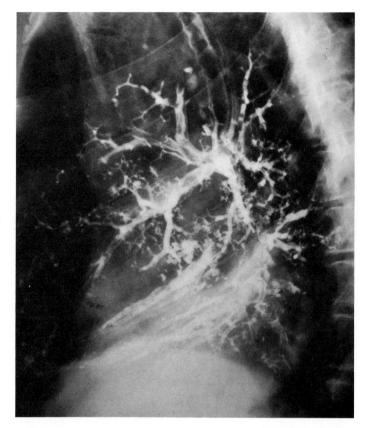

Figure 3–61. DOUBLE LESION SIGN

Collapse of the RML and anterior and medial basal segments of the RLL. A tumor in the intermediate bronchus should cause collapse of the *entire* lower lobe. Slowly resolving pneumonia.

3–61); RUL plus the RLL (either the entire lobes or individual segments) without involvement of the RML (Fig. 3–62); and the LLL and LUL except for the lingula. Others can be predicted from Figure 3–59.

Since these combinations are only slightly more likely to represent primary malignancy than if the two lesions were in opposite lungs, I have selected the term *double lesion sign* to denote this practical rule.[326] Its application requires only a superficial knowledge of the segmental anatomy of the lung. The sign has frequent application and for practical purposes may be relied upon to exclude bronchogenic carcinoma.

But bilateral primary bronchogenic carcinomas do occur.[152] So one must keep in mind possible exceptions: (1) multicentric neoplasms; (2) separate areas of collapse, one produced by the primary neoplasm and one by a metastasis; (3) extension of a primary bronchial neoplasm through a fissure to involve another large bronchus; (4) a tumor in one location and an unrelated inflammatory lesion in another; (5) anatomic variation in the distribution of the bronchi, e.g., a lingular arrangement in the right lung; and (6) a channel through an intrabronchial neoplasm, so situated that some of the bronchial orifices are patent while others are occluded. Totaled together, though, these exceptions are still rare and merely provide a counterpoint of caution.

The double lesion sign is almost as reliable with multiple infiltrates without collapse. It does not apply to involvement of several segments *within* a lobe, since if there is no interlobar septum to intervene, carcinoma readily extends across lung parenchyma. A tumor may fortuitously "pick off" several segmental bronchi while sparing others (Fig. 7–7B).

One should not be dogmatic in interpreting the double lesion sign. I have myself been guilty of overselling this sign and, after encountering some failures, have lost a little of my original enthusiasm for it. Two of the errors occurred in cases of bron-

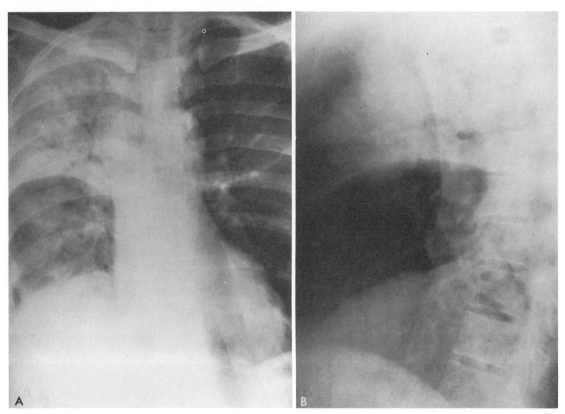

Figure 3–62. DOUBLE LESION SIGN

The entire RUL and RLL are consolidated and partially collapsed. Absence of middle lobe involvement weighs heavily against the diagnosis of a bronchial lesion. Lobar pneumonia.

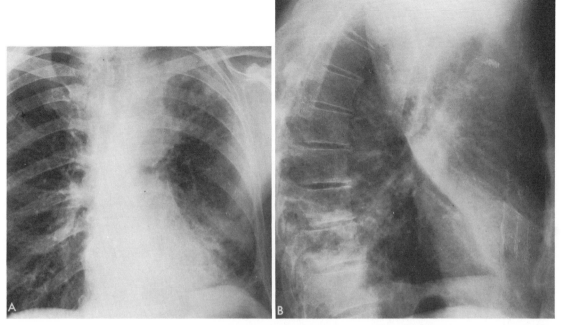

Figure 3–63. FAILURE OF THE DOUBLE LESION SIGN

There is mild collapse of much of the LUL, especially the lingula, and an area of infiltrate in the posterior basal segment of the LLL. Bronchogenic carcinoma was found in the LUL bronchus. The LLL infiltrate subsequently cleared.

chogenic carcinoma in which the RUL and RML were collapsed. One proved to be a carcinoma in the RUL bronchus with an apparently unrelated pneumonia of the RML. In the other, the carcinoma involved the right main stem bronchus, but an air passage through the tumor permitted the RLL to remain expanded. LeRoux has had a similar experience.[724] Another failure is illustrated in Figure 3–63. In all fairness, however, the sign has proved reliable in nearly all cases.[325] Figure 3–64 depicts an interesting example of multiple benign intrabronchial papillomas.[290, 477, 844, 1031, 1041, 1131]

LOBAR ENLARGEMENT

Enlargement of a lobe is easily recognized roentgenologically by the outward bulging of its septa (Fig. 3–65). Except in the RUL (Fig. 3–66), demonstration of lobar enlargement requires the lateral view. Even when all the segments of a lobe are not affected, a septum may still bulge if the con-solidation occupies the region adjacent to it. Lobar enlargement can be mimicked to a certain degree by encapsulated interlobar fluid. The latter, however, shows a sharply defined biconvex shadow; whereas lobar enlargement shows only a single, sharp, convex border at the surface adjoining the fissure.

There are few pathologic conditions capable of causing lobar enlargement and these can usually be readily differentiated by clinical and laboratory findings. In 1949, we reported lobar enlargement in five of eight patients with Friedländer's pneumonia,[349] and we have since encountered many others. This roentgen finding is readily explained at the autopsy table by the voluminous lobe packed tightly with inflammatory exudate.[605, 690]

Lobar enlargement is not to be considered a pathognomonic sign of Friedländer's pneumonia, since it is also encountered in a small percentage of patients with pneumococcal and other severe forms of pneumonia, tuberculosis,[607] and lung abscess and is not rare in bronchogenic carcinoma (Fig.

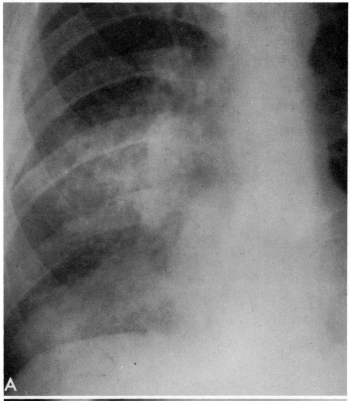

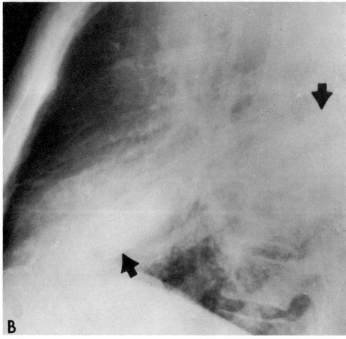

Figure 3–64. MULTIPLE BRON-
CHIAL PAPILLOMAS CAUSING
DOUBLE LESION SIGN

A and *B*, Collapse of the medial segment of the RML and superior segment of the RLL (arrows).

(*Figure continued on opposite page.*)

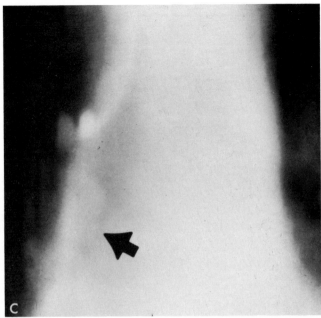

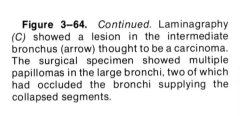

Figure 3–64. *Continued.* Laminagraphy *(C)* showed a lesion in the intermediate bronchus (arrow) thought to be a carcinoma. The surgical specimen showed multiple papillomas in the large bronchi, two of which had occluded the bronchi supplying the collapsed segments.

3–21). However, about half the patients with a bulging septum who presented signs and symptoms of acute pneumonia in our institution had Friedländer's pneumonia.

Of course, lobar enlargement can also result from the various forms of hyperaeration. The roentgen recognition of this form of lobar enlargement depends on the demonstration of the displaced fissures, increased radiolucency of the affected lobe, and, when present, thin walled bullae. The value of respiratory techniques in the study of patients with emphysema has already been discussed (Chap. 1).

It is well known that the central form of obstructive overinflation is caused by incomplete obstruction of a major bronchus. As with collapse, the constriction may be caused by an intrinsic mass or stenosis, extrinsic pressure (e.g., a large heart), or bronchial plugging (e.g., a foreign body). Apart from the typical mediastinal shift to the side of the lesion on inspiration (Fig. 1–4), there is increased radiolucency and decreased vascularity of the affected lung, with retention of its radiolucency on expiration(Fig. 3–67) and restricted motion of the ipsilateral hemidiaphragm (Fig. 1–4). The minor fissure may move more with respiration than the diaphragm in RLL hyperinflation, whereas the reverse is the rule in RUL emphy-

sema.[728] Obstructive lobar hyperinflation may be overlooked in the presence of adjacent lobar collapse or mistaken for compensatory overdistention (Fig. 3–68).

It is my belief that there is also a peripheral form of obstructive hyperinflation analogous to the peripheral form of pulmonary collapse. Examples of this condition are encountered in idiopathic unilateral hyperlucent lung,[792] in acute "bronchiolitis" of infants, during asthmatic attacks, and in some cases of chronic pulmonary emphysema.[257] In these conditions, bronchography reveals normal patency of the large bronchi, but the contrast medium fails to enter the smallest bronchial twigs in the involved areas even though the alveoli are distended with air (Fig. 5–34). The process may be confined to just a portion of a lobe or may involve an entire lobe or one lung, or may be diffuse and bilateral.

The lobar enlargement of congenital lobar emphysema is difficult to explain (Fig. 3–69). In this serious condition of the newborn, a lesion of the lobar bronchus is usually but by no means always present.[558] An anomaly of the cartilage rings, a web, stricture, or anomalous vessel may account for the overinflation.[202, 687, 1199] However, in an appreciable number of patients there is no lesion at all to explain the progressive

(*Text continued on page 142.*)

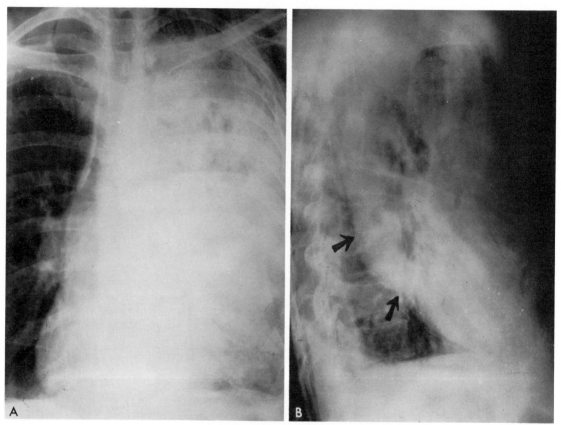

Figure 3–65. LUL ENLARGEMENT IN FRIEDLÄNDER'S PNEUMONIA

A, The heart and midline structures are displaced to the right. There is early breakdown within the pneumonic process. *B,* The left lateral view shows a marked posterior bulge of the major fissure (arrows). (From Felson, B., Rosenberg, L. S., and Hamburger, M., Jr.[349]; reproduced with permission of Radiology.)

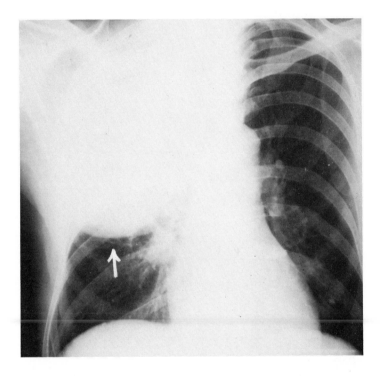

Figure 3–66. ENLARGED RUL IN FRIEDLÄNDER'S PNEUMONIA

There is a downward bulge of the minor fissure (arrow). (From Felson, B., Rosenberg, L. S., and Hamburger, M., Jr.[349]; reproduced with permission of Radiology.)

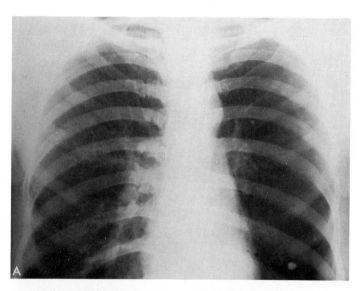

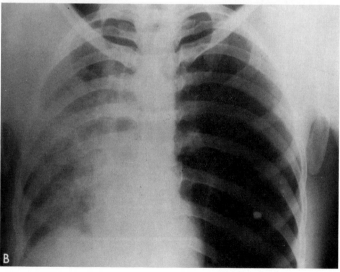

Figure 3–67. OBSTRUCTIVE HYPERAERATION OF THE LUNG

A, Inspiration. Although the right hilum is larger and more opaque, the carcinoma was in the left main bronchus. Impaired vascularity of the left lung accounts for the hypervascularity on the right. Otherwise the chest appears normal. *B,* Expiration. Marked shift of the mediastinum to the right.

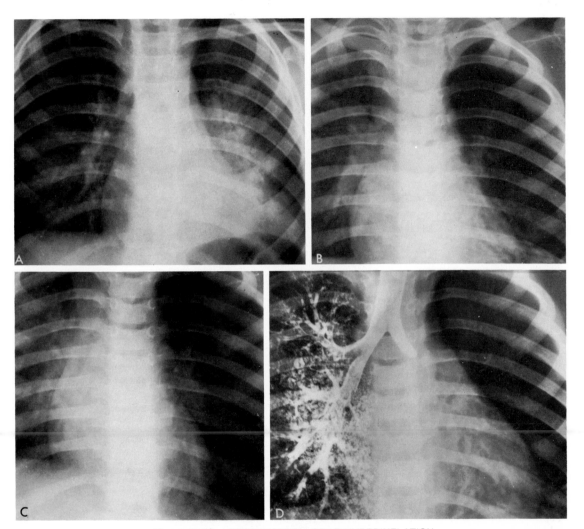

Figure 3–68. OBSTRUCTIVE LOBAR HYPERINFLATION

A, Pneumonia in lingula and LLL. *B*, 3 months later. There is now collapse of the LLL and obstructive overdistention of the LUL. *C*, 1 month later. Obstructive hyperinflation of the entire left lung is now present. *D*, Bronchogram shows intrinsic stenosis of the left main stem bronchus. The appearance of complete obstruction is attributed to the viscosity of the contrast medium. Inflammatory stenosis. The cause was not ascertained.

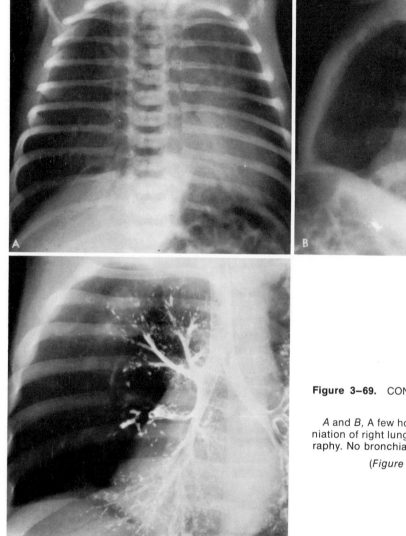

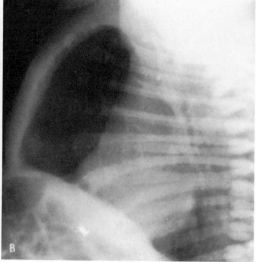

Figure 3–69. CONGENITAL EMPHYSEMA OF
RML

A and *B*, A few hours after birth. Moderate herniation of right lung into left thorax. *C*, Bronchography. No bronchial lesion is evident.

(*Figure continued on opposite page.*)

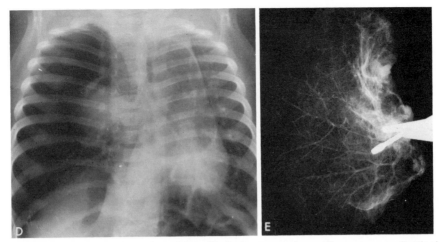

Figure 3–69. *Continued. D,* Few days later. Marked progression with severe mediastinal herniation. *E,* Roentgenogram of operative specimen. The lobe did not collapse when unclamped.

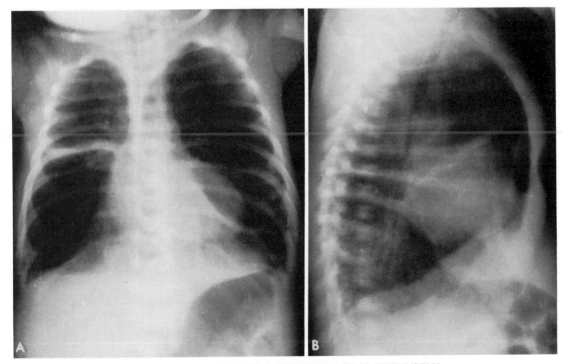

Figure 3–70. BILATERAL CONGENITAL LOBAR EMPHYSEMA

Age 15 days. The LUL and RML had to be resected. Note the compression collapse of the adjacent lobes and the partial inversion of both leaves of the diaphragm. The infant had been ill for two days.

lobar enlargement.[8, 509, 559, 677, 709, 857, 1131] Hislop and Reid have demonstrated an increased number of alveoli in a congenitally emphysematous lobe.[547] In some infants, the lobar emphysema is preceded by opacity of the overexpanded lobe.[311]

Compression collapse of adjacent lobes occurs and mediastinal herniation may be striking (Fig. 3–69C). I have been shown several infants in whom the lesion was not apparent at birth but appeared at about two weeks of age after a bout of pneumonia. Is it sometimes an acquired condition? Figure 3–70 is an example of bilateral lobar emphysema which required resection of the LUL and RML. Congenital lobar emphysema may disappear spontaneously, but I have no idea how often this occurs.

CHAPTER 4

THE SEGMENTS

Studies of the anatomy of the lung by Abey, Ewart, Huntington, and others laid the anatomic foundations for our present understanding of the pulmonary segments.[106] In recent years there has been a revival of interest in this subject. This has come about through the demonstration by Churchill and Belsey that the bronchopulmonary segments are surgical units and consequently resectable,[188] and through the careful anatomic and clinical studies of Jackson and Huber,[592] Brock,[128] Foster-Carter and Hoyle,[395, 396] and Boyden.[109]

Detailed knowledge of the segmental anatomy is obviously important to the bronchoscopist for the identification of the various bronchial orifices for localization of a tumor or extraction of a foreign body; to the surgeon for the operative localization of a pulmonary lesion and the conservation of lung tissue; and to the internist for postural drainage. However, this information is even more important in chest roentgenology,[918] and it is my conviction that any physician unwilling to study it should not attempt to interpret chest films.

Many disease processes may be segmental in distribution. Among these are such common conditions as neoplasm, pneumonia,* bronchiectasis,[25] lung abscess, tuberculosis,[1088] aspirated foreign body, and pulmonary infarct. Some of these conditions show a predilection for particular segments and spare other segments. For example, lung abscess frequently occurs in the poste-

rior segment of the upper lobe or in the superior or posterior basal segment of the lower lobe, especially on the right side.[128] Sequestration of the lung almost invariably involves the posterior basal segment of a lower lobe.

The recognition of segmental collapse depends on a thorough familiarity with the size, shape, and distribution of the normal segments. Since the arteries of the lung closely parallel the bronchi, the diagnosis of pulmonary infarction may also be facilitated by noting its segmental or subsegmental distribution. Differentiation of pleural or mediastinal disease from a pulmonary lesion may also be aided by a knowledge of segmental anatomy.

Observations based on an understanding of the segmental anatomy have elucidated the pathogenesis of a number of diseases. The sequelae of bronchial tuberculosis and the nature of so-called epituberculosis[582, 1088] have been clarified, in part, from such information. The realization that central pneumonia, a frequent roentgen diagnosis of the past, is not central at all but lies in the superior segment of a lower lobe is also based on this knowledge. We are now familiar with the common pattern of spread of bronchogenic carcinoma, which causes larger and larger areas of collapse as it extends proximally into the major bronchi.[998] For these reasons, the importance of a complete comprehension of segmental anatomy cannot be overemphasized.

---

*As Fraser and Wortzman,[403] Dornhorst and Pierce,[266] and Simon[1121] have pointed out, however, segmental distribution is often simulated in lobar pneumonia when not actually present. Pierce[940] has even stated that if a pneumonia appears to be perfectly segmental, one should suspect an underlying bronchial lesion.

NORMAL SEGMENTAL ANATOMY

Figures 4–1 and 4–2 illustrate the segmental bronchi and Figures 4–3 to 4–8 show (*Text continued on page 147.*)

143

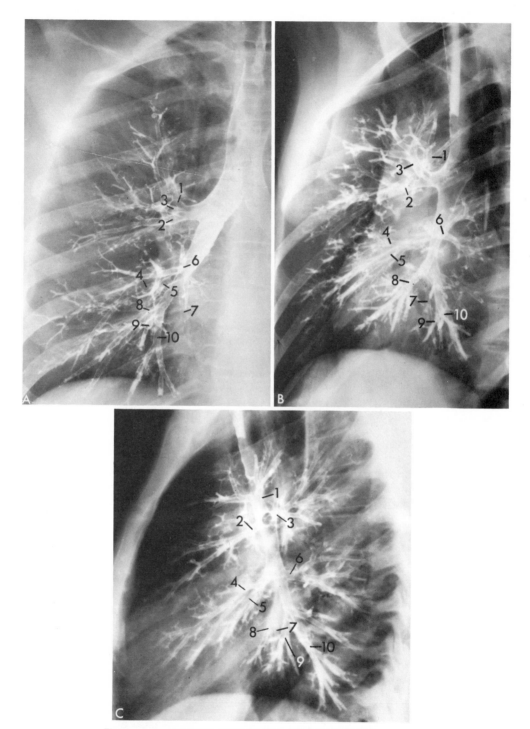

Figure 4–1.   NORMAL SEGMENTAL BRONCHI OF RIGHT LUNG

Patient 1. *A*, AP view. *B*, Right posterior oblique view. *C*, Right lateral view. On all illustrations in this chapter, the numbers refer to Boyden's nomenclature (Table 4–1). All are recumbent Bucky films.

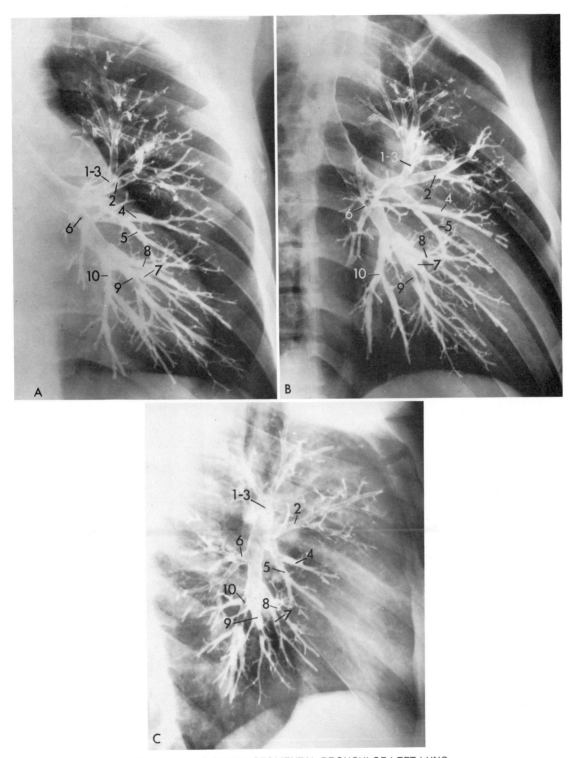

Figure 4–2. NORMAL SEGMENTAL BRONCHI OF LEFT LUNG

Patient 2. *A*, AP view. *B*, Left posterior oblique view. *C*, Left lateral view. The superior division bronchus of the LUL is not quite trifurcated.

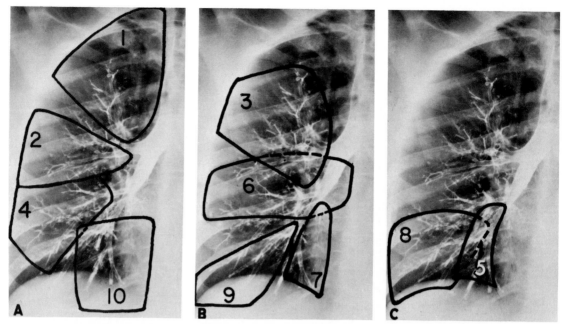

Figure 4–3. NORMAL RIGHT PULMONARY SEGMENTS, FRONTAL VIEW

Patient 1. In Figures 4–3 to 4–9, multiple prints are used to avoid confusion from superimposition. In each illustration, the segmental outlines follow as closely as possible the *visible* bronchographic distribution of the respective bronchi.

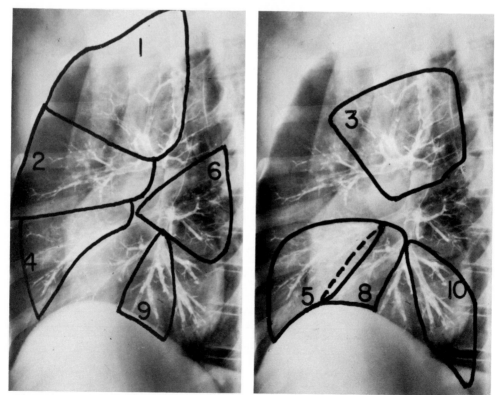

Figure 4–4. NORMAL RIGHT PULMONARY SEGMENTS, RIGHT POSTERIOR OBLIQUE VIEW

Patient 1. The medial basal segment bronchus could not be recognized in this view.

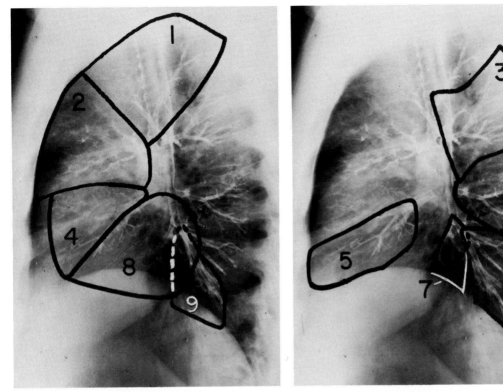

Figure 4–5. NORMAL RIGHT PULMONARY SEGMENTS, LATERAL VIEW
Patient 1.

the pulmonary segments in two representative normal patients. The right side of one patient and the left side of the other are shown. Because of the wide variation in the size and distribution of the bronchi and their segments among different individuals, these illustrations should be considered to be examples rather than rigid patterns. Furthermore, the degree of rotation greatly influences the appearance and position of the segments in the oblique views. It should also be emphasized that identification of individual bronchi and delineation of the spatial arrangement of the segments on bronchograms are often extremely difficult and sometimes almost guesswork. Several of the diagrammed segments illustrated in my first book[330] were modified for this presentation because readers called attention to discrepancies. Although a roentgen approach may not be as accurate as one utilizing anatomic techniques, it seems more practical for our purposes.

Because a clearer concept of segmental anatomy can be obtained from such illustrations, a word description seems superfluous, especially since it is available elsewhere. Attention is called to the excellent presentations on segmental anatomy by Borman,[98] Boyden,[106] Boyden and Tompsett,[118] Brock,[128] Di Rienzo,[257] Esser,[304] Foster-Carter,[394] Jackson and Huber,[568,592] Kane,[621] Krause and Lubert,[671] Lehman and Crellin,[713] Temple and Evans,[1203] and Zsebök.[1346]

Several systems of nomenclature of the bronchopulmonary segments have been devised. In 1960, at the Seventh International Congress of Anatomists meeting in New York, a nomenclature which is today receiving wide acceptance was adopted for the segments and their blood supply.[112] This system, which I prefer because of its clarity, is shown in Table 4–1 (in English rather than the original Latin version). The Boyden numbering system can be utilized for brevity.

There is considerable difference of opin-

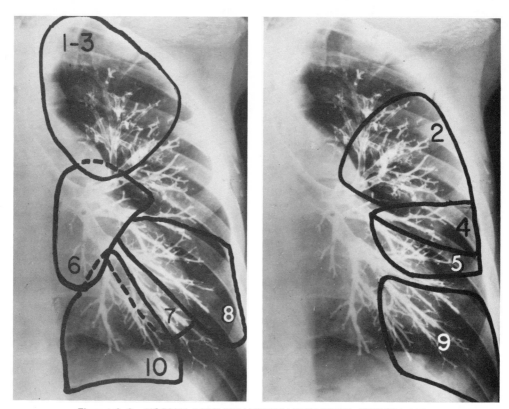

Figure 4–6. NORMAL LEFT PULMONARY SEGMENTS, FRONTAL VIEW

Patient 2.

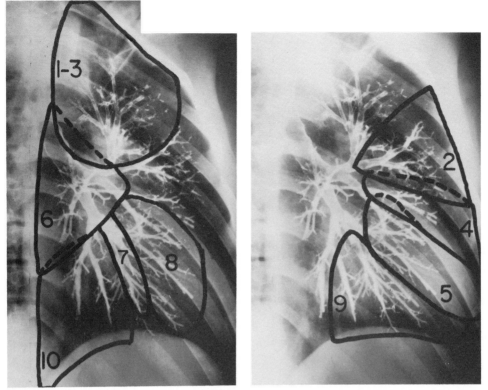

Figure 4–7. NORMAL LEFT PULMONARY SEGMENTS, LEFT POSTERIOR OBLIQUE VIEW

Patient 2.

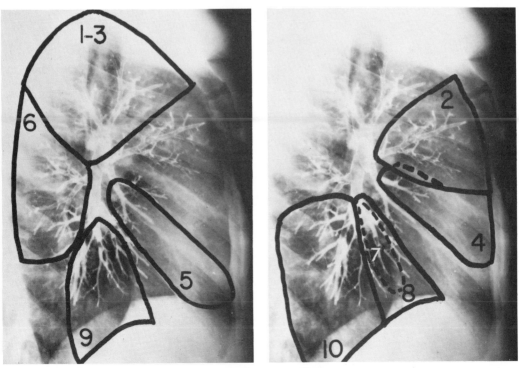

Figure 4–8. NORMAL LEFT PULMONARY SEGMENTS, LATERAL VIEW

Patient 2.

TABLE 4–1. Nomenclature of Bronchopulmonary Segments*

Right Lung

Upper lobe	Apical	B1
	Anterior	B2
	Posterior	B3
Middle lobe	Lateral	B4
	Medial	B5
Lower lobe	Superior	B6
	Medial basal	B7
	Anterior basal	B8
	Lateral basal	B9
	Posterior basal	B10

Left Lung

Upper lobe		
Upper division	Apicoposterior	B1–3
	Anterior	B2
Lower (lingular) division	Superior	B4
	Inferior	B5
Lower lobe	Superior	B6
	Medial basal	B7
	Anterior basal	B8
	Lateral basal	B9
	Posterior basal	B10

*Modified from that of Seventh International Congress of Anatomists, New York, 1960; with Boyden numbering system.

ion concerning several aspects of the terminology because of the frequency of normal variants. For example, Boyden[106] and Hardie-Neill and Gilmour[505] pointed out that there is ample justification to include a subsuperior segment in the lower lobes, and Jackson and Huber joined the anterior and medial basal segments of the LLL into one segment.[592] Brock divides the superior division of the LUL into three instead of two segments: the apical, posterior, and anterior.[128] Be this as it may, no system of nomenclature can be expected to suit everyone's taste. If you are familiar with the basic pattern and its most frequent variations you have gained an adequate understanding of the subject.

Boyden,[106] Fiser,[364] Huizinga and Smelt,[575] and Esser[304] have studied the major *subdivisions* of each bronchopulmonary segment in detail, but these are so variable and complex that only the more constant of them will be discussed. These are included in the next section. My own at-

tempts to identify the subsegments on bronchograms and on abnormal chest roentgenograms have been disheartening, to say the least.

SEGMENTAL AND SUBSEGMENTAL VARIATIONS

As already indicated, there are innumerable variations from the prevailing patterns. Many of these are rare and only the commoner ones, some of which reach an incidence of almost 50 per cent, will be considered here.

It should first be noted that each segment and subsegment has its own bronchus and that slight developmental migration of the origin of one of these bronchi may greatly alter the size and distribution of its segment. For example, a slight upward shift of the takeoff of the posterior division of the posterior basal bronchus (so that it arises from the stem bronchus) is responsible for the subsuperior segment of the lower lobe (Fig. 4–19). This segment, in turn, encroaches on the superior segment, which is consequently reduced in size. Mechanisms such as this account for the conspicuous variation in volume of a segment among different individuals. In many situations, trifurcations occur where bifurcations are expected, and vice versa. Brock has aptly stated, "Trifurcations are often really two rapidly occurring bifurcations."[128] A supernumerary fissure may partly or completely separate any segment or subsegment from its neighbors. These fissures have been discussed in the preceding chapter.

Right Upper Lobe

The RUL bronchus, which usually leaves the main stem at the level of the carina,* divides quickly into its segmental bronchi, which in turn subdivide into subsegmental bronchi. A fairly common pattern is: apical and posterior rami of the apical segment, posterior and lateral rami of the posterior segment, and anterior and lateral rami of the anterior segment (Fig. 4–9). Trifurcation of

---

*In children this takeoff is frequently a little lower.

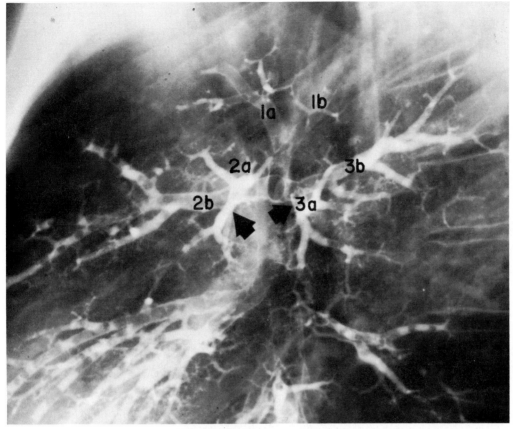

Figure 4–9. SUBSEGMENTAL BRONCHI, RUL

Lateral view. Posterior *(1a)* and apical *(1b)* rami of the apical segment; lateral *(2a)* and anterior *(2b)* rami of the anterior segment; and lateral *(3a)* and posterior *(3b)* rami of the posterior segment. The two lateral (axillary) rami (arrows) are well developed. There is trifurcation of the lobar bronchus.

the lobar bronchus is not as common as bifurcation. When a bifurcation occurs, any two of the three segments may arise from either of the two divisions (Fig. 4–10). Occasionally there are four segments, the extra one usually resulting from a double origin of the posterior bronchus, one of which supplies the lateral (axillary) region. This is seen in about 15 per cent of individuals (Fig. 4–20). Consolidation involving this so-called axillary segment, recognizable in the lateral view from its position astride the junction of the minor and major fissures (Fig. 4–11), is a frequent occurrence.[252, 625] It has been explained by the presence of the fourth segment, described above, or by overdevelopment of the lateral subdivision of either the anterior or posterior segment. The upper limit of the anterior segment may lie almost anywhere along the anterior margin of the upper lobe. At times, it extends quite low and occupies an area anterior to the RML (Fig. 4–12).

Occasionally, an anomalous bronchus arises from the right side of the trachea above the RUL bronchus and extends into the lung (Figs. 4–13 and 4–22). It is said to occur normally in certain primates.[643] In the human, it usually represents a displaced branch of the apical segmental bronchus, although rarely it has been shown to be a true supernumerary bronchus.* It

---

*A displaced bronchus supplies a normally located pulmonary segment or subsegment; a supernumerary bronchus supplies additional or abnormally located lung tissue.

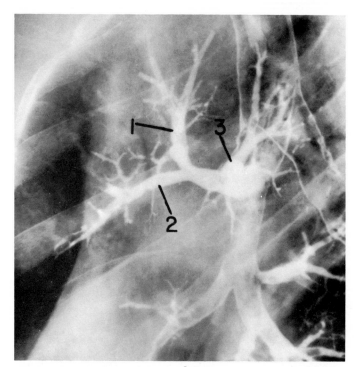

Figure 4–10. BIFURCATION OF RIGHT UPPER LOBE BRONCHUS

The apical and anterior segments (*1* and *2*) arise from one division and the posterior segment *(3)* from the other.

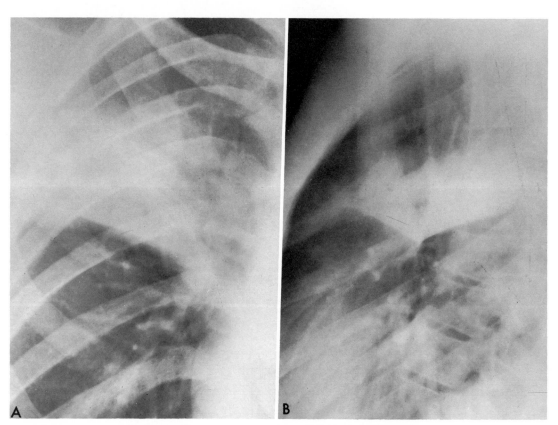

Figure 4–11. RIGHT "AXILLARY SEGMENT" PNEUMONIA

The infiltrate appears delimited by the minor septum in the PA view *(A)*, simulating anterior segmental involvement. In the lateral view *(B)*, it straddles the junction of the major and minor septa. There is slight collapse.

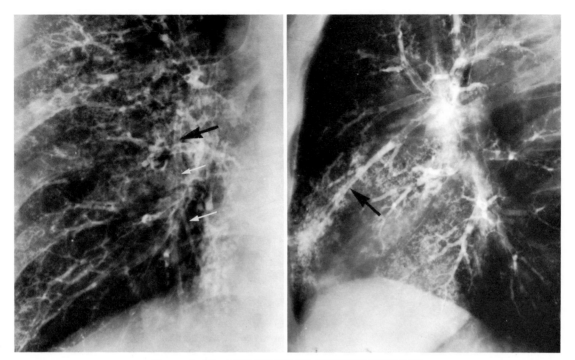

Figure 4–12. LOW RAMUS OF ANTERIOR SEGMENT

AP and lateral bronchograms. A subdivision of the anterior segment supplies an area anterior to the RML (arrows).

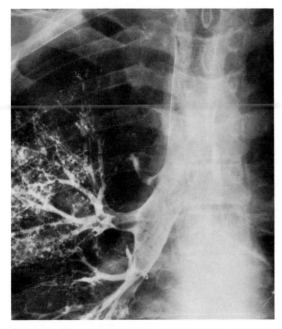

Figure 4–13. ANOMALOUS BRONCHUS ARISING FROM RIGHT SIDE OF TRACHEA

It appears to represent a displaced branch of the apical segment bronchus.

may end blindly in anomalous pulmonary tissue.[237, 440, 486, 518, 794] A branch of the right pulmonary artery accompanies the bronchus.[678] Figure 4–14 shows a rare instance of two RUL bronchi of equal size arising adjacent to each other from the main stem bronchus.[118, 557, 575, 611] Three separate bronchi to this lobe have been recorded.[1035]

Right Middle Lobe

Division of the RML into medial and lateral segments of approximately equal size is seen in about 60 per cent of all individuals. A common variant is that of a small lateral segment and a large medial one, although the reverse may occur. In 10 to 20 per cent, the arrangement of the two segments is the same as that in the lingula, i.e., superior-inferior (Fig. 4–15). Once in a while there are three segments (Fig. 4–16). Rarely, union of the RML bronchus or one of its segments with the adjacent anterior segment bronchus of the RUL or the anterior basal bronchus of the RLL[118, 608] occurs (Fig. 4–17).

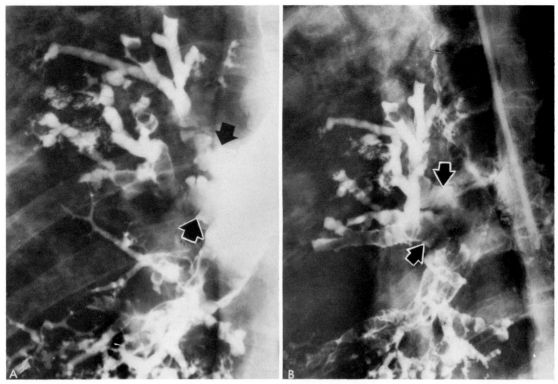

Figure 4–14.   TWO EQUAL SIZED RUL BRONCHI

AP (A) and left anterior oblique *(B)* views. The upper bronchus (top arrow) appears to include the apical segment bronchus and a large anterior subdivision; the lower division (bottom arrow) supplies the posterior and part of the anterior segment. Bronchiectasis is present. The patient also showed tracheobronchomegaly.

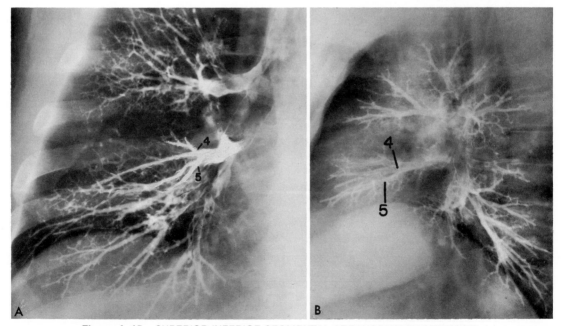

Figure 4–15.   SUPERIOR-INFERIOR SEGMENTAL ARRANGEMENT IN THE RML

A, PA view. The RML bronchus has been retouched. *B,* Lateral view. *4,* Superior segment. *5,* Inferior segment.

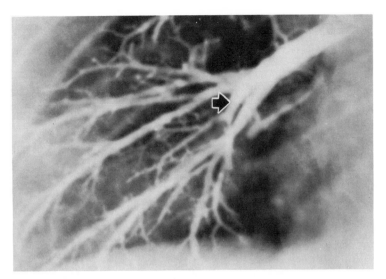

Figure 4-16. RML WITH PROBABLY THREE SEGMENTAL BRONCHI

The additional bronchus (arrow) arises from a trifurcation and supplies the lateral portion of the medial segment. Presumably, it represents an "early" division of the medial segment bronchus. AP view of selective RML bronchogram.

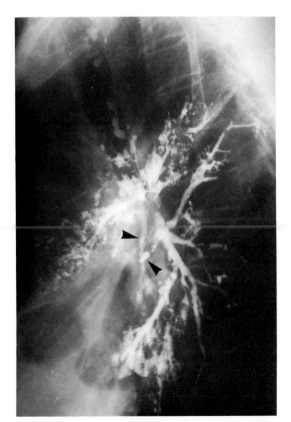

Figure 4-17. RML SEGMENT SUPPLIED BY RUL BRONCHUS

The anomalous bronchus (upper arrowhead) is a displaced lateral segment bronchus (B4). The medial segment (lower arrowhead) is supplied by the RML bronchus.

Right Lower Lobe

The bronchus to the superior segment of the RLL arises from the posterior aspect of the intermediate bronchus, almost invariably at the level of the takeoff of the RML bronchus. In most cases, the segment sits transversely on the basal segments, although sometimes the arrangement is oblique. The size of the superior segment varies considerably. In about 75 per cent of individuals, it occupies more than half the height of the lobe. It has three rather constant subdivisions—the medial, superior, and lateral—often recognizable on bronchography (Fig. 4-18). However, the relative volume of these subsegments varies greatly from patient to patient. The superior segment may arise from two separate bronchi equidistant above and below the normal site[106] (Fig. 4-19).

As implied earlier, a subsuperior segment sandwiched between the superior and the basal segments is frequently present. Its bronchus arises from the posterior surface of the RLL bronchus 1 to 3.5 cm distal to the takeoff of the superior segment bronchus (Figs. 4-18 and 4-20). Brock encountered this variation in 52 per cent of his patients,[128] and Boyden in 61 per cent.[106] On the basis of its prevalence, a strong case has been made by Boyden for adding this segment to the nomenclature.[106, 128, 625] I'm for my friend Edward Boyden. In the absence

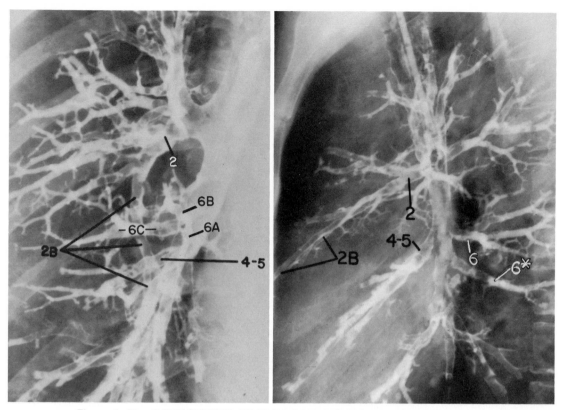

Figure 4–18. SUBSEGMENTAL BRONCHI OF THE SUPERIOR SEGMENT OF RLL

AP and lateral bronchograms. Medial *(6A)*, superior *(6B)*, and lateral *(6C)* rami. *2B* is a low ramus of the anterior segment bronchus supplying an area anterior to the middle lobe. There is also a subsuperior bronchus *(6*)*.

of a subsuperior bronchus, the same area may be supplied by a high branch of the posterior basal bronchus, but more often it is incorporated into the superior segment.

The four basal segment bronchi of the RLL arise from the stem bronchus about a centimeter apart, in the following order: medial, anterior, lateral, and posterior. Although their origins are fairly constant, there is considerable variation in their branching and distribution. The medial basal segment parallels the posterior portion of the right heart border. Sometimes it is partly a subdivision of the anterior segment, and rarely it arises from the intermediate bronchus.[790] It is absent in about 15 per cent of individuals.[89, 106, 119, 575] The anterior basal segment is remarkably constant in position. The stem bronchus, after giving off these two branches, continues for a variable distance before its final bifurcation into lateral and posterior segmental branches. The lateral segment may be absent; the posterior segmental bronchus then supplies its area.

Left Upper Lobe

The length of the left main stem bronchus before it divides into upper and lower lobe bronchi varies from 1.5 to 3.5 cm. The LUL bronchus bifurcates into superior and lingular divisions in about 75 per cent of individuals. In the remainder, a trifurcation occurs, with a modified superior division above, the lingula below, and the anterior bronchus between. In some, the anterior bronchus is in the exact middle of the three; in others, it favors either the upper division (Figs. 4–2 and 4–45) or the lingula (Fig. 4–21). The trifurcate arrangement is caused either by a downward displacement of the anterior segment bronchus, which merely arises lower than normal, or by its splitting into two parts with the larger inferior branch undergoing downward displacement and the upper branch remaining at the usual site.[118] It is often difficult to identify these variable bronchi on bronchograms or on anatomic dissections. For example, what may appear to be an inferiorly displaced or "split" anterior segmental bronchus might just as easily represent an overdeveloped superior lingular division.

The apicoposterior bronchus runs a variable length before it divides into its two components. Occasionally a trifurcation of the superior division of the LUL occurs so that the pattern is identical to that in the RUL. Figure 4–2A almost qualifies. Boyden found a lateral-medial instead of the normal superior-inferior arrangement in the lingula in 15 per cent of anatomic dissections. Figure 7–7G illustrates what must be the longest lingula in the world. A tracheal bronchus on the left is about as common as

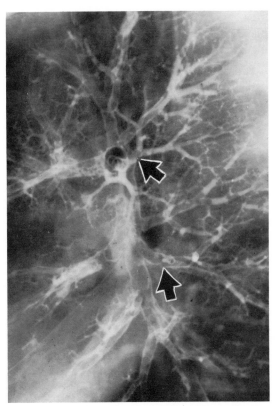

Figure 4–20. RIGHT SUBSUPERIOR SEGMENT

This accessory segmental bronchus (lower arrow) is present in more than half of normal persons. In this patient, there are also four segmental bronchi in the RUL, the apical and posterior (arising from a common stem), the anterior (showing almost no lateral ramus), and a lateral or axillary bronchus (upper arrow). Right lateral view.

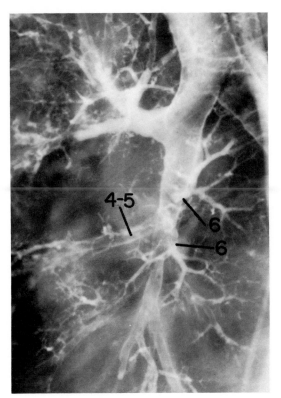

Figure 4–19. VARIATION OF SUPERIOR SEGMENTAL BRONCHUS OF RLL

There are two divisions (6), the upper arising above the level of origin of the RML bronchus and the lower arising below it.

priapism in the old men's home. An anomalous bronchus arising from the left main stem and extending into the apical region of the LUL[557] is demonstrated in Figure 4–22.

Left Lower Lobe

Unlike the right side, the superior segment of the LLL rests obliquely on the basal segments in about 90 per cent of cases. It extends about two thirds of the distance to the diaphragm in nearly 50 per cent. Its bronchus originates about a centimeter beyond the origin of the lobar bronchus and about 5 cm distal to the carina. Rarely the superior segment bronchus arises at the bifurcation of the main stem bronchus, or even from the LUL bronchus (Fig. 4–23). A

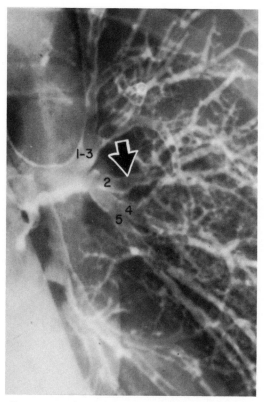

Figure 4–21. TRIFURCATION PATTERN OF LUL

The anterior segment bronchus (arrow) favors the lingular rather than the upper division. Right anterior oblique view.

true subsuperior segment is encountered in about 30 per cent.[89, 106]

The basal segment bronchi of the LLL arise close together on the stem bronchus. In most people, the basal trunk bifurcates into an anteromedial and posterolateral division, although a trifurcation is not rare. In nearly all individuals, the medial basal arises in conjunction with the anterior basal, although occasionally it has a separate origin, as on the right side. Boyden states that, unlike its counterpart in the right lung, the medial basal bronchus is a more constant branch than the anterior basal. The posterior basal segment supplies a larger area than on the right, often at the expense of the lateral basal segment, which may even be entirely absent.

From a large number of bronchograms, I selected 30 examples of excellent bronchial delineation of each lobe for study of the roentgen anatomy and variations. This proved to be a frustrating experience, since the overlap and variations were extremely confusing, notwithstanding the availability of three projections. This was especially true of the lower lobes.

Among the 30 bronchograms of the RUL, three showed one unusually small segment. In one it was the anterior segment, in the second it was the posterior, and in the third

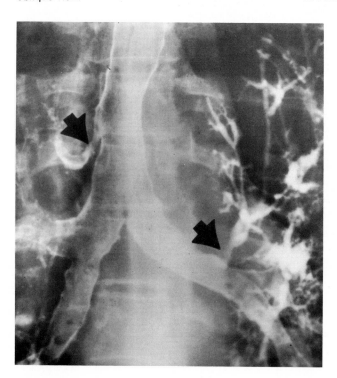

Figure 4–22. ANOMALOUS BRONCHI

A tracheal bronchus (upper arrow) ramifies in the apical portion of the RUL. I couldn't tell whether it was displaced or supernumerary. Another anomalous bronchus (lower arrow) arises from the left main stem just proximal to the LUL–LLL bifurcation and supplies a portion of the apical subsegment of the LUL. AP view.

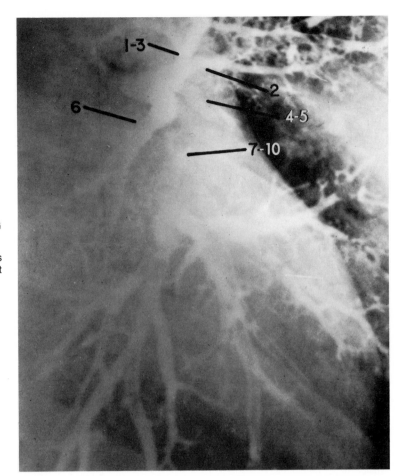

Figure 4–23. SUPERIOR SEGMENT BRONCHUS ARISING FROM LUL BRONCHUS

The bronchus *(6)* originates near the lobar bifurcation. Right oblique view.

the apical segment. In another instance, four segmental bronchi were visible (Fig. 4–20). One patient appeared to have two upper lobe bronchi, equal in size, arising from the right main bronchus (Fig. 4–14). In another, a branch of the anterior segment bronchus extended far forward and downward, occupying a tongue of tissue in front of the upper part of the RML (Fig. 4–12). Lesser degrees of this variation were common.

Of the 30 RML bronchograms, two showed a complete superior-inferior pattern of the segments (Fig. 4–15), and in three others this arrangement was partial. A trifurcation of the middle lobe bronchus appeared to be present in three patients (Fig. 4–16). In one patient, the RML bronchus arose from the intermediate bronchus about 1 cm distal to the superior segment of the LLL; in another, a branch of the medial seg-

ment extended upward well into the territory usually occupied by the anterior segment of the RUL.

In the RLL, there was one instance in which the superior segment was supplied by two bronchi, one arising above the level of the RML orifice and the other below it (Fig. 4–19). A subsuperior bronchus arising directly from the posterior aspect of the stem bronchus was seen in six cases (Fig. 4–18). In ten others, the subsuperior zone was supplied from a posterior branch of the posterior basal bronchus. In the remainder, the area was supplied by the superior segment bronchus. The medial basal bronchus appeared to be absent in three cases and extremely small in one. The lateral basal bronchus seemed to be absent in one.

Among the 30 LUL bronchograms, the lobar bronchus showed a definite trifurcation in two, the divisions representing the apicoposterior, the anterior, and the lingular segments (Fig. 4–21). In seven others, there appeared to be downward displacement of part or all of the anterior segment bronchus so that there were two quickly occurring bifurcations. A medial-lateral arrangement of the lingula was seen in one patient. In another, a branch arising from the superior lingular segment bronchus seemed to extend into the posterior segment.

Of the 30 bronchograms of the LLL, the superior segment bronchus arose from the LUL bronchus near its junction with the LLL bronchus in one instance (Fig. 4–23). The subsuperior region was supplied by a separate subsuperior bronchus in four patients, by a posterior branch of the posterior basal segment in ten, and by a branch of the lateral basal in one. In the remainder, it was part of a large superior segment. In one case, the medial segment bronchus seemed to arise directly from the lower lobe bronchus; in the remainder it was thought to have a common stem with the anterior basal. In two, the anterior and lateral basals originated from a common stem.

It should again be emphasized that the naming of these lower lobe bronchi was often uncertain and that conventional bronchography is surely not as reliable as anatomic methods in elucidating segmental anatomy.

A discussion of segmental variations would not be complete without mention of the common anomaly *pulmonary sequestration*.

THE MANY FACES OF PULMONARY SEQUESTRATION

Pulmonary sequestration is surprisingly common for a disease that was hardly known 25 years ago.[136, 237, 420, 1329] As often happens with the newly resurrected, it received a good deal of attention and soon its features were concisely defined. Today the roentgen diagnosis is suggested and confirmed with regularity. But not all cases fall into the usual mold. I have encountered a variety of roentgen patterns in this condition and believe that they merit attention.[341]

To begin with, sequestered lung is a congenital mass of aberrant pulmonary tissue that has no *normal* connection with the bronchial tree or the pulmonary arteries. It is supplied by an anomalous artery arising from the aorta. Its venous drainage is via either the azygos system, the pulmonary veins, or the inferior vena cava.[519]

Intralobar sequestration is confined within the lung, almost invariably lying in the substance of the posterior basal segment of a lower lobe, although it often extends into adjacent segments. It is intimately connected with the adjacent lung—no pleural envelope exists.[20, 513, 679, 795, 1141, 1296] Extralobar sequestration is thought by some to be unrelated embryologically to the intralobar variety,[110] but there is one case reported in which the two coexisted in the same lung.[641] The extralobar variety is found between the lower lobe and the diaphragm, within the substance of the diaphragm, or in the upper portion of the abdomen. It is enclosed in a pleural sheath of its own.[87, 117, 439, 618]

The anomalous artery almost always arises from the lower descending thoracic aorta or upper abdominal aorta* and has the elastic nature of a normal pulmonary artery rather than the muscular structure of an aortic branch. The anomaly is attributed to failure of the systemic arterial connections to the base of developing fetal lung to obliterate, preventing normal inosculation of the main pulmonary arteries into the primitive pulmonary arterial plexuses.[156, 296] Thus, the anomalous pulmonary tissue is "captured" by the artery and "sequestered" from the bronchial tree. It sounds reasonable, if a bit Galahadian.

Sequestration is usually asymptomatic but infection may supervene at any age—I have seen it develop in a 65 year old man. Infection seldom if ever occurs with extralobar sequestration. I have also seen two patients with severe persistent hemothorax from rupture of the anomalous artery, one caused by trauma and the other spontaneous. Both patients recovered after surgical repair (Fig. 4–24).

The tissue sequestered within the lung usually consists of pulmonary parenchyma or a cyst. Air may enter from the surrounding lung via the pores of Kohn or through small parenchymal or bronchial leaks related to infection. The blind bronchi within the sequestered lung often become

---

*Occasionally it is a branch of a subclavian, intercostal, or phrenic artery.[59]

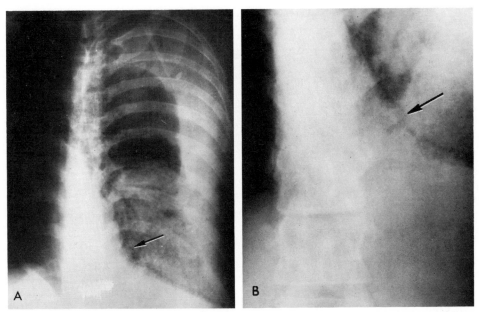

Figure 4–24. TRAUMATIC AVULSION OF THE SYSTEMIC ARTERY TO A PULMONARY SEQUESTRATION

Pleural bleeding could not be controlled in this young victim of a cycle accident. The triangular shadow in the left costovertebral angle (arrows) proved at operation to be sequestered pulmonary tissue. The air bronchogram seen all through the LLL is attributed to pulmonary contusion. (Courtesy of Dr. Patrick A. Lynch, Yakima, Washington.)

distended with trapped mucus secreted by bronchial glands.

Each of these pathologic variations has its roentgen counterpart and they account for the multifaceted radiographic patterns of this disease. The nonaerated parenchyma produces a solid, ill-defined opacity; the cyst presents a sharply defined fluid and/or air filled shadow (Fig. 4–25). Still another pattern is that of the pulmonary bronchogenic cyst, which results from a mucus filled blind bronchus, outlined by air that has entered from the adjacent lung via collateral drift (Fig. 4–26).

Occasionally the anomalous artery itself can be visualized on the PA film or on tomography as a fusiform or branching shadow joining the aorta to the inferior medial margin of the sequestration (Fig. 4–27). The vessel has been seen under the left hemidiaphragm after induced pneumoperitoneum.[519, 541] One case is reported in which rib notching was related to the anomalous artery.[283] Hard to explain is the occasional instance of radiologically demonstrated and surgically proved sequestration in which earlier plain films revealed no abnormality (Fig. 4–28).

In view of this divergence of roentgen patterns, it is apparent that any indolent lesion involving a posterior basal segment should raise the likelihood of intralobar sequestration.

Extralobar sequestration is more difficult to recognize. I have seen it only three times: once as a small bump on the left diaphragm, once as a left inferior paravertebral lesion (Fig. 4–29), and once associated with an intrathoracic left kidney.

Additional roentgen procedures often confirm the diagnosis, but may create some new faces of their own. For example, barium swallow will occasionally reveal a bronchus-like structure connecting the esophagus or stomach to the anomalous pulmonary tissue. This is the so-called *esophageal lung* (Fig. 4–30). It may be seen with either intra- or extralobar sequestration, and some think it an inherent part of the malformation.[76, 439, 693] I don't; it seems to me that esophageal lung is the result of incomplete separation of the esophagus and trachea combined with sequestration. Boyden thinks that there are two forms of sequestration, the "capture" type and the esophageal (or gastric) type.[107, 117]

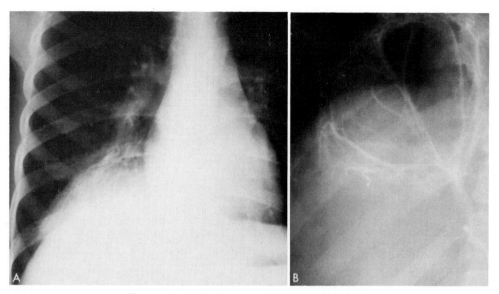

Figure 4–25. SEQUESTRATION, CYSTIC TYPE

A, Note the lesion involving the posterior basal portion of the RLL. *B,* Selective injection of an anomalous artery that arises from the abdominal aorta and supplies the pulmonary lesion. See also Figure 4–28. (Courtesy of Dr. Richard L. Clark et al.[195] and Dr. John P. Dorst; reproduced with permission of Charles C Thomas, Publisher.)

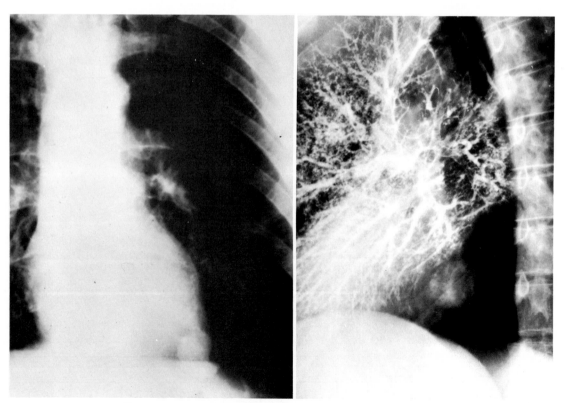

Figure 4–26. SEQUESTRATION WITH BRONCHOGENIC CYST

The rounded nodule in the posterior basal segment represents a blind mucus filled bronchus surrounded by hyperaerated pulmonary tissue, demarcated by the bronchogram. See also Figure 4–31. (Courtesy of Dr. Marvin Rassell.)

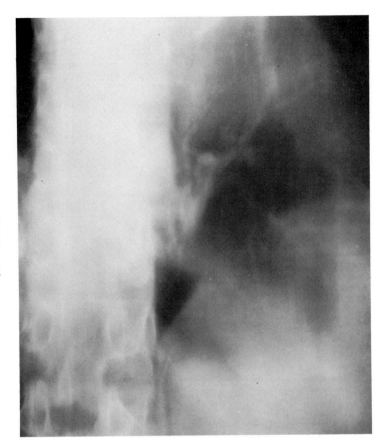

Figure 4–27. SEQUESTRATION WITH VISIBLE ANOMALOUS ARTERY

Tomogram shows the anomalous vessel arising from the descending thoracic aorta and extending into a hyperaerated posterior basal segment of the LLL. Unproved, but the patient's identical twin had a similar lesion confirmed at operation.

The diagnosis of sequestration can often be made by bronchography. Normal bronchi do not enter the lesion but are draped around it. The visible bronchi do not terminate abruptly at its margins, as with tumor, cyst, or other obstructive lesions, but branch normally down to the finest twigs, which then frame the sequestered lung[133] (Fig. 4–31). Rarely, contrast medium will leak into the malformed segment[1337] (Fig. 4–30).

Thoracic aortography will establish the diagnosis by demonstrating one or more anomalous arteries from the descending aorta just above or below the diaphragm entering the lung (Figs. 4–24, 4–30, 4–32, 4–33). Rarely the anomalous artery may arise from the ascending aorta, the aortic arch, the subclavian artery, or even the innominate or celiac. Selective injection of the anomalous artery has been performed but it hardly warrants the attempt.

Venous drainage of intralobar sequestration is usually via pulmonary veins, whereas that of the extralobar form is generally through the azygos system. However, the reverse is not uncommon. I have been unable to find any reference to bilateral sequestration, although I have seen one likely case, until recently.[300a] Figure 4–32 may be an example of another.

Sequestration may be associated with other abnormalities. Figure 4–33 shows sequestration in total situs inversus, probably representing a variant of Kartagener's syndrome. It is also encountered with diaphragmatic hernia[59] and in the congenital pulmonary venolobar syndrome (p. 87). Infection of the sequestered tissue or the lung around it may give rise to the typical appearance of a lung abscess, fungus ball,[158] or bronchiectasis. Even without sequestration, severe acquired bronchiectasis is often associated with large "bronchial" arteries arising from the descending aorta.[742] Differentiation from sequestration is made by demonstrating bronchographically that the dilated bronchi are branches of normal lobar and segmental bronchi.

(*Text continued on page 168.*)

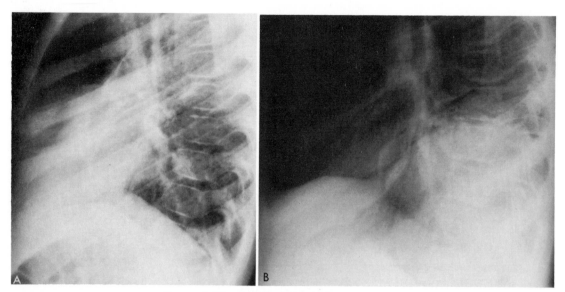

Figure 4-28. "ACQUIRED" SEQUESTRATION

A, Right lateral view. The patient presented with RML pneumonia. Note that the RLL is normal. *B,* Same view approximately a year later. There is now an extensive density involving most of the basal segment of the RLL. Same patient as in Figure 4-24.

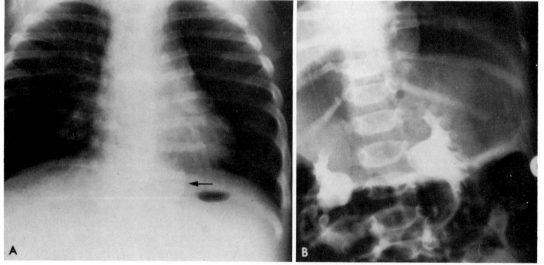

Figure 4-29. EXTRALOBAR SEQUESTRATION

A, There is a left inferior paravertebral lesion with a sharp lateral border (arrow). *B,* The juxtavertebral lesion is better seen on this urogram. At operation the lesion was separate from the LLL and had its own pleural sheath.

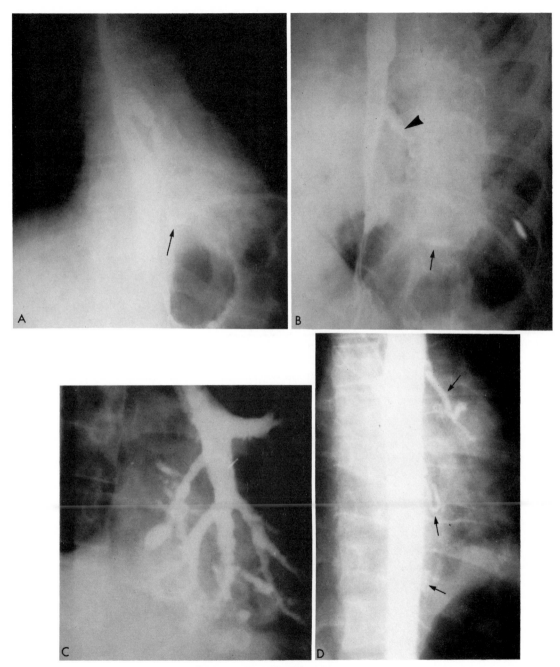

Figure 4–30. ESOPHAGEAL LUNG

A, Barium swallow. Barium leaves the middle third of the esophagus via a "bronchus" and enters the LLL infiltrate, filling small cystlike pockets (arrow). *B,* Left oblique esophagram. The esophageal bronchus (arrowhead) opens into multicystic cavities (arrow). *C,* Conventional bronchogram. Contrast medium leaked into the cystic sequestration from the sides, but there is no normal posterior basal bronchus. Bronchiectasis is present in the adjacent segments of the LLL. *D,* Thoracic aortogram. Three aortic vessels (arrows) supply the sequestered segment. (Courtesy of Dr. Harold G. Jacobson.)

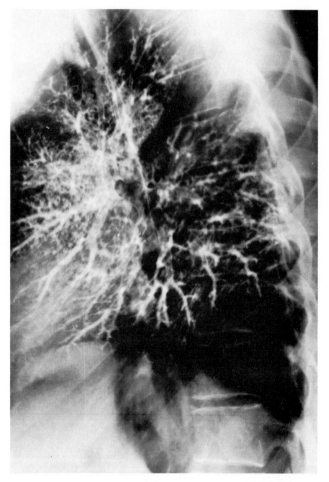

Figure 4–31. DIAGNOSTIC BRONCHO-
GRAM IN SEQUESTRATION

Same patient as Figure 4–26. Off-lateral projection. Normal bronchi are draped around the
hyperaerated segment in the LLL. The small
bronchi that frame the sequestered lung are
terminal twigs normally seen at the periphery
of the lung. There is no suggestion of displacement of the bronchi as by a bulla, cyst, or
other expanded lesion.

A

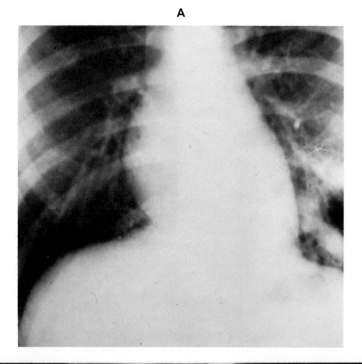

B

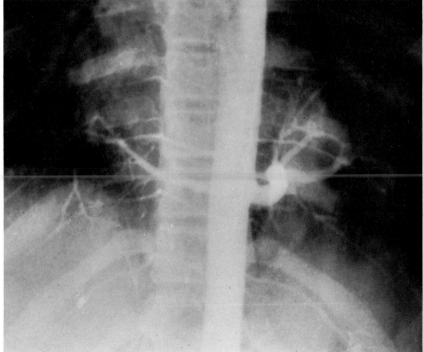

Figure 4–32. BILATERAL SEQUESTRATION?

A, Bronchogenic cyst at the left base. Note the signs of mucoid impaction. The right base appears normal. *B,* The aortogram shows bilateral anomalous arteries supplying the posterior basal region of both lower lobes. No surgical confirmation. If there were a visible lesion in the RLL, the diagnosis of bilateral sequestration would be secure. (Courtesy of Dr. Charles F. Mueller.)

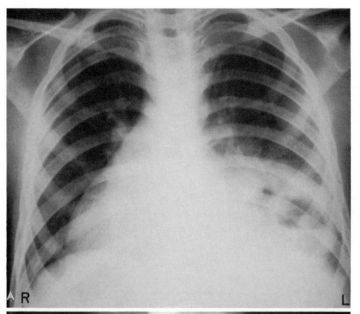

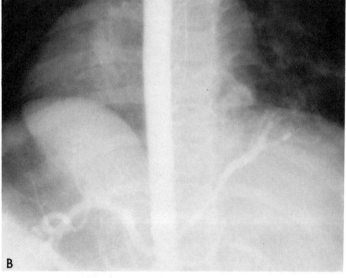

Figure 4–33. SEQUESTRATION IN TOTAL SITUS INVERSUS

The right testis was lower than the left. *A,* Extensive infiltrate in LLL with several air-fluid levels. *B,* Aortography. An artery arising from the abdominal aorta near the celiac supplies the lesion. The patient also had severe chronic sinusitis. Is this Kartagener's syndrome with bronchiectasis and *acquired* aortic blood supply, or is it sequestration with *congenital* artery? I'm not sure.

SEGMENTAL COLLAPSE

Because it is merely another expression of the anatomy which has already been discussed and illustrated, the roentgen appearance of segmental consolidation will not be described. On the other hand, a discussion of the pulmonary segments would not be complete without the inclusion of segmental collapse.

Collapse of a segment, as of a lobe, may be the result of obstruction of the segmental bronchus itself or of multiple small peripheral bronchi within it.[304] The causes of segmental collapse are essentially the same as those of lobar collapse. The roentgen signs, too, are similar, with one notable exception. The decrease in volume, as indicated by the size of the radiopacity, the displacement of septa, and the secondary signs, may be minimal or even unrecognizable. There are several reasons for this: (1) the considerable normal variation in size of the segments; (2) the similarity in size and configuration between a consolidated subsegment and collapse of its parent segment; (3) the relatively small portion affected compared with the total bulk of the lobe, requiring little spatial rearrangement. Crowding of the vascular markings and of the air filled bronchi, when apparent, is certainly useful in the detection of segmental collapse, as is the silhouette sign. Segmental collapse is usually more easily recognized on tomography and bronchography than on conventional films.

Roentgen Signs

A number of excellent descriptions of the roentgen signs of collapse of the individual segments are available.[621, 671, 1019, 1123, 1203] Certain roentgen details peculiar to segmental collapse are emphasized in the following section.

RIGHT UPPER LOBE

The apical segment of the RUL often collapses toward the mediastinum. Depending on the degree of collapse, its radiopacity may be inconspicuous in the frontal projection. On the lateral view, the region is generally entirely obscured by the shoulders. In some patients, then, the only evidence of collapse on conventional films may be a fuzzy lateral border of the right superior mediastinum and loss of definition of the upper right margin of the ascending aorta. The minor fissure may be elevated. Tracheal displacement is often absent (Figs. 3–34 and 4–34).

In the frontal view, the collapsed anterior segment shows a sharp border at the minor fissure, which is bowed upward. The bandlike shadow seldom reaches the major fissure on the lateral view (Figs. 2–7, 4–35 and 14–4). More complete collapse of this segment

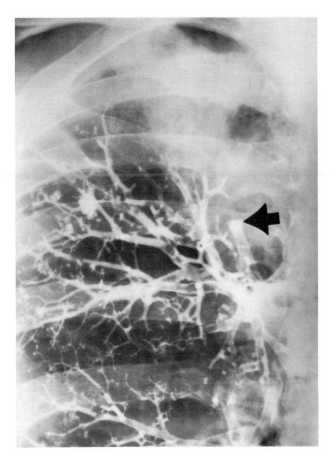

Figure 4–34. COLLAPSE OF THE APICAL SEGMENT OF THE RUL

There is no significant displacement of the trachea or hilum. Carcinomatous obstruction (arrow) is shown bronchographically.

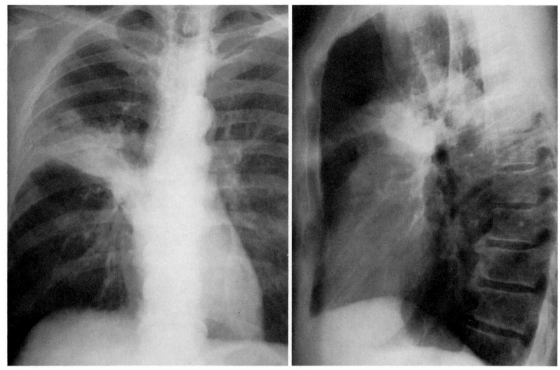

Figure 4–35. COLLAPSE OF ANTERIOR SEGMENT OF RUL

The minor fissure is bowed upward. The lateral subsegment is well developed. Bronchogenic carcinoma.

may result, on frontal projection, in a parahilar opacity, usually with a straight lower border. The right hilar shadow is denser than the left. The right border of the ascending aorta is obliterated (Fig. 4–36).

In the frontal view, the collapsed posterior segment is located somewhat laterally. It may present a sharp lower border if its lateral subdivision is well developed and abuts on the minor fissure (Fig. 4–11). In the lateral view, its posterior border is sharply delineated by the major fissure which may bow forward. The roentgen appearance is similar to that of collapse of the posterior subsegment of the LUL (Fig. 4–43).

RIGHT MIDDLE LOBE

Segmental collapse in the RML (Fig. 4–37) is probably fairly common.[500] Typically, the lateral segment is sharply defined by the minor fissure, which may show little or no downward displacement. The heart border is not obliterated, since the infiltrate does not make contact with it. On the lateral

projection, there is considerable variation in the position of this segment. Most often it appears to occupy the superior portion of the lobe, extending along the minor fissure for a variable distance and usually reaching the angle between the junction of the major and minor fissures, which are often bowed toward each other. The density does not extend to the anterior chest wall. So many different patterns are encountered on the lateral view that it is advisable to rely mainly on the frontal projection for differentiating lateral from medial segmental collapse.

The medial segment of the RML collapses against the heart, producing the silhouette sign on the frontal view. Again, the minor fissure is often visible at its normal level. As implied earlier, in the lateral view this segment does not show a consistent position in relation to the fissures (Fig. 4–38); however, it does extend to the anterior chest wall. Because of their medial-lateral arrangement, considerable superimposition of the shadows of the two RML segments nearly always occurs on the lateral view. Consequently, consolidation or collapse of

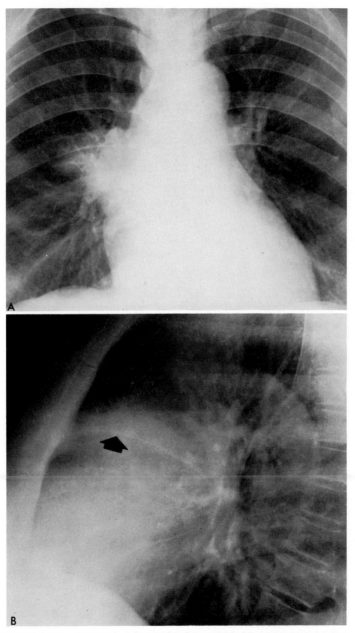

Figure 4–36. MARKED COLLAPSE OF ANTERIOR SEGMENT OF RUL

A, The right hilum is denser than the left and there is a parahilar opacity. The right border of the ascending aorta is obliterated. *B*, Right lateral view. The minor fissure is elevated and the infiltrate has a sharp lower border (arrow). Subsiding pneumonia.

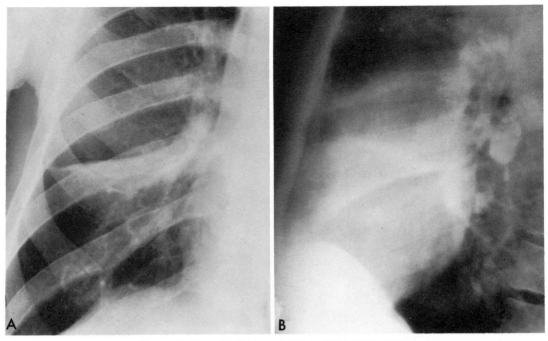

Figure 4–37.   LATERAL SEGMENT COLLAPSE, RML

Pneumonia with slow resolution. *A*, PA view. Note the preservation of the right heart border. The minor fissure is slightly depressed. *B*, Lateral view. The lesion appears to occupy the posterior two thirds of the lobe and extends between the two septa.

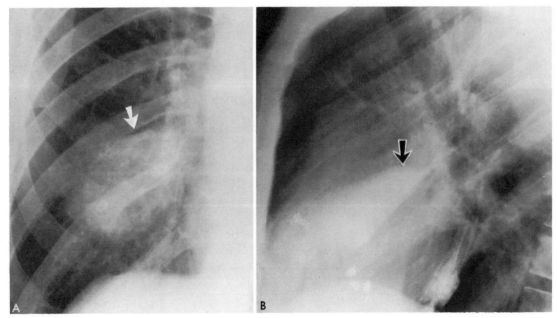

Figure 4–38.   MEDIAL SEGMENT COLLAPSE, RML

A, The heart border is obliterated and the minor fissure is slightly depressed (arrow). *B*, Lateral view. The opacity extends from the chest wall anteriorly to the junction of the minor (arrow) and major fissures posteriorly. Slowly resolving pneumonia.

either segment may appear to occupy almost the entire middle lobe in this projection.

Medial segment collapse may be mimicked closely by collapse of the entire RML (Figs. 1–14 and 3–42). In several cases presumed to be medial segment collapse because the lateral segment appeared normally aerated and the minor fissure was clearly visible in normal position, the lordotic view demonstrated that the radiopacity extended all the way out to the lateral chest wall, indicating collapse of the entire lobe. In such cases, I believe the collapsed lateral segment is so thin in AP diameter that it casts little shadow. I have no idea how frequently this occurs, but perhaps collapse confined to the medial segment of the middle lobe is not as common as we have been led to believe.

RIGHT LOWER LOBE

Collapse of the superior segment of the RLL is usually seen in frontal projection as a wedge shaped parahilar opacity. It does not obliterate the cardiovascular border, a point of differentiation from collapse of the anterior segment of the RUL. Occasionally the major fissure is so depressed that the roentgen beam strikes it tangentially, simulating the minor fissure in collapse of the RML (Fig. 3–40). The distinction is readily made by the retention of the cardiac silhouette. The right hilum often shows an increased density because of the opaque lung behind it. In the lateral projection, the upper portion of the major fissure may be displaced backward and downward (Fig. 14–3). The appearance is similar to that of collapse of its counterpart on the left side (Fig. 4–46).

Isolated collapse of a subsuperior segment is extremely rare. It presents as a pancake opacity extending transversely across the lobe between the superior and the basal segments.

The collapsed medial basal segment overlaps the right heart border. Although obliteration of the heart border in the frontal view has been noted by others, I have not seen it. In the lateral view, it appears as a narrow band extending from the midportion of the diaphragm toward the hilum. Its anterior margin may touch the major septum (Fig. 4–39).

Anterior basal segmental collapse is seen in frontal projection as a density in the lateral lung base. The costophrenic angle is often involved. In the lateral projection, the collapsed segment is represented by a narrow band extending from the diaphragm toward the hilum, sharply defined anteriorly by the oblique septum, which shows posterior displacement (Fig. 4–40).

The collapsed lateral basal segment gives an appearance similar to anterior basal segmental collapse on the frontal view, but lies more posteriorly in the lateral view. It does not contact the major septum, which shows little posterior displacement. Figure 4–41 illustrates a normal sized lateral basal segment. I could find no good example of isolated collapse of this segment in my material.

The collapsed posterior basal segment occupies the region of the medial costophrenic sinus in the frontal view. It does not obliterate the heart border, but extends considerably below the other segments so that it is often visible through the diaphragm well below the dome. On the lateral view, it extends from the region of the posterior costophrenic sinus toward the hilum (Fig. 4–42). In consolidation or collapse of this segment, the large posterior basal vessels are obscured on the well-penetrated AP or PA film. If these vessels remain visible, the disease lies in the medial basal segment or in the middle lobe.[1280]

LEFT UPPER LOBE

Segmental collapse in the left lung generally causes roentgen changes similar to those seen on the right; therefore, only the differences will be emphasized here. The collapsed apicoposterior segment of the LUL occupies the medial portion of the lung above the hilum and obliterates the aortic knob. On the lateral view, it is sharply delineated posteriorly by the major fissure, which is usually bowed forward.

Isolated collapse of the posterior subsegment of the LUL is not rare (Fig. 4–43). The left heart border and aortic knob remain visible, while the left pulmonary artery is usually obliterated. In the frontal view, it closely resembles a lesion in the superior segment of the LLL. The latter, however, does not obliterate the pulmonary artery. A collapsed apical segment (Fig. 4–44A and B) obliterates the aortic knob in the frontal

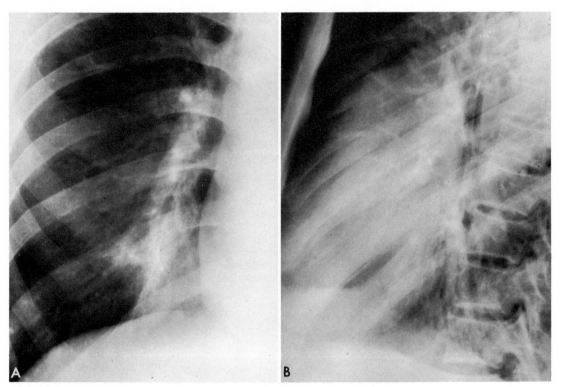

Figure 4–39. COLLAPSE OF MEDIAL BASAL SEGMENT OF RLL

A, Frontal view. The heart border is not obscured. *B*, Lateral view. The anterior border reaches the displaced major septum. The air filled bronchi are crowded together. Pneumonia.

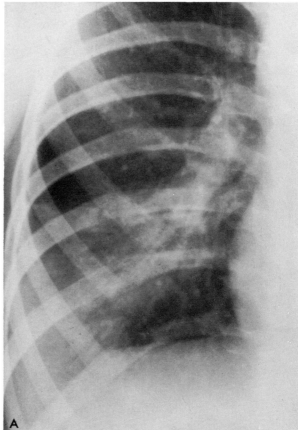

Figure 4–40. ANTERIOR BASAL SEGMENT
COLLAPSE OF RLL

A, PA view. Note the lateral position of this
segment. *B*, Lateral view. Abutment on the posteriorly displaced major fissure is shown. The
sharp posterior margin is spurious and represents overlap of the posterior portion of the
heart. Bronchogenic carcinoma.

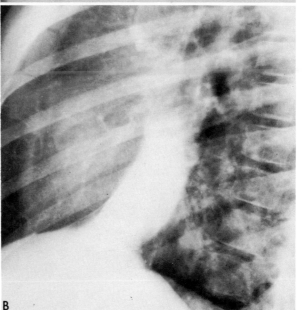

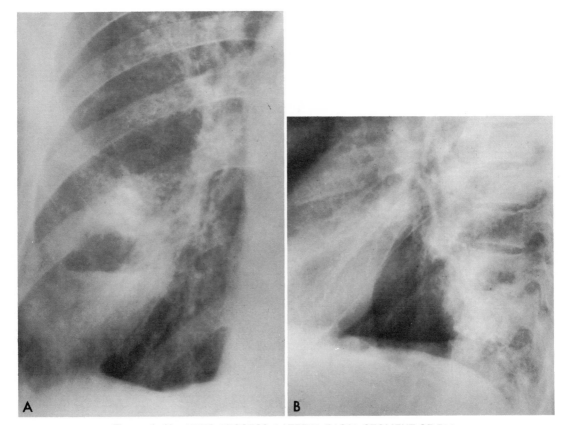

Figure 4–41. LUNG ABSCESS, LATERAL BASAL SEGMENT OF RLL

A, In the frontal projection, the opacity lies laterally and is indistinguishable from anterior segment involvement. Compare with Figure 4–40. *B,* Lateral view. The lesion lies posteriorly, projected over the posterior basal segment.

view. In the lateral, it extends vertically to the extreme apex of the lung.

Collapse of the anterior segment (Figs. 2–12 and 4–44*A* and *B*) does not present as sharp a lower border as in the RUL because of the absence of a minor fissure. Collapse of the superior division of the LUL presents a summation of the above signs (Fig. 4–44*C* and *D*).

Segmental collapse is uncommon in the lingula. It can be differentiated from collapse of the entire lingula by the smaller zone of obliteration of the left heart border on the frontal view and by the smaller extent of the opacity on the lateral view (Figs. 4–43 and 4–45).

LEFT LOWER LOBE

The collapsed superior segment (Fig. 4–46) and individual basal segments of the

LLL (Figs. 4–47 to 4–49) resemble their counterparts on the right, except that the greater obscuration by the left side of the heart sometimes makes it difficult to recognize their presence on the PA teleroentgenogram.

Collapse of multiple segments produces findings equivalent to the sum of the individual segments involved. Although the *open bronchus sign* (see p. 124) applies as well to segmental collapse as it does to lobar collapse in eliminating the possibility of bronchogenic carcinoma, the same does not hold for the *double lesion sign* (see p. 128). There is no septal barrier to the extension of a tumor within a lobe; thus a carcinoma may obstruct several bronchi whose orifices are not adjacent to each other (Fig. 7–7*B*). The sign does apply, of course, to multiple segments of collapse in different lobes.

Experimental obstruction of a segmental bronchus does not cause collapse because (*Text continued on page 180.*)

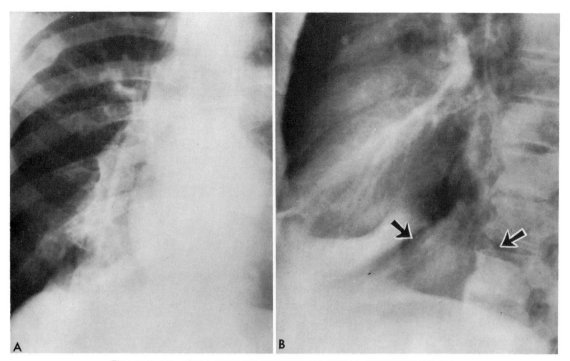

Figure 4–42. COLLAPSE OF POSTERIOR BASAL SEGMENT OF RLL

On the PA projection *(A)*, the heart border is preserved and the pulmonary opacity extends behind the heart to the medial border of the base of the right lung. On the lateral view *(B)*, the posterior inferior angle of the lower lobe is involved (arrows). Adenocarcinoma. (Courtesy of Dr. E. Robert Heitzman.)

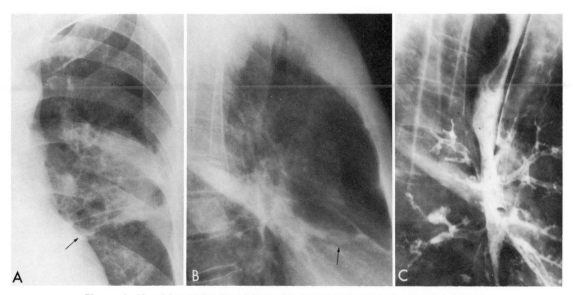

Figure 4–43. COLLAPSE OF POSTERIOR SUBSEGMENT AND LINGULA OF LUL

On frontal projection *(A)*, the heart border is preserved over the upper infiltrate but obliterated by the lower (arrow). Note obliteration of the left pulmonary artery shadow by the posterior subsegmental disease. On the lateral view *(B)*, the collapsed posterior subsegment borders the major septum, which is not displaced. Collapse is also seen in the superior lingular segment (arrow). *C,* Lateral bronchogram confirms the presence and location of the collapse. Slowly resolving pneumonia.

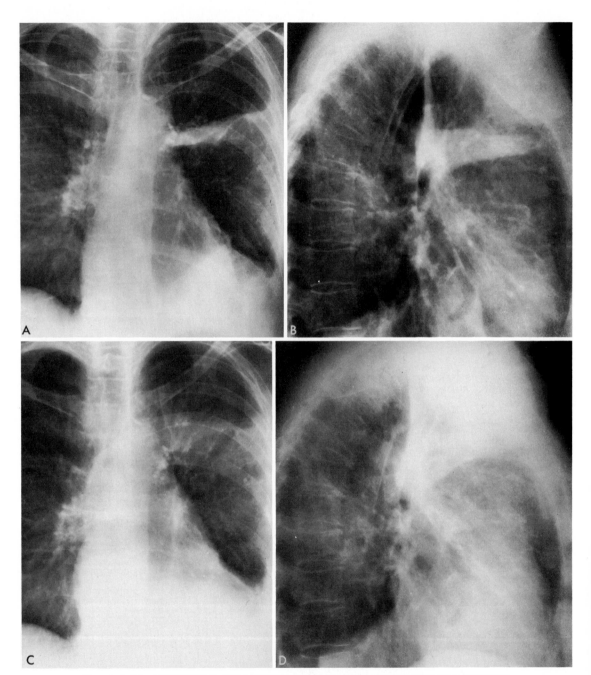

Figure 4–44. SEGMENTAL COLLAPSE IN THE LUL FROM RADIATION PNEUMONITIS

A and *B*, Collapse of apical subsegment and anterior segment of the LUL. The upper and left borders of the aortic knob are obliterated by the apical involvement. The lower border of the anterior segment is not "fissure sharp." *C* and *D*, Three weeks later. The entire superior division of the LUL is now involved. The overdistended LLL reaches almost to the pulmonary apex. Pleural reaction at left base. The patient had recently completed a postoperative course of radiation therapy for carcinoma of the breast.

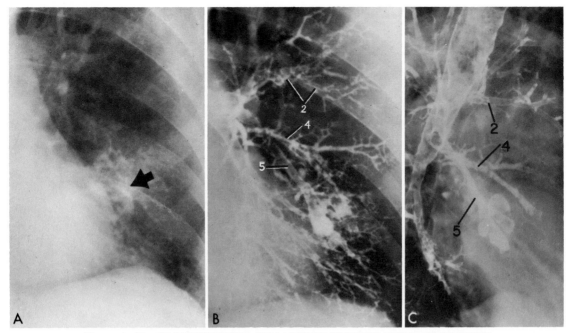

Figure 4–45. BRONCHIECTATIC COLLAPSE OF INFERIOR LINGULAR SEGMENT

The opacity (arrow) on the teleroentgenogram *(A)* obliterates a short segment of the heart border. Bronchography *(B and C)* shows saccular bronchiectasis almost entirely confined to the inferior lingular segment *(5)*. The superior lingular bronchus *(4)* is displaced slightly downward. The anterior segment bronchus *(2)* of the LUL has a high takeoff.

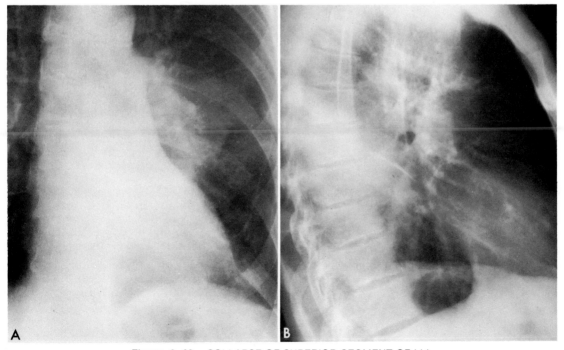

Figure 4–46. COLLAPSE OF SUPERIOR SEGMENT OF LLL

The left heart border and left pulmonary artery are preserved in the frontal view *(A)*. The upper part of the left side of the heart appears more opaque than the lower. In the lateral view *(B)*, the collapsed segment is poorly defined and obscured by the vertebrae. Note the increase in radiopacity of the midthoracic vertebral bodies compared with the upper and lower ones. The major fissure is displaced posteriorly. Bronchogenic carcinoma.

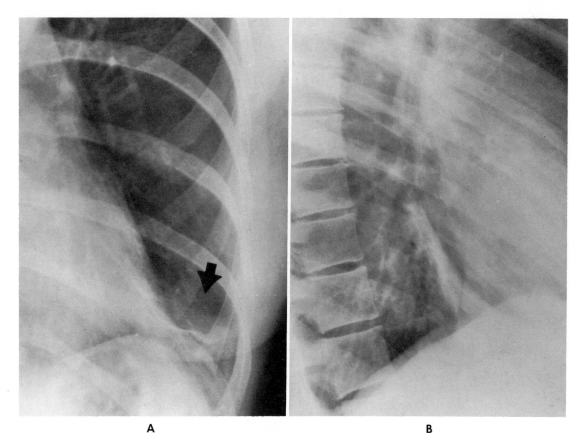

A   **B**

Figure 4–47. COLLAPSE OF ANTERIOR BASAL SEGMENT OF LLL

The heart border is not obliterated by the lesion (arrow) in the frontal view *(A)*. In the lateral view *(B)*, the infiltrate borders the major fissure, which is displaced posteriorly. Pneumonia.

of so-called *collateral air drift*, i.e., the passage of air across the parenchyma from one segment to the next.[24, 214, 973, 1240] Collapse does occur if an interlobar septum intervenes between the two segments. Collateral air drift is attributed, at least in part, to the presence of tiny interalveolar openings, the *pores of Kohn*,* and bronchiolar-alveolar communications, the *channels of Lambert*[668, 669] (Fig. 7–23). This cross ventilation, however, seldom prevents segmental col-

*In *Fundamentals of Chest Roentgenology* I misspelled the name *Cohn*. I received a letter from a Czech reader stating that it should have been *Ghon* and that my reference #297 should have been *Věšína*, not *Vêŝin*. I checked both references and wrote him that he was wrong on both counts. He replied, "You may be right about Kohn, but Věšína is my cousin!"

lapse.[574] It is theorized that the associated inflammation occludes these tiny orifices, sealing off the obstructed segment.[223] Rarely, however, complete obstruction of a segmental bronchus may occur without collapse.[266] This accounts for the occasional case in which enlarged bronchi are visible distal to an occluded segmental bronchus. I have seen it in bronchial adenoma (Fig. 4–50), in congenital segmental bronchial atresia[226] (Fig. 7–15), and in bronchogenic cyst[219] (Fig. 7–16). The bronchi are usually distended with inspissated mucus or pus. The dilated bronchi are recognized by their branching fusiform structure of water density, sometimes containing bubbles of entrapped air,[971] best seen on tomography. This finding is more commonly seen in

(*Text continued on page 184.*)

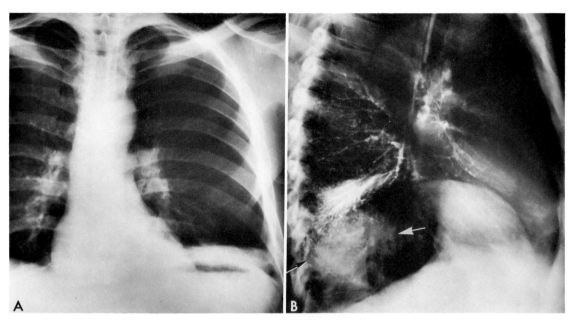

Figure 4–48. LATERAL BASAL SEGMENT COLLAPSE OF THE LLL

The heart border is preserved. In the PA view *(A)* it appears similar to anterior segment involvement (see Fig. 4–47*A*), but in the lateral projection *(B)* the lesion (arrows) looks like posterior segment disease (compare with Fig. 4–49*B*). Bronchographic flooding of the subsuperior segment has occurred. *B* is a recumbent right lateral Bucky film, which explains the high right hemidiaphragm (see p. 12).

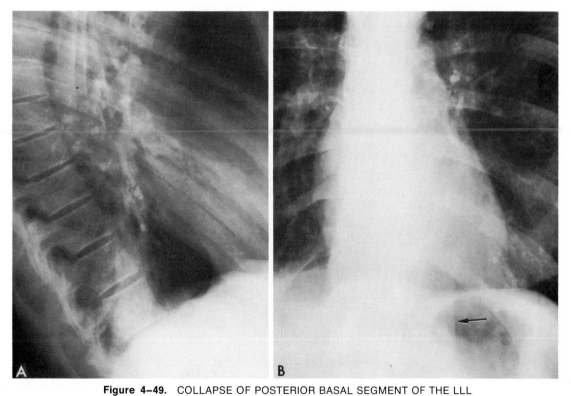

Figure 4–49. COLLAPSE OF POSTERIOR BASAL SEGMENT OF THE LLL

The infiltrate is partly hidden by the heart in the PA view. Note its low position (arrow). Pneumonia.

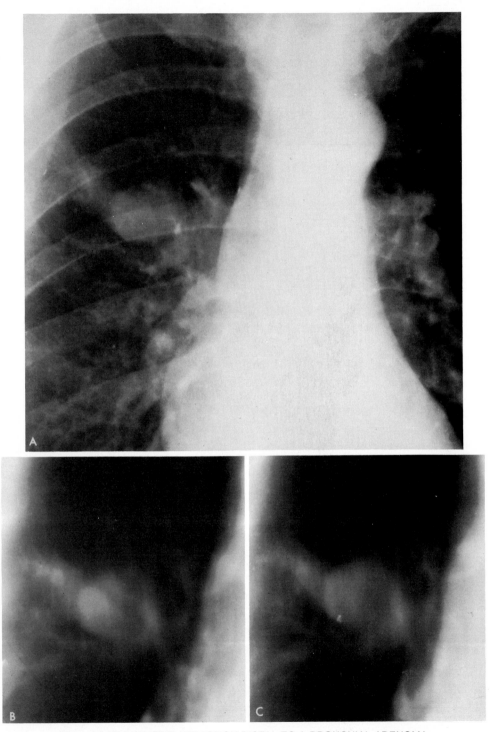

Figure 4–50.   MUCOID IMPACTION DISTAL TO A BRONCHIAL ADENOMA

A, Teleroentgenogram. *B* and *C,* Tomograms. The obstructing tumor in the anterior segment bronchus of the RUL is not visible. The dilated bronchi distal to it are clearly outlined by air that has entered the segment via collateral ventilation.

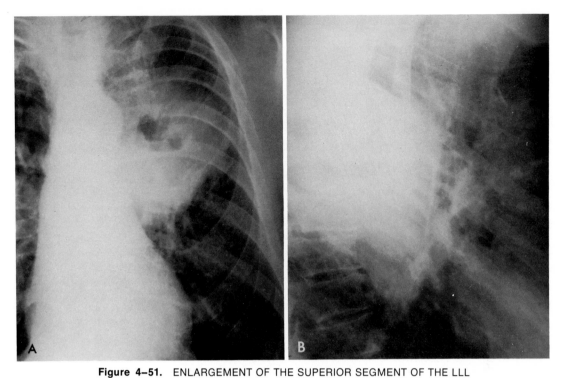

Figure 4–51. ENLARGEMENT OF THE SUPERIOR SEGMENT OF THE LLL

There is a central cavity with fluid level. Note persistence of the aortic knob and heart shadow. Tuberculosis.

Figure 4–52. SEGMENTAL ENLARGEMENT IN FRIEDLÄNDER'S PNEUMONIA

The lateral basal segment on the left is enlarged. Note the sharp bulging superior margin (arrow). (From Felson, B., Rosenberg, L. S., and Hamburger, M., Jr.[349]; reproduced with permission of Radiology.)

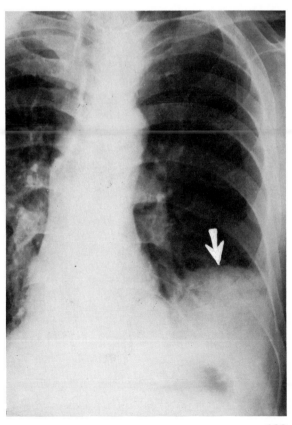

bronchial adenoma than in carcinoma. Mucoid impaction, a condition occurring in asthmatics and other patients with chronic pulmonary symptoms, may produce a similar pattern *without* bronchial obstruction[162] (Fig. 7–17). In many such cases, *Aspergillum fumigatus* has been demonstrated in the sputum.[1307]

The differential diagnosis of segmental collapse is essentially the same as that of lobar collapse and will not be repeated. Disk atelectasis will be discussed in Chapter 12.

A round form of nonsegmental collapse is said to occur in pleural effusion. The edge of the compressed lung may become airless and roll up in a ball. When the fluid clears, the rest of the lung may aerate first, leaving the rounded area no room to expand.[503] I have never recognized this interesting phenomenon but am patiently watching for it.

SEGMENTAL ENLARGEMENT

Enlargement of a segment is recognized by the bulging of the interlobar septum adjacent to it (Fig. 4–51). Even on the side of the lesion not facing the septum, the enlarged segment may be sharply outlined because of the abrupt transition between it and the adjacent compressed normal lung. Segmental enlargement has the same connotation as lobar enlargement, which was discussed in the preceding chapter. It accounts for the so-called "cannonball" opacities sometimes seen in Friedländer's (Fig. 4–52) and other pneumonias.[349]

Segmental enlargement seldom occurs in emphysema,[223] except in the bullous variety. Obstructive emphysema due to constriction of a segmental bronchus is much less frequent than its lobar counterpart, probably because of collateral air drift.

CHAPTER 5

THE HILA AND PULMONARY VESSELS

The vascular alterations that frequently occur in intrathoracic disease often provide a major clue to diagnosis. Recognition of pulmonary congestion will often steer the course of differential diagnosis in the proper direction. Even minimal changes in the vascular structures, if detected, may lead to earlier diagnosis of such serious lesions as pulmonary hypertension or embolism.[1130, 1179] So it is essential that you closely study the vascularity of the lung on every chest roentgenogram.

There are five vascular systems in the thorax that are or may become visible on the chest film: pulmonary artery, pulmonary vein, bronchial artery, azygos vein, and lymphatic. Each of these systems has its specific roentgen pattern, usually clearly distinguishable from all other patterns and involving the hilum, mediastinum, or lung, alone or in combination. These circulations will be dealt with individually in this and in the next chapter, but let's begin with the hila.

THE HILA

The Normal Hila

First a word about the word. In the manuscript of my book *Fundamentals of Chest Roentgenology*, I used *hilum/hila* throughout. The copy editors were inclined to change every *hilum* to *hilus* and every *hila* to *hili*, claiming some obscure Latin rule. Having no classical language background and not wishing to delay publication over a trivial semantic problem (I'm antisemantic, anyway), I yielded. Then I received a com-

munication from my friend Dr. Harold Rosenbaum of Lexington, a radiologist and frustrated lexicographer, berating me for the scriptural *faux pas*. I referred him to the real culprits, and the subsequent heated polemics-by-mail ended in what I judged to be a draw. So I'm back to *hilum/hila*, simply because *hili* sounds to me like a Basque game played in Florida.

The hila are composed of the pulmonary arteries and their main branches, the upper lobe pulmonary veins, the major bronchi, and the lymph glands. The lower lobe pulmonary veins do not cross the hila in their course to the left atrium and therefore do not contribute to the hilar shadows. The bronchi account for little of the hilar opacity, since they are filled with air, and the normal lymph nodes are too small to add to the size or density. Therefore, the normal hilar shadows consist mostly of the large pulmonary arteries and upper lobe veins (Fig. 5-1).

The undivided pulmonary artery, 4 to 5 cm in length and about 3 cm in diameter, lies entirely within the pericardial sac, as does its bifurcation. The right pulmonary artery remains within the pericardium until it gives off its first branch, the artery to the RUL. This vessel lies medial to the upper lobe veins which form most of the profile of the upper half of the right hilum. The pulmonary artery continues as the descending or inferior division to supply the RML and RLL. It accounts for the lower half of the right hilum.[265, 536, 703] The lateral angle between the upper and lower portions of the right hilum is formed by the superior pulmonary vein above and the descending pulmonary artery below.[703] The medial portion

185

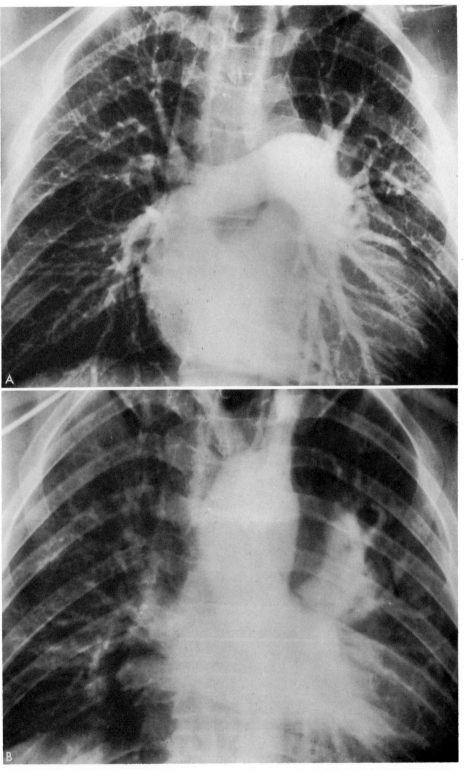

Figure 5–1. See opposite page for legend.

of the horizontal fissure often terminates at this angle. The RUL bronchus lies above the right pulmonary artery and is therefore *eparterial.*[108]

The left pulmonary artery lies intrapericardially for a short distance before entering the lung. Instead of a single anterior trunk, as on the right, there are usually one or more smaller LUL branches arising anterosuperiorly. The lingular and the superior and basilar segmental arteries of the LLL arise from the continuation of the pulmonary artery (the interlobar portion).[108] If the left pulmonary artery divides within the pericardium, as it occasionally does, it forms at least a portion of the pulmonary arc on the cardiac outline and two or more branches emanate from the lateral border of the arc (Fig. 5–1A). If the division occurs outside the pericardium, the middle arc is formed by the undivided pulmonary artery and the main left pulmonary artery is seen entering the lung and quickly branching (Fig. 5–2). The left main bronchus enters the lung below the left pulmonary artery *(hyparterial).*

The dimensions of the normal hila vary considerably from one individual to another, and the two sides often differ in the same individual. In those cases in which the left pulmonary artery shadow blends with that of the main pulmonary artery, forming a part or all of the pulmonary arc segment of the heart, a smaller left hilum usually results. Because of these variations, accurate measurements are difficult. On teleroentgenograms, the transverse diameter of the normal descending branch of the right pulmonary artery at its widest point is 10 to 16 mm in men and 9 to 15 mm in women.[173, 824]

The size of the hilar shadows was graded on teleroentgenograms of the chest in 1000 apparently healthy soldiers, most of whom were between the ages of 20 and 35. Although wide differences were noted, in only three (0.3 per cent) were they of such a size that pathologic enlargement was suggested. Comparison of the widths of the two hila was also made. In 84 per cent the hila were equal in size. In 8 per cent the right hilum appeared distinctly larger than the left; in 8 per cent the reverse was noted (Chap. 15).

Attempts have been made to set a maximal numerical measurement for the normal hilum in the hope of facilitating the detection of carcinoma of the lung.[1009] However, because of the wide range of overlap between the normal and abnormal, I do not believe that actual measurements are practical.

On adequately penetrated films, the two hilar shadows are generally of about equal radiopacity. Their relative opacity was studied in 1500 normal adults of various ages (Chap. 15). The two sides were equal in 91 per cent, the right was slightly denser than the left in about 6 per cent; the left was slightly denser than the right in 3 per cent. In only four individuals (0.3 per cent) was there a moderate difference in the hilar densities, the right being greater in density than

Figure 5–1. ANGIOGRAM SHOWING THE NORMAL HILAR VASCULATURE (Opposite)

A, Arterial phase. The right pulmonary artery gives off the RUL division before it reaches the right hilum. The inferior division accounts for the lower half of the right hilar shadow. The left pulmonary artery forms part of the left middle arc in this patient, and its first generation branches emanate from several areas along this arc. *B,* Venous phase. The right upper pulmonary vein forms the upper half of the contour of the right hilum. Most of the left upper pulmonary vein lies behind the pulmonary artery so it accounts for little of the left hilar contour. The inferior pulmonary veins lie well below the hila and do not contribute to their shadows.

the left in all four. Films showing scoliosis, patient rotation, or a rib, transverse process, or dilated descending aorta overlapping a hilum were excluded.

As each pulmonary artery shadow is traced medially to its cardiovascular intersection, it sometimes is seen to obliterate the left heart border or the right lateral border of the ascending aorta. I found this to be true on the right side in about one fourth of 500 normal chests, and on the left in about three fourths. A number of films had to be excluded because the area in question was inadequately demonstrated (Chap. 15). A normally positioned pulmonary arc and origin of the left pulmonary artery tend to rule out transposition of the great vessels.

Additional examinations are often required to clarify a suspected hilar lesion. These include well-penetrated Bucky films to confirm the differences in density and to demonstrate other mediastinal node bearing areas;[443] films made with slight degrees of patient rotation (preferably under fluoroscopic control) to differentiate between the truly round or oval shadow of lymph nodes or other masses and the foreshortened shadow of a pulmonary artery on end; routine lateral and oblique films to provide additional views of the area; the Valsalva maneuver to bring out the "lumpy" shadow of lymph nodes as the hilar vessels shrink; barium studies to demonstrate impingement on the esophagus by additional lymph

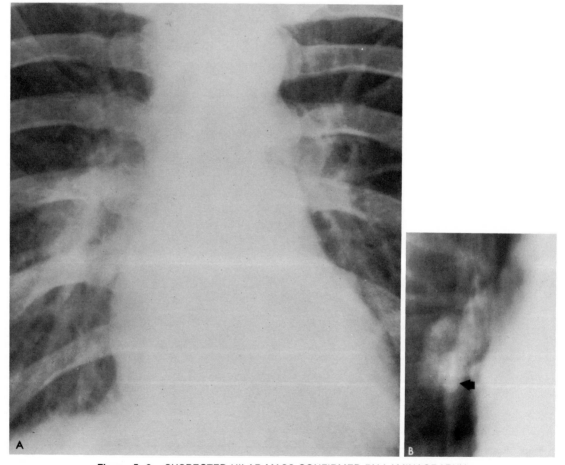

Figure 5–2. SUSPECTED HILAR MASS CONFIRMED BY LAMINAGRAPHY

The plain film *(A)* shows fullness and increased density of the right hilum. The main left pulmonary artery forms much of the left hilum. *B,* Laminagraphic cut just behind the pulmonary artery shows a mass containing stippled calcium. The overlying right inferior pulmonary artery (arrow) is out of focus. Probable enlarged lymph node.

node masses, particularly in the carinal region (Fig. 1–8); and laminagraphy in frontal and in lateral projection to bring out the hilar details and to delineate other masses (Fig. 5–2). Occasionally, bronchography and angiocardiography are useful.

In our own hands the Bucky film, barium esophagram, and laminagram have been the most helpful. To avoid a great deal of time consuming studies, considerable judgment must be exercised in the selection of patients for intensive work-up. I have relied, in the borderline case, on abnormal hilar density and shape rather than size alone.

In the lateral view, the hilar structures are, of course, more difficult to discern, and it is particularly hard to distinguish right from left. However, displacement secondary to collapse[1286] or to left atrial dilatation,[692] enlargement by tumor, obliteration by adjacent lesions, and venous dilatation in pulmonary hypertension[174] can sometimes be recognized.[1251] Since the changes are subtle, a high quality film in true lateral position, determined by the appearance of the sternum and spine, is essential (Fig. 5–3). A Bucky technique is preferable. Either lateral, right or left, is adequate for the purpose, since the two hila are close enough to each other that differential magnification and distortion do not occur.

The RUL bronchus is higher than the left and its end-on projection presents in the lateral view as a small circle superimposed over the lower trachea. About 2 cm below this is the similar projection of the LUL bronchus. It is seen more clearly than the right because it is surrounded by vessels— above by the pulmonary artery and below by the veins. The carina is visible as an increased blackening at the lower end of the trachea.

The right pulmonary artery lies anterior to the carina, and the right pulmonary veins lie inferior to it. The left pulmonary artery extends behind the carina, often parallel with the aortic arch but well below it. The left pulmonary veins converge in front of the lower portion of the hilum to enter the back of the left atrium. It's easy to remember that the RUL bronchus lies higher than the left and that the left pulmonary artery lies higher and more posterior than the right.

Hilar Abnormalities

INCREASED DENSITY

A distinct increase in density of one hilum as compared with the other (in the absence of extensive calcification) often indicates an abnormality in the hilum itself or in the lung in front of or behind it (Figs. 4–36, 5–2, and 5–4). This is not to imply that all pathologic hila will show such an increase in radiopacity, but rather that in the borderline case a difference in the relative density of the two hila is an indication for further study. Similarly, a lack of sharpness of the lateral border of a hilum should be looked upon with suspicion because of the implications of the silhouette sign. The *hilum overlay* and *hilum convergence* signs are variations of this principle (p. 39).

THE SMALL HILUM

Bilateral small hila generally indicate congenital heart disease, particularly the cyanotic forms associated with infundibular pulmonary stenosis or displacement or absence of the main pulmonary artery. These include tetralogy of Fallot (Fig. 5–33), tricuspid atresia, truncus arteriosus, and transposition of the great vessels. The *T's* serve as a mnemonic. Central pulmonary embolism partially obstructing the undivided pulmonary artery or its right and left main branches may also reduce the size of both hila (Fig. 5–5).

Sometimes only one hilum will appear to be small. This is seen in such conditions as congenital absence[7, 782, 1110, 1171, 1328] or hypoplasia[52, 787] of a pulmonary artery (Fig. 5–6), pulmonary embolism (Figs. 5–7 and 5–38), neoplastic involvement of a pulmonary artery (Fig. 5–8), obstructive overdistention (Fig. 1–4), idiopathic unilateral hyperlucent lung (also called Macleod's or Swyer-James syndrome) (Fig. 5–37), and marked lobar collapse in which the hilum is displaced behind the heart (Fig. 3–35). In all these conditions, the intrapulmonary branches of the pulmonary artery on the affected side appear sparse and inconspicuous, usually with evidence of overcirculation on the normal side. The lung on the involved side

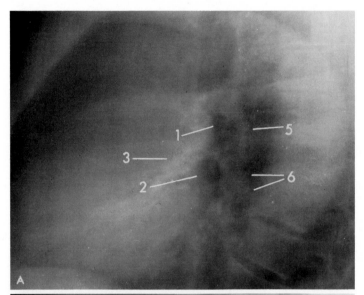

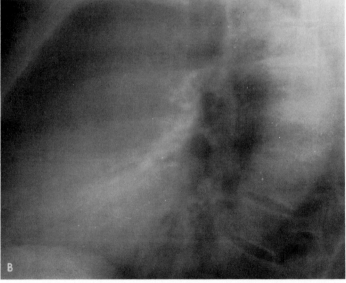

Figure 5–3. LATERAL VIEW OF THE HILA

A heavy *(A* and *B)* and a thin *(C* and *D)* patient. *(1)* RUL bronchus (end-on). *(2)* LUL bronchus (end-on). *(3)* Right pulmonary artery. *(4)* Right pulmonary veins. *(5)* Left pulmonary artery. *(6)* Left pulmonary veins.

(Figure continued on opposite page.)

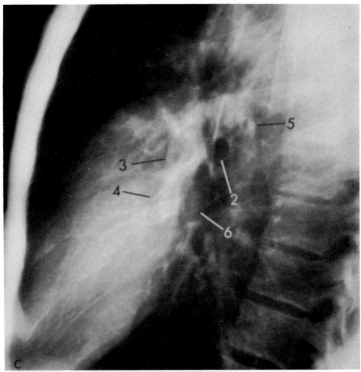

Figure 5–3. *Continued.*

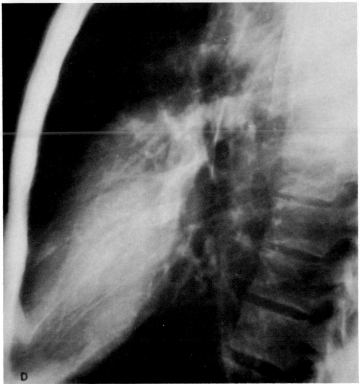

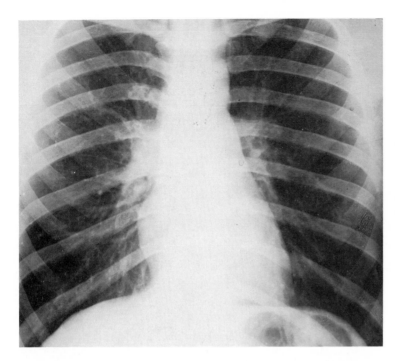

Figure 5–4. INCREASED DEN-
SITY OF RIGHT HILUM

Later films showed obvious
lymph node enlargement which
eventually subsided spontaneously. Probable histoplasmosis.

often appears more radiolucent than normal, simply because it contains less blood.
Depending on the cause, the affected lung
may show increased, normal, or diminished
volume.

THE LARGE HILUM

Bilateral hilar enlargement is usually
caused by lymphadenopathy or vascular dilatation secondary to heart disease, such as
congenital left to right shunts, cor pulmonale, left ventricular failure,[265] or mitral
valve disease. Table 5–1 gives a more
complete listing. In cor pulmonale, the
large hila are often more conspicuous because they are less obscured by the heart,
and better contrasted by the overinflated
lung[1123] (Fig. 5–9).

Unilateral hilar enlargement results from
neoplasm,[1212] herniation of the pulmonary
artery through a congenital pericardial defect, pulmonary artery thromboembolism[501, 630, 631, 1206] (Fig. 5–10), aneurysm
(Figs. 5–11 and 5–12), idiopathic congenital
dilatation,[623] and valvular pulmonary stenosis (Fig. 5–13). In the last named condi-

tion, the poststenotic dilatation[561] often appears to extend well into the left pulmonary
artery but never into the right.[135, 1143] This
causes a distinct asymmetry of the two pulmonary arteries, a sign almost diagnostic of
this condition. This dilatation has been attributed to a leftward direction of the jet
emanating from the constricted valve.[181, 182]
However, on angiography, there is central
dilatation of the right pulmonary artery as
well, but the dilated segment lies hidden in
the mediastinum.[1049]

Unilateral or bilateral main pulmonary artery dilatation is almost always accompanied by enlargement of the pulmonary
trunk and of the right ventricle. The mere
presence, then, of distended central pulmonary arteries is good evidence for right heart
and main pulmonary artery dilatation. The
certainty is enhanced if the middle left arc
is enlarged on the frontal view (Fig. 5–9) or
the lower anterior clear space is encroached
upon in the lateral.

It is extremely important to note the relative position of the two hila in the chest
roentgenogram. This has already been discussed in connection with lobar collapse in
Chapter 3.

(Text continued on page 201.)

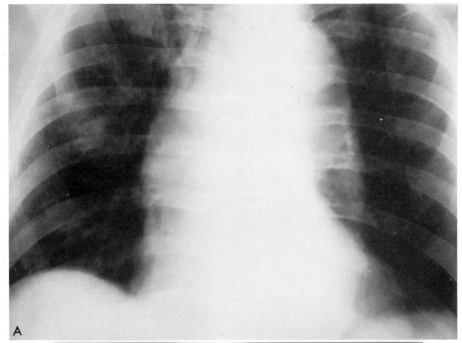

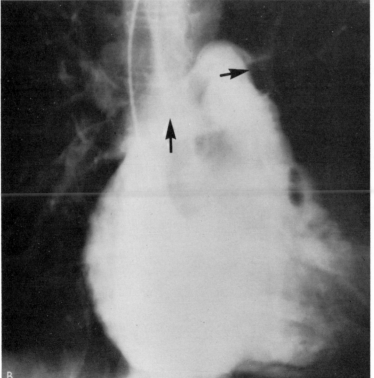

Figure 5–5. CENTRAL PULMONARY EMBOLISM

A, The hila, partly hidden by the dilated aorta, are small. The vascularity is greatly diminished in both lungs. At autopsy, both pulmonary arteries just beyond the bifurcation of the undivided pulmonary artery were almost completely obstructed by emboli. (Courtesy of Dr. Emil Guttman.) *B,* Angiogram in another patient. A large embolus is visible in the right pulmonary artery (vertical arrow), extending into its superior and inferior divisions. A second embolus is seen in the central portion of the left pulmonary artery (horizontal arrow). The hila were small and the lungs oligemic.

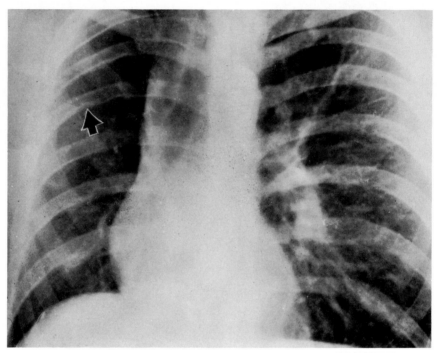

Figure 5–6.   LACK OF RIGHT HILUM IN CONGENITAL ABSENCE OF RIGHT PULMONARY ARTERY

   The mediastinal structures are shifted into the right thorax, which is smaller than the left. The left lung shows increased vascularity because it receives all the blood from the right heart. The unilateral notching of the ribs (arrow), a rare finding in this condition, is attributed to collateral circulation to the right lung via the intercostal arteries. There was no evidence of heart disease. Unproved. (Courtesy of Dr. Norman Magid.)

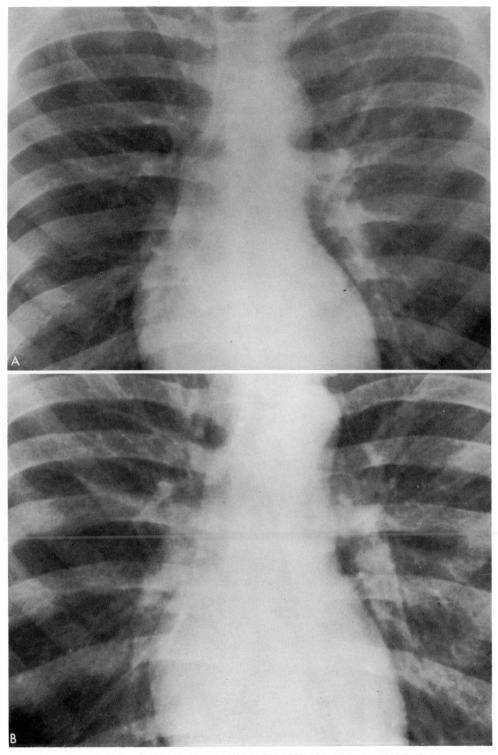

Figure 5–7.   SMALL RIGHT HILUM IN PULMONARY ARTERY EMBOLISM

This young man had a classic episode of pulmonary embolism, with recovery. *A,* Immediately after acute onset. Note the small right hilum and decreased circulation to the right lung. Infarction did not occur. *B,* 17 days later; the lungs now appear normal. (Courtesy of Dr. Lee S. Rosenberg.)

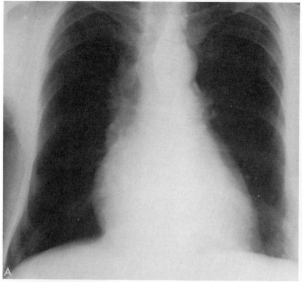 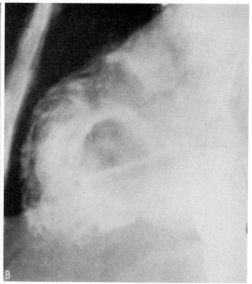

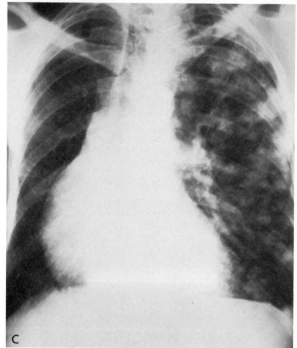

Figure 5–8. MALIGNANT TUMOR BLOCKING
PULMONARY ARTERY

A, PA teleroentgenogram. The hila are very
small, the lungs strikingly oligemic. *B,* Lateral
dextroangiogram shows the tumor. Metastatic
sarcoma phyllodes from the breast. (Courtesy of
Dr. Owen Brown.) *C,* Primary cardiac angio-
sarcoma blocking right pulmonary artery
and then metastasizing to left lung. (Courtesy of
Dr. J. J. McCort.)

*TABLE 5–1. Conditions Resulting in
Bilateral Enlargement of Hilar Shadows*

Common
  Congenital heart disease (left to right shunts)
  Expiration film
  Lymphadenopathy (see Table 6–1)
  Pulmonary embolism
  Pulmonary hypertension, arterial (cor pul-
    monale) or venous

Rare
  Polycythemia

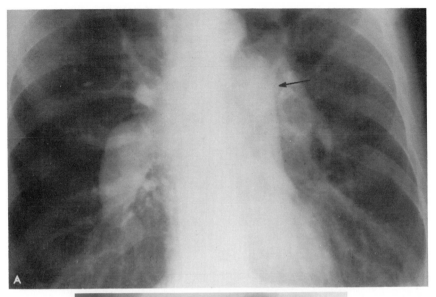

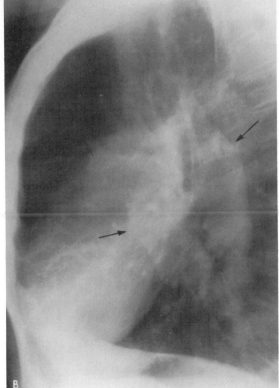

Figure 5–9. BILATERAL HILAR ENLARGEMENT IN COR PULMONALE

A, There is also enlargement of the undivided pulmonary artery, accounting for the convexity of the middle cardiac curve on the left (arrow). *B,* In the lateral view, the left pulmonary artery (upper arrow) lies considerably posterior to the right (lower arrow).

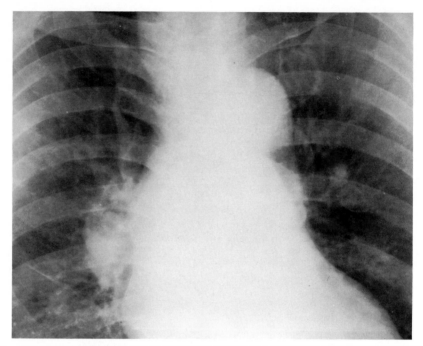

Figure 5–10. ENLARGED RIGHT HILUM IN CHRONIC RIGHT PULMONARY ARTERY THROMBOEMBOLISM

There is an abrupt transition between the large right pulmonary artery and its diminutive branches, producing an "amputated" appearance. An identical appearance was seen 7 years later. Proved at autopsy.

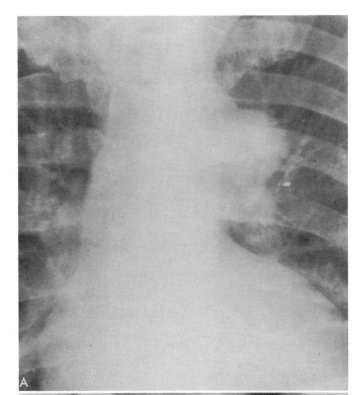

Figure 5–11. POSTTRAUMATIC PUL-
MONARY ARTERY ANEURYSM CAUSING
HILAR ENLARGEMENT

A, Gunshot wound of the left chest was
followed by enlargement of the superior
pole of the left hilum. *B,* Angiocardiogram
shows filling of the aneurysm (arrow)
from the pulmonary artery. A false aneurysm was found at operation.

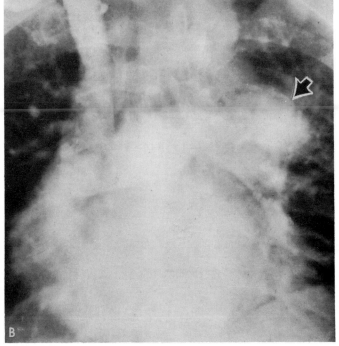

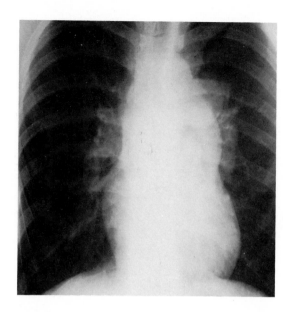

Figure 5–12. PULMONARY ANEURYSM FOLLOW-
ING POTTS OPERATION

The main and left pulmonary artery are markedly
dilated many years after the aortopulmonary shunt.
The patient was found wandering about aimlessly with
a loaded revolver at a Governors' conference.

Figure 5–13. ENLARGED LEFT
HILUM IN CONGENITAL PULMO-
NARY VALVULAR STENOSIS

An incidental finding at autopsy in an 82 year old man. The
converging intrapulmonary vessels mark the hilar mass as a
dilated left main pulmonary artery.

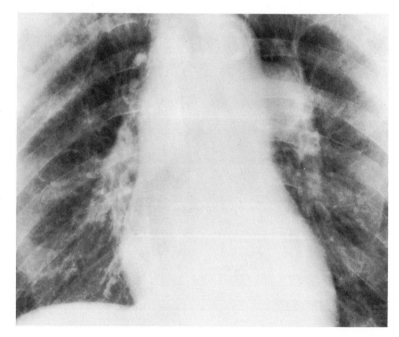

THE INTRAPULMONARY ARTERIES AND VEINS

The Normal Pulmonary Vasculature

The normal pulmonary vessels are particularly well seen in the medial portion of the base of the right lung. In the outer third of the lungs, the vessels become rapidly attenuated and seldom measure more than a millimeter or two in width. In fact, sharply defined branches in the outer zone are uncommon, occurring in about 5 per cent of normal adults (Chap. 15). There are wide differences in the appearance of the pulmonary vasculature, depending not only on individual variation but also on film quality, body habitus, and age.[863] I compared the upper to the lower lobe vessels in 1000 adults, covering the hilum with my thumb to avoid optical bias. The upper lobe vessels appeared smaller than the lower in 63 per cent, the two groups were equal in 34 per cent, and the upper vessels were larger than the lower in about 3 per cent (Chap. 15). The latter figure should be taken into account when evaluating chest films for early congestive failure, as discussed later.

The effect of respiration on vessel size and pulmonary radiolucency is well known (Fig. 1–5). However, not all individuals show significant pulmonary alteration with respiration. Inspiration and expiration films were available from a chest survey in slightly less than 300 normal individuals (Chap. 15). Unless the two films showed a distinct difference in the diaphragm level, confirming that a reasonably deep breath was taken, I excluded them. Alterations in heart size and shape were ignored; only the lungs were studied. In 25 per cent, little or no difference in pulmonary vascularity or aeration could be detected between the two films. In 46 per cent, a moderate amount of basal clouding and enlargement of lower lobe vessels occurred on expiration. In 25 per cent, severe opacification was seen, simulating the pattern of congestive failure.

THE PULMONARY VEINS

It is extremely desirable to distinguish between the intrapulmonary branches of the arteries and veins on the plain roentgenogram, but this is no simple matter. Laminagrams and, of course, angiograms are much better suited for this purpose.

There are generally two main pulmonary veins on each side. The superior one on the right is formed by the apical, posterior, and anterior veins of the RUL and the RML vein; the LUL is similarly drained. In the lower lobes, the superior and inferior basal veins unite to form the common basal vein which then joins the vein of the apex of the lower lobe and the medial vein close to the left atrium.[265, 510, 711]

The segmental pulmonary veins do not parallel the arteries or bronchi, since they lie at the periphery of the segments.[112] The inferior veins on the right are often recognized because they converge toward the left atrium rather than toward the hilum[1169] (Figs. 5–1 and 5–14). The LLL veins are not so often visible because the heart usually obscures this area.

The normal veins are slightly larger and less well defined than the arteries and in the upper lobes usually lie lateral to them.[145] They take a wider arc to the hilum and are straighter and have fewer branches than the arteries.[828] In the upper lobes, the veins coursing to the left atrium are usually lost in the maze of the hilum. At times they may be recognized when they meet the main pulmonary artery trunk at an angle inconsistent with entry into it. The bilateral course of the upper pulmonary veins has been likened to the mustache of a British sergeant major, and the lower lobe arteries to that of a Chinese mandarin. But in these times, hirsutism is superfluous.

I reviewed a series of PA teleroentgenograms of healthy adult men to determine the frequency of recognition of the larger pulmonary veins in the lower lungs. The sole criterion for their identification was the ability to demonstrate vascular shadows passing toward the left atrium. For the right side 500 films were studied. Pulmonary veins were identified definitely in 48 per cent, questionably in 40 per cent, and not at all in 12 per cent. Corresponding figures on the left side for 350 films were 15, 36, and 49 per cent. Attempts to differentiate upper lobe arteries and veins proved futile. A similar but more detailed study of

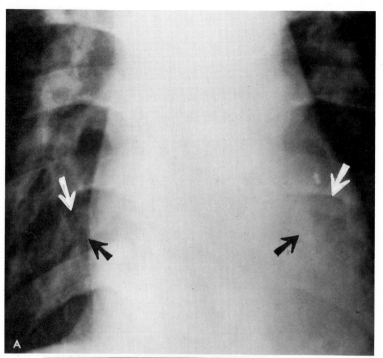

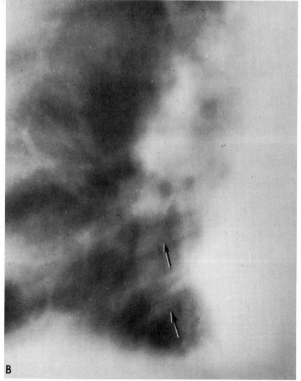

Figure 5–14. PULMONARY VEINS

A, The lower lobe veins (arrows) are often recognizable on the normal chest film by their convergence toward the left atrium. *B,* AP laminagram of a patient with bronchogenic carcinoma. The normal right inferior pulmonary veins stand out clearly (arrows).

the visibility of the pulmonary veins and arteries was made by Lodge.[751]

A rather frequent finding on the normal PA roentgenogram is an opacity visible through the heart just to the right of the spine. It is similar in location and appearance but smaller than the enlarged left atrium so commonly seen through the heart in mitral stenosis (Fig. 5–15). I looked for it in 175 normal chest films in which the area was adequately penetrated. In 68 per cent, a double shadow could not be seen. In 27 per cent it was questionably shown; in 5 per cent it was clearly visible (Chap. 15). There has been considerable speculation concerning the anatomic basis of this shadow. From laminagraphic, angiographic, autopsy, and other studies, it is now apparent that this shadow represents the confluence of several large right pulmonary veins outlined by pulmonary air just before they enter the pericardium (Figs. 5–16 and 5–17). I have not seen it in the left lung, possibly for the

same reason that the left side of an enlarged left atrium is so seldom visible on the frontal film: it blends with the rest of the heart and does not present an abrupt margin to the central beam.

Even the double shadow on the right seen in mitral stenosis need not always be that of the left atrium itself. The central pulmonary veins are also enlarged in this disease and their confluence may sometimes account for the edge of the abnormal density. This, of course, is not the case when the left atrium is voluminous.

A variation of entry of the left superior pulmonary vein into the left atrium is illustrated in Figure 5–18. The patient shown in A had mild dysphagia, and I considered the anterior esophageal defect to be an intramural extramucosal tumor. I felt a bit silly in the operating room when shown what appeared to be a normal pulmonary vein accounting for the defect. As I thought about it later, I realized that a normally located left

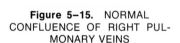

Figure 5–15. NORMAL CONFLUENCE OF RIGHT PULMONARY VEINS

The density seen through the right heart shadow (arrow) resembles an enlarged left atrium, but the barium filled esophagus (inset) shows no indentation or displacement.

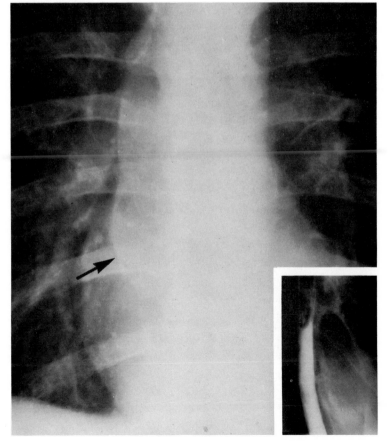

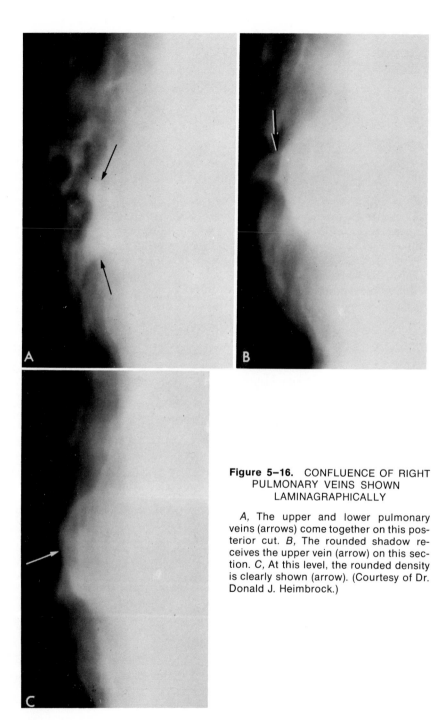

Figure 5–16. CONFLUENCE OF RIGHT PULMONARY VEINS SHOWN LAMINAGRAPHICALLY

A, The upper and lower pulmonary veins (arrows) come together on this posterior cut. *B,* The rounded shadow receives the upper vein (arrow) on this section. *C,* At this level, the rounded density is clearly shown (arrow). (Courtesy of Dr. Donald J. Heimbrock.)

upper pulmonary vein should not lie in front of the esophagus; it must have entered the back rather than the side of the left atrium in this patient. Years later, I saw this particular variant on a pulmonary angiogram in another patient (Fig. 5–18B) and was able to predict the indentation on the front of the esophagus shown in Figure 5–18C.[594, 864]

THE PULMONARY ARTERIES

The intrapulmonary arteries supply the segments of the lung in a manner similar to the bronchi insofar as the prevailing patterns are concerned, but variations are frequent.[112] Rarely, the right pulmonary artery branching mirror-images the left, i.e., it is epibronchial. Its normal comma shape is lacking and it lies at the same level as the left. There is a uni- or bilobed right lung with no middle lobe[993] (Fig. 3–12). Associated anomalies include polysplenia, symmetrical liver, atrioventricular communis defect, and abnormal inferior vena cava pattern. The converse of this, bilateral hypobronchial pulmonary arteries with three lobes of each lung, also shows a consistent syndrome pattern: asplenia, symmetrical liver, right-sided stomach, pulmonary stenosis or atresia, transposition of great vessels, atrioventricular communis defect, and total anomalous pulmonary venous return.[690a] Another variation is that of a RUL artery dividing into an apical posterior and an anterior division.

The pulmonary arteries have distinctly more branches than their venous counterparts and follow the bronchi more closely. The sum of the diameters of the branches is always greater than the diameter of the parent artery.[1319]

Congenital Anomalies of the Pulmonary Vessels

ARTERIAL ANOMALIES

There are a variety of congenital anomalies of the pulmonary arteries. *Absence of the right pulmonary artery* (Fig. 5–6) is generally not associated with a congenital heart anomaly; *absence of the left* is nearly always associated with tetralogy of Fallot.[456, 1110] However, I have seen several exceptions to this rule (Fig. 5–40). Congenital hypoplasia of a pulmonary artery may be difficult to distinguish from acquired unilateral pulmonary oligemia, as in pulmonary embolism.

Pulmonary artery coarctation may be central, peripheral, or both. The peripheral form is usually multiple and involves a number of the larger pulmonary artery branches. Complete occlusion of the affected vessels may occur, but more often there is a weblike constriction with poststenotic dilatation. The central form, which involves the undivided pulmonary artery and its right and left main divisions, usually shows a longer segment of narrowing.

At times, the poststenotic dilatation can be recognized by its nodularity along the course of the affected vessels or as lumpiness in the hilum itself (Fig. 5–19). However, more often than not, the lesion is picked up incidentally at angiography performed because congenital heart disease is suspected. The patient may actually have a ventricular septal defect or supravalvular aortic stenosis as a concomitant of the lesion; but sometimes the unusual murmurs caused by the arterial constriction falsely suggest a cardiac lesion.

Pulmonary coarctation is also encountered in the rubella syndrome and in idiopathic hypercalcemia.[296, 314, 399] The possibility has been raised that these constrictions represent organized pulmonary emboli, acquired in utero or postnatally. Certainly emboli can produce tags and webs in the tiny peripheral pulmonary branches,[909] so why not centrally?

The term *pulmonary sling* has been applied to aberrant origin of the left pulmonary artery from the main pulmonary trunk. Or you might say that the left pulmonary artery arises from the right, which is the same thing. The pulmonary bifurcation occurs to the right of the trachea near the carina. At this point, the left pulmonary artery arises, passes over the right main stem bronchus, and courses between the trachea and the esophagus to reach the left hilum. In so doing, it compresses the right bronchus (rarely the left), sometimes causing obstructive emphysema or collapse of the right lung. The right side of the trachea is indented in the frontal projection, but the anomaly is more readily recognized on the lateral view by the rounded density of the

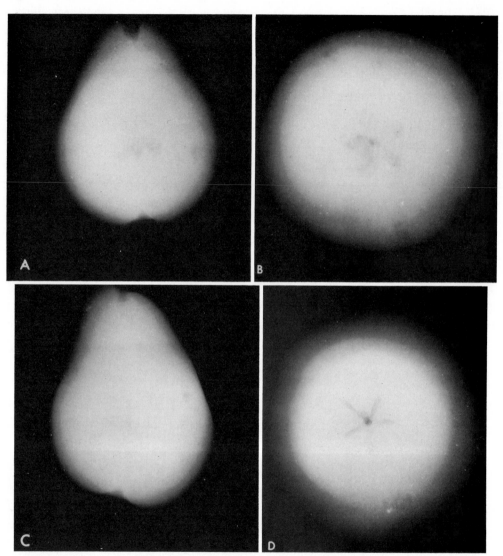

Figure 5–17. EXPLANATION OF THE DOUBLE DENSITY SEEN THROUGH THE HEART

A, Roentgenogram of a pear, side view. *B,* The same pear, end view, slightly enlarged. *C,* Side view of another pear in which the neck has been pinched slightly, creating a shallow ledge. *D,* End-on view of this pear, slightly enlarged. A double shadow is seen, whereas in *B,* because there is no ledge, only one shadow is seen.

(Figure continued on opposite page.)

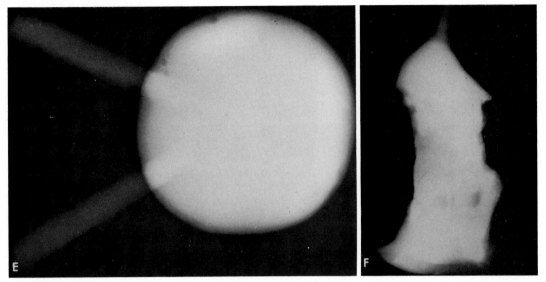

Figure 5–17. *Continued. E,* Two carrots have been stuck into the pear. The carrots, like the pulmonary veins, are visible only before they enter the pear (i.e., the left atrium). *F,* 3 minutes later.

aberrant vessel seen end-on between the esophagus and the trachea (Fig. 5–20). The diagnosis is easily confirmed by angiography.[296, 617]

ARTERIOVENOUS SHUNTS

Anomalous origin of a pulmonary artery from the aorta may occur without pulmonary sequestration[156, 303] (Fig. 4–32). Usually the vessel arises from the descending thoracic aorta, but it may originate from the ascending, transverse, or abdominal aorta, the subclavian, innominate, or celiac artery. Generally the artery has the characteristic elasticity of a normal pulmonary artery rather than the muscular pattern of an aortic branch. It has been assumed that some of the systemic arterial connections to the developing fetal lung fail to obliterate and this prevents the normal inosculation of the main pulmonary arteries with the primitive pulmonary arterial plexuses.[156, 296]

Pulmonary arteriovenous fistula is a well-known anomaly associated with congenital familial telangiectasia (Rendu-Osler-Weber's disease) in about half the patients. It often presents roentgenographically as an intrapulmonary nodular or sinuous opacity connected to the hilum by one or more enlarged arteries and draining via enlarged pulmonary veins to the left atrium. Fluoroscopically, abnormal pulsations can often be identified, and shrinkage with the Valsalva maneuver is the rule. Multiple lesions are common. The vascular nature of the anomaly is readily demonstrated by laminagraphy and, of course, by angiography (Fig. 5–21). A "micronodular" form has also been described. However, in a recent case of familial telangiectasia, Dr. Robert J. Ritterhoff demonstrated by serial sectioning that these tiny vessels were arterial and perhaps capillary, i.e., telangiectases, and not arteriovenous. The angiogram illustrated in Figure 5–22 seems to confirm this finding in another patient. This fact deserves a special niche in your repository of useless information.

Other intrathoracic extracardiac shunts are less frequent. Communication between an intercostal artery and a pulmonary artery or vein may occur in chest wall arteriovenous malformation and may give rise to rib notching. An acquired systemic-pulmonary arterial shunt may develop following destructive infection of the chest wall, as in the severe granulomatous disease secondary to white blood cell antibody abnormality in children. Appropriate systemic arteriography will demonstrate the pulmonary vascular connections. Some-

(*Text continued on page 213.*)

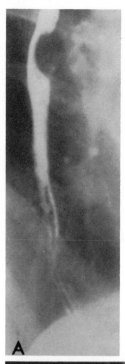

Figure 5–18. PULMONARY VEIN VARIATION

A, The indentation on the front of the esophagus was found at operation to be caused by a left pulmonary vein. *B*, A different patient. Pulmonary angiogram shows a left superior pulmonary vein entering the superomedial aspect of the left atrium (arrow). *C*, The esophagram shows an anterior indentation (arrow) produced by the pulmonary vein variant shown in *B*.

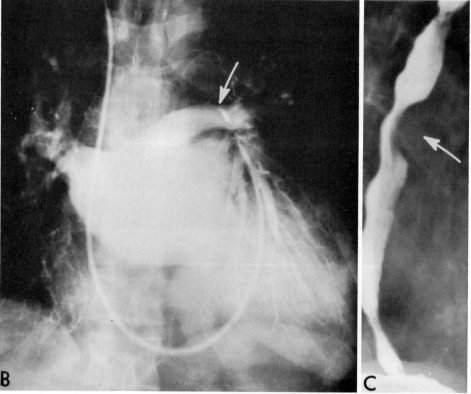

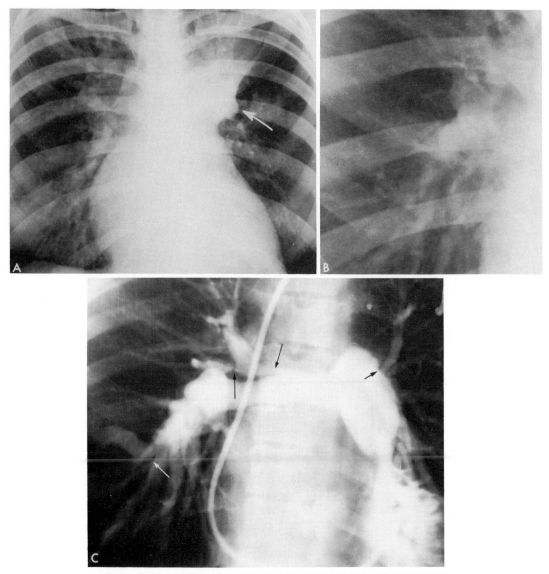

Figure 5–19. TWO CASES OF PULMONARY ARTERY COARCTATION

A, There is a nodularity adjacent to the right hilum. The superior division of the LUL is collapsed as a result of compression of the bronchus by the dilated pulmonary artery (arrow) distal to a constriction. Confirmed at operation. *B,* A lumpy right hilum in another patient. *C,* Pulmonary arteriogram of *B.* The right main pulmonary artery is diffusely constricted. There are multiple peripheral coarctations (arrows) with poststenotic dilatation.

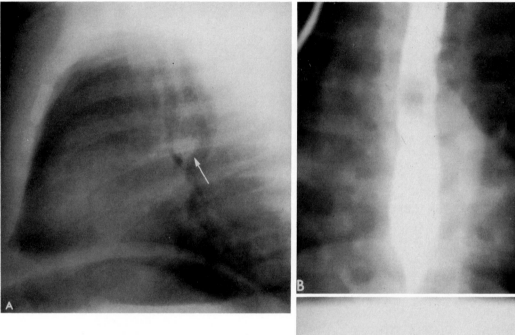

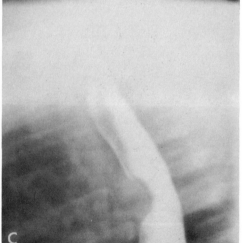

Figure 5–20. PULMONARY ARTERY "SLING"

The frontal view of the chest was normal. *A*, Right lateral view shows a large oval density between the lower trachea and the air filled esophagus (arrow). *B* and *C*, AP and lateral views of the esophagus show an extrinsic defect just above the carina. There were no pulmonary signs or symptoms. At operation, the left pulmonary artery arose to the right of the trachea and passed between the trachea and esophagus to reach the left hilum.

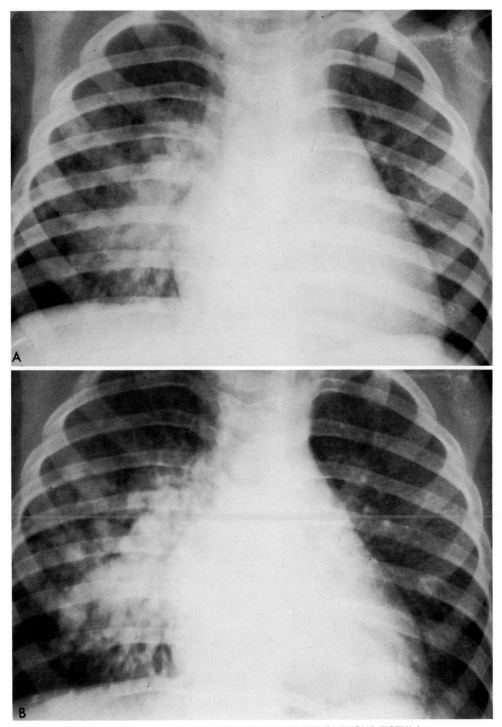

Figure 5–21. CONGENITAL PULMONARY ARTERIOVENOUS FISTULA

Cyanotic infant with a cardiac murmur. *A*, Teleroentgenogram shows a Medusa-head shadow in the right lung. *B*, The pulmonary angiogram demonstrates its vascular nature. RML resection resulted in clinical cure.

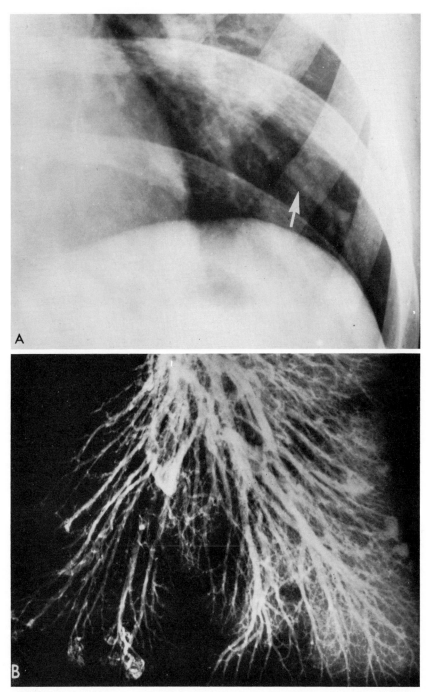

Figure 5–22.   SMALL NODULAR CONGENITAL PULMONARY TELANGIECTASES

    A, Plain films show a large vessel (arrow) terminating in a small nodule at the left base. Several other finely nodu-
lar shadows are present nearby. The patient died of brain abscesses. *B,* Postmortem pulmonary artery injection of
the left lung. Multiple small vascular collections, probably telangiectases, are demonstrated. The patient also had
congenital telangiectases of the skin and other viscera.

times retrograde flow in a major pulmonary artery is seen. In fact, if on a pulmonary arteriogram one of the larger pulmonary arteries fails to fill, consider not only obstruction but also a systemic shunt with reversed flow.

Similar communications may occur through a pleural symphysis or from a surgical procedure, such as a superior vena cava-pulmonary artery anastomosis in congenital heart disease.[195] Communications between the systemic and pulmonary veins may be found in superior vena caval syndrome. Likewise, in hepatic cirrhosis, many minute pulmonary arteriovenous fistulas and even portopulmonary venous shunts may occur, producing fine nodularity in the lungs and resulting in cyanosis.[72, 485, 1024, 1246]

ANOMALOUS PULMONARY VENOUS RETURN AND OTHER ABERRANT VEINS

Anomalous connection of one or more of the large pulmonary veins is a common entity.[361, 426] It may be part of a more complex congenital cardiac condition or represent an isolated lesion. In partial or total anomalous pulmonary venous return, the vessels may drain into one or more of the following structures: the vertical vein (left superior vena cava), coronary sinus, right superior vena cava, right atrium, portal vein (or one of its tributaries), ductus venosus, hepatic vein, or inferior vena cava.

The vertical vein, an anomalous persistence of the left anterior cardinal vein, is an interesting structure. Sometimes it conducts blood toward the heart, sometimes away from it. In some individuals it is merely a normal variant, transporting blood from the left innominate vein to the coronary sinus and thence into the right atrium. In this case, it may represent one of paired superior vena cavas or the *only* superior vena cava. It usually receives the hemiazygos vein. A left superior cava is encountered in about 5 per cent of patients with congenital heart disease and in about 0.5 per cent of normal individuals.[426] Occasionally, the left superior vena cava connects with the left atrium, producing a right to left shunt,[426, 1200, 1310] but once in a while the blood goes the other way.[82]

The vertical vein lies in the same coronal plane as the right superior vena cava and therefore fairly far anteriorly. On the right side, the superior vena cava shadow blends with the ascending aorta, also an anterior structure; but on the left, the aorta lies posteriorly and thus the vertical vein can be seen as a separate shadow,[171, 335] disappearing at the lower border of the clavicle because it enters the neck (Fig. 2–23).

When pulmonary venous blood returns from the lung via the vertical vein, the flow may be "downhill" to the coronary sinus, but more often it is "uphill" to the left innominate vein. If *all* the pulmonary blood takes the latter route, there is prominence of the left upper border of the cardiovascular silhouette (a large vertical vein), and marked enlargement of the right superior vena cava because it is carrying the blood from the lungs as well as that from the upper portion of the body. This accounts for the "figure 8" or "snowman" cardiovascular configuration of total anomalous pulmonary venous return (Fig. 5–23), a contour seldom seen in infancy. With partial anomalous venous return via this route, the snowman has relative microcephaly.

Drainage of anomalous pulmonary veins below the diaphragm is not uncommon. The vessels may coalesce into a single channel, enter the abdomen through the esophageal hiatus, and drain into the portal vein. A few examples of indentation of the anterior surface of the lower end of the esophagus by the anomalous vessel have been reported.

With *total* anomalous pulmonary venous return below the diaphragm, as a result of stenosis at the site of emptying into the systemic vein and perhaps the higher systemic venous pressure there is marked interstitial and alveolar pulmonary edema at birth. This results in pronounced Kerley's lines and a mottled appearance of the lungs. The heart is often normal in size. The rare total pulmonary drainage into a partially obstructed vertical vein will produce identical changes (Fig. 5–24).

Partial anomalous venous return below the diaphragm is much more common on the right, with drainage of the right inferior pulmonary vein into the abdomen, often through the diaphragm itself. This has already been discussed under the heading of scimitar syndrome (p. 87).

Anomalous entry of a pulmonary vein into

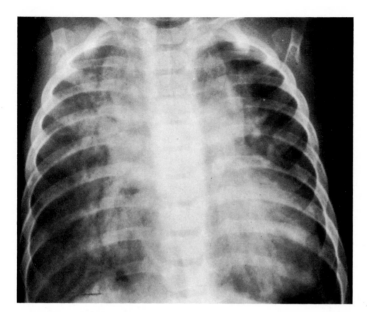

Figure 5–23. TOTAL ANOMALOUS PULMONARY VENOUS RETURN WITH "SNOWMAN" HEART

The left upper prominence is formed by the vertical vein, the right by the distended superior vena cava.

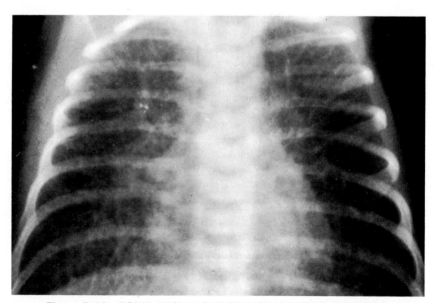

Figure 5–24. TOTAL ANOMALOUS PULMONARY VENOUS RETURN

In this infant, the veins drained into a constricted vertical vein. Note the marked interstitial and alveolar pulmonary edema and normal sized heart. An identical roentgen appearance is seen with total anomalous pulmonary venous return below the diaphragm.

the right superior vena cava or right atrium, often associated with atrial septal defect, can occasionally be suspected by noting that a pulmonary vessel in the right upper lung takes an unusual course.

Total anomalous venous return may occur in an individual via several of the routes previously described. Laminagrams are useful in delineating and studying all these anomalous vessels but, of course, pulmonary angiography is more definitive.

Pulmonary Hypertension

Here is a classification of pulmonary hypertension offered by the late Paul Wood, one of the world's great cardiologists:[1322]

1. Hyperkinetic, due to increased pulmonary blood flow
   Example: left to right shunt
2. Vaso-occlusive, due to closing of the vascular pathways, however caused
   a. obstructive — by conditions outside or within the vessels
      Example: multiple embolism
   b. obliterative — by strictural disease of the vessels themselves
      Example: cor pulmonale from emphysema
   c. vasoconstrictive — by functional contraction of the muscular arteries
      Example: acute asthma
3. Passive, due to high pulmonary venous pressure
   Example: mitral stenosis

INCREASED PULMONARY FLOW AND HYPERKINETIC HYPERTENSION

With increased pulmonary flow resulting from congenital heart conditions associated with left to right shunts, the intrapulmonary arteries are usually visibly enlarged (Fig. 5–25), whether or not hyperkinetic hypertension is associated. So are the pulmonary veins, of course, since they must drain away the increased flow. In the lateral view, the hila appear enlarged, with tentacles of enlarged arteries and veins emanating from them.

Certain ancillary signs of arterial overcirculation may also be present. The configuration of the heart, particularly prominence of the pulmonary artery segment and enlargement of the hila, is helpful. Of even greater importance is the fluoroscopic demonstration of exaggerated pulmonary artery

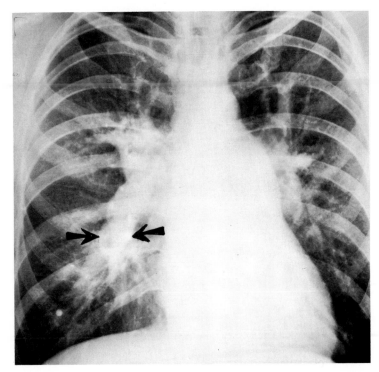

Figure 5–25. GROSS ENLARGEMENT OF INTRAPULMONARY ARTERIES IN LEFT TO RIGHT SHUNT

There is convergence of the enormous pulmonary artery branches toward the hila. The peripheral vessels are also prominent. The right inferior pulmonary artery (arrows) showed striking intrinsic pulsation. Proved atrial septal defect.

pulsation. Image amplification and cine are not essential for a satisfactory examination of these pulsations but certainly facilitate the study.[429]

The term *hilar dance* is a misnomer for this sign. Don't look for it in the hilum and don't expect a jig. Many congenital and acquired cardiac conditions without increased pulmonary flow may cause prominent hilar pulsation, including even isolated pulmonary stenosis.[428] However, if one looks more peripherally, particularly along the right inferior pulmonary artery (arrows in Fig. 5–25), pulsation takes on a more specific connotation.[157, 427] Intrinsic pulsation here can be recognized by the simultaneous outward thrust of the two sides of the vessel or by the pulsatile movement of the medial border of this vessel in a direction opposite to that of the adjacent right heart border (this excludes pulsation transmitted from the heart). Other intrapulmonary arteries may also show this type of expansile pulsation or, if viewed end-on, may be seen to increase in diameter with each cardiac systole, but I find it easier to interpret in the right lower artery.

This form of abnormal pulsation of the pulmonary artery branches, in my experience, is encountered in a limited number of cardiac conditions, mostly congenital. These include atrial septal defect, in which the finding is remarkably constant; many but not all cases of ventricular septal defect, total anomalous pulmonary venous return, most cases of transposition of the great vessels, some cases of truncus arteriosus, coronary arteriovenous fistula and anomalous coronary artery, and intracardiac rupture of congenital sinus of Valsalva aneurysm. I have personally observed examples of each of these. Surprisingly, these exaggerated pulsations are not seen in patent ductus arteriosus, probably because the increased pulmonary flow is relatively constant throughout the cardiac cycle.

Development of pulmonary hypertension does not seem to cause the disappearance of the abnormal pulsations. In two of three cases of atrial septal defect that did not show abnormal pulsation, cardiac catheterization revealed a concomitant pulmonary stenosis.

Increased pulmonary flow can also occur as an acquired condition. High output states such as exercise, pregnancy, anemia, fever, and hyperthyroidism may exaggerate the flow. However, roentgen changes, including intrinsic pulsation, are generally absent or so mild that they can be recognized only when earlier or subsequent normal studies of the same patient are available.[1130]

Leakage of an aortic aneurysm into the pulmonary artery will produce tremendous pulmonary flow and intrinsic pulsation. I saw one once and the whole fluoroscopic room pulsated. I have had the opportunity of examining only one patient with pure pulmonary insufficiency and he showed abnormal pulsation. Not one of the many patients with acquired cor pulmonale whom I've fluoroscoped showed intrinsic pulsation.

INCREASED VASCULAR RESISTANCE AND VASO-OCCLUSIVE HYPERTENSION

Pulmonary arterial hypertension of significant degree is attributable to increase in the pulmonary arterial resistance.[1178] The upper limit of the normal pulmonary artery pressure is approximately 30/15 mm Hg, with a mean pressure up to 20 mm. Pulmonary arterial hypertension generally does not manifest itself radiologically until the pressures reach 50/25. Increase in pulmonary vascular resistance may be caused by diffuse lung disease, such as emphysema, interstitial fibrosis, and various types of hypoventilation syndrome (cor pulmonale); pulmonary arterial disease, such as embolism, arteritis, and arteriolar sclerosis; left ventricular failure and severe mitral stenosis,[238, 384] and certain forms of congenital heart disease associated with increased pulmonary flow, such as septal defect and patent ductus.[633] In some patients the cause of the pulmonary hypertension is not apparent (essential pulmonary hypertension).

Among the patients with congenital left to right shunt, the obstruction at the precapillary level may be so severe that the shunt is reversed (Eisenmenger's physiology). Persistence of the fetal type of small pulmonary artery branches may be the cause of the increased pulmonary vascular resistance in some children with left to right shunt.[354] In these, pulmonary hypertension is present early in life and may not improve when the shunt is surgically corrected.

Roentgenologically, the pulmonary artery

trunk, the right and left main branches, and their larger central subdivisions are frequently dilated, whereas the more peripheral vessels, usually in the outer halves of the lungs, decrease abruptly in caliber[3] (Figs. 5–9 and 5–26). The roentgen appearance is similar in all forms of increased pulmonary resistance, congenital or acquired. Even in diffuse microembolization of the lungs,[908] where you might expect the vessels in the middle third of the lung also to be enlarged, the cor pulmonale pattern is more likely to be found.[781, 870]

I don't believe anyone can quantitate the pulmonary resistance or predict the size of a shunt from the chest film with any useful degree of accuracy.[736, 903, 1032] Many patients with severe pulmonary resistance do not even show peripheral oligemia. In fact, films made before and after the development of pulmonary hypertension may show little or no visible change in the pulmonary circulation. Furthermore, equal diminution in peripheral vascularity may occur with mild and with severe pulmonary hypertension.

In regard to the roentgen signs of pulmonary arterial hypertension, then, the following statements appear valid:

1. A roentgen pattern of normal pulmonary vascularity does not preclude the presence of increased flow.
2. Increased pulmonary arterial vascularity is reliable evidence of increased flow.
3. Increased arterial vascularity extending to the periphery of the lungs does not exclude the presence of high vascular resistance.
4. Pruning of the peripheral pulmonary vessels is reliable evidence of increased vascular resistance, congenital or acquired. However, the *degree* of pruning does not correlate well with the actual level of the pulmonary hypertension.[903]
5. From the pulmonary vascular pattern alone you cannot distinguish between congenital and acquired pulmonary hypertension. However, expansile arterial pulsation is overwhelming evidence of a congenital lesion.
6. One additional point: calcification in the walls of the major pulmonary arteries is reliable evidence of severe (systemic level) and long-standing pulmonary hypertension, congenital or acquired (Fig. 14–12).

PASSIVE (VENOUS) HYPERTENSION

Pulmonary venous (postcapillary) hypertension is a reflection of a rise in left atrial pressure significantly above the normal level of 5 to 10 mm Hg. It occurs acutely in left ventricular failure and chronically in mitral stenosis. Other causes are rare and include left atrial thrombus or tumor, congenital or acquired pulmonary vein obstruction, congenitally hypoplastic left heart, and polycythemia.[727, 825] Transmission of the elevated left atrial pressure into the valveless pulmonary veins takes place. Eventually, the back pressure jams the capillary system, resulting in secondary pulmonary arterial hypertension.

On the roentgenogram, the pulmonary veins may enlarge. This can occur throughout the lungs, but dilatation in the upper pulmonary zones with constriction in the lower is often seen[268, 837, 1124, 1130, 1179] (Fig. 5–27). This is particularly well shown in the lateral projection. The pulmonary arteries follow suit. The flow through the upper zone vessels is much greater and much faster than through the lower zones. This redistribution of flow has been confirmed many times on lung scans and by angiography[459] (Fig. 5–28), but is absent in many patients.[145, 904]

As stated on page 500, I found the upper lobe vessels distinctly larger than the lower in 3 per cent of normal chest films. Yet Lavender et al. had no such examples in 50 normal controls.[705] They encountered upper lobe venous prominence in 80 per cent of 36 patients with mitral stenosis and in 39 per cent of 43 with left ventricular failure.

The explanation for the upper lobe-lower lobe vascular discrepancy is not clear. Gravity seems to play a role, since the vascularity may equalize when the patient is recumbent.[838] 'Tis said that inversion of the mitral stenosis patient may cause prominence of the lower lobe vessels! Has anyone ever radiographed a bat in cardiac failure?

Other roentgen signs of venous pressure elevation consist of convexity of the outer border of the upper right hilum[265, 704] (Fig.

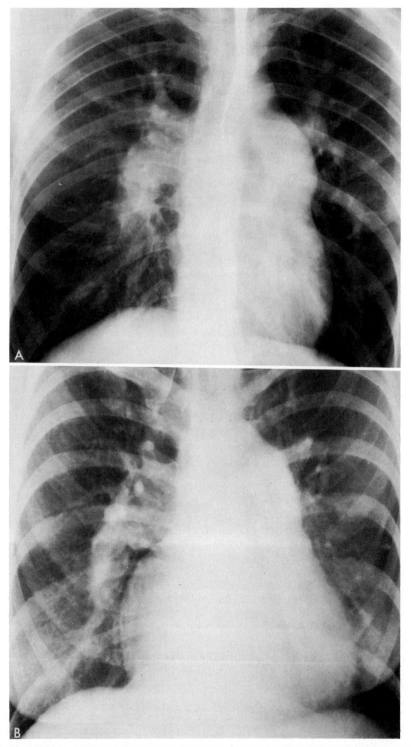

Figure 5–26.   ATRIAL SEPTAL DEFECT WITH INCREASED PULMONARY VASCULAR RESISTANCE

Two different patients. The central arteries are huge. The left pulmonary artery is incorporated in the left middle arc. There is an abrupt decrease in arterial caliber in the midlung; the peripheral branches are constricted. Cyanosis developed in both patients.

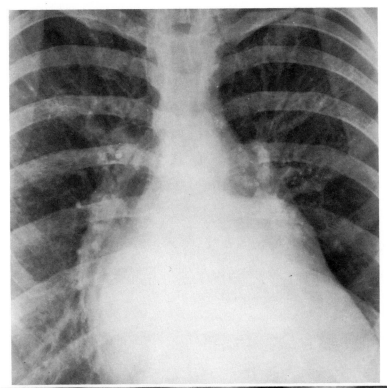

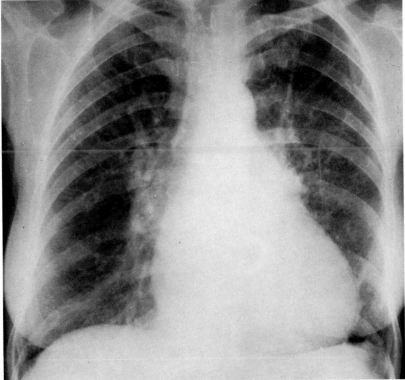

Figure 5–27.   TWO EXAMPLES OF PULMONARY VENOUS HYPERTENSION IN MITRAL STENOSIS

The upper pulmonary veins appear engorged, the lower constricted. The intrapulmonary branches of the pulmonary arteries are relatively small.

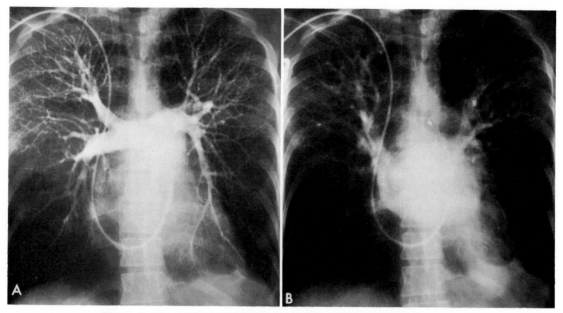

Figure 5–28.   MITRAL STENOSIS WITH PULMONARY HYPERTENSION

A, Pulmonary contrast injection, arterial phase. *B,* Venous phase. Note the distribution of the bulk of the vascular flow through the upper pulmonary vessels. Passive hypertension.

5–29), perihilar clouding or frank pulmonary edema, and Kerley's lines. Signs of pulmonary arterial (precapillary) hypertension may also be present as a result of the transmitted back pressure.[837, 1247]

Measured pulmonary pressure levels are not proportional to the degree of the roentgen changes nor does absence of the signs necessarily signify normal venous pressure.[904, 1129, 1289] As implied earlier, I feel that the accuracy of recognizing and evaluating venous alterations on conventional chest films leaves much to be desired. I know that many experienced observers place considerable reliance on these changes. I do, too, but only when the signs are pretty obvious and more than one are positive. I tested a colleague who claimed he could predict the pressure readings in mitral stenosis. He is now convinced that we don't know how to measure pulmonary venous pressure in Cincinnati. I am forced into the awkward position exemplified by my young son when he declared, "I'm not going to fight with girls anymore. There's no place to hit 'em."

By the way, there is a clear distinction between pulmonary congestion and edema, and the one shouldn't be equated with the other. Congestion is simply venous dilatation, often recognizable as such on the film (Fig. 5–27). Edema may be interstitial, usually apparent as Kerley's lines and occasionally as peribronchial cuffing (Figs. 5–54 and 5–56), and intraalveolar, with its extensive alveolar pattern (Chap. 7). Although they frequently coexist (the edema then usually hides the congestion),[1004] either may occur alone. Witness the pure congestion of polycythemia vera[551, 943, 992, 1045] and the interstitial edema of a drug reaction (Fig. 5–55). Nonetheless, pulmonary congestion seen radiographically is, in general, a reliable sign of impending cardiac failure.

The pulmonary veins also enlarge in congenital or acquired left to right shunts. The veins simply reflect the flow through the lungs—the larger the shunt, the larger the veins.[906]

In infants with septal defect, venous congestion localized to the RUL is occasionally encountered (Fig. 5–30). The mechanism for this distribution is not clear. Indeed, there is some difference in opinion as to whether the roentgen changes actually represent congestion or pneumonia.[248, 670]

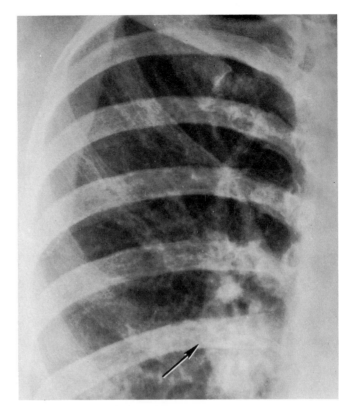

Figure 5–29. PULMONARY   VENOUS
HYPERTENSION IN MITRAL STENOSIS

There is a convex lateral border of the
upper right hilum (arrow) formed by the
dilated superior pulmonary vein.

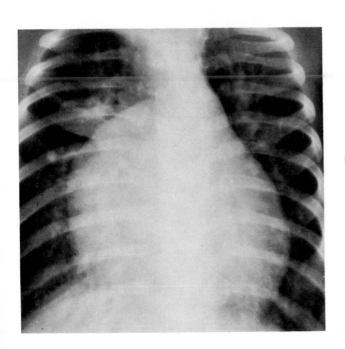

Figure 5–30. RUL VENOUS CONGESTION
AND COLLAPSE IN SEPTAL DEFECT

Mongoloid with septum primum defect.

In mitral stenosis or insufficiency, the left atrial back pressure may occasionally cause severe dilatation of a major pulmonary vein, which can be mistaken for a tumor nodule[138] (Fig. 5–31). The same mechanism may result in a pulmonary varix [463] (Fig. 5–32).

However, pulmonary varix may also be congenital in origin.[479, 493, 873] In some patients the dilated vein pulsates; it shrinks during the Valsalva procedure. Angiography is the only reliable way to differentiate it from pulmonary arteriovenous fistula.

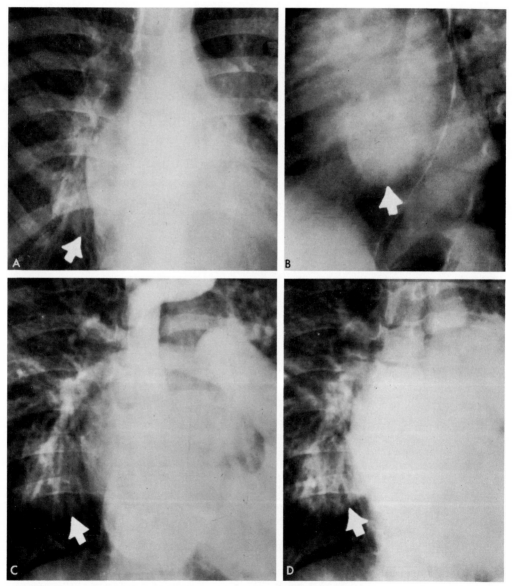

Figure 5–31. MARKED ENLARGEMENT OF A MAJOR PULMONARY VEIN IN MITRAL STENOSIS

A and *B*, Frontal and left anterior oblique views. The intrapulmonary mass (arrow) was first thought to represent a tumor. *C*, Angiocardiogram at 2 seconds. No opacification of the lesion. *D*, Angiocardiogram at 5 seconds shows filling of the dilated vessel with contrast medium during the pulmonary venous phase.

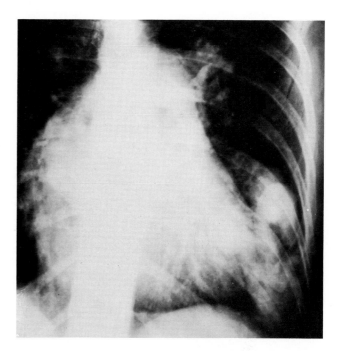

Figure 5-32. PULMONARY VARIX IN MI-
TRAL STENOSIS

The plain film showed a multilobular opacity
in the region of the lingula which pulsated on
fluoroscopy. It had not changed in 4 years.
Angiocardiogram, venous phase, shows the
lingular lesion filled with contrast medium. It
did not opacify during the arterial phase. Autopsy confirmation. (Courtesy of Gottesman,
L., and Weinstein, A.[463]; reproduced with permission of Dis. Chest.)

Pulmonary Oligemia

Pulmonary arterial undercirculation associated with decreased pulmonary flow
occurs frequently in the cyanotic forms of
congenital heart disease, notably in those
with pulmonic stenosis and right to left
shunt (Fig. 5-33). The pulmonary vascularity may appear strikingly diminished and
both lungs abnormally radiolucent. The
pulmonary arc may be concave or convex,
but the hila are generally small. This is
especially apparent in the lateral view. Bilateral oligemia of the lung is also found
with various types of diffuse emphysema,[276,
400] pulmonary thromboembolism,[481] primary
pulmonary hypertension,[1204] and even cardiac tumor[815] (Figs. 5-8 and 5-34).

Unilateral undercirculation is encountered in absence (Fig. 5-6), hypoplasia, or
thromboembolism of the right or left pulmonary artery[374, 481, 1132, 1218] (Fig. 5-35); in pulmonary neoplasm (Fig. 5-36); in unilateral
pulmonary emphysema and obstructive hyperinflation (Fig. 1-4); and in idiopathic
unilateral hyperlucent lung.

The latter condition, also known as
Swyer-James and Macleod syndrome[780, 952,
979] has now been established as an acquired
disease, a sequel of severe unilateral
pneumonia.[224, 232] Evidence points to a peripheral form of obstructive emphysema as
the cause for the radiolucency and diminished vascularity.[221, 792] The classic findings
of unilateral obstructive overinflation, bronchiectasis, and hypovascularity (Fig. 5-37)
securely establish the diagnosis. Collapse of
a lower lobe with compensatory expansion
of the upper lung has been mistaken for this
entity, but bronchography will reveal the
collapsed lobe and show that the expanded
lobe is not bronchiectatic. Simon studied a
resected lobe in unilateral hyperlucent lung
by fixing it and injecting barium into the
bronchial tree. He demonstrated peripheral
obstruction of the terminal bronchioles by
scar formation.[1121]

Unequal vascularity may be seen in the
lungs in tetralogy of Fallot and in left to
right shunts, the left lung often being the
less vascular.[1294, 1308] This undervascularity
is simulated by the relative hyperlucency
seen with congenital or surgical absence of
the pectoral muscles,[1166, 1255] scoliosis or
poor positioning, pleural disease on the
contralateral side, and in certain normal individuals. In a review of about 500 well-
positioned PA teleroentgenograms, I found
both lungs equally radiolucent in 72 per
cent, one lung locally darker than the other
to a slight degree in 25 per cent, and distinctly so in 0.5 per cent, one lung slightly

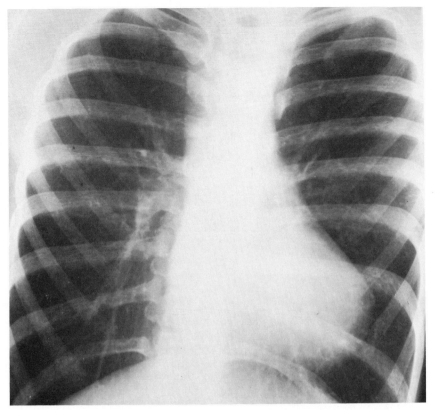

Figure 5–33. SMALL HILA AND SEVERE PULMONARY OLIGEMIA IN TETRALOGY OF FALLOT

There is a right aortic arch. Some of the juxtahilar vessels are bronchial arteries.

but diffusely more radiolucent than the other in 1.2 per cent, and distinctly blacker in 0.8 per cent. No explanation for these "normal" differences in the opacity of the two lungs was apparent.

Westermark noted localized oligemia in pulmonary embolism without infarction.[1279] The sign is not infrequent but is difficult to elicit unless comparison can be made with earlier or later roentgenograms[501, 630, 631, 647, 661] (Fig. 5–38). It is sometimes accompanied by a plump hilar shadow, representing the thrombus itself or cor pulmonale secondary to the embolization.[375, 501, 647] The pulmonary scan and obviously the angiogram are more reliable methods of showing oligemia. The angiogram also demonstrates other signs of embolism: defect in the arterial lumen, abrupt termination of the vessels, pruning of side branches, prolonged arterial perfusion, and diminished capillary flow.

Localized oligemia also occurs with pulmonary artery obliteration by tumor, primary or metastatic (Fig. 5–39).

Roentgen evaluation of the status of pulmonary blood flow is not always reliable.[736] I was one of three "guinea pigs" subjected to the "acid test" by Arnois, Silverman, and Turner.[15] A number of children's chest films, covered with black paper except for the peripheral two thirds of the right lung, were shown to each of us and we were instructed to record whether the arterial circulation was increased, normal, or decreased. The tests were repeated on three separate occasions, except that the third time we were allowed to view the entire film. No significant difference among readers or readings was noted. All performed well with the cases of pulmonary overcirculation, but our accuracy was poor in distinguishing undervascularity from the normal.

(*Text continued on page 230.*)

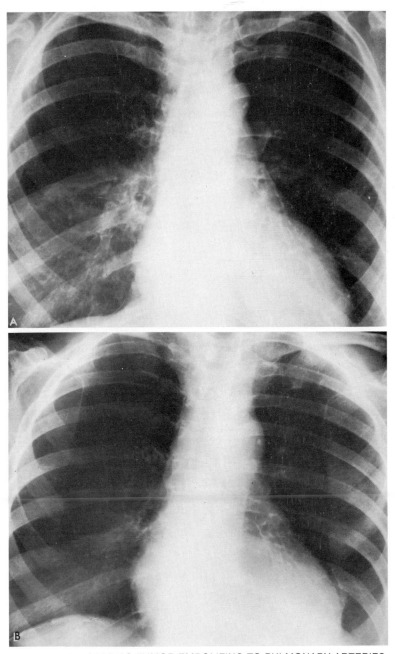

Figure 5–34. CARDIAC TUMOR EMBOLIZING TO PULMONARY ARTERIES

A, The left lung and upper half of the right are severely oligemic. *B,* 3 months later. The right lower lung is now also affected. Polypoid hemangioendothelioma of right atrium with tumor emboli to lung. The larger bronchi show incidental mural calcification.

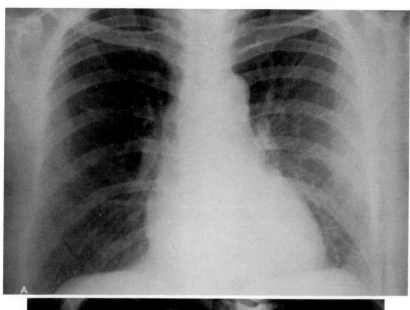

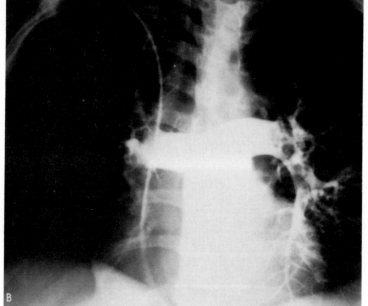

Figure 5–35. PULMONARY ARTERY EMBOLISM

A, The right lung is oligemic. *B,* Angiogram. The right pulmonary artery is almost totally occluded by clots. The left shows many nonocclusive emboli.

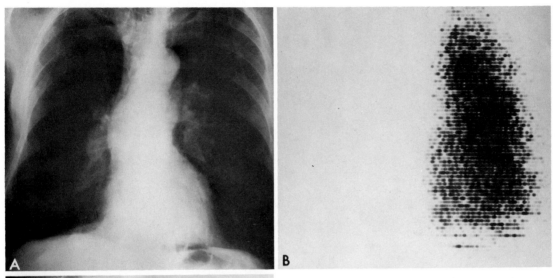

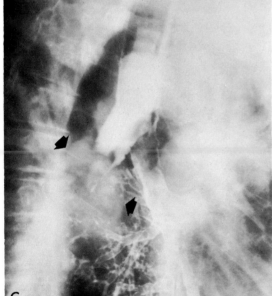

Figure 5–36. BRONCHOGENIC CARCINOMA
COMPRESSING RIGHT PULMONARY ARTERY

A, PA film. The right lung is oligemic. (The left is
overpenetrated!) There were roentgen signs of obstructive hyperinflation on the right. *B*, Lung scan
shows complete absence of flow to the right lung. *C*,
Bronchogram in right oblique projection. The right
main bronchus is occluded by a moderate sized mass
(arrows). (Courtesy of Dr. Kenneth Woodman.)

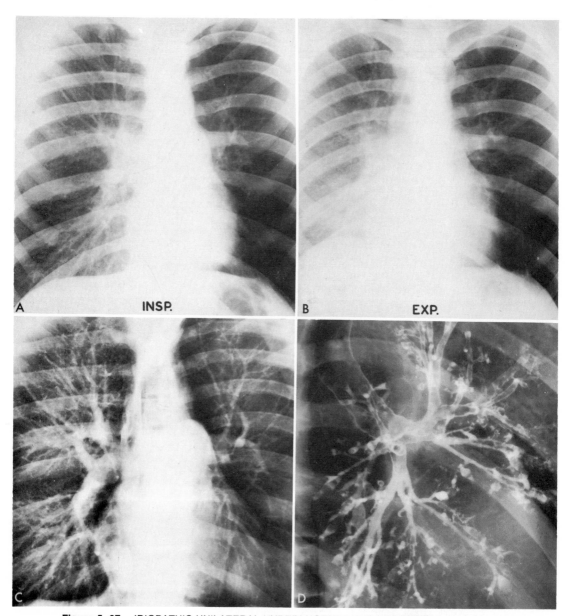

A   INSP.   B   EXP.

C   D

Figure 5–37.   IDIOPATHIC UNILATERAL HYPERLUCENT LUNG WITH SMALL LEFT HILUM

A and *B,* Inspiration and expiration films. The hyperlucency of the left lung persists on expiration. The heart shifts toward the left on inspiration and the left hemidiaphragm shows poor excursion. These are the signs of obstructive emphysema. *C,* The pulmonary angiogram shows marked decrease in size of the left main pulmonary artery and its branches, with compensatory increased flow on the right. *D,* The left bronchogram shows a peculiar form of diffuse bronchiectasis with absence of "alveolar" filling. This suggests a peripheral form of obstructive emphysema. The right bronchogram was normal. (From Margolin, H. N., Rosenberg, L. S., Felson, B., and Baum, G.[792]; reproduced with permission of Charles C Thomas, Publ.)

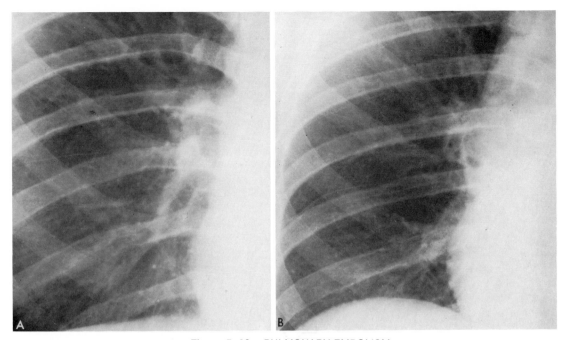

Figure 5–38. PULMONARY EMBOLISM

A, Before embolic episode. *B*, After embolism. The hilar shadow appears amputated distally and there is a central zone of avascularity lateral to it. Proved at autopsy.

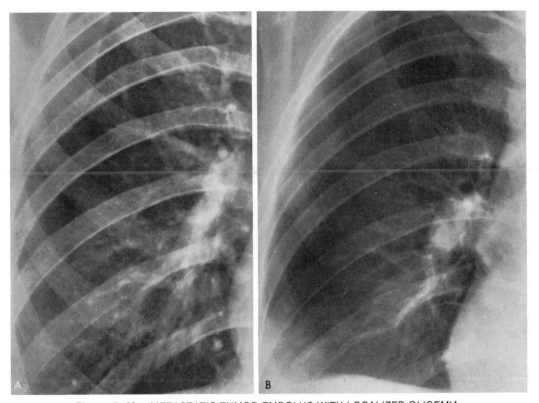

Figure 5–39. METASTATIC TUMOR EMBOLUS WITH LOCALIZED OLIGEMIA

A, Normal chest. *B*, 4 years later. There is marked diminution in the arterial vascularity of the right lung and the hilum appears amputated. An infarct is seen in the right costophrenic angle. Metastasis from the pelvis to the heart with occlusion of the right main pulmonary artery and basal infarct were found at autopsy.

It was concluded that in children with congenital heart disease it is much easier to recognize increased than decreased pulmonary flow.

THE BRONCHIAL CIRCULATION

The bronchial arteries, which constitute a low volume-high pressure vascular system that nourishes the airways, usually originate from the descending aorta at the level of the fifth or sixth vertebral body (Fig. 5–40). Occasionally they arise from the internal mammary or brachiocephalic arteries instead. They vary greatly, not only in origin but also in number and distribution.[113] Most often there are two branches to the left lung and one to the right, but this occurs in only about 40 per cent of individuals.[170] They often arise from a common trunk with an upper intercostal artery.

They have many juxtahilar branchings which intercommunicate with branches of the subclavian, internal mammary, and mediastinal arteries. Corrosion studies reveal that the bronchial arteries, two per bron-

chus, follow the bronchi distally at least as far as the respiratory bronchioles, extending to about 1 cm from the periphery of the lung. The normal bronchial arteries anastomose with the pulmonary arteries along the distal bronchial tree.[216, 953]

The bronchial veins form as minute plexuses in the bronchiolar walls and intercommunicate freely with the pulmonary veins. They empty through mediastinal venous plexuses into the azygos system.[1246] However, much of the bronchial arterial capillary flow is drained by the pulmonary veins. The bronchial veins do not normally fill at bronchial arteriography but are sometimes visible in fibrotic pulmonary conditions.[216]

The bronchial arteries are not visible in the normal state on the plain roentgenogram. Dilatation often occurs in the form of collateral channels to the lungs when pulmonary arterial flow is greatly reduced,[1155] as in tetralogy of Fallot and truncus arteriosus with severe pulmonary stenosis or atresia.[742] The bronchial artery branches may then be seen on the plain PA and lateral films as multiple small nodular opacities in the hila or short tortuous linear shad-

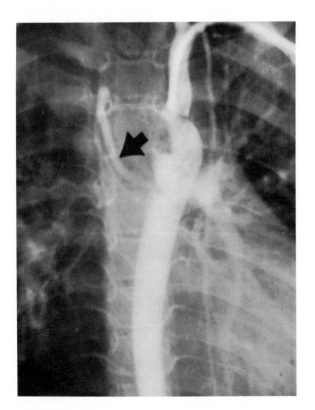

Figure 5–40. RIGHT BRONCHIAL ARTERY ON AORTOGRAM

Countercurrent left subclavian artery injection. Tetralogy of Fallot and patent ductus with absent right pulmonary artery. The left pulmonary artery fills via the ductus. The enlarged right bronchial artery (arrow) arises from the upper descending aorta, passes superiorly to the clavicular level, then inferiorly to the right hilum, where its branches enter the right lung. The intercostal arteries are prominent bilaterally. Compare the pulmonary arteries on the left with the bronchial arteries on the right.

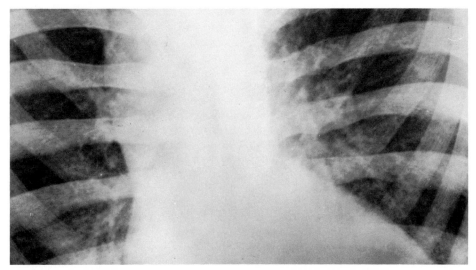

Figure 5–41. BRONCHIAL ARTERIES IN PSEUDOTRUNCUS

The delicate linear and nodular (end-on) vessels in the hila and lungs indicate bronchial arterial collaterals. The larger vessels have no hilar connections. A right aortic arch is present.

ows within the proximal lung fields[752] (Figs. 5–33 and 5–41). Sometimes a large bronchial artery will notch the posterior wall of the esophagus.

However, the enlargement that occurs secondary to lung disease—emphysema, inflammatory lesions, bronchiectasis, embolism, or carcinoma—requires bronchial arteriography for demonstration. For a time, it was hoped that this procedure would provide a reliable method for the diagnosis of bronchogenic carcinoma (Fig. 5–42), since the blood supply of this tumor generally comes from the bronchial circulation.[1245] But other pulmonary lesions alter the bronchial arteries to a similar degree[774] and carcinoma itself does not always do it, so bronchial arteriography is no longer used for this purpose.

The status of the pulmonary artery circulation clearly affects the bronchial circulation. In pulmonary hypertension, the bronchial arteries often become moderately enlarged and tortuous. They may be quite dilated distal to a pulmonary artery embolus. Communication, direct or via capillaries, may take place with the pulmonary veins in pulmonary suppuration and with the pulmonary arteries in chronic inflammation,[99] bronchiectasis, and destructive granulomas.[1246]

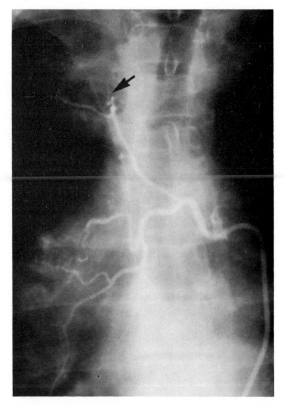

Figure 5–42. SELECTIVE RIGHT BRONCHIAL ARTERIOGRAM IN BRONCHOGENIC CARCINOMA

A small collection of tumor vessels is seen in the right apex (arrow).

Other systemic vessels may penetrate the lung.[1246] The artery to sequestered lung falls into this category. Intercostal artery flow to the lung may reach such proportions in congenital pulmonary stenosis or atresia as to notch the ribs (Fig. 5–6). As stated earlier, in destructive granuloma of the chest wall, the subclavian and intercostal arterial flow may shunt into a pulmonary artery, reversing its flow.[239]

THE AZYGOS SYSTEM

The azygos circulation is an important though often overlooked source of informa-

tion on the chest roentgenogram. Derived from the cardinal system, it forms a deep group of veins that interconnect the important venous structures of the body (Fig. 5–43). It is all but invisible in the normal plain roentgenogram, but typical in configuration and behavior when enlarged.

The only part of the azygos system seen in the healthy chest is the arch of the azygos vein, which extends forward from the spine to its entry in the superior vena cava. Its end-on projection is seen on the frontal film as a round or oval shadow in the crotch between the takeoff of the RUL bronchus and the right tracheal border, where it creates a miniature silhouette sign along the tracheal wall. It is invariably present in the recum-

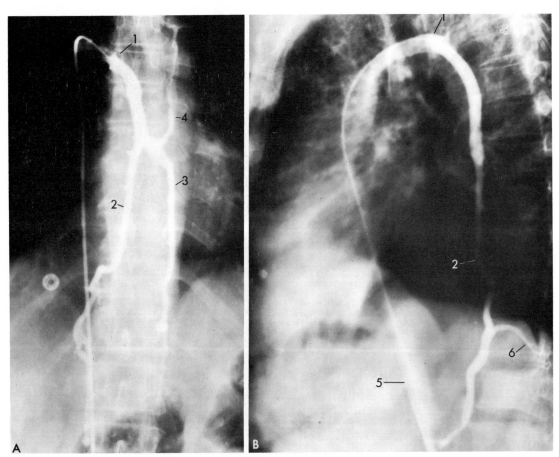

Figure 5–43.   AZYGOGRAPHY VIA THE FEMORAL VEIN

The catheter traverses the inferior cava, right atrium, and superior cava to enter the azygos orifice. *A,* AP view. *B,* Lateral view. *(1)* azygos arch, *(2)* azygos vein, *(3)* hemiazygos vein, *(4)* accessory hemiazygos, *(5)* reflux into inferior cava via a collateral from the lower azygos vein, *(6)* vertebral vein. (Courtesy of Dr. Owen L. Brown.)

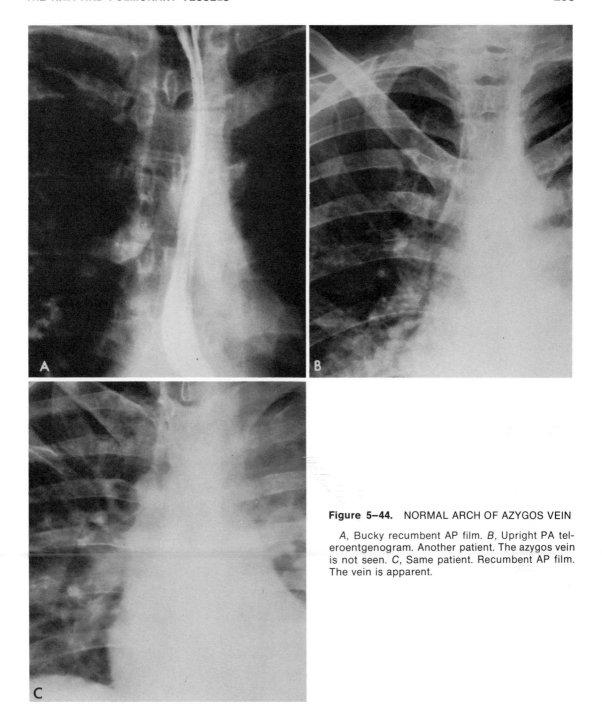

Figure 5–44.   NORMAL ARCH OF AZYGOS VEIN

A, Bucky recumbent AP film. *B*, Upright PA teleroentgenogram. Another patient. The azygos vein
is not seen. *C*, Same patient. Recumbent AP film.
The vein is apparent.

bent position, beautifully depicted on
Bucky films (Fig. 5–44A) and tomograms. It
is said to measure up to 17 mm in diameter
on inspiratory tomograms.[706] However, it is
frequently invisible on the erect film (Fig.
5–44B, C).

I looked for the azygos vein shadow in

1000 normal upright PA teleroentgenograms. In 60 per cent the angle did not show
well, so no conclusions could be drawn. Of
the remaining 400 chests in which the right
lower border of the trachea was visible, 76
per cent did not show an azygos vein at all.
In 15 per cent there was slight thickening of

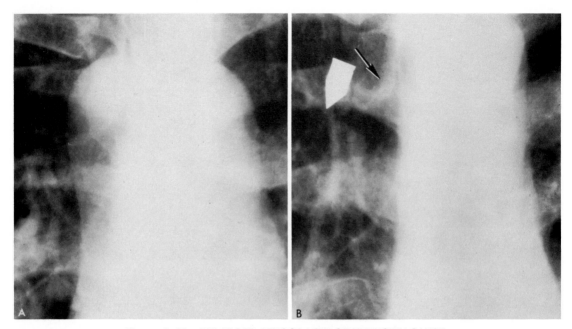

Figure 5–45.   ENLARGED AZYGOS VEIN OF UNKNOWN CAUSE

A, Supine view. The right border of the trachea is obliterated by the greatly enlarged azygos vein. *B,* Upright spot film a few moments later, during Valsalva maneuver (indicated by metal marker). All that remains of the huge azygos vein is a slight thickening along the right side of the trachea (arrow).

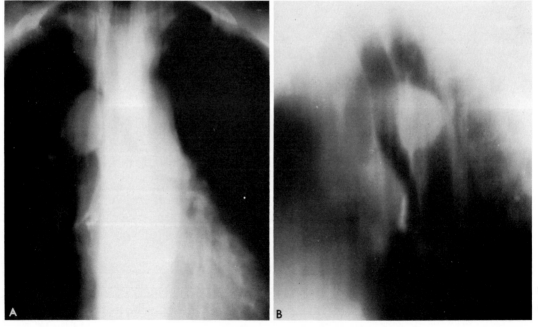

Figure 5–46.   TOMOGRAMS OF AN ENLARGED AZYGOS VEIN

A, AP view. *B,* Lateral view. The azygos vein bridges the space between the vertebral column and the superior vena cava just below the aortic arch. Suspected inferior cava obstruction.

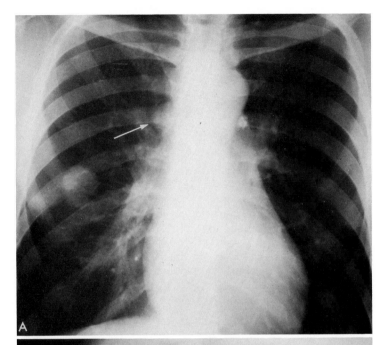

Figure 5–47. METASTASES TO THE AZYGOS LYMPH NODE

A, Bronchogenic carcinoma in the RML. Note the small rounded nodule at the site of the azygos arch (arrow). *B,* Lateral view. The lower arrow points to the pulmonary lesion. The upper arrows point to the azygos node. Compare with Figure 5–46*B.* The node lies in front of the trachea, the vein behind the trachea.

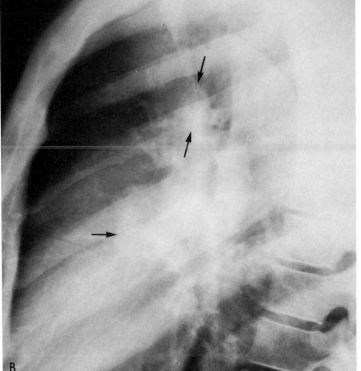

the angle; in 8 per cent a round or oval shadow was visible, but it never measured more than 1 cm in diameter. A second series of about 500 chest films gave almost identical results. Keats et al. found it in 56 per cent of teleroentgenograms and noted that it was larger during pregnancy.[634] Wishart found it in 65 per cent of all children, 19 per cent in infants up to 6 months and 80 per cent in children 8 to 14 years.[1312] With right aortic arch, the azygos prominence often can be seen to the right of the knob.[365] The presence of an azygos lobe adds some interesting variations (p. 74).[264] The right paraesophageal line deviates to the right over the azygos vein at the level of the right main bronchus (Fig. 11–25).

The normal or abnormal azygos vein always shrinks dramatically when the patient assumes the upright position, takes a deep inspiration, or performs the Valsalva maneuver. The shadow appears oval or round, depending on the angle of projection of the venous arch. It may be distorted, displaced, or obliterated by pulmonary collapse, consolidation, or pneumothorax.

The enlarged azygos arch may reach considerable size,[785, 1181] but the effects of position and respiratory maneuvers are still striking (Fig. 5–45). The enlarged vessel may be visible in oblique and lateral projections as a rounded density or as an arcuate shadow just below and parallel to the aortic arch, extending from the spine to the superior cava (Fig. 5–46). Azygography by rib injection or by catheterization via the inferior cava, right atrium, and superior cava (Fig. 5–43) is advocated as a method of deciphering abnormal azygos flow.[1159, 1217, 1299] I believe these methods are seldom indicated, since conventional films and fluoroscopy, supplemented by simple femoral or brachial vein contrast injection for patients with caval obstruction, will provide the required information. For example, lymph node enlargement in the azygos region (Fig. 5–47) is readily distinguished by its failure to shrink with the Valsalva maneuver.

Table 5–2 lists the causes of azygos vein enlargement. Figure 5–48 is an example of rheumatic heart disease in which the azygos vein dilated during a bout of failure, and Figure 5–49 illustrates a traumatic false aneurysm of the azygos vein. In congestive failure and pericardial disease, the dilated

TABLE 5–2. *Causes of Azygos Vein Enlargement*

Common
  Portal hypertension (Fig. 5–50)
  Congestive failure (Fig. 5–48)
  Occlusion of superior vena cava (Figs. 5–51 and 5–52)
  Absence or occlusion of inferior vena cava (Fig. 2–25)
  Pregnancy[634]
  Idiopathic (Fig. 5–45)

Rare
  Constrictive pericarditis
  Pericardial effusion
  Traumatic aneurysm of azygos vein (Fig. 5–49)
  A–V fistula

superior vena cava[172] often obscures or obliterates the shadow of the enlarged vein.

Since the valves of the azygos vein are seldom competent,[1217] most of the conditions enumerated in Table 5–2 enlarge not only the arch but the rest of the azygos system as well, though this is seldom evident on plain films. However, in superior vena cava obstruction, an enlarged collateral, a branch of the accessory hemiazygos, is sometimes seen as a rounded shadow obliterating a short segment of the aortic knob[63, 1173] (Fig. 5–52). However, Hanke recorded it in 7 per cent of 7500 chest films in a tuberculosis hospital and considered it a normal finding (Fig. 5–52C).[502] In portal hypertension (Fig. 5–50), superior caval obstruction (Fig. 5–52), and congenital absence of the inferior vena cava[9, 264, 901] (Fig. 2–24), the greatly enlarged azygos and hemiazygos veins may be visible in the lower mediastinum through the heart shadow.*[1148] Absence of the shadow of the inferior vena cava at the posterior border of the heart on the lateral chest film is said to be a reliable sign of azygos continuation of the cava.[530]

In chronic superior vena cava obstruction, the esophageal veins, connecting the azygos with the systemic and portal venous systems, often enlarge, commonly producing "downhill" varices[347] (Fig. 5–51). Interest-

(*Text continued on page 241.*)

---

*A curious combination of anomalies, including congenital heart disease, is seen in some patients with absence of the hepatic portion of the inferior cava. If the stomach bubble is on the right, polysplenia is nearly always present (Fig. 3–19).

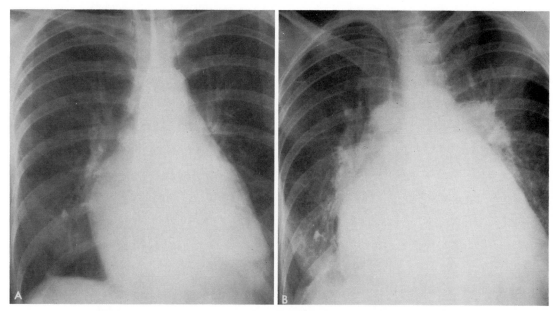

Figure 5–48. AZYGOS VEIN ENLARGEMENT IN CONGESTIVE FAILURE

A, Compensated rheumatic heart disease. *B*, 1 year later. The patient is now in cardiac failure. Both films are upright teleroentgenograms.

Figure 5–49. TRAUMATIC ANEURYSM OF THE AZYGOS VEIN

The patient had injured his chest 2 weeks earlier. Operation disclosed a tear in the azygos vein with a false aneurysm. (Courtesy of Dr. Ross O. Hill.)

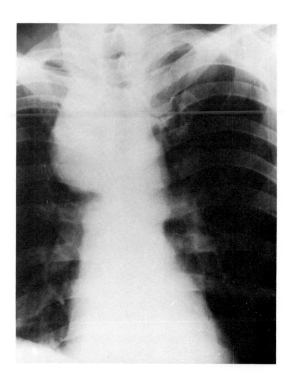

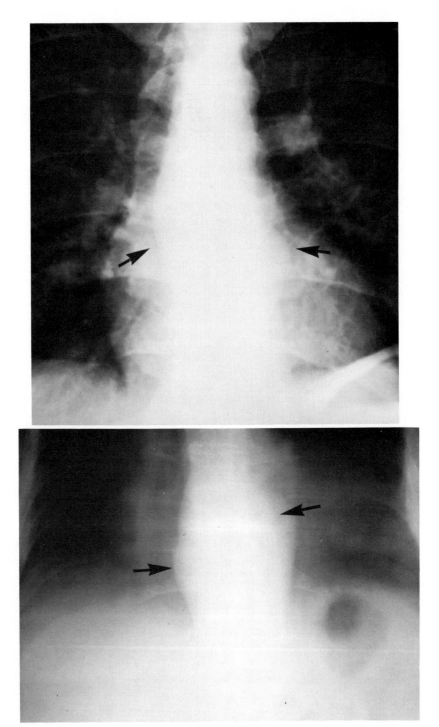

Figure 5–50. ENLARGED AZYGOS AND HEMIAZYGOS VEINS IN PORTAL HYPERTENSION

Two different patients. Note the wavy margin of both the right and left vertical juxtaspinal shadows (arrows), a characteristic finding.

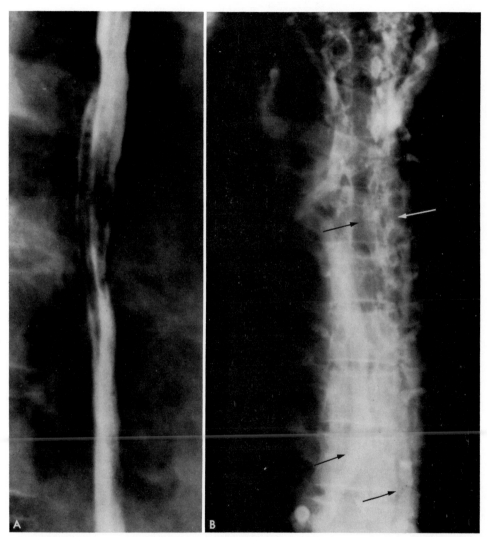

Figure 5–51. "DOWNHILL" VARICES IN SUPERIOR VENA CAVAL OBSTRUCTION

A, The varices are confined to the upper half of the esophagus. *B,* Bilateral brachial venography shows extensive filling of mediastinal collaterals, including esophageal varices (between upper arrows). The azygos and hemi-azygos veins are delineated by the contrast medium (lower arrows). Bronchogenic carcinoma.

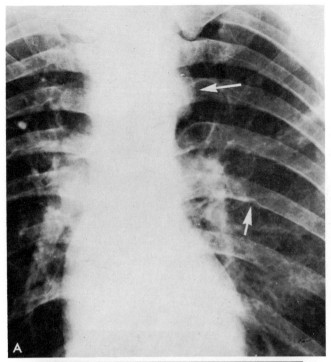

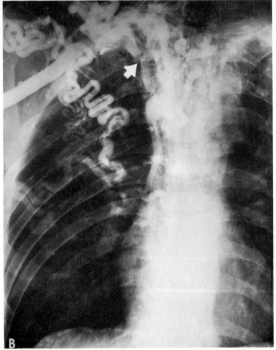

Figure 5–52. SUPERIOR VENA CAVAL OBSTRUCTION WITH RIB NOTCHING

A, The left 8th rib is notched (vertical arrow). An enlarged branch of the accessory hemiazygos vein juts out from the aortic knob (horizontal arrow). *B,* Right brachial venogram shows obstruction of the superior vena cava (arrow) with extensive collaterals, including a tortuous intercostal vein which is notching the right 5th rib. Enlarged nonopacified azygos and hemiazygos veins are seen through the heart in the lower mediastinum. At autopsy, fibrocalcific mediastinitis was found obstructing the cava.

(Figure continued on opposite page.)

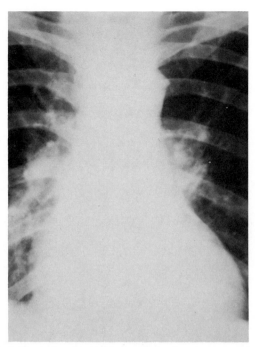

Figure 5–52. *Continued. C,* Normal patient with accessory hemiazygos vein adjacent to aortic knob.

ingly, the dilated veins are confined to the upper esophagus in carcinomatous obstruction, but involve the entire esophagus in the more chronic type of superior caval syndrome caused by mediastinal fibrosis. Similarly, the enlarged intercostal venous collaterals associated with superior caval obstruction may occasionally indicate their presence by notching the ribs as they make their tortuous way to the azygos vein (Fig. 5–52).

THE LYMPHATIC VESSELS

The lung possesses an extraordinary profuse network of lymphatics to drain the lymph that originates from both the alveoli and capillaries.[212] The lymphatic vessels extend as far as the alveolar ducts but do not enter the alveolar walls.[835] They run with the pulmonary veins along the septa between the secondary lobules. The lymphatics drain centrally from the pleura and parenchyma through the deep lymphatic system within the lung to the hila (Fig. 5–53). Valves within the lymphatic vessels control the direction of flow.

The pulmonary lymphatics, normal or abnormal, are not ordinarily visible on the roentgenogram. However, the effects of their engorgement can frequently be seen. Kerley described three types of linear shadows which he related to lymphatic dilatation: (A) thin nonbranching lines several inches in length, radiating from the hila, and not following the course of the arteries, veins, or bronchi; (B) transverse lines up to an inch long, seen best in the lateral portion of the lung bases and extending to the pleura; and (C) fine interlacing lines throughout the lung, producing a spiderweb appearance.[644, 645] These subsequently became known as Kerley's A, B, and C lines. The B lines have been discussed more widely than the A and C lines, probably because of their greater frequency and ease of recognition.[345, 469]

The B lines have been definitely shown to conform to the interlobular septa. There is general agreement that the transient form is caused by interstitial edema, but opinions differ as to whether the more permanent lines indicate dilatation of the lymphatics, chronic interstitial edema, hemosiderin or dust deposition, or interstitial fibrosis.[382, 386, 464, 468, 729] It is likely that more than one of these play a role in their development.

The B lines are short, thin, faint, linear shadows 1 to 3 cm in length and 1 to 2 mm

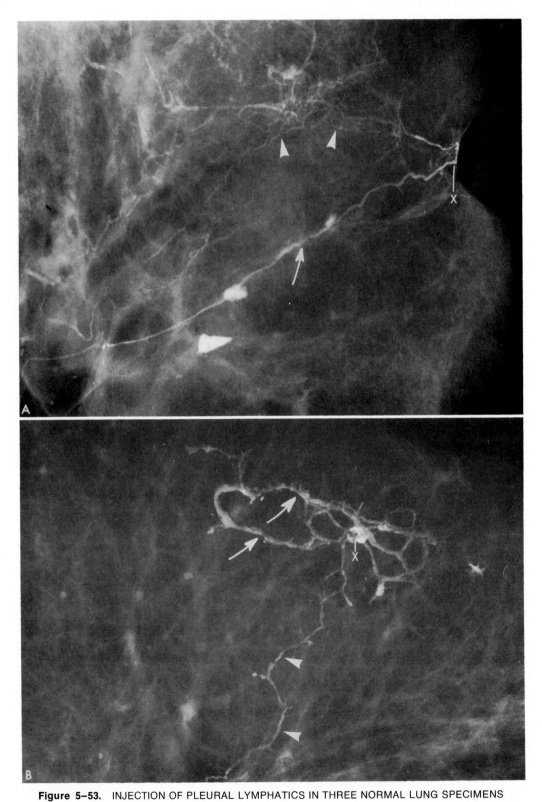

Figure 5–53.   INJECTION OF PLEURAL LYMPHATICS IN THREE NORMAL LUNG SPECIMENS

X marks the site of injection. Arrowheads indicate intrapulmonary lymphatics, arrows indicate pleural lymphatics.

(Figure continued on opposite page.)

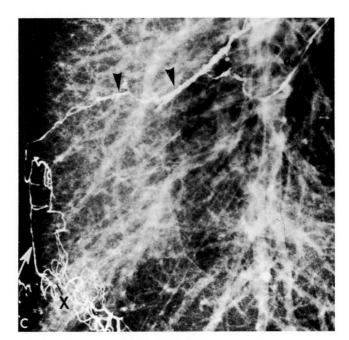

Figure 5–53. *Continued. C* is a copy of Trapnell's case.

in width. They are arranged in a horizontal stepladder pattern, 0.5 to 1.0 cm apart usually along the lower lateral lung margins. They are seen best in the costophrenic angles, occasionally occurring along the mediastinum, diaphragm, or pulmonary apices. Whatever the location, the lines are always perpendicular to the nearest pleural surface[382, 1114] (Fig. 5–54).

The distribution of B lines is almost certainly related to the fact that the pulmonary lobules are well developed in these areas, whereas they are poorly developed in the central and posterior portions of the lung.[529] Only those thickened septa that are parallel to the beam will show. Since each septum circumnavigates its pulmonary lobule and is therefore annular in shape, turning the patient slightly does not cause the B line to disappear. This helps to distinguish it from a blood vessel, scar, or disk of atelectasis, any of which will foreshorten or disappear on rotation.

The A lines have also been attributed to thickening of the interlobular septa around larger lobules oriented in nonhorizontal directions.[529] My feeling, based on lymphatic injection of lungs at autopsy by Trapnell[1223] and in our own department by Dr. Yahya Berkmen (Fig. 5–53), is that both A and C lines represent dilated anastomotic lymphatics. See for yourself the striking resemblance between Figures 5–53 and 5–55. Curiously, Trapnell no longer holds this view but has accepted the interlobular theory, even after seeing Figure 5–55.[1228] So does Heitzman.[522]

Like the Australian bushman who wanted a new boomerang but never found out how to throw the old one away, I find it difficult to discard long held concepts. So I looked further and found a spectacular movie prepared by Dr. Marceau Servelle of Paris. He injected the pleural lymphatics with Visciodol-chlorophyll during operation on patients with severe mitral stenosis and took color movies and roentgenograms of the lungs during and after injection. He showed *absolutely, unequivocally, and incontrovertibly* that you can easily see dilated lymphatics with the naked eye and roentgenographically; that they conform to the size, shape, pattern, and location of Kerley's A and C lines; and that the B lines are mostly lymphatics with a slight amount of perilymphatic leakage. So there!

A note of caution should be raised concerning the interpretation of B lines: on normal chest roentgenograms of good contrast and detail, similar lines may occasionally be

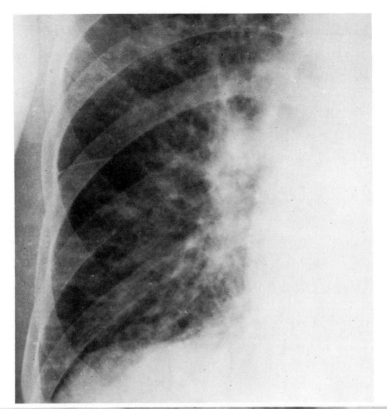

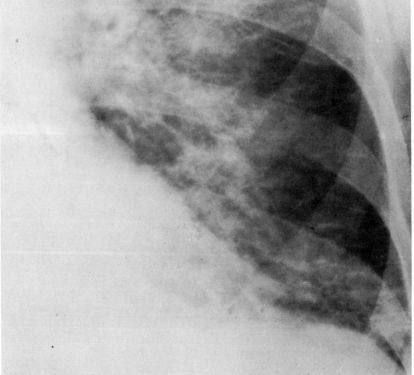

Figure 5–54. KERLEY'S B LINES

Two patients with acute left ventricular failure. The lines disappeared as cardiac compensation was restored.

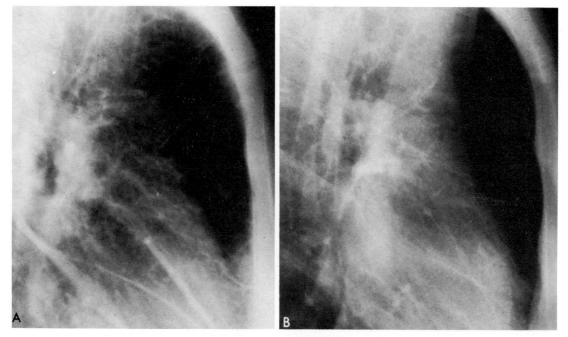

Figure 5–55. KERLEY'S A AND C LINES FROM PENICILLIN REACTION

A, Lateral view shows long A lines and spiderweb B lines. Note the thickened interlobar fissures, representing either pleural edema or interlobar fluid. *B,* 2 days later the chest is normal.

seen in the vicinity of the lateral costophrenic angles. Chest teleroentgenograms of 1000 healthy adult men were studied for transverse lines in this region. Each lung was studied in 500 cases. I found a few transverse lines in the costophrenic regions (probably representing fine arterial branches) in 17 per cent on the right side and in 19 per cent on the left. The transverse lines were even more numerous, although still relatively thin, in 1.6 per cent on the right and 3.2 per cent on the left. The right lung in one patient and the left in three others showed a pattern indistinguishable from that described by Kerley. These findings indicate that you should be conservative in interpreting these shadows in borderline cases.

Kerley's lines may be transient or persistent (Table 5–3). The transitory lines are frequently present in left ventricular failure (Fig. 5–56), disappearing as compensation is restored. In these cases, they represent the interstitial component of pulmonary

TABLE 5–3. Causes of Kerley's Lines (A, B, and C)

TRANSIENT
Common
    Pulmonary edema (any cause)[236]
Rare
    Pneumonia (Fig. 5–60)
    Pulmonary hemorrhage
    Transient respiratory distress of newborn

PERSISTENT
Common
    Lymphangitic metastases[602, 730, 884, 885, 1225]
        (Fig. 5–61)
    Pneumoconiosis[883, 1226] (Fig. 5–62)
    Rheumatic mitral valve disease
Rare
    Alveolar cell carcinoma
    Congenital heart disease
    Interstitial fibrosis of any cause
    Lymphoma
    Mineral oil aspiration[129]
    Obstruction of thoracic duct
    Pulmonary lymphangiectasis
    Pulmonary venous occlusive disease[1074]
    Sarcoidosis[883, 1227]
    Scleroderma
    Tumor of left atrium

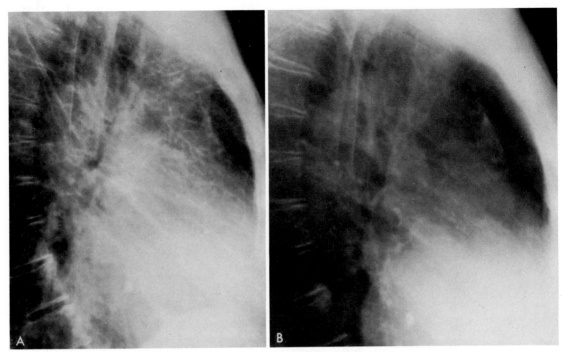

Figure 5–56. KERLEY'S B LINES IN LATERAL PROJECTION

A, During a bout of congestive failure. *B*, After recovery.

edema. This is often associated with "cuffing" around the larger bronchi and vessels and with transient pleural thickening, which may also indicate interstitial edema.[444] Of course, alveolar edema often accompanies the interstitial form. In fact, pulmonary edema of any cause is often associated with Kerley's lines. Curiously, about half the patients in whom the A and C lines are predominant are suffering a bout of sensitivity to penicillin, Myleran, nitrofurantoin, or other drugs.[247, 876, 1305] (Figs. 5–55 and 5–57). In cardiacs, the A lines are probably related to the rapid development of pulmonary edema or very high venous pressure.[528]

Persistent Kerley's lines are frequently seen in mitral valve disease (Fig. 5–58), with elevated pulmonary venous pressure[163, 469, 528, 1114] but there is no close correlation between the level of the mean left atrial pressure and the presence of the lines,[212, 820] as is commonly implied. The lines disappear after successful valvular surgery. They are seldom encountered in congenital heart disease, and then mainly with those types that cause myocardial failure (e.g., endocardial fibroelastosis) or obstruction to flow through the left heart, such as total anomalous pulmonary venous return (Fig. 5–24), pulmonary vein stenosis, or mitral or aortic stenosis or atresia. Rarely the lines are confined to one portion of a lung, a finding probably indicative of localized venous or lymphatic compression[8] (Fig. 5–59). Table 5–3 and Figures 5–24 to 5–62 include all the conditions I could think of that are associated with Kerley's lines.

The lymphatics of the lung may occasionally be visualized during life by lymphangiography. Contrast medium injected into a lower extremity normally makes its way slowly to the cisterna chyli in the epigastrium and thence via the thoracic duct into the venous circulation at the junction of the left subclavian and internal jugular veins. Blockage of the thoracic duct by tumor, infection (e.g., filariasis), lymphangiomatous malformation, operative or other trauma, thrombosis of the left subclavian vein, congenital anomalies, or from unknown causes may result in chylothorax

(*Text continued on page 250.*)

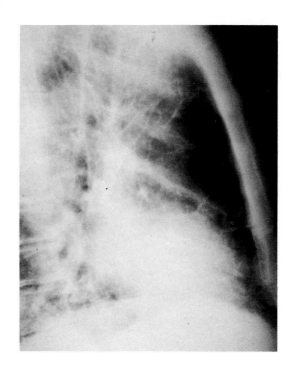

Figure 5–57. KERLEY'S LINES DURING MYLERAN THERAPY FOR LYMPHOMA

A and C lines are present. The interstitial pulmonary edema cleared after therapy was stopped and recurred when the drug was resumed.

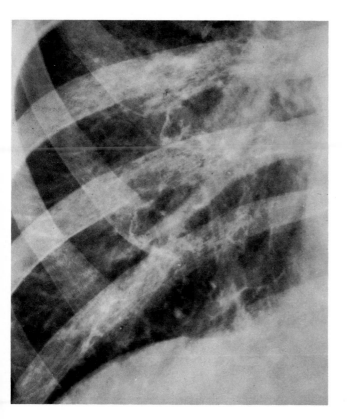

Figure 5–58. PERSISTENT B LINES IN MITRAL STENOSIS

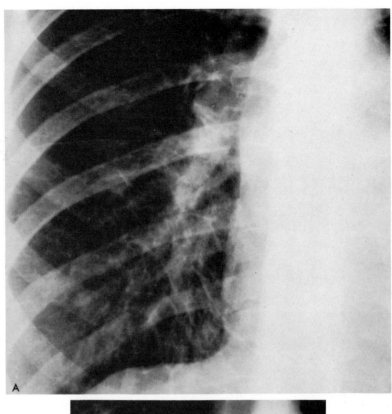

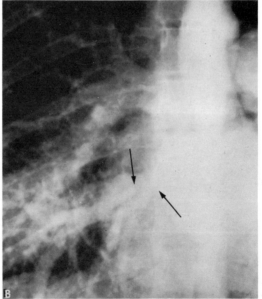

Figure 5–59. LOCALIZED KERLEY'S LINES

A, A and C lines are confined to the right juxtacardiac region. Other films showed a large, partly calcified, carinal lymph node. *B,* Pulmonary angiogram shows partial obstruction of the right interior pulmonary veins (arrows) from compression by the large node. (Courtesy of Dr. Morton Ziskind.)

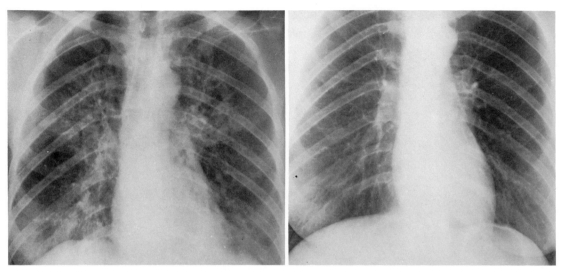

Figure 5–60.   KERLEY'S LINES (A and C) IN ACUTE VIRUS PNEUMONIA

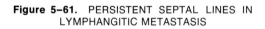**Figure 5–61.**   PERSISTENT SEPTAL LINES IN
LYMPHANGITIC METASTASIS

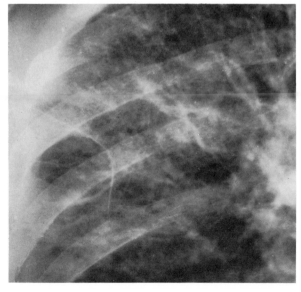

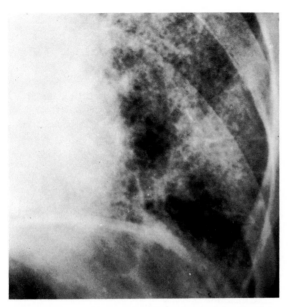

Figure 5–62. PERSISTENT KERLEY'S B LINES IN SILICOSIS

and dilatation of the lymphatics within the lung.[1042] Under such circumstances, a pedal lymphangiogram may occasionally demonstrate the site of the leak, communication with the pulmonary lymphatics or with the pleural space, and sometimes even the cause[180, 702, 892, 1100, 1293] (Fig. 1–20). I suspect that in at least some of the patients with so-called congenital lymphangiectasia, the thoracic duct is obstructed by one of the above conditions. Servelle and Soulie showed extensive lymphatic leakage into the pleura in hydrothorax as well as into the lung in pulmonary edema.[1101]

CHAPTER 6

THE LYMPH NODES

ANATOMY

Based on the work of Rouvière, Engel, and others,[297, 657, 1039] a practical anatomic classification of the intrathoracic lymph nodes is diagrammed in Figure 6–1* and illustrated in part in Figures 6–2 to 6–4.

---

*I have simplified some of the terms so that they are easier to remember: tracheal = paratracheal; bronchial = tracheobronchial; lobar = lobar and interlobar; carinal = bifurcation; esophageal = paraesophageal and retrotracheal; anterior mediastinal = prevascular.

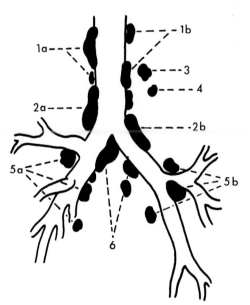

Figure 6–1. DIAGRAM OF MEDIASTINAL LYMPH NODES

(1a) and *(1b)*, Right and left tracheal nodes. *(2a)* and *(2b)*, Right and left bronchial nodes. The azygos node is the lowermost of this group on the right side. *(3)*, Aortic nodes. *(4)*, Ductus node. *(5a)* and *(5b)*, Right and left hilar nodes. *(6)*, Carinal nodes. The posterior and anterior mediastinal and parenchymal nodes are not shown. After Engel[300] and Rouvière.[1039]

The nodal areas are grouped as follows:
(1) right and left tracheal nodes
(2) right and left bronchial nodes, including on the right the azygos node
(3) aortic nodes, lying along the aortic knob and descending aorta
(4) the ductus node
(5) right and left hilar nodes, including the lobar nodes
(6) carinal nodes
(7) esophageal nodes
(8) posterior mediastinal nodes
(9) anterior mediastinal nodes
(10) parenchymal nodes
(11) right and left diaphragm nodes

There is an anecdote in connection with Figure 6–2, which happens to be my own chest. At the outbreak of World War II, this much calcium on a chest film meant automatic disqualification for entry into the Army. When I reported for my physical examination and chest film at an Army hospital, I stopped in the radiologist's office and told him of the calcium, expressing the hope that I would not be rejected. He told his technician to hit the film 15 KV light and, my calcium invisible, I passed the examination.

My first assignment was to the very same radiology department; my benefactor was to be shipped out to the Far East. As I reported to him I said, "Hello, you good samaritan." He said, "Goodbye, you bastard!"

LYMPH CIRCULATION

The lymphatics of the thorax are drained by the thoracic duct and right and left bronchomediastinal trunks. The thoracic duct enters the venous circulation at or near the junction of the subclavian and jugular veins, or rarely via a jugular lymph sac (Fig. 13–12).

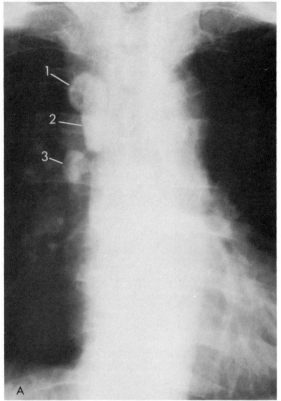

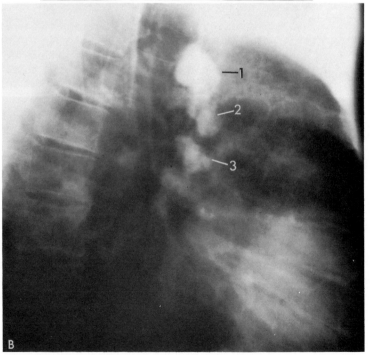

Figure 6–2. LYMPH NODE
ANATOMY

A and *B*, Calcified nodes. *(1)*,
Right tracheal. *(2)*, Right bronchial.
(3), Azygos node.

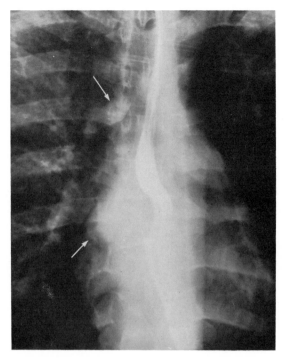

Figure 6–3. BUCKY FILM SHOWING CARINAL ADENOPATHY

The soft tissue mass of nodes is visible through the heart on this well-penetrated recumbent film (lower arrow). There is also an indentation of the right side of the esophagus. The normal azygos vein is visible (upper arrow). The enlarged nodes later spontaneously disappeared. Probable histoplasmosis.

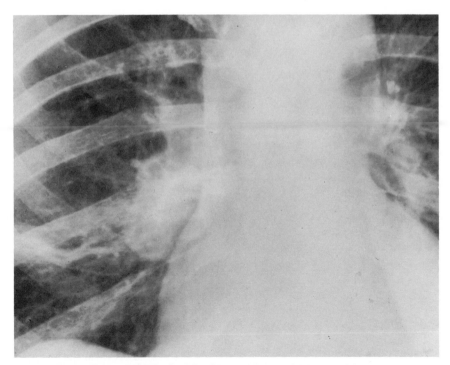

Figure 6–4. RIGHT LOWER LOBAR LYMPH NODE ENLARGEMENT

The nodes appear to lie within the lung at the lower edge of the right hilum. Proximal to the enlarged nodes the hilum appears normal. There is an associated lesion in the right lower lung. Lymphatic leukemia.

The bronchomediastinals empty independently or after variable anastomosis into the corresponding subclavian-jugular junction. Rouvière concluded from his studies that the right tracheal nodes ultimately drained the entire right lung as well as the lower half of the left lung.

Whether due to variations in the lymphatic drainage or to blockage of the flow by clogged nodes, these pathways are not necessarily the ones followed by a spreading pathologic process. McCort and Robbins, in a study of surgical material for metastases from cancers arising in the various lobes of the lung, noted many exceptions to the expected patterns.[810] In general, the hilar nodes draining the involved lobe appeared to be the first line of defense. In tumors of the RUL, the right bronchial and tracheal nodes appeared to be the next group affected, occasionally with associated involvement of the right anterior mediastinal and carinal nodes. The right tracheal nodes were also involved in the two patients with RML carcinoma. RLL carcinoma often metastasized to the carinal nodes; in addition, the anterior mediastinal nodes were sometimes affected, but only occasionally was tumor found in the right tracheal group. The LUL drained chiefly into the anterior mediastinal region, the left or right tracheals seldom being involved. Tumors in the inferior portion of the LUL metastasized mainly to the carinal nodes. The LLL appeared to drain into the carinal and anterior mediastinal nodes; extension to the right or left tracheals was less common.

Nohl stated that right-sided carcinoma never metastasizes to the left supraclavicular nodes, but that carcinoma of the left lung often spreads to the right supraclavicular.[885] Others say that any bronchogenic carcinoma may metastasize to either supraclavicular region. Carinal node metastases drain to the azygos and right tracheal nodes.[886] Esophageal nodes are found in about half the autopsied cases of bronchogenic carcinomas.[1158] Obviously, at least in the case of carcinoma of the lung, there seems to be no consistency in the pattern of thoracic lymphatic drainage, and considerable deviation from the pathways described by Rouvière is seen.[1039]

ROENTGEN SIGNS OF NODAL ENLARGEMENT

Moderate enlargement of individual nodes or groups of nodes is often demon-

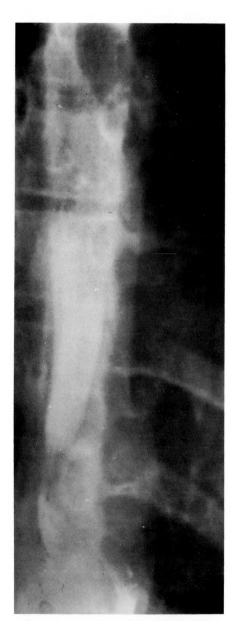

Figure 6–5. ESOPHAGEAL-AORTIC NODES

Bucky AP esophagram showing a soft tissue mass obliterating the left margin of the descending aorta and indenting the esophagus. At operation, the node was adherent to the esophageal wall. Histoplasmosis. (Courtesy of Dr. Lee S. Rosenberg.)

strable by conventional roentgen methods, including teleroentgenograms in the frontal, lateral, and oblique projections.[715] However, additional studies are frequently helpful in their recognition. Well-penetrated Bucky, high kilovoltage,[1235] or tomographic AP films are extremely valuable for demonstrating enlarged nodes hidden by the spine and mediastinal structures, especially the carinal, esophageal, and aortic groups[326, 443, 809] (Figs. 6–3 and 6–5). In the lateral view, poorly defined or lobulated margins of the right or left pulmonary artery are often seen with hilar nodes (Fig. 6–6).

On fluoroscopy, slight rotation of the patient and the Valsalva procedure, as described in Chapter 1, are helpful in distinguishing vascular prominence from hilar adenopathy, the nodes maintaining a lumpy rounded appearance while vessels become foreshortened. Barium swallow is essential to the recognition of juxtaesophageal lymph nodes.

Bronchography has also been recommended to demonstrate nodal pressure on the trachea and bronchi. Many authors have advocated pulmonary angiography and azygography for the diagnosis and determination of operability of broncho-

genic carcinoma, but I have had little personal experience with these techniques.[490, 637, 1078, 1175, 1330]

The silhouette sign is often useful in recognizing and localizing lymphadenopathy. Obliteration of a segment of the descending aorta, right tracheal border, or pulmonary artery by large lymph nodes is common. The cervicothoracic sign may be applicable to upper mediastinal node enlargement. Similarly, anterior mediastinal nodes may obscure a segment of a border of the heart or ascending aorta.

Carinal Node Enlargement

Of considerable importance is the recognition of enlargement of the carinal nodes. Fleischner and Sachsse pointed out that since the esophagus passes in close proximity to these node bearing areas, a barium swallow will often reveal nodal enlargement as a shallow indentation, narrowing, or displacement of the esophagus just caudal to the carina.[383] Although the left oblique position is usually best for this purpose (Fig. 6–7), I have encountered several examples in which the changes were appar-

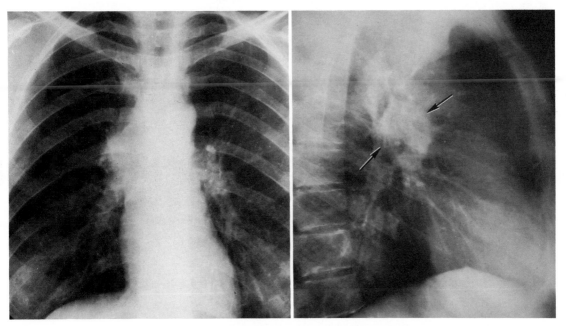

Figure 6–6. RIGHT HILAR NODE ENLARGEMENT
The lateral view is often helpful in differentiating the various groups of enlarged nodes. Metastatic carcinoma.

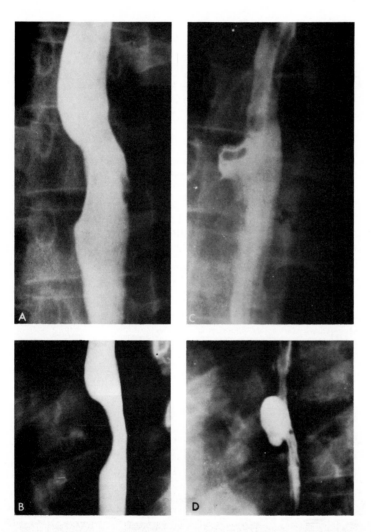

Figure 6-7. CARINAL NODE IM-
PRINT ON THE ESOPHAGUS

A and *B,* Frontal and left anterior
oblique spot films of the carinal area
with barium in the esophagus. Note
the typical extrinsic defect produced
by the enlarged carinal nodes. *C* and
D, Similar views obtained 8 months
later. A traction diverticulum has now
appeared at the site of the defect.
Histoplasmosis seems probable on
the basis of skin test conversion.
(From Felson, B.[326]; reproduced with
permission of Charles C Thomas,
Publisher.)

ent only in the frontal projection or right oblique (Fig. 6–8).

Of course, any mediastinal mass may produce identical findings. The intact esophageal mucosa and sloping margins of the imprint distinguish it from intrinsic tumor of the esophagus. This does not hold true for the occasional instance when a lymph node mass becomes adherent to the esophageal wall and indents it in the manner of an intra-

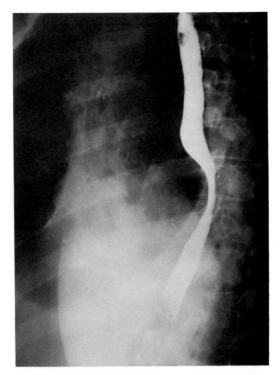

Figure 6–9. POSTERIOR RETRACTION OF ESOPH-AGUS BY ELONGATED AORTA

Since the esophagus and aorta lie in the same sheath, the elongated and tortuous atherosclerotic aorta often pulls the middle third of the esophagus backward and toward the left. This may simulate a carinal mass *pushing* the esophagus.

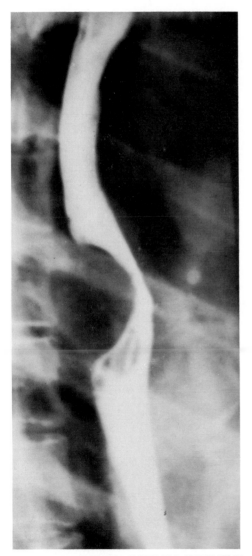

Figure 6–8. CARINAL NODE ENLARGEMENT

The esophageal indentation was visible only in the frontal and in this right oblique view. The angular margins indicate that the node is probably adherent to the esophageal wall. No diagnostic proof. (Courtesy of Dr. Eli Rubenstein.)

mural extramucosal tumor (Fig. 6–8). The carinal node imprint may also be simulated by enlargement of the left atrium and by posterior retraction of the esophagus by an elongated aorta. Differentiation from dilated left atrium is easily made from the high location and relatively small size of the carinal imprint. In esophageal retraction, the posterior wall of the esophagus parallels the descending aorta (Fig. 6–9).

Middlemass stated that all patients presenting a lung shadow of unknown etiology should be investigated for carinal lymphadenopathy.[829] The demonstration of carinal nodes in such cases strongly favors the diagnosis of carcinoma of the lung in the older patient and primary tuberculosis[1161] or histoplasmosis in the young[329] (Fig. 1–8). Study of the carinal area is also useful in confirming the presence of lymphadenopathy when one or both hila show borderline enlargement. The esophagram is thus helpful in the diagnosis of such conditions as lymphoma and bronchogenic carcinoma, in which the detection and treatment of all areas of lymph node involvement are of obvious importance.[326]

Hilar Node Enlargement

The lobar nodes lie within the lung fields. Their involvement can often be recognized by an enlargement at the outer edge of the hilum extending into the affected lobe (Figs. 6–4 and 6–10). In bronchogenic carcinoma, these nodes often blend inseparably with the primary lesion in the lung and are thus easily overlooked. The main hilar nodes lie within the hilum (Fig. 6–6A).

Tracheal and Bronchial Node Enlargement

Tracheal and bronchial node enlargement often coexist. They are seen as a lobulated

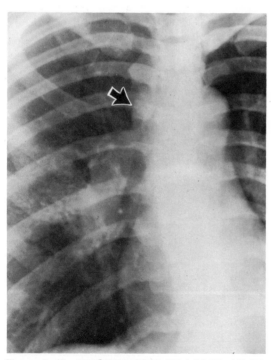

Figure 6–10. ENLARGEMENT OF LOBAR, HILAR, AND AZYGOS NODES

The pulmonary infiltrate is in the apex of the RLL. The azygos node (arrow) lies in the angle between the trachea and right main stem bronchus. Probable primary tuberculosis.

density projecting laterally from the superior mediastinum (Fig. 6–11). The tracheal nodes often appear to extend a short distance above the clavicles, through which they remain visible. On the right side, they always obliterate the tracheal border. They often indent the trachea and may partially obstruct it (Fig. 6–12). The position of these nodes is roughly the same as that occupied by an intrathoracic goiter; differentiation depends on demonstrating enlargement of other groups of lymph nodes.

The lowermost node in the right bronchial chain, the azygos node, lies in the angle between the trachea and the right main stem bronchus (Figs. 5–47 and 6–10). It may be mistaken for the rounded end-on shadow of the azygos vein itself, normal or enlarged, which is found in the same location on well-penetrated plain or Bucky films[291, 385, 714, 1080] (Fig. 6–3). Differentiation is simple: change in size with respiratory maneuvers and recumbency is an infallible sign of the venous structure. Lesions in other planes may present in the azygos area on frontal projection,[94] but they seldom obliterate the right lower tracheal margin.

The left tracheal and bronchial nodes, less often enlarged than the right, are located medial and anterior to the shadow of the aortic knob and can usually be seen through it (Fig. 6–13). Considerable enlargement is required before the nodes project laterally beyond the knob.

The ductus node near the left pulmonary artery is not infrequently enlarged and may occasionally be identified obliterating the cardiac silhouette above the left pulmonary artery. Though it lies a slight distance from the left main bronchus it might readily be included in the left bronchial group, since the two often enlarge together (Fig. 6–13).

Other Lymph Node Enlargement

Enlarged esophageal nodes may occasionally be seen through the trachea or heart in the frontal view (Fig. 6–5). They often impinge on the esophagus from the side or from behind. Intramural lymph nodes are not supposed to be present in the esophagus, but Figure 14–5 appears to indicate a unique exception to this rule. As with the carinal nodes, involved esophageal

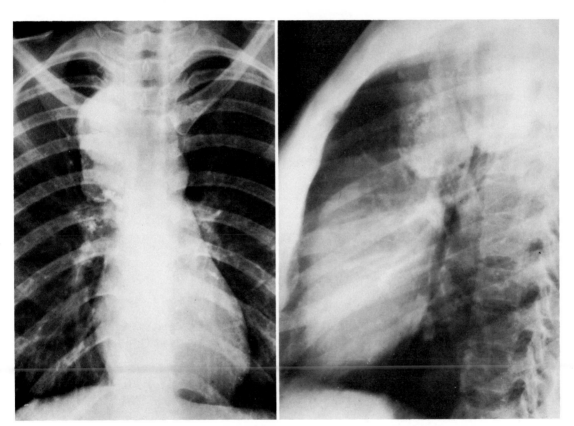

Figure 6–11. RIGHT TRACHEAL AND BRONCHIAL NODES

Note extension above the clavicle in the frontal view. Inactive histoplasmosis.

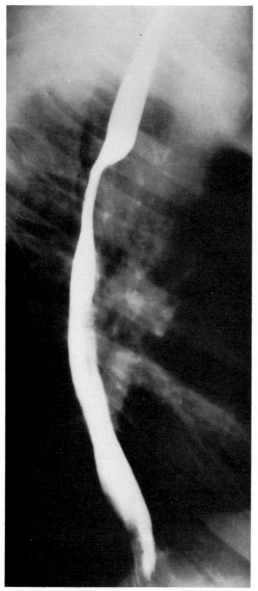

Figure 6–12. TRACHEAL OBSTRUCTION BY HISTOPLASMIC LYMPHADENITIS

Emergency surgical intervention was necessary in this 4 year old boy.

nodes may attach to the esophageal wall and present as an intramural extramucosal lesion, sometimes even causing dysphagia. Embarrassingly, I have made a diagnosis of esophageal neoplasm in several such instances. It made me feel like the time my

wife came downstairs and announced, "The baby just had a bowel movement in bed."

I responded, "Why tell me about it?"

"It's your bed!"

The anterior mediastinal (prevascular) chains, right and left, lie in front of the heart but, if greatly enlarged, may project lateral to it (Fig. 6–14). Enlarged diaphragm nodes are occasionally seen in the right or left cardiophrenic angle.[167]

The aortic nodes are uncommonly enlarged. They obliterate the adjacent margin of the descending aorta, requiring well-penetrated films, preferably Bucky, for their demonstration[443] (Fig. 6–5). Posterior mediastinal nodes lie in the region of the paravertebral gutter and are seldom visibly enlarged. They usually displace the posterior mediastinal lines (Chap. 11). Rarely, an aggregate of normal lymphoid tissue is found well out in the lung, presenting roentgenographically as a pulmonary nodule.[476, 1106, 1224]

CLINICAL SIGNIFICANCE OF LYMPH NODE ENLARGEMENT

The recognition of enlarged lymph nodes is of obvious importance. It may suggest the correct diagnosis of a pulmonary lesion, as in primary tuberculosis in the child and bronchogenic carcinoma in the adult; or it may represent the sole roentgen manifestation of disease, as in sarcoid, lymphoma, or metastatic malignancy. In carcinoma of the lung, demonstration of nodal involvement may influence the decision to operate or determine the boundaries of the portals to be irradiated.

In some diseases, there is a predilection for involvement of certain groups of lymph nodes, for example, the lobar nodes in erythema nodosum[316] and in sarcoid. In this situation, a clear uninvolved zone may be visible between the nodes and central hila (Fig. 6–15). The lobar, hilar, and right bronchial and tracheal nodes are commonly involved together in lymphoma as well as in sarcoid (Fig. 6–16). The anterior mediastinal nodes are seldom visibly enlarged in sarcoid,[1298] but they often are in lymphoma[307, 366, 379] (Fig. 6–14), especially

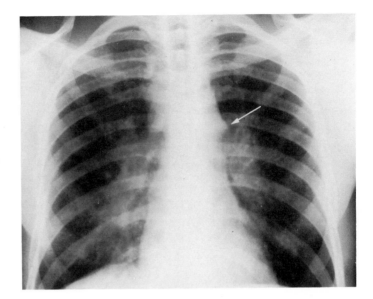

Figure 6–13. DUCTUS NODE (arrow)

Bilateral bronchial and hilar adenopathy is also present. Sarcoid.

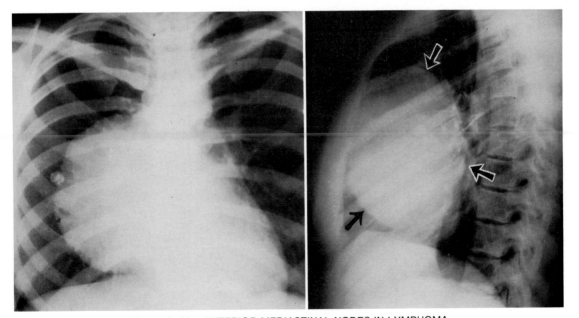

Figure 6–14. ANTERIOR MEDIASTINAL NODES IN LYMPHOMA

A huge mass (arrows) of lymph nodes involving the right anterior mediastinal chain was found at operation.

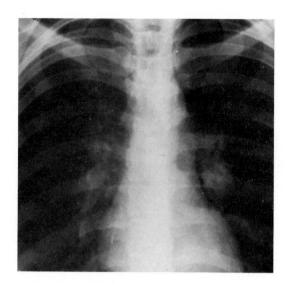

Figure 6–15. LOBAR NODE ENLARGEMENT IN SARCOIDOSIS

A clear zone is visible medial to the enlarged nodes.

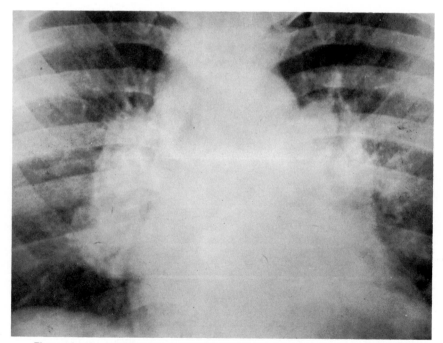

Figure 6–16. WIDESPREAD LYMPH NODE ENLARGEMENT IN LYMPHOMA

Lobar, hilar, and right bronchial and tracheal node enlargement.

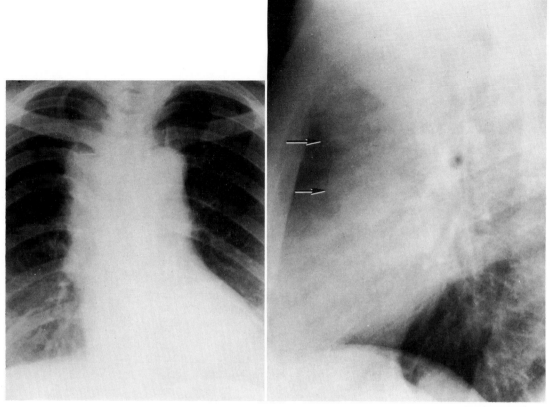

Figure 6–17. ANTERIOR MEDIASTINAL NODES IN HODGKIN'S DISEASE (arrows)
There is a cervicothoracic sign.

Hodgkin's disease (Fig. 6–17). In fact, extension of this nodal involvement into the anterior chest wall about the sternum is almost diagnostic of Hodgkin's disease. Unilaterality favors tuberculosis, histoplasmosis, or cancer. Table 6–1 lists conditions that cause roentgenologic lymph node enlargement.

Lymph node disease may cause lobar or segmental collapse. The collapse may result either from compression of the bronchus by enlarged nodes or from distortion by fibrotic ones. Certain bronchi seem to be more vulnerable than others in this respect. The RML bronchus is often compressed or distorted by fibrotic or fibrocalcific lymph nodes caused by past tuberculosis or histoplasmosis[329] (Fig. 6–18). In like manner,

TABLE 6–1. Causes of Thoracic Lymph Node Enlargement

Common
  Primary tuberculosis
  Histoplasmosis
  Lymphoma
  Sarcoid
  Metastatic malignancy
  Pneumoconiosis

Rare
  Other fungus diseases
  Reticuloses
  Wegener's granuloma
  Infectious mononucleosis
  Tularemia
  Erythema nodosum
  Idiopathic
  Nonspecific inflammatory lymphadenitis

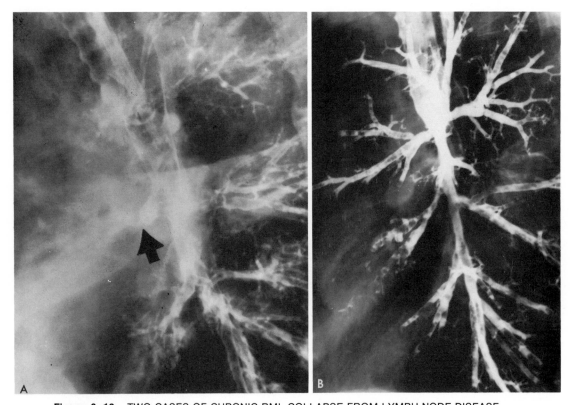

Figure 6–18. TWO CASES OF CHRONIC RML COLLAPSE FROM LYMPH NODE DISEASE

A, Contracted, quiescent, tuberculous, or histoplasmic node obstructs the RML bronchus (arrow). *B,* An enlarged granulomatous node has compressed the bronchus, causing RML collapse and bronchiectasis.

any lobar or segmental bronchus may be occluded.

The pull exerted by fibrous contraction of healing granulomatous mediastinal nodes is the cause of traction diverticula of the esophagus (Fig. 6–7). Intranodal neoplasm or perinodal fibrosis may also cause obstruction of the superior vena cava (Fig. 5–52) or of a pulmonary vein (Fig. 5–59). The nature and complications of calcification within these inflamed lymph nodes is discussed in Chapter 14.

CHAPTER 7

THE PULMONARY AIRWAYS

The air passages of the lung include, in sequence, the larynx, trachea, bronchi, bronchioles, alveolar ducts, alveolar sacs, and alveoli. Apart from the trachea and main stem bronchi, the airway components as such are invisible on the normal plain film. When surrounded by alveolar infiltrate, however, the lumens of lobar, segmental, and smaller bronchi may become visible as an air bronchogram (Chap. 2). Even so, the details of a bronchial lesion are seldom well depicted on the plain film. Tomography also has its limitations in this regard. It will never attain the position of bronchography as a tool for bronchial visualization, al-though its innocuousness offers a considerable advantage.

But why bronchography? In many clinics, the procedure has seldom been performed since the days when bronchiectasis was rampant. Yet bronchography is still a valuable procedure and can often provide information not otherwise available. Among its more important indications are the demonstration and elucidation of a bronchial lesion inaccessible to the bronchoscope* (Fig. 7–1); the exclusion of carcinoma on the

---

*The development of fiberoptic bronchoscopy and brush biopsy techniques has made this less of an indication.[352a, 849]

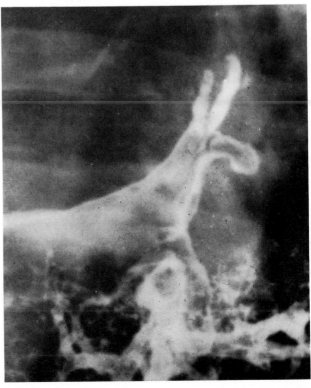

Figure 7–1. BRONCHOGRAPHY IN BRONCHIAL CARCINOMA

Right anterior oblique view. Obstruction of the individual segmental bronchi in the collapsed LUL. Their side branches are occluded. The bronchi are distended. So is the moose. Unretouched.

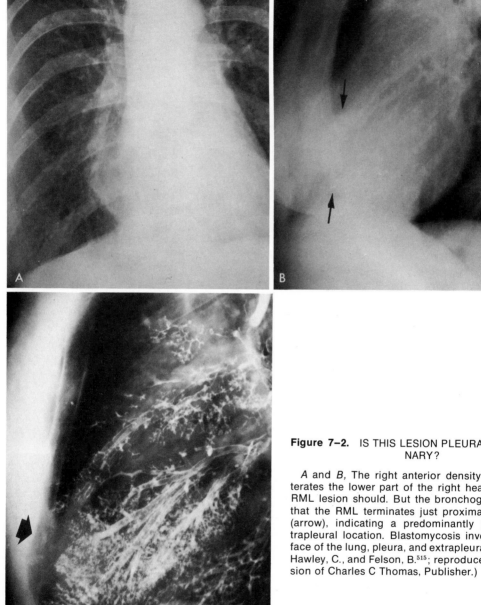

Figure 7-2. IS THIS LESION PLEURAL OR PULMO-
NARY?

A and *B,* The right anterior density (arrows) obliterates the lower part of the right heart border as a
RML lesion should. But the bronchogram *(C)* shows
that the RML terminates just proximal to the lesion
(arrow), indicating a predominantly pleural or extrapleural location. Blastomycosis involving the surface of the lung, pleura, and extrapleural tissue. (From
Hawley, C., and Felson, B.[515]; reproduced with permission of Charles C Thomas, Publisher.)

basis of a *patent bronchus* or *double lesion sign* (Chap. 3); the identification of such congenital anomalies as agenesis and sequestration (Chaps. 3 and 4); and the clarification of confusing intrathoracic shadows, e.g., pleural versus pulmonary location (Fig. 7–2).

Bronchography as performed at present has been too bothersome to attain its potential. This is why I have become excited about the inhalation method using tantalum or barium. I believe this will soon replace conventional bronchography.[363, 542, 610, 748, 862, 1112] Just imagine finding a lesion on a chest film and, before the patient leaves the radiology department, placing a mask over his face and spraying atomized contrast medium into the appropriate bronchi, depicting an endobronchial tumor. This is not a pipe dream—it will become reality before long (Fig. 1–19).

THE LARYNX

Radiology of the larynx and other cervical structures is outside the scope of this book but not beyond the domain of the chest roentgenologist. Lesions in the various structures of the neck, vocal cord paralysis, and other structural and functional alterations of the pharynx and larynx are important manifestations or causes of thoracic disease. As an example, let's just discuss one topic.

The Vallecular Sign

Vallecular sign is the name applied by Arendt and Wolf to the retention of barium sulfate in the pockets of the valleculae and pyriform sinuses after swallowing.[13] It is the roentgen counterpart of clinical dysphagia and is of importance in chest roentgenology because of its relationship to aspiration pneumonitis and to laryngeal nerve involvement from an intrathoracic neoplasm.

The sign is encountered with local disease in the vicinity of the larynx and pharynx, carcinoma of the esophagus or gastric fundus, and mediastinal neoplastic and inflammatory conditions. More significantly, it is consistently present in pharyngeal paresis and paralysis caused by a variety of neurologic and muscular disorders, including cerebral hemorrhage, poliomyelitis, pseudobulbar palsy, and myasthenia gravis.[783, 1090, 1282] A similar finding is occasionally encountered in debilitated elderly patients in whom atony of the pharyngeal muscles interferes with normal deglutition.

The sign is elicited best with a fluid barium mixture. In the normal patient the barium disappears almost completely from the hypopharynx a moment after swallowing. A positive vallecular sign is indicated by the retention of a significant amount of barium in the hypopharynx for a prolonged period. Dilatation of the pharyngeal cavity and absence of effective contraction during swallowing also occur. In myasthenia gravis, no retention of barium occurs at first, but the sign may become apparent after repeated swallowing attempts. It will often disappear after appropriate medication for the myasthenia.

THE TRACHEA

The normal tracheal dimensions vary considerably with respiration. On expiration, the trachea decreases about 10 per cent in width and 20 per cent in length,[556] and the carina moves upward about 1 cm. The carinal angle, which normally averages about 60 degrees, increases 10 to 15 degrees on inspiration and a similar amount on recumbency. The trachea collapses conspicuously on cough and during the Valsalva maneuver.[648, 1333]

These respiratory alterations have some practical importance. The distal tip of an intratracheal tube may appear in satisfactory position on an inspiratory film, but on expiration may extend into the right main stem bronchus and block the left bronchial orifice. This normal variability of the carinal angle detracts from its value as a detector of left atrial enlargement or carinal lymphadenopathy.

Abnormal dilatation—the trachea may even attain the width of the vertebral column—is usually associated with dilatation of the large bronchi. This rare condition is called *tracheobronchiomegaly* or *Mounier-Kuhn syndrome*. Although generally considered congenital, it is seldom found in children. In some individuals it seems to have a cause and effect relationship with severe chronic tracheobronchial infection, and no one seems sure which came first. It has been called bronchomalacia. On bronchography, the trachea and bronchi often show scalloping or diverticulum-like protrusions between the tracheal rings or trans-verse muscle bundles. The condition is sometimes associated with cystic bron-chiectasis [566, 629] (Figs. 4–14 and 7–3).

An abnormal degree of collapse of the trachea on respiration is sometimes encoun-tered among children. *Inspiratory collapse* at the cervicothoracic junction, a rare find-ing, is seen with laryngeal obstruction,

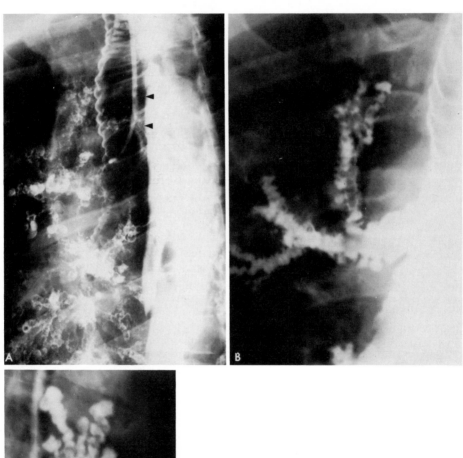

Figure 7–3. TRACHEOBRONCHIOMEGALY

A, Catheter bronchogram, left oblique view. The ar-rowheads touch the left posterior tracheal wall. The trachea is almost as wide as the spinal column. Note the scalloped protrusions between the tracheal rings. *B* and *C,* Severe, widespread chronic bronchitis and cystic bronchiectasis. The large bronchi show nu-merous diverticula. (Courtesy of Dr. Daniel Mc-Farland.)

infantile larynx, and idiopathic infantile stridor. Severe *expiratory collapse* of the intrathoracic portion of the trachea is more common. It results from diffuse peripheral bronchiolar obstruction, as in asthma and bronchiolitis.[1316] Buckling and deviation of the trachea to the side opposite the aortic arch on expiration is a common normal finding.[176]

A tracheal mass or foreign body may result in bilateral diffuse pulmonary hyperaeration. On expiration, because of the normal reduction in tracheal caliber, the mass more nearly fills the lumen and prevents free egress of air from the lungs. Interestingly, the heart then appears to shrink on expiration rather than on inspiration. This paradoxic alteration in heart size may also be seen during an acute asthmatic attack and in severe bilateral diffuse pulmonary emphysema (Fig. 1–6). Table 7–1 lists a variety of intra- and juxtatracheal masses, benign and malignant, and Figures 7–4 and 7–5 illustrate some examples of these.

Tracheal deformity often results from an indwelling tracheotomy tube, especially of the cuff type.[432, 599] Stenosis or web formation in the trachea may be congenital, inflammatory, or traumatic.[1199]

Tracheal fistula extending into the esophagus, mediastinum, or lung is not very common. The congenital variety of tracheoesophageal fistula is usually associated with esophagus atresia. The isolated *H* type fistula is best demonstrated in the prone position with the esophagus filled (via catheter) with aqueous contrast medium.[850, 1131] In the adult, tracheal or tracheoesophageal fistula may be congenital[694] (Fig. 7–6) but is usually an acquired lesion—carcinomatous, traumatic, or inflammatory.[1277, 1327] The latter is generally attributable to quiescent fibrocalcific histoplasmosis or tuberculosis of the mediastinal nodes with erosion into the trachea.

THE LARGE BRONCHI

The bronchographic configuration of an obstructing bronchial lesion is often highly suggestive of its diagnosis. Further, the absence of a lesion in the bronchus supplying an area of pulmonary collapse (open bronchus sign) excludes neoplasm as a cause of the collapse.

Bronchogenic Carcinoma

Primary carcinoma commonly gives a tapered, funnel or V shaped defect (Fig. 7–7A), occasionally with a slightly curled slender termination, the so-called *rat-tail* (Fig. 7–7B). In my personal experience, the rat-tail deformity has proved to be diagnostic of carcinoma and the V shaped contour almost so. Irregularity of the obstructed bronchus (Fig. 7–7C) is also an indication of malignancy but by no means an infallible one. Other signs of bronchogenic carcinoma, less secure in my eyes, include annular constriction, solitary or multiple mural indentations ("thumbprinting") (Fig. 7–7D), invasion or spreading apart of the bronchi adjacent to an obstructed bronchus, failure of the side branches of the blocked bronchus to fill (Fig. 7–1), and marked bending of a bronchus.[28, 800, 842, 1309]

Commonly, a carcinoma will amputate a bronchus (Fig. 7–7E), sometimes flush with its takeoff, so that the lesion is easily missed[891, 1008, 1014] (Fig. 7–7F, G). Such an oversight is prevented by obtaining spot films or movies of the bronchus under suspicion in many projections. In fact, I believe that movies or television tape is the ideal way to record a bronchographic exploration for tumor. Not only can the affected bronchus be delineated in infinite projections, but complete respiratory fixation of the bronchial tree and lung in the vicinity of the lesion can be demonstrated, strongly supporting the diagnosis of carcinoma.[257, 1313]

TABLE 7–1.   Causes of a Tracheal Mass[387, 570]

Aberrant thyroid tissue	Invasion from adjacent malignant tumor (thyroid, esophagus, lung)
Amyloid	
Bronchial adenoma (carcinoid, cylindroma)	
Chondroma, hamartoma	Leiomyoma
Extrinsic mass (tumor, aneurysm, etc.)	Metastatic tumor
	Papilloma
Fibroma	Primary malignant neoplasm (carcinoma, lymphoma, sarcoma)
Hemangioma	
Inflammatory granuloma (tuberculosis, fungus, Wegener's)	Scleroma
	Tracheopathia osteoplastica
	Vascular ring
	Xanthoma

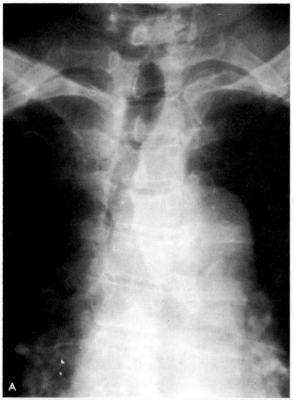

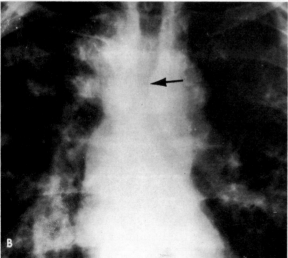

Figure 7–4. TRACHEAL CARCINOMA

A, Bucky film. *B*, Teleroentgenogram of another patient presenting with multiple aspiration lung abscesses. The carcinoma (arrow) involves the carinal region. (Courtesy of Dr. Chapin Hawley.)

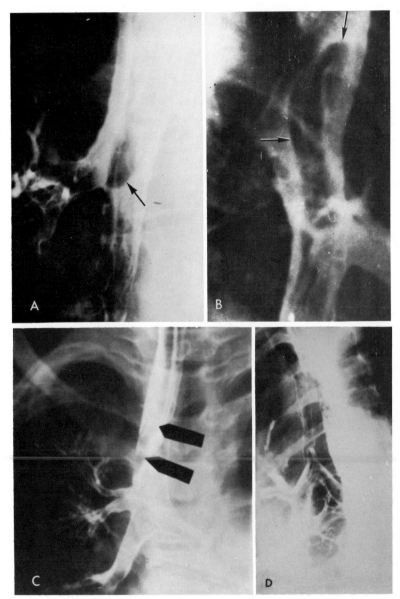

Figure 7–5. BENIGN LESIONS OF THE TRACHEA

A and B, Adenomatous polyp. A pedunculated lesion (arrows) is apparent on frontal and oblique views. The patient had recurrent bouts of pneumonia on the right. C, Cylindroma. A small defect is outlined by large arrows. (Courtesy of Dr. Charles J. Karibo.) D, Amyloidosis of trachea. (Courtesy of Dr. Dale H. Myers.)

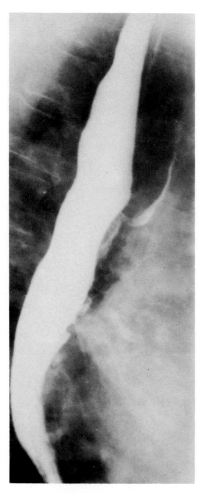

Figure 7–6. TRACHEOESOPHAGEAL FISTULA

Note the absence of a mass. At operation two fistulas were found with no surrounding inflammation. The patient was an elderly woman with chronic symptoms. Congenital?

Relative fixation is seen with inflammatory lesions, bullous emphysema,[319] and after thoracoplasty or radiation therapy, but a completely frozen pattern adjacent to an obstructed bronchus usually means malignancy.

Carcinoma of the lung doesn't always produce *localized* bronchial obstruction. As indicated elsewhere (Fig. 3–56), submucosal extension of alveolar cell and, rarely, other types of carcinoma causes diffuse constriction of the bronchi in the collapsed segment. They are squeezed to almost threadlike caliber and few of the small side branches are filled (Fig. 7–7H).

Other Bronchial Lesions

A smooth, rounded, bronchial filling defect, convex toward the hilum, usually indicates a bronchial adenoma (Fig. 7–8), sarcoma, metastatic neoplasm (Fig. 7–9), or hamartoma[203, 419, 438, 800, 1056, 1086, 1205] (Fig. 7–10). However, bronchogenic carcinoma may also sometimes cause this type of defect (Fig. 7–7I). Bronchial adenoma is said to expand the lumen of the obstructed bronchus, but this is rare in my experience. Multiple rounded defects with or without obstruction, an infrequent finding, generally indicate papillomatosis of the respiratory passages[290, 477, 1031, 1041, 1131] (Fig. 3–64), fibroepithelial polyposis,[616] amyloidosis, or neoplasm metastatic to the bronchial mucosa.[438]

An inflammatory bronchial lesion caused by tuberculosis, fungus disease, or other granuloma may exactly duplicate a carcinoma (Figs. 3–36 and 7–11) but generally produces a longer constriction. Bronchial obstruction may also occur in some cases of organized pneumonia.[65] If the bronchus proximal to an obstructing lesion is dilated or if contrast medium readily enters a cavitary lesion, inflammation is strongly suggested. Severe distortion or perforation may occur in some patients with actinomycosis[391] (Fig. 7–12) and Wegener's granuloma,[342] but in others the bronchogram is normal.

A smooth, round-bottomed termination of a large bronchus occurs in three conditions: bronchial aplasia[897] (Fig. 3–13), surgical resection, or fractured bronchus[143, 562, 803] (Fig. 3–24). The latter may be associated with a fistulous tract.

In silicosis and coalworkers' pneumoconiosis (they may even be the same disease), the large opacity, also called *conglomerate mass* or so-called *progressive massive fibrosis*, is consistently associated with an occluded bronchus (Fig. 7–13). In one patient, I mistook the bronchographic obstruction for cancer, with tragic results. I have since had the opportunity to examine a number of such lesions bronchographically and at autopsy and in not a single instance could I demonstrate a patent bronchus entering a conglomerate mass.[332] Others have had similar experience.[298, 642, 895]

An extrinsic lesion must also be considered when bronchial displacement, indentation, or complete occlusion is demonstrated.[120] Aneurysm, lymphadenopathy (Fig. 6–18), or mediastinal tumor usually causes a smooth, broad, excentric narrowing, often with displacement. Sometimes an apparently extrinsic deformity is the result of proximal peribronchial invasion by a peripheral bronchogenic carcinoma. In this situation bronchoscopic biopsy will usually be negative.

Table 7–2 is a gamut of the causes of bronchial occlusion.

Bronchial Rearrangement

In congenital absence, collapse, or surgical resection of a portion of the lung, the bronchi are displaced as the remaining pulmonary tissue accommodates itself to the vacant space. Curiously, the large bronchi rearrange themselves to simulate the pattern of the normal segmental anatomy. But because they extend over a larger area than they were designed to, the bronchi are smaller in caliber than normal segmental bronchi (Fig. 3–14).

Mucoid Impaction

Inspissated secretions, commonly mucus and inflammatory products, frequently accumulate distal to a bronchial obstruction. The bronchi distended with these secretions are generally not visible simply because the surrounding lung is collapsed and airless. The pathologist commonly sees the bronchial changes but takes them for granted and turns his attention to the obstructing lesion.

In the case of an occluded *segmental* bronchus, the lung distal to the obstruction may retain some air. The distended bronchi may then be visible as fusiform, round, or oval structures which often show branching. A bubble or two of air may be entrapped. The lesions are particularly well demonstrated by tomography.

The nature of the underlying obstruction is variable but generally of long duration. Bronchogenic carcinoma (Fig. 7–14), bronchial adenoma (Fig. 4–50), congenital bronchial atresia[435, 1198, 1252] (Fig. 7–15), and bron-chogenic cyst (Figs. 4–26 and 7–16) are the most common. The term *bronchocele* or *bronchial mucocele* has been applied to the latter two lesions.[718, 1198]

Mucoid impaction is also seen without obstruction in such chronic pulmonary conditions as bronchial asthma and other allergic states. It has been attributed to an Arthus reaction. Aspergillus sensitivity has often been found in this group[162, 808, 1307, 1335] (Figs. 7–17 and 7–18). In these sensitivity states, the mucous plugs are expectorated at intervals and new ones may appear in other parts of the lung. The emptied pockets may persist as bronchiectasis, usually of the varicose variety (Fig. 7–18C). Bronchography will sometimes bathe a mucous plug with contrast medium, outlining it in the manner of an endobronchial tumor.

In the patients with bronchial obstruction, hyperinflation of the lung may occur around the mucous impaction (Figs. 7–15 and 7–16). The reason for this, I believe, is explained by what I call the *Culiner theory.* This is a good time to discuss it.

THE CULINER THEORY

This theory, presented by Culiner and Reich in 1961,[223] is based on the following experiment:

At thoracotomy in a dog, the intact LLL was lifted through the incision and its segmental bronchi were surgically isolated. Since the endotracheal tube was open to the atmosphere, the lobe completely deflated. Partial inflation of the lobe was obtained by ventilating it through a single patent segmental bronchus under a pressure of 20 cm of water for a period of 10 minutes. The other segmental bronchi of the lobe were then clamped and totally occluded. Ventilation of the segment with the patent bronchus with a pressure of 20 cm of water again expanded it, but the occluded segments remained collapsed.

When a pressure of 40 cm of water was applied with a cycled respirator, complete aeration of both the obstructed and nonobstructed segments of the lobe was demonstrated. Obviously this must have occurred across the intersegmental plane through the collateral channels.

Finally, one of the occluded segmental
(*Text continued on page 280.*)

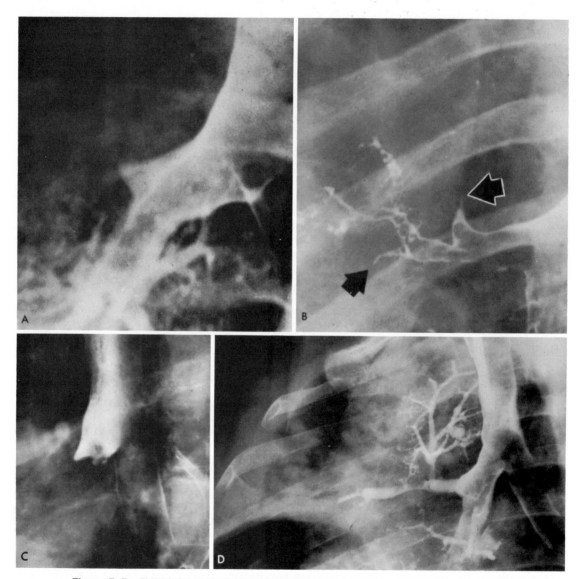

Figure 7–7. TYPES OF BRONCHOGRAPHIC DEFECT IN BRONCHOGENIC CARCINOMA

A. V shaped obstruction of RUL bronchus. *B,* Rat-tail involvement of bronchi of RUL (arrows). *C,* Irregularity with V shaped component occluding right main bronchus. *D,* Mural indentation of RUL bronchus.

(Figure continued on opposite page.)

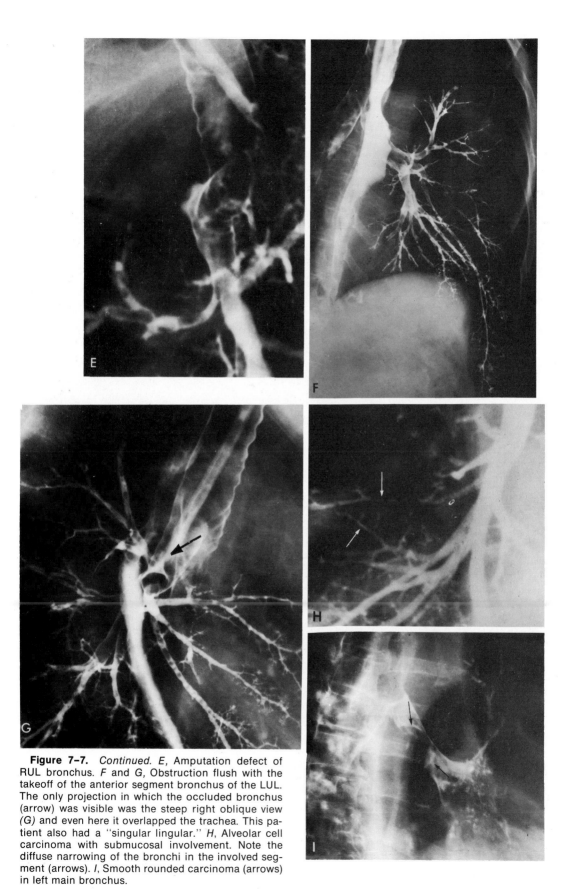

Figure 7–7. *Continued. E,* Amputation defect of RUL bronchus. *F* and *G,* Obstruction flush with the takeoff of the anterior segment bronchus of the LUL. The only projection in which the occluded bronchus (arrow) was visible was the steep right oblique view *(G)* and even here it overlapped the trachea. This patient also had a "singular lingular." *H,* Alveolar cell carcinoma with submucosal involvement. Note the diffuse narrowing of the bronchi in the involved segment (arrows). *I,* Smooth rounded carcinoma (arrows) in left main bronchus.

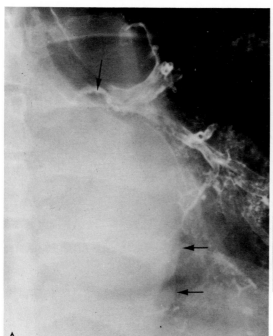

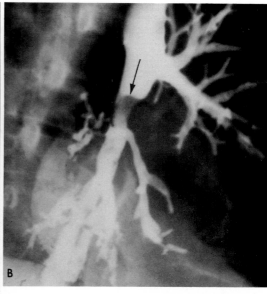

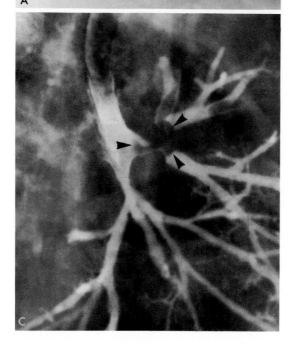

Figure 7–8.   THREE EXAMPLES OF BRON-
CHIAL ADENOMA

A, "Iceberg" tumor with a small component in
the left main stem bronchus (upper arrow) and a
huge extrabronchial mass in the LLL (lower
arrows). (Courtesy of Dr. S. Robert Graham.) *B,*
Nonobstructing adenoma in LLL bronchus
(arrow) with moderate bronchiectasis. *C,* Round
tumor in LUL bronchus (arrowheads) without obstruction. There is also extrinsic compression of
the proximal LLL bronchus.

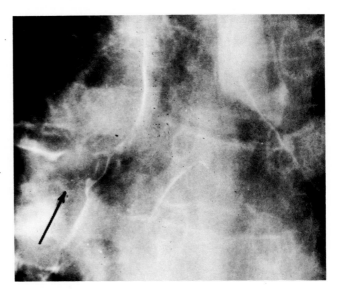

Figure 7–9. METASTATIC HYPER-
NEPHROMA IN THE RUL BRONCHUS
(arrow)

No pulmonary abnormality could be seen.

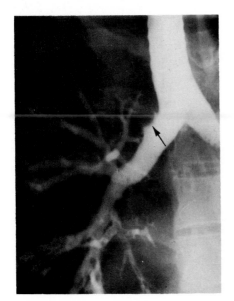

Figure 7–10. INTRABRONCHIAL HAMARTOMA

The smooth rounded defect at the takeoff of the RUL bronchus
(arrow) is associated with marked lobar collapse.

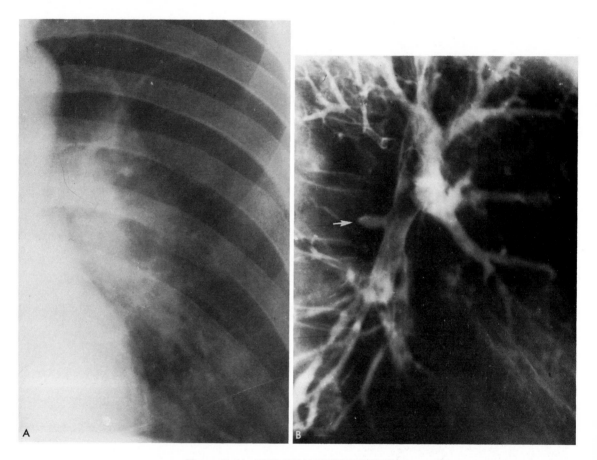

Figure 7-11.   INFLAMMATORY STRICTURE

A, Collapse of superior segment of LLL. Note preservation of pulmonary artery and left heart border. *B*, Lateral view of left bronchogram. The superior segment bronchus is occluded (arrow).

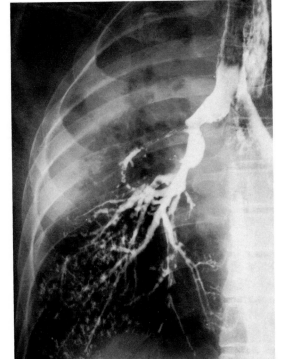

Figure 7–12. ACTINOMYCOSIS

Severe distortion of the intermediate bronchus and occlusion of the RUL bronchus. (From Flynn, M. W., and Felson, B.[391]; reproduced with permission of Charles C Thomas, Publisher.)

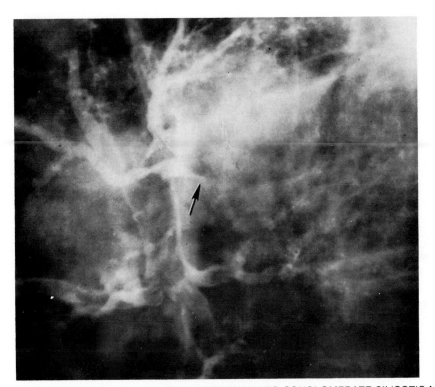

Figure 7–13. BRONCHIAL OBSTRUCTION SECONDARY TO CONGLOMERATE SILICOTIC MASS

Lateral view. The posterior segment bronchus of the RUL shows a tapered occlusion at the base of the conglomerate mass (arrow).

TABLE 7–2. *Causes of Bronchial Defect*

Common
  Agenesis
  Carcinoma
  Extrinsic pressure by lymphadenopathy,
    mediastinal tumor, aneurysm, etc.
  Inflammatory stricture or granuloma
    (tuberculosis, fungus, etc.)
  Silicotic conglomerate mass
  Surgical amputation

Rare
  Amyloidoma, plasmacytoma
  Bronchial adenoma, polyp
  Broncholith
  Foreign body, parasite
  Fractured bronchus
  Intrabronchial hamartoma
  Lymphoma, chloroma
  Mesenchymal tumor (neurofibroma, leiomyoma,
    lipoma, hemangioma, myoblastoma, etc.)
  Metastatic tumor
  Mucous plug, mucoviscidosis
  Organized pneumonia
  Papilloma
  Rhinoscleroma
  Sarcoma

bronchi was opened. This nonobstructed segment collapsed but *the obstructed segments remained inflated.* Obviously some sort of check-valve mechanism had occurred at the pores of Kohn and channels of Lambert. Marked compression had to be exerted upon these segments to cause the contained gas to escape through the collateral channels.

A similar mechanism might explain localized pulmonary hyperaeration in man. Since straining or coughing often raises the pulmonary pressure above 40 cm of water, it is possible that under the clinical circumstance of an occluded segmental bronchus, the momentarily elevated pressure might permit air to hyperdistend the blocked segment via collateral ventilation. The escape of the air might then be inhibited by the check-valve mechanism.

Culiner subsequently applied his theory to obstructive emphysema, bullous emphysema, idiopathic unilateral hyperlucent lung (Swyer-James syndrome), and bron-

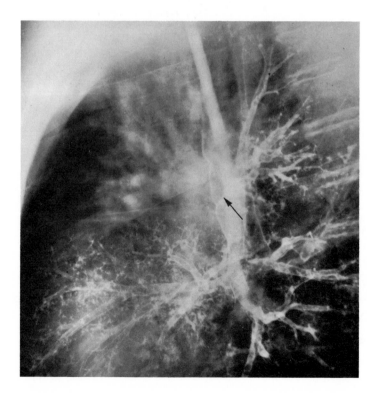

Figure 7–14. DISTENDED BRONCHI DISTAL TO A BRONCHOGENIC CARCINOMA

The anterior segment bronchus is blocked (arrow), but the segment shows neither collapse nor airlessness.

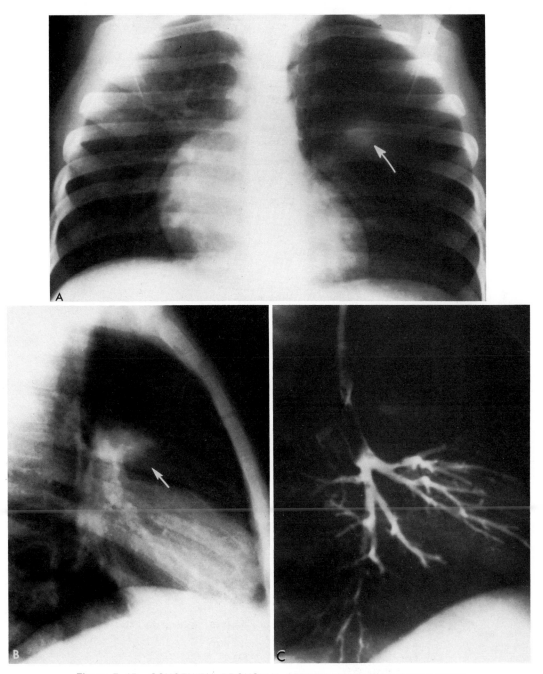

Figure 7–15.   CONGENITAL BRONCHIAL ATRESIA WITH MUCOID IMPACTION

A and *B*, The upper portion of the LUL is overdistended and the mediastinal structures are shifted to the right. Note the rounded shadow within the overinflated pulmonary tissue (arrows). *C*, Bronchogram shows congenital absence of the superior division bronchus of the LUL with overdistention of its segments. Right oblique projection. (Courtesy of Dr. John P. Dorst.)

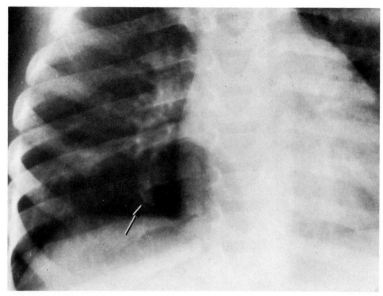

Figure 7–16. BRONCHOGENIC CYST

The mucoid impaction (arrow) lies within an aerated cyst which occupies most of the base of the RLL. At operation, no aortic vessel supplied the area. See also Figure 4–26.

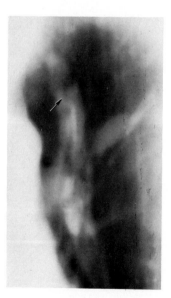

Figure 7–17. MUCOID IMPACTION WITHOUT BRONCHIAL OBSTRUCTION

The patient had intermittent episodes of an allergic nature. The tomogram shows distended branching bronchi with a few trapped air bubbles (arrow). (Courtesy of Dr. Marvin J. Rassell.)

chial cyst.[219-222] Based as it is on segmental intercommunication, the theory cannot (and need not) apply to lobar bronchial obstruction, except perhaps when an interlobar septum is incomplete. It readily explains the hyperventilation and mucous impaction seen with some cases of segmental obstruction. If the pores of Kohn are not shut off by the inflammatory changes associated with the obstruction, free access during coughing and straining permits overdistention of the lung distal to the occluded bronchus. The mucous glands, continuing their function in the bronchi beyond the obstruction, distend it with mucus.

Culiner's theory does not explain the mucoid impaction in nonobstructed bronchi. It is presumed that the excessive mucus produced by *Aspergillus fumigatus* and in allergic situations accumulates in the bronchi and inspissates in situ.

The theory is obviously a simplistic one, but it does appear to fit essentially every situation, and no other hypothesis that I'm aware of, including the newer surfactant theories, does.

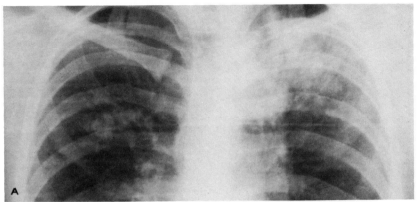

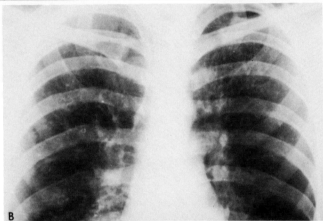

Figure 7–18. MUCOID IM-
PACTION IN ASPERGILLUS
SENSITIVITY

A, Infiltrate in both upper
lungs. Note the lobulated appearance on the right. *B,* Several months later the upper
lungs have cleared, leaving faint
radiolucencies. There are now
lobulated lesions in the midthird of the right lung laterally.
C, Bronchogram, showing varicose bronchiectasis in the RUL.
(Courtesy of Dr. G. S. Maresh.)

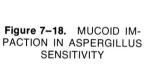

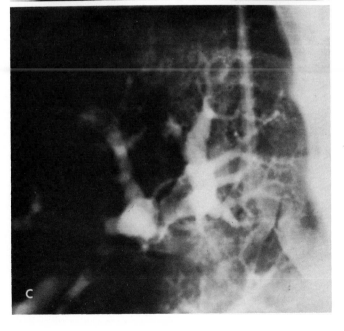

THE SMALL BRONCHI

This section deals with bronchi of a diameter of 2 or 3 mm and less. Although occlusion of bronchi of this size by carcinoma and other lesions does occur, the site and configuration of the obstruction is almost impossible to see on bronchography.

Bronchiectasis

Bronchiectasis comes in a variety of shapes and sizes. And classifications. So far as I am concerned, there are only five types of bronchiectasis: cylindrical, saccular, cystic, varicose, and bronchiolar.

CYLINDRICAL BRONCHIECTASIS

Also called *tubular and fusiform*, this type of bronchiectasis shows little change in caliber as the bronchi subdivide. Thus, each affected branch is about the same width as its parent, and its lumen is of more or less uniform diameter throughout its extent. Each dilated bronchus appears occluded at its distal extremity so that there is no "alveolization" (Fig. 3–27).

Cylindrical bronchiectasis may revert to normal and so, depending on your definition, may not be bronchiectasis at all, at least when it is impermanent. If you consider *bronchiectasis* to mean dilatation of a bronchus, then *reversible bronchiectasis* is an acceptable term. If you include infection in your definition, then call this form *pseudobronchiectasis*.[78]

The cause of the dilated bronchi in reversible bronchiectasis is related to the associated pulmonary collapse. What happens to bronchi in segmental or lobar collapse? Obviously they must shorten to accommodate to the smaller size of the affected lung. In so doing, they become wider and yet retain their cylindrical configuration (Fig. 3–28). There is a children's puzzle called "Chinese Torture" which illustrates this clearly. When the child inserts a finger in each end of the woven tubular toy, he cannot extract them by pulling since the tube then elongates and narrows, gripping the two fingers more tightly. When he shortens the tube by pushing his hands together, the lumen widens and permits him to extricate his fingers.

SACCULAR BRONCHIECTASIS

This form is associated with severe bronchial infection, often with expectoration of foul smelling pus. In pre-antibiotic days, there were many unfortunate sufferers, and surgical resection was their only salvation. In fact, the "lung-mapping" bronchographic technique was developed to demonstrate the extent and location of the disease for the surgeon. Today we seldom see severe saccular bronchiectasis.

The diameter of the saccules is distinctly greater than that of the normal caliber parent bronchus. Again, bronchographic filling of the finer lung structure distal to the dilated bronchi is never seen (Figs. 2–47 and 7–19).

CYSTIC BRONCHIECTASIS

Cystic bronchiectasis is probably always an acquired disease; at least I've never heard of it in the newborn and have watched it develop as a sequela of histoplasmosis and tuberculosis. Furthermore, it is much more frequent in adults than in children. It is seldom associated with severe pulmonary suppuration, although milder in-

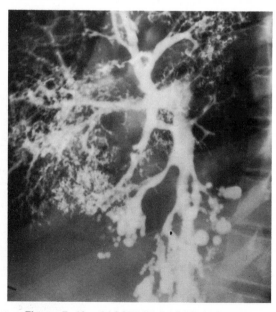

Figure 7–19. SACCULAR BRONCHIECTASIS

The RML and RLL are collapsed. No "alveolar" filling is seen distal to the dilated bronchi. The apparent constriction in the RML bronchus was inconstant.

fection is frequently present. The cystic cavities, which may be very large, are fed by normal bronchi and often look like balloons on a stick (Figs. 7–3 and 7–20). Often there is a small amount of fluid in some of the cysts. There is striking dilatation of the bronchi on inspiration and collapse on expiration [257, 401, 589, 1333] (Fig. 1–7). Bullae, with which bronchiectatic cysts are readily confused, neither fill with contrast medium nor alter significantly on respiration.

VARICOSE BRONCHIECTASIS

In this type, the dilated bronchi assume a beaded, ampullary, or irregular contour, like varicose veins. It affects predominantly the segmental and subsegmental bronchi and often spares the small peripheral branches (Fig. 7–21). Thus, there is a normal bronchial pattern distal to the bronchiectasis.[401, 852] I used to believe, along with Fleischner, that bronchiectatic bronchi were always obstructed distally. Varicose bronchiectasis is an obvious exception to this rule.

The cause of this uncommon form of bronchiectasis is unknown. It may be associated with emphysema and chronic bronchitis, and is the rule in unilateral hyperlucent lung (Swyer-James syndrome) (Fig. 5–37).

BRONCHIOLAR BRONCHIECTASIS (BRONCHIOLECTASIS)

This will be discussed in the next section.

THE DISTAL AIRWAYS

Chronic Bronchitis

Chronic bronchitis is considered a disease entity by British physicians, and their concepts have been widely accepted in the United States. It is currently defined as a clinical condition associated with severe chronic cough, expectoration of large quantities of mucus, and progressive dyspnea.

The plain film findings, consisting of mild overinflation, "increased markings," and

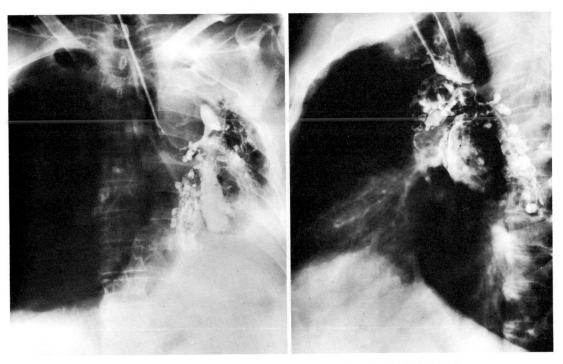

Figure 7–20. CYSTIC BRONCHIECTASIS IN INACTIVE TUBERCULOSIS

The entire left lung is greatly shrunken. The heart and overexpanded right lung extend far into the left thorax. The patient had severe fibrocavitary tuberculosis many years ago.

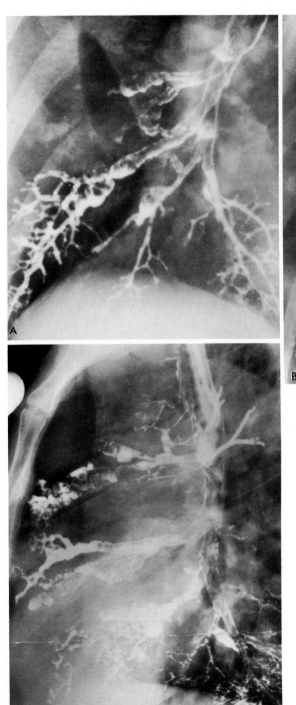

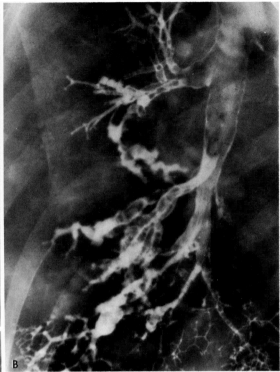

Figure 7–21.   VARICOSE BRONCHIECTASIS

Left oblique and lateral projections. Some of the bronchi show ampullary or irregular dilatation *(A and B)*, others have a beaded appearance *(C)*. Note that the dilatation is confined to the larger bronchi and that the smaller distal bronchi are normal.

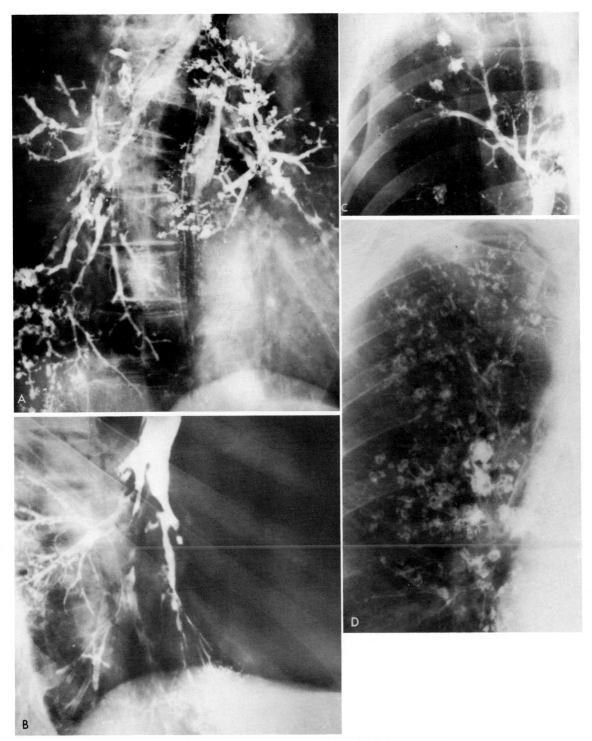

Figure 7–22. FOUR EXAMPLES OF CHRONIC BRONCHITIS

A, "Broken bough" and "hanging fruit" patterns are shown. There is mild varicose bronchiectasis in the RUL. *B,* Huge bullae occupy much of the lung, interfering with peripheral filling. *C,* "Mimosa" pattern in the RUL. Is a mimosa a starfish? *D,* "Flower" pattern in most of the right lung. It looks more like alphabet soup to me (with a few matzo balls added).

"tramlines," are vague and unreliable. The bronchographic picture (Fig. 7–22) has been described by many writers, often in terms replete with botanical references.[41, 186, 253, 277, 721, 868, 949, 967, 968, 977, 1309, 1326] The findings include:

(1) Multiple serrations or diverticulum-like projections along the wall of the trachea and larger bronchi, attributed either to filling of mucous glands or to inter-cartilaginous atrophy of smooth muscle folds (Fig. 7–3).

(2) Decreased caliber of the larger bronchi, poor peripheral filling, and the "broken bough" appearance (Fig. 7–22A and B). These are caused by irregular distribution of the contrast medium in the bronchial tree because of spasm, mucus, and emphysema.[721]

(3) Varicose bronchiectasis with a rosary pattern[949, 967] (Fig. 7–21). Cylindrical, saccular, or cystic bronchiectasis may be present, but some think it is coincidental (Fig. 7–3).

(4) Bronchiolectasis, appearing as tiny round or oval pools of contrast medium that hang like fruit or acorns from the smaller twigs of the bronchial tree[1326] (Fig. 7–22A).

(5) Small irregular globs of contrast medium—the *mimosa, lily of the valley,* or *flower pattern*[253, 721] (Fig. 7–22C and D)—said to represent pooling in pockets of centrilobular emphysema.[977]

(6) Overdistended lungs and/or emphysema (Fig. 7–22B).

The assumption that these signs are reliable evidence of symptomatic chronic bronchitis worries me because I have encountered a number of incidental examples during bronchography for carcinoma and other conditions. Admittedly, these patients may have had preexisting bronchitis overlooked by the history taker, but I have personally checked with several patients and could not elicit a story of significant chronic cough, expectoration, or dyspnea.

THE BRONCHIOLO-ALVEOLAR SYSTEM

Anatomy

This section deals with the finer anatomic structures of the lung. I would like to begin by quoting a beautifully lucid, unpublished description by Dr. Longstreet C. Hamilton, written in 1967 when he was Chief of Radiology at Walter Reed Hospital:[496]

"The primary or respiratory lobule is the unit of functioning tissue of the lung. It cannot be neatly packaged, and it is strange that many hot anatomical arguments have raged over this respiratory lobule. One begins with a lobar bronchus which divides into smaller and smaller branches until the terminal bronchiole is reached—the last part of the bronchial tree lined with cuboidal epithelium, having no cartilage and giving off no alveoli.[953] The desire in most orderly minds for this division to occur in a strict succession of symmetrical dichotomies may account for some confusion, because the bronchial tree does not do this. A very large second order bronchus may sprout tiny bronchi, branching immediately into terminal bronchioles which eventuate in primary lobules of varying sizes, on a "space available" basis, quite close to the hilum. The same process occurs also in the succeeding third to sixth order bronchi. At this stage, all the airways are reaching terminal bronchiole size (about 1 mm) and this marks the end of the supporting or conducting bronchus. Reid has shown with bronchograms and histologic sections of the periphery of the lung that when little branches begin to occur within 2 mm of each other they are usually terminal bronchioles.[980]

"Each terminal bronchiole (Fig. 7–23A and B) gives rise to 2 or 3 respiratory bronchioles, so named because they have functional alveoli within their walls. Depending on available space, the respiratory bronchiole may branch 2 or 3 times, each branch having 2 or more alveolar ducts. Each duct has 2 to 6 air sacs from which the alveoli hang like grapes from a stem. The single respiratory bronchiole with its alveolar ducts, air sacs, and alveoli comprise the primary lobule.[835] However, disproportionate space-available branching of bronchi results in wide variability of pattern of these ultimate units of respiratory tissue.

"The secondary lobules vary in size and tend to be larger and more uniform in the periphery of the lobes of the lung. The lobules are roughly pyramidal in shape, and measure a centimeter, more or less, across the base, and a centimeter in height. Those in the periphery may reach 2 or 3 cm in height, and are further distinguished by the fact that they have fairly complete and regular septa bounding them. The central ones are more irregular in shape and volume and are jumbled up with large bronchi and blood vessels. If there is much in the way of functional septa in these central lobules, they are hard to find."

Each secondary lobule contains three to five acini.[524, 954, 1066] The acinus is about a half centimeter in diameter and generally contains four to five primary lobules. The alveoli are about 0.2 mm in diameter.[111, 116, 970, 974] The alveoli have many intercommunications via the pores of Kohn, occasional connections with bronchioles via the channels of Lambert (Fig. 7–23C and D), and rare interacinar anastomoses.[114, 115]

The peripheral part of the airway in a normal bronchogram consists of eight to ten subdivisions of segmental bronchi, each branch occurring at an interval of 2.5 to 1.0 cm until at the very periphery branching occurs every 2 to 3 mm. Reid and Simon call these the *centimeter* and *millimeter* patterns, respectively.[977] The centimeter pattern represents bronchi and larger bronchioles while the millimeter pattern represents the terminal bronchioles.

The Disseminated Alveolar Pattern

From a roentgen standpoint, widespread pulmonary disease usually presents one of four basic patterns: *vascular, alveolar, interstitial,* or *destructive.* Pure vascular involvement—further divisible into arterial (pulmonary, bronchial), venous, and lymphatic—is usually readily recognized (Chap. 5). The same applies to many cases in the destructive group (Chap. 8), in which there is contiguous involvement of the alveoli, interstitial tissue, bronchi, and vessels. Here cavitation and irregular destruction of the gross architecture indicate the *en bloc* nature of the lesion. On the other hand, interstitial involvement often goes unrecognized, even though fine sharp nodulation or a honeycomb appearance is reliable indication of its presence (Chap. 8). As to the roentgen pattern in alveolar diseases, only a few serious attempts have been made to lay down criteria for its recognition.

The importance of being able to distinguish between these types of distribution becomes apparent when you consider that there are several hundred different diseases capable of producing disseminated lesions in the lung.[21, 140, 323, 352, 466, 653] With so many possibilities, what's the chance of a useful differential diagnosis? The only hope is to apply a discriminatory approach, to subdivide into patterns, and thereby reduce the long list of possibilities. Such an approach is particularly applicable to the alveolar diseases. I base this precept on my conviction that it is usually possible to identify alveolar involvement roentgenographically. A number of roentgen signs have proved reliable in this respect.

ROENTGEN SIGNS

The margins of alveolar infiltrates are fluffy and ill defined, like cotton candy, except where they abut upon a pleural surface. The wispy edges fade imperceptibly into the surrounding normal lung (Fig. 7–24). The fluffiness is attributable to irregular interdigitation of completely involved groups of alveoli with adjacent partially involved or normal groups.

Rarely, a similar fluffiness is seen with metastatic neoplasm. Metastases ordinarily originate in the interstitial tissue and enlarge concentrically, nearly always remaining sharply outlined as they compress rather than infiltrate the adjacent alveoli. However, certain tumors, particularly metastatic choriocarcinoma, sometimes liberate an endocrine substance, perhaps a gonadotropin,[308] which incites a halo of hemorrhage in the surrounding lung. And where is this hemorrhage? In the alveoli, of course; and this is what is responsible for the fluffy outline (Fig. 7–25).

Coalescence is another important feature of alveolar disease (Figs. 7–25 and 7–26). Individual small or large lesions blend with adjacent ones as the intervening alveoli become involved. Although coalescence may also occur with interstitial lesions, it is not so striking and is a late phenomenon. The coalescence of destructive lesions is attributable, at least in part, to the alveolar component.

At times, the widespread pulmonary process may involve a segment or a lobe completely. While the interstitial tissues and vessels may be involved concomitantly,

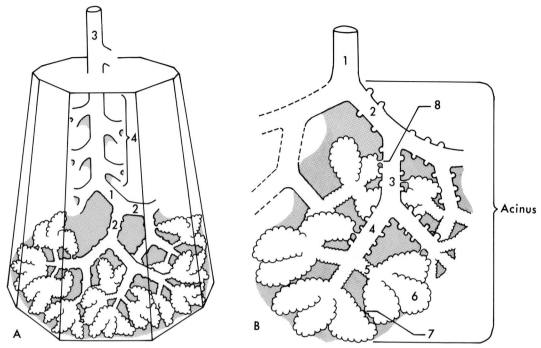

Figure 7–23. ANATOMIC STRUCTURE OF LUNG

A, Diagrammatic representation of a secondary pulmonary lobule and its contents. (1), Terminal bronchiole. (2), Respiratory bronchiole, first order. (3), Lobular bronchus. (4), Intralobular bronchioli. B, Diagrammatic representation of an acinus. (1), Terminal bronchiole. (2) to (4), Respiratory bronchiole, first, second, and third orders. (5), Alveolar duct. (6), Alveolar sac. (7), Pore of Kohn. (8), Channel of Lambert.

(Figure continued on opposite page.)

the preponderant lesion must be alveolar, since, after all, what is a segment or lobe if not a mass of alveoli? Relevant to the present discussion, then, recognizable segmental or lobar distribution is another sign of alveolar disease (Fig. 7–27).

The "butterfly" or "bat's wing" shadow (Figs. 7–24 and 7–27) is a widespread, bilaterally symmetrical infiltration which is prominent in the central portion of each lung and fades toward the periphery. The apex, base, and lateral margin of each lung are relatively spared. There may be clear areas on both sides of the minor fissure and adjacent to the superior mediastinum.[552, 955, 987] (Fig. 7–28).

This roentgen sign is extremely common. The reason for the central distribution is not clear. It has also been demonstrated in the lateral projection (Fig. 7–29) but some disagree on this point.[444] I have in several instances confirmed the central location at the autopsy table.[36, 378, 537, 646]

The butterfly shadow is not always ho-

mogeneous but often consists of large, blotchy, ill-defined, coalescent densities interspersed with relatively small areas of normal lung tissue. The infiltrate presents the same fluffy outline as other forms of alveolar disease. Rarely the sign may be unilateral, a one-winged butterfly as it were[875] (Fig. 7–30). The butterfly wings often extend to the pulmonary periphery in some areas; sometimes both lungs appear *totally* involved. Occasionally, the shadows are confined to the upper or lower half of the two lung fields (Fig. 2–42).

The classic butterfly shadow used to be considered pathognomonic of uremic pulmonary edema. This is obviously a false presumption; it is not even diagnostic of pulmonary edema, although this is by far its commonest cause. It signifies one thing and one thing only: extensive alveolar disease.

The presence of an *air bronchogram* (Chap. 2) provides another reliable sign for the recognition of alveolar disease, and a common one[7, 25, 26] (Figs. 7–27 and 7–28). It (*Text continued on page* 295.)

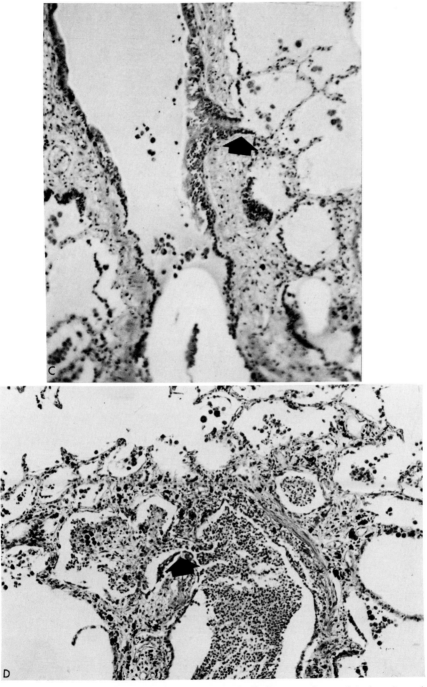

Figure 7–23. *Continued. C,* Channel of Lambert (arrow). *D,* Pneumonic exudate in a bronchiole passing through a channel of Lambert (arrow) into a peribronchial alveolus. (Courtesy of Recavarren, S., Benton, C., and Gall, E. A.[970]; reproduced with permission of Seminars in Roentgenology.)

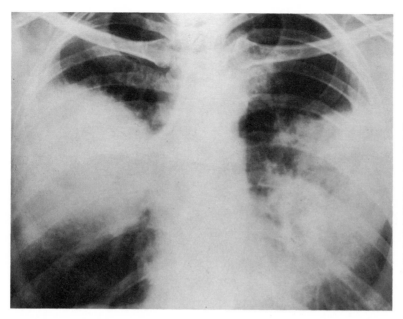

Figure 7–24. ALVEOLAR LYMPHOMA WITH FLUFFY MARGINS

The wispy, ill-defined borders are a common sign of alveolar disease. The butterfly is flitting across the page. Its left wing is marked by an air bronchogram. The patient received a course of radiation therapy and remained in good health for 8 years, finally succumbing to disseminated lymphoma. (From Felson, B.[333]; reproduced with permission of Seminars in Roentgenology.)

Figure 7–25. METASTATIC CHORIOCARCINOMA WITH FLUFFY MARGINS

Hemorrhage into the alveoli surrounding the metastatic nodules accounted for the ill-defined margins and coalescence. (Courtesy of Dr. Robert N. Berk.)

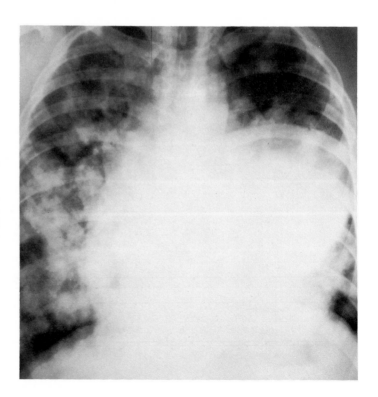

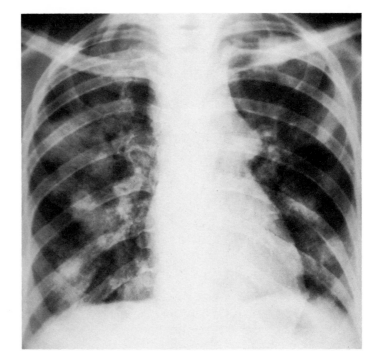

Figure 7–26. COALESCENCE IN THE ALVEOLAR FORM OF SARCOID

The large densities show fluffy outlines as well. Mediastinal lymphadenopathy is present.

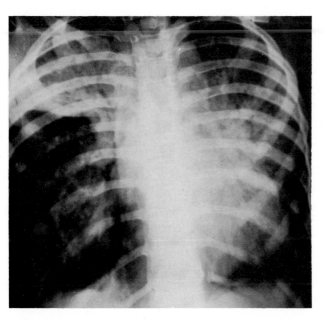

Figure 7–27. LOBAR INVOLVEMENT WITH DISSEMINATED PNEUMONIA

This child also had severe congenital heart disease and chickenpox. The RUL is completely consolidated. Note also the fluffy margins and butterfly distribution of the pneumonia elsewhere in the lungs, and the air bronchogram. Autopsy revealed a bacterial pneumonia. (From Felson, B.[333]; reproduced with permission of Seminars in Roentgenology.)

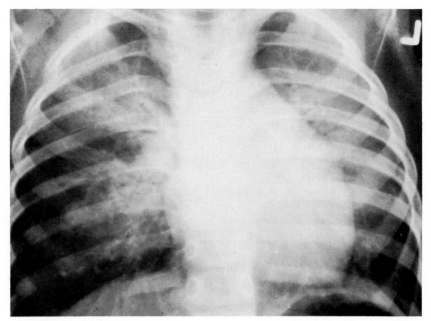

Figure 7–28. CLASSIC BUTTERFLY PATTERN IN ALVEOLAR PROTEINOSIS IN A CHILD

Note again the fluffy margins and the faint air bronchogram. The infiltrate fades peripherally in the apices, bases, and lateral lung margins. The areas on both sides of the minor fissure and adjacent to the superior mediastinum also show relatively less involvement. Autopsy proof.

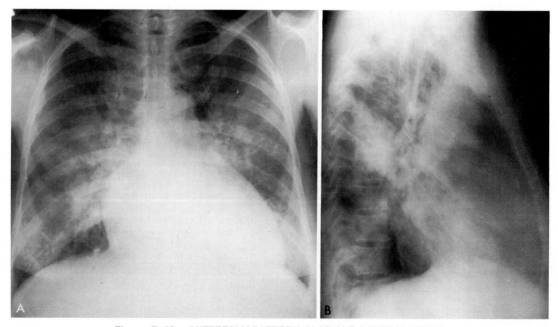

Figure 7–29. BUTTERFLY PATTERN IN AP AND LATERAL VIEWS

Note the central location of the pulmonary edema in both views. Congestive failure.

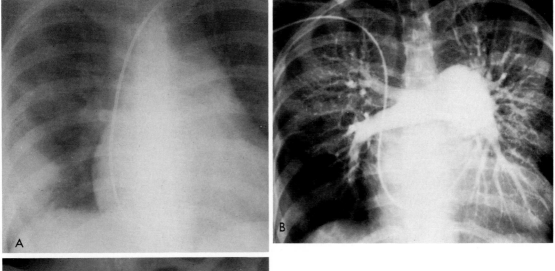

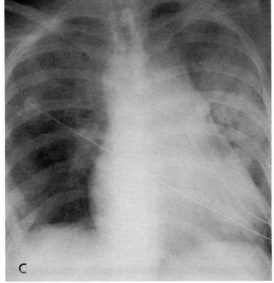

Figure 7–30. UNILATERAL PULMONARY EDEMA

A, Right pulmonary infarct. *B*, Pulmonary angiogram showing blocked branches of right inferior pulmonary artery. *C*, 2 weeks later. Terminal episode of acute pulmonary edema sparing most of the right lung. Autopsy confirmation.

results when air filled bronchi become surrounded by infiltrate. And what surrounds bronchi? Alveoli, of course.

To carry this concept one step further, small areas of uninvolved lung interspersed between involved groups of alveoli are often visible as irregular radiolucencies within the infiltrate, giving a mottled appearance. This *air alveologram* (Chap. 2) is most typically seen in resolving pneumonia, but is common in other forms of alveolar disease as well (Figs. 2–51 and 7–31). Tiny areas of lung destruction, dilated bronchi, honeycombing, and preexisting small bullae surrounded by infiltrate all may simulate

the air alveologram.[569, 1105, 1343] Therefore, only when the sign is quite definite do I consider it indicative of alveolar involvement. It is commonly associated with an air bronchogram, which is a more reliable sign.

Ziskind, Weill, and Payzant have called attention to what they term the *acinus nodule* as an indicator of alveolar disease.[1345] This refers to the acinus of Loeschcke,[755] defined as a unit of lung composed of a single terminal bronchiole and all its subdivisions, including several orders of respiratory bronchioles and their alveolar ducts, sacs, and alveoli (Fig. 7–23). There are said to be 80,000 acini in the human lung.[115] The

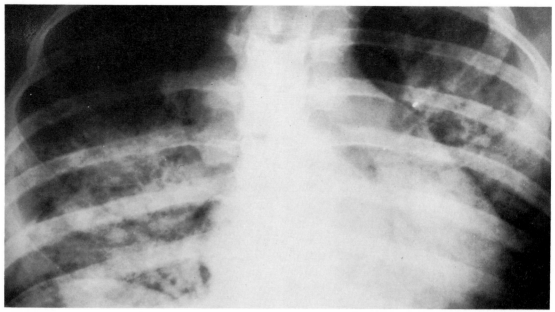

Figure 7-31. THE AIR ALVEOLOGRAM IN WIDESPREAD PNEUMONIA

Finely branching air filled bronchi are also evident.

acinar lesion was described pathologically many years ago by Aschoff in connection with tuberculosis. He noted in this disease that the acinar nodule represented an exudative alveolar lesion.[18]

The roentgen counterpart of the acinar lesion is typically illustrated by the so-called "alveolar flooding" which occurs during bronchography (Fig. 7–32). Ziskind and his group believe that the small, ill-defined, rosette-like collections of contrast medium usually represent acini.*[1345]

The presence of nodules of this size and configuration has proved to be a frequent and reliable indication of alveolar disease. I have, with Ziskind, assumed them to be acinar lesions. However, Recavarran, Benton, and Gall of my own institution have presented strong evidence that these nodular densities are often not related to the acini at all but represent peribronchiolar consolidations[970] (Fig. 7–33). Although true acinar nodules must actually occur, as in the

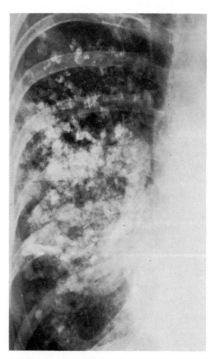

Figure 7-32. ALVEOLAR FLOODING FOLLOWING NORMAL LIPIODOL BRONCHOGRAPHY

The small nodular aggregates of contrast medium are believed to represent acini.[1345]

---

*However, Reid and Simon[977] have demonstrated that the bronchographic medium usually stops in the terminal bronchioles and seldom enters the acini.

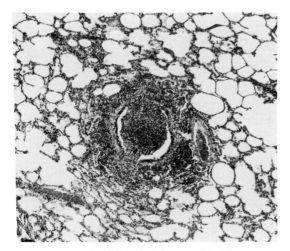

Figure 7–33. ALVEOLAR NODULE

There is a peribronchiolar arrangement and irregular involvement of the marginal alveoli surrounding the bronchiole. (Courtesy of Recavarren, S., Benton, C., and Gall, E. A.[970]; reproduced with permission of Seminars in Roentgenology.)

aspiration of contrast media or other substances, they are apparently uncommon. Henceforth, I plan to be noncommital and call these densities *alveolar nodules*.

The nodules range in diameter from about 1.0 to 1.5 cm and have ill-defined margins. They are often visible in the thinner, peripheral regions of widespread alveolar infiltrates but sometimes constitute the predominant lesion (Figs. 7–34 and 7–35). Alveolar nodules are considerably larger and show a greater tendency to coalesce than do so-called *interstitial nodules* as seen in pneumoconiosis, miliary tuberculosis, and histoplasmosis.

The "timing" of acute alveolar lesions is often different from that of acute interstitial lesions; that is to say, the time between the onset of symptoms and the first roentgen appearance of infiltrate is shorter with alveolar disease.[999] The best explanation for this is that the alveolar air is *replaced* by alveolar exudate, whereas the alveoli are *compressed* by intramural (interstitial) exudate. Replacement obliterates the alveolar air more readily and more completely than compression, so that water density in the affected area appears earlier with alveolar than with interstitial disease. This also probably explains why alveolar involvement generally appears to be more radiopaque than interstitial involvement and

why its extension and regression seem to be demonstrated sooner.

To take an example, in alveolar pneumonia, positive roentgen findings appear earlier after the onset of symptoms, change more rapidly, and are more striking than in acute miliary tuberculosis. However, so seldom is a chest roentgenogram obtained in the early stages of disease that the value of this sign is limited.

Table 7–3 summarizes the roentgen signs that constitute the alveolar pattern. Several of them are usually present in the individual patient, but almost any one of them, properly interpreted, can stand alone as reliable evidence of alveolar involvement.

The recognition of the alveolar signs requires films of good technical quality with adequate penetration of the diseased areas. Oblique and lateral views and especially Bucky films are helpful; tomography is occasionally of value. The thinner areas and peripheral margins of the infiltrate should be scrutinized, as they often provide the key findings.

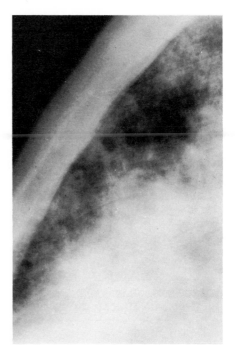

Figure 7–34. PERIBRONCHIOLAR NODULES IN ALVEOLAR PROTEINOSIS

The poorly defined nodules measure from 0.5 to 1.0 cm in diameter. There is extensive coalescence. An air alveologram is seen within some of the densities.

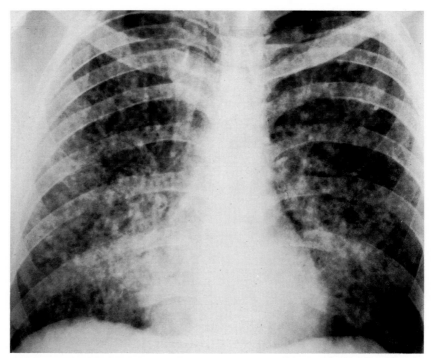

Figure 7–35. PERIBRONCHIOLAR NODULES IN CHICKENPOX PNEUMONIA IN AN ADULT

The nodules are larger than those of miliary tuberculosis or other interstitial granulomas. Except for debilitated children, especially those receiving steroids, radiation therapy, chemotherapy, or antibiotics, chickenpox pneumonia is a disease of adults.

Problems in differentiating the alveolar from the interstitial and mixed patterns do arise, and rather often. The normal lung spaces between closely packed alveolar or interstitial lesions may resemble honeycombing, and it is sometimes difficult to decide which are the lesions, the opacities or the lucencies. Similar problems arise in distinguishing small alveolar nodules from large interstitial ones. Further, interstitial nodules may break into alveoli, producing coalescence and making the distinction from primary alveolar disease impossible.

TABLE 7–3. Roentgen Signs That Indicate Alveolar Disease

Fluffy margins
Early coalescence
Segmental or lobar distribution
Butterfly shadow
Air bronchogram or alveologram
Alveolar nodules
Rapid timing

As stated earlier, the air alveologram may be simulated by a variety of other pulmonary radiolucencies surrounded by infiltrate. One more caution: the alveolar pattern often obscures a concomitant interstitial or vascular involvement; for example, the signs of alveolar edema usually overshadow those of interstitial edema and of pulmonary venous congestion.

To avoid mistakes, one is well advised to disregard any individual alveolar sign which is atypical or uncertain. If you're not sure, don't commit yourself! Despite the difficulties, however, a broad experience with clinical cases plus a relatively limited experience with histologic correlation indicate to me that when the alveolar signs are clear-cut they have a high degree of reliability.

The attempt to distinguish the alveolar pattern from other patterns is a fascinating game with practical implications. The differential diagnosis of disseminated pulmonary diseases often depends on the accuracy with which the alveolar pattern can be identified. Relatively few conditions produce it and these will now be briefly discussed.

DISSEMINATED ALVEOLAR DISEASES

Widespread alveolar involvement is encountered in a variety of unrelated diseases.[478, 807] I have found it quite useful to classify these diseases into acute and chronic subdivisions and to group similar conditions together (Table 7–4).

CAUSES OF WIDESPREAD ACUTE ALVEOLAR INVOLVEMENT

Pulmonary Edema. Of the acute conditions, pulmonary edema is by far the most common. There are many causes of pulmonary edema (Table 7–5) and the alveolar pattern may be seen with any of them. One cannot reliably diagnose the cause of the edema on the basis of the pulmonary pattern alone. We once reviewed the chest films of 15 unselected patients with unquestionable pulmonary edema, of whom six had uremia. We were unable to predict from the roentgen appearance alone which ones had azotemia. Cardiac enlargement was present in some of the uremics; the butterfly distribution was just as classic among the nonuremics. The roentgen changes in uremia did not parallel the nitrogen retention level.

TABLE 7–4. Disseminated Alveolar Diseases

ACUTE
  Common
    Pulmonary edema
    Pneumonia of unusual etiology
    Hyaline membrane disease, aspiration syndrome, transient tachypnea of the newborn
  Rare
    Pulmonary hemorrhage (trauma, anticoagulants, idiopathic hemosiderosis, Goodpasture's syndrome, etc.)
CHRONIC
  Not-so-rare
    Sarcoidosis
    Tuberculosis, fungus disease
    Alveolar cell carcinoma
    Lymphoma
    Alveolar proteinosis
  Rare
    Hair spray pneumonia
    Desquamative pneumonitis, lymphocytic interstitial pneumonitis
    Mineral oil aspiration
    Alveolar microlithiasis
    Histiocytosis X

TABLE 7–5. Some Causes of Pulmonary Edema[36, 467, 506, 847, 875, 1303]

Common
  Agonal
  Aspiration
  Cardiac—congestive failure, pulmonary venous obstruction, hypoplastic left heart syndrome, etc.
  Cerebral disorders[990] (stroke, head trauma, epilepsy, postictus,[175, 571] brain tumor)
  Drug reactions[124] (nitrofurantoin,[590, 858] Myleran, penicillin)
  Excessive parenteral fluids
  Fat embolism,[71] lymphography[236]
  Inhalation of noxious gases[282, 663, 805]
  Poisoning,[85, 991] intravenous narcotics[4a, 148]
  Pulmonary embolism or infarction
  Thoracic trauma, "shock lung"[495a]
  Uremia

Rare
  Allergic reactions
  Connective tissue disorders (periarteritis, lupus)
  Hanging and suffocation
  High altitude[506]
  Hypoproteinemia
  Malaria
  Near drowning
  Oxygen toxicity
  Pneumothorax with thoracentesis
  Thyroid storm[1010]
  Transfusion reaction

In several instances, the edema cleared despite progressive elevation of the serum urea nitrogen.

Occasionally, the infiltrate in pulmonary edema is blotchy, miliary, or nodular[847] (Fig. 7–36). When associated with signs of allergy, the latter has been called *pulmonary hives.*[1258] As already noted, the edema may be confined to the upper or lower lung fields on the roentgenogram (Fig. 2–42). Upper lobe distribution seems to occur more often with cerebral conditions.[321] A monolobar edema is also occasionally found.

Unilateral distribution of pulmonary edema has been attributed to underperfusion of the nonedematous lung because of embolism (Fig. 7–30), emphysema, or preexisting pleural disease, or to lying on the affected side during a bout of congestive failure.[33, 374, 421] Another interesting cause is the rapid aspiration of a large quantity of air or fluid from the pleural sac[1229] (Fig. 7–37).

Pulmonary venous congestion does not necessarily coexist with edema. When both are present, a cardiac origin of the edema is likely. As already noted, the congestion may be obscured by the alveolar edema. Simi-

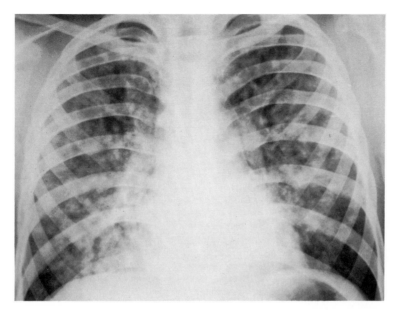

Figure 7–36. NODULAR PUL-
    MONARY EDEMA

Several hours after a transfusion reaction. The signs and
symptoms of acute pulmonary
edema were present. Two days
later the chest was normal.

larly, other related conditions, such as infarction, are often hidden.

Interstitial edema often portends the
development of widespread alveolar
edema.[345, 468, 473] The interstitial edema is
recognizable by the presence of Kerley's
lines, peribronchial and perivascular cuff-

ing, and diffuse thickening of the
pleura.[444, 516]

Pulmonary edema usually develops and
disappears quickly. In nonfatal cases, clearing generally begins at the periphery and is
usually complete within three to nine days.
Roentgen improvement is distinctly faster

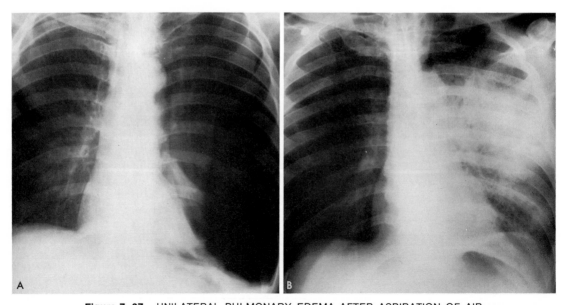

Figure 7–37. UNILATERAL PULMONARY EDEMA AFTER ASPIRATION OF AIR

A, Spontaneous left pneumothorax. *B,* Left pulmonary edema the day after removal of the pleural air.

than in pneumonia. The rapid, almost day-to-day change in the roentgenogram is very helpful in differential diagnosis, but pneumonia complicating the edema may slow down the rate of clearing.[1023] Physical findings may be meager and the widespread roentgen alteration sometimes comes as a complete surprise to the clinician.

Pneumonia. Pneumonia is also a common cause of widespread acute alveolar disease. Interestingly, these extensive pneumonias are usually of "off-beat" etiology, i.e., they are not caused by the common pneumonia producing organisms (Table 7–6). Thus, in the acutely ill, febrile patient with widespread alveolar pattern, a diagnosis of pneumonia of unusual type can be made with reasonable assurance. It often represents an opportunistic infection following suppression of the immune mechanisms by congenital, induced, or acquired disease, or after intensive treatment with antibiotics, chemotherapeutic agents, cortisone, or radiation. The specific causative factor of the pneumonia can usually be established on clinical or laboratory grounds (Fig. 7–38). A reversal of the butterfly pattern, i.e., alveolar infiltrate peripherally and clear lung centrally, has been reported in eosinophilic pneumonia,[165, 1021] the so-called PIE or pulmonary infiltrate with eosinophilia. I have seen several such cases, cause unknown, which responded almost miraculously to cortisone (Fig. 7–39). If the steroid is discontinued too early, recurrence will take place in the original location. The belief that viral pneumonia is interstitial in location is widely held but fallacious. Although this type of pneumonia may *start* as an interstitial process, by the time it becomes radiologically apparent, it is mainly alveolar.[446]

Other Causes. In the newborn, hyaline membrane disease,[431, 508, 807] aspiration syndrome, and transient tachypnea*[680, 1192, 1276] commonly present a widespread alveolar pattern. I have had little experience with hyaline membrane disease in the adult, although we have seen it in some of our patients receiving high concentration of oxygen via the respirator.[849]

Extensive hemorrhage in the lung may occur from a variety of causes,[478, 807] including direct thoracic trauma,[1301] blast injury, cardiac operations,[404] a bleeding respiratory tract lesion, newborn stress,[804] an-

---

*Recently, Steele and Copeland raised doubts concerning the validity of this syndrome.[1164]

TABLE 7–6. *The Diffuse Pneumonias*[323, 807, 1345]

Influenza[511]
Pseudomonas[987a, 1213]
Salmonella[586]
Shigella
Asthmatic[344]
Pneumocystis[160, 201, 313, 318, 392, 1022, 1292]
Löffler's[756, 1285]
Allergic[940] (farmer's lung,[573, 840] pigeon breeder's
  lung[505a, 1187a, 1260a])
Cytomegalic inclusion virus[1015]
Other viral[204, 1343]
Hydrocarbon[606]
Mucoviscidosis
Leptospirosis[1119]
Varicella[1065, 1150]
Herpes simplex[1343]
Measles (giant-cell)
Primary atypical (Eaton agent, mycoplasma)
Infectious mononucleosis

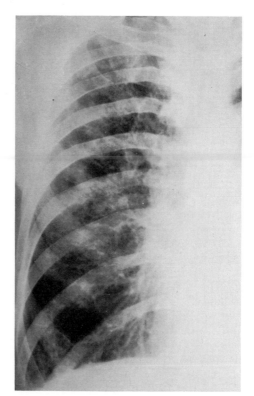

Figure 7–38. ACUTE DIFFUSE PNEUMONIA OF ASTHMATICS[344]

Note the coalescent alveolar nodules.

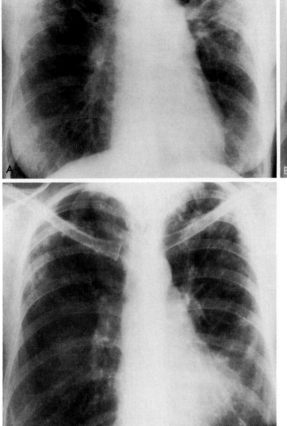
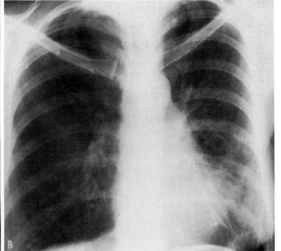

Figure 7–39. PULMONARY INFILTRATE WITH EOSINOPHILIA (PIE)

A, Peripheral infiltrate. Biopsy 3 weeks later showed eosinophilic pulmonary infiltrate. *B,* Clearing subsequent to a month of cortisone therapy. *C,* Recurrence 2 weeks after cortisone was discontinued. The infiltrate cleared after further therapy. Note the reversed butterfly pattern in *A* and *C.*

ticoagulants[131] (Fig. 7–40), leukemia, idiopathic hemosiderosis,[588, 650] Goodpasture's syndrome[159, 458, 758, 1193, 1232] (Fig. 7–41), and from unknown causes. The fresh blood and the resultant pulmonary reaction to it consistently produce an alveolar pattern. The blood is usually quickly absorbed, in a matter of days.[1302] The hemorrhage is often recurrent and more persistent in idiopathic pulmonary hemosiderosis and in Goodpasture's syndrome. Terminally, interstitial fibrosis may supervene and replace the alveolar pattern.[255, 475] In view of the acute episodic nature of the bleeding in these conditions and despite the overall chronic course of some of them, I have elected to place all types of pulmonary hemorrhage

under the category of *acute* alveolar diseases.

CAUSES OF WIDESPREAD CHRONIC ALVEOLAR INVOLVEMENT

Sarcoid. Of the *chronic* causes of the disseminated alveolar pattern, sarcoid is the most common in our institution, which has a large Negro population. Although it may not be as frequent as the interstitial nodular form of the disease, I have seen well over 25 cases of this alveolar form[327] (Fig. 7–26). Some doubt has been raised as to whether this roentgen pattern is associated with a similar pathologic distribution of the sarcoid lesions.[1062] Dr. Gary A. Podolny and I studied five patients in whom a lung biopsy had been performed at the time a roentgen-

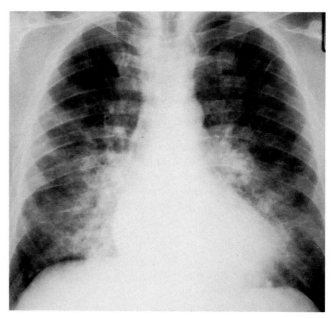

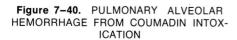

Figure 7–40. PULMONARY ALVEOLAR HEMORRHAGE FROM COUMADIN INTOX-ICATION

The lungs cleared a few days after discontinuing the drug. (Courtesy of Drs. Owen L. Brown and Charles A. Stern.)

ogram revealed the typical alveolar sarcoid pattern. These slides were reviewed by Dr. On Ja Kim, of our Pathology Department, and later by Dr. David G. Freiman, Professor of Pathology at Harvard Medical School and author of a classic monograph on sarcoid.[763] Dr. Freiman found that the alveolar spaces in many foci were partially or completely obliterated, undoubtedly contributing to the alveolar pattern seen on the roentgenogram. However, he attributed the obliteration to marked *interstitial* cellular infiltration and granuloma formation. He felt that the alveolar component represented an incursion into the alveolar space by an inflammatory mass arising in the interstitium, showing varying degrees of disruption of the epithelial lining. Dr. Kim agreed with these views.

In other words, the roentgen appearance in alveolar sarcoid is the result of encroachment on and obliteration of the air spaces by an interstitial process and not by a diffuse involvement confined to alveoli. As stated earlier, an alveolar roentgen pattern will obscure an interstitial one. I guess that's what happens in this form of sarcoid. I'm still troubled by the fact that both pathologists stated that these cases showed the ordinary and usual histologic appearance seen in other roentgen forms of sarcoid.

Other Granulomatous Diseases. Tuberculosis and fungus disease may also pro-

duce a subacute or chronic disseminated alveolar pattern.[4, 478] Although other roentgen manifestations are far more frequent in these diseases, the alveolar form occurs sufficiently often to include them here. At one time called "galloping consumption," this widespread pneumonic form of tuberculosis implies lower resis-

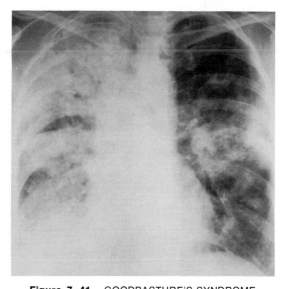

Figure 7–41. GOODPASTURE'S SYNDROME

Asymmetrical alveolar hemorrhage. Confirmed at autopsy.

tance (Fig. 7–42). The same applies to fungus diseases, such as the alveolar forms of histoplasmosis, torulosis, and aspergillosis. They often occur as an opportunistic infection during the course of lymphoma or after an organ transplantation. They might logically also be listed under the acute group.

Malignant Neoplasm. The roentgen manifestations of alveolar cell (bronchiolar) carcinoma are highly variable and often indistinguishable from those of other types of primary pulmonary carcinoma.[54, 64, 1261] However, despite its name, only occasionally does it have an alveolar distribution. The disseminated alveolar form of the disease (Fig. 7–43) is considered by some to be multicentric in origin and by others to represent bronchogenic spread from a single focus.[565]

The alveolar form of lymphoma[425, 1018] presents either as a primary lesion of the lung or as part of a disseminated disease. Surprisingly, the primary form, localized or extensive, may run a relatively benign course[39] (Fig. 7–24). In fact, the term *pseudolymphoma*[581] may include some of these patients.[1270]

Alveolar Proteinosis. Alveolar pro-

teinosis nearly always presents the typical roentgen pattern of diffuse alveolar disease[210, 240, 951, 960, 1030] (Figs. 7–28, 7–34). I have encountered many patients with this fascinating condition, all of whom showed widespread alveolar roentgen signs. Recently, an entity called *silicoproteinosis* has been reported among sandblasters.[139] The lungs appear radiologically and histologically similar to alveolar proteinosis but contain much silica. The disease runs a short course and has a fatal outcome (Fig. 7–44).

Other Causes. The existence of hair spray pneumonia (thesaurosis) as an entity has been questioned.[140, 494] However, cases have been recorded of individuals exposed to hair spray and other preparations containing synthetic resins who presented a widespread chronic alveolar pattern which cleared after the exposure was terminated.[62] I have seen but two examples, one a lady who was diagnosed by a radiologist when he observed her blowing up a storm with her hair spray can in his waiting room. Her chest film showed improvement after she was weaned, but worsened when her addiction recurred. That's why I believe that thesaurosis is a disease.

Desquamative pneumonitis is considered

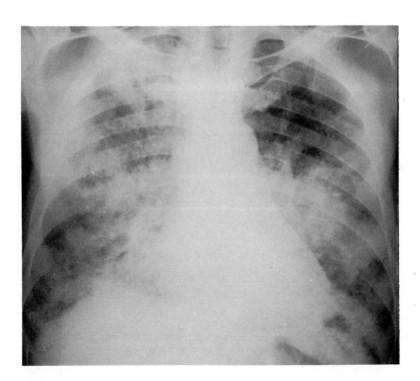

Figure 7–42. ALVEOLAR FORM OF DISSEMINATED TUBERCULOSIS

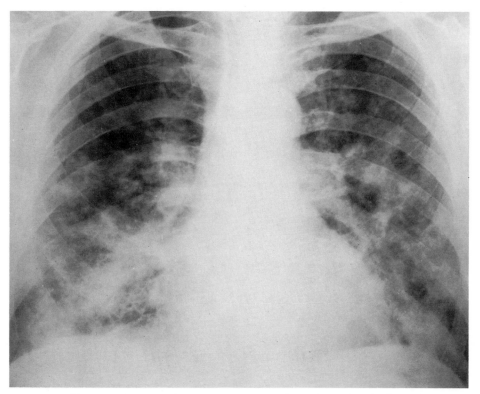

Figure 7–43.   ALVEOLAR FORM OF ALVEOLAR CELL CARCINOMA

to be interstitial *in origin*. However, since the alveolar-lining cells desquamate into the alveolar spaces, the resulting roentgen pattern is usually at first of the alveolar type[140, 414, 741, 743] (Fig. 7–45), later becoming interstitial. Lymphocytic interstitial pneumonitis and giant cell pneumonitis may show a similar sequence.

A diffuse alveolar pattern may appear soon after the aspiration of a considerable amount of mineral oil[1269] (Fig. 7–46). This represents the oil itself and the alveolar reaction to it. Later on, the pattern usually changes to an interstitial or mixed one, the result of fibrotic reaction to the phagocytized oil that has been transported into the interstitial tissues.

Alveolar microlithiasis is a disease in which there are tiny calculi within innumerable alveoli.[29, 1147] In case you're interested, a number of instances have been reported among snuff-dippers in Thailand.[183] As might be expected, the roentgen picture is clearly alveolar (Fig. 14–19). An

alveolar form of histiocytosis X has also been reported.[1265]

As is apparent from Table 7–4, once the alveolar pattern is recognized, relatively few conditions need be considered. It is significant that in the last 100 or so proved cases of widespread alveolar disease I have seen, each of the diagnoses ultimately established was found listed in this table.

Localized Alveolar Involvement

Most of the roentgen criteria of disseminated alveolar disease apply equally well to localized alveolar disease. One or more of the signs is consistently found in connection with acute and chronic localized pneumonia,[1343] pulmonary infarction,[93, 377] and segmental and lobar collapse. Alveolar cell carcinoma[54, 64, 457] (Fig. 2–44) and lymphoma[917] and pseudolymphoma should be added to the list. The localized alveolar conditions are also visible early and change

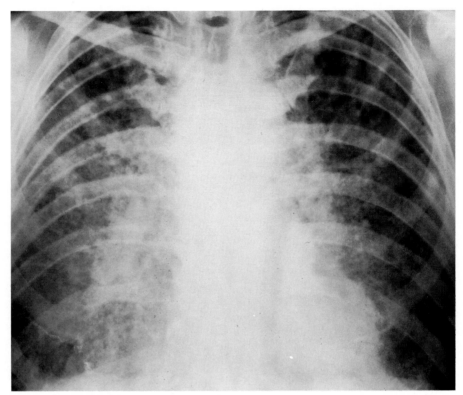

Figure 7–44. SILICOPROTEINOSIS IN A SANDBLASTER

(Courtesy of Dr. Stephen A. Kieffer.)

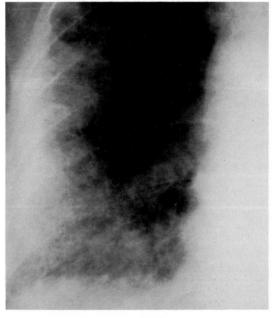

Figure 7–45. DESQUAMATIVE PNEUMONITIS

Close-up of right lung. The left lung showed a similar appearance. There is a predilection for the lung bases.

quickly. Perhaps related to the recently emphasized lobular distribution of thromboembolic disease,[525] a pulmonary infarct usually clears by "melting" from the circumference.[1317] Pneumonia, on the other hand, usually resolves by uniform mottling and then fading away.

It should be emphasized that it is by no means always possible to recognize the alveolar pattern on the basis of the signs enumerated. Confusion with mixed patterns and even with interstitial disease does occur. Hence, the attitude should be adopted that the signs must be definite before reliance is placed upon them. Nonetheless, when clearly present, the alveolar roentgen pattern is highly accurate in predicting histologic alveolar involvement and is thus extremely helpful in the differential diagnosis of diffuse pulmonary diseases.

Emphysema

For years, most radiologists glibly diagnosed emphysema on the basis of a combi-

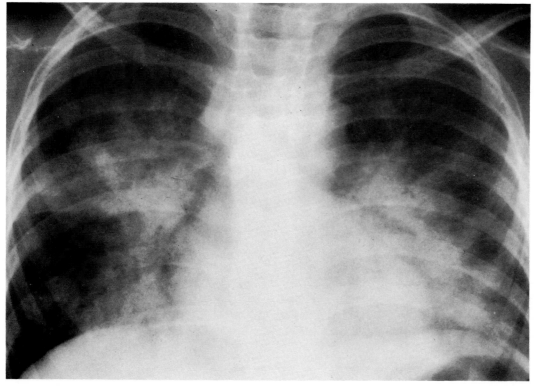

Figure 7–46. MINERAL OIL PNEUMONITIS IN AN INFANT

(Courtesy of Dr. William H. McAlister.)

nation of roentgen signs. We felt so secure in our conclusions that we didn't even bother to check them out at the bedside or autopsy table. But then the pulmonary physiologists burst our bullae by pointing out an extremely poor correlation of the roentgen diagnosis with the clinical findings, pulmonary function studies, or gross and microscopic appearance of the lungs. Many of the same roentgen signs were seen in the absence of emphysema and, conversely, significant clinical, physiologic, and pathologic emphysema often occurred in patients with a normal appearing roentgenogram.[454, 707, 839, 846, 976] Attempts to redefine the roentgen criteria of emphysema are under way,[454] but in this interim period the results have so far been disappointing.

In the remarks to follow, I will try to relate only facts and keep speculation at a minimum. You, the reader, will have to supply the missing information as it becomes available in the future.

The World Health Organization modifica-

tion of a CIBA symposium definition of emphysema is a good solid place to start:

"Emphysema is a condition of the lung characterized by increase beyond the normal in the size of air spaces distal to the terminal bronchiole, with destructive changes in their walls."[190]

The useful and authoritative National Tuberculosis Association classification of emphysema and related conditions[868] is shown in Table 7–7. The definitions that go with

TABLE 7–7. Classification of Pulmonary Emphysema and Related Conditions[868]

Chronic bronchitis
Asthma
Pulmonary emphysema
  Paracicatricial
  Lobular
    centrilobular
    panlobular
    unclassified
Pulmonary overinflation
  Obstructive (formerly *localized obstructive emphysema*)
  Nonobstructive (formerly *compensatory emphysema*)

this classification are also helpful. *Chronic bronchitis* is a condition characterized by excessive mucous secretion, cough, and dyspnea. *Asthma* is a disorder characterized by an increased responsiveness of the trachea and bronchi to various stimuli and manifested by a widespread narrowing of the airways that changes in severity, spontaneously or as a result of therapy. Clinically, it presents with episodes of dyspnea, cough, and wheezing.

Paracicatricial emphysema refers to overdistention of air spaces and alveolar wall destruction adjacent to fibrotic lesions of the lung, gross or microscopic. *Centrilobular* emphysema is distention and destruction of alveolar walls surrounding the central respiratory bronchioles within the secondary pulmonary lobule. In *panlobular emphysema* there is generalized dilatation and destruction of the air spaces of the secondary lobule. In *unclassified lobular emphysema*, the original location of the lesion within the secondary lobule cannot be defined because of extensive destructive changes, often manifested by bullae. Any of these forms of emphysema may be diffuse or localized to one or several portions of the lung.

Pulmonary overinflation (hyperaeration, overdistention) is defined as an abnormal increase in the size of the air spaces distal to the terminal bronchiole without destructive changes in the alveolar walls. *Obstructive overinflation*, as caused by a foreign body or neoplasm, was previously called obstructive emphysema or check-valve obstruction. *Nonobstructive overinflation*, formerly called compensatory emphysema, is associated with nearby collapse or resection of pulmonary tissue.

Senile emphysema is a poor and misleading term. It usually refers to pulmonary changes accompanying thoracic cage alteration with age. Since diaphragm excursion remains good and airway resistance is not increased, there is no significant pulmonary function impairment.[284, 846] *Bullous emphysema* refers to the large, thin walled, cystic air spaces formed by the breakdown of many alveoli and interlobular septa, often associated with a check-valve bronchial communication. A *bleb* is a small superficial bulla. *Pneumatocele* carries the connotation of temporary status and an origin in an inflammatory process.

Rarely, emphysema is associated with *alpha₁ antitrypsin deficiency.* The mechanism is as yet unclear. There is nonbullous panacinar emphysema usually involving both lung bases.[488, 975]

ROENTGEN SIGNS

A large number of roentgen findings have been attributed to emphysema. Logically, most have been based on the assumption that emphysema means overinflation—after all, the Greek root of the word emphysema means *to inflate.* These signs include pulmonary hyperlucency, the presence of bullae, increased AP diameter of the chest, kyphosis, anterior bowing of the sternum, increased retrosternal space, small vertical heart, cor pulmonale, a low flat diaphragm, visible phrenocostal attachments, diminished diaphragmatic excursion, and my own little secret—paradoxical diminution of the heart size on expiration rather than on inspiration.

More recently, the pulmonary vasculature has come into focus, and to the above signs of emphysema has been added prominent pulmonary arteries at the hila with abrupt attenuation in caliber of the branches in the central pulmonary zones. Diminished size and number of the vessels in the lung periphery, diffuse or local, may accompany it. Nordenström claims that the aortic knob is larger in emphysematous patients than in matched controls.[887]

Few of these signs are reliable.[846] Pulmonary hyperlucency on the roentgenogram is partly a function of individual variation, development of chest musculature, and technical factors of film exposure and processing, as well as of overinflation. Bullae, limited or extensive, are not clearly related to diffuse emphysema as the pathologist sees it and commonly exist as an isolated finding.[707]

In the lateral projection, increase in the AP thoracic diameter, kyphosis, and sternal bowing, mainly encountered in the elderly, have been shown to be a function of weight loss; the smaller abdomen makes the chest appear relatively large.[651] The dimensions of the retrosternal space and heart also vary with body build.

The pulmonary vasculature is highly variable in normal individuals and is altered by a variety of nonemphysematous conditions. A low flat diaphragm is commonly seen in skinny people, in whom it is also not unusual to see the muscle-rib attachments. I consider it a waste of time to count the ribs to determine diaphragm level because of the remarkable variation from one healthy individual to the next.

So where does all this leave us? As far as I am concerned, minimal or even moderate pulmonary emphysema is not a roentgen diagnosis, even with a lateral view at hand. A few roentgenologists take exception,[839] but I've given too many well people a reading of emphysema and too many emphysematous ones a normal chest report to accept their view.

Advanced diffuse pulmonary emphysema is another story. It can usually be detected radiologically[879, 1123] (Fig. 7–47). The signs I place most faith in are (1) decreased excursion of the diaphragm, (2) diminished vascularity of the central and peripheral portions of the lung fields (particularly if disproportionate to the enlarged hilar vessels), and (3) increase of considerable degree in the retrosternal clear space. Of course, signs of cor pulmonale, when present, are helpful. Decrease in the transverse diameter of the heart on expiration instead of on inspiration is a highly reliable sign but, unfortunately, is only occasionally present (Fig. 1–6). Distinct downward concavity of the diaphragm is certainly evidence of hyperinflation, if not of diffuse emphysema.[402] Basal bullae may indent the diaphragm and even invert it.

I consider fluoroscopy an essential part of the examination for emphysema. Diminished diaphragm excursion is more reliable when demonstrated fluoroscopically than with films. The same applies to paradoxical alteration of heart size. Localized air trapping and bullae are also often more apparent fluoroscopically. Tomography, bronchography, and angiography may elicit local or general hypovascularity, bullae, air trapping, and some of the signs of associated bronchial disease.

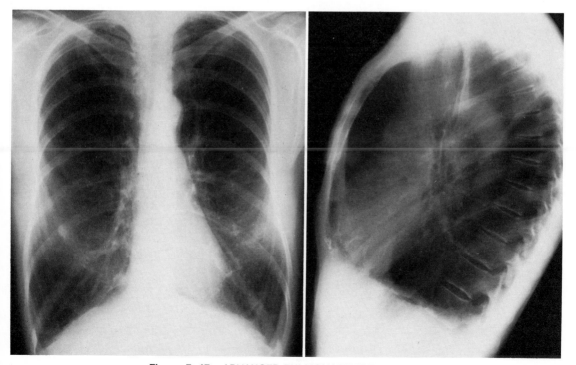

Figure 7–47. ADVANCED PULMONARY EMPHYSEMA

The lungs show diminished vascularity in the central and peripheral zones, the pulmonary arc is slightly convex, the retrosternal space is significantly widened, and the diaphragm has a slight downward concavity. Fluoroscopy revealed a minimal diaphragmatic excursion.

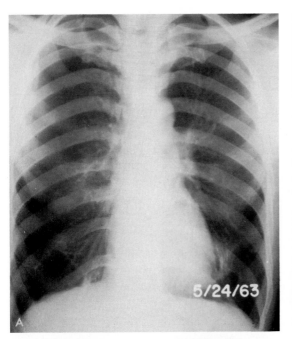

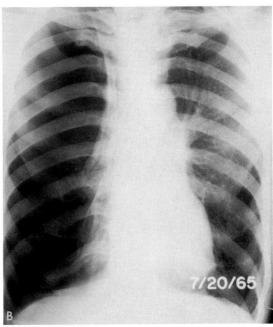

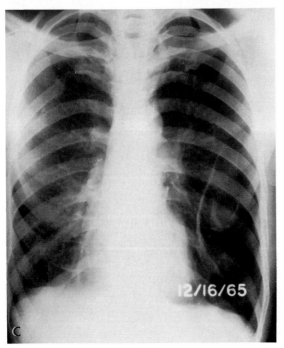

Figure 7–48. PROGRESSIVE BULLOUS
EMPHYSEMA SURGICALLY TREATED

A, Moderate bullous emphysema at right base. *B*,
Large right-sided bullae compress the right lung. The
patient was moderately dyspneic. *C*, 3 months after
right bullectomy. There is now enlargement of the
bullae on the left. The patient is still dyspneic.

As already stated, absence of all these signs still does not exclude the possibility of emphysema of significant import, nor does their presence provide infallible evidence of diffuse emphysema, particularly in the elderly. The more of the signs that are present, however, the better the correlation will be with the clinical, physiologic, and pathologic findings.

Efforts are being made to distinguish clinically and roentgenologically between centrilobular and panlobular emphysema.[402, 841] The term "blue bloater" is said to describe the clinical prototype of the severe chronic bronchitic with centrilobular emphysema who shows increased pulmonary vascularity and cor pulmonale; "pink puffer" is supposed to typify the patient with severe diffuse panlobular emphysema who has pulmonary overdistention and clear lungs.[402] I can't speak for the reliability of these clinical patterns, but the colorless radiographic emulsion has difficulty enough in revealing emphysema at all, let alone distinguishing between its hues. I am reminded of the birds and bees lecture I was giving my youngest son when his older brother interrupted with, "Gee, Pop, he can't even tell time yet!"

BULLOUS EMPHYSEMA

A further word on bullae. As noted, they are by no means a constant manifestation of diffuse emphysema. Conversely, extensive bullae may be present in the absence of significant centrilobular or panlobular emphysema. Patients with severe dyspnea and even cyanosis secondary to extensive bullous disease may improve tremendously after resection of the bullae, thereby permitting expansion of the surrounding compressed lung (Fig. 7–48). Unfortunately, how to predict which patient will benefit from operation is unclear. Surgical therapy was withheld from an incapacitated foreign political figure for years because sophisticated pulmonary function tests indicated that his bullae were accompanied by diffuse panlobular emphysema. His condition became so hopeless that he insisted on operation, and resection of the bullae resulted in a spectacular recovery. His chest physician considered emigration.

If you put a needle into a bulla, it will often develop a persistent leak which may even result in tension pneumothorax. This indicates a free bronchial communication or wide open collateral ventilation.

A localized area of avascularity on the plain film may represent the site of a bulla whose wall is invisible, but remember that the chest film of normal young people may show a local radiolucency (p. 499). Tomography, angiography, and bronchography will often outline bullae that are not visible on the plain film (Fig. 7–49).

PULMONARY OVERINFLATION

In hyperinflation, the walls of the alveoli, ducts, and sacs are not broken, but merely stretched. Overinflation may take a variety of forms. The large lungs of athletes may be included in this category. Roger Bannister, the miler and himself a physician, is often mentioned as the prototype. Compensatory overinflation adjacent to pulmonary collapse or resection is also an example.

Lobar emphysema of infants (Figs. 3–69 and 3–70), when associated with a bronchial lesion, results from air trapping secondary

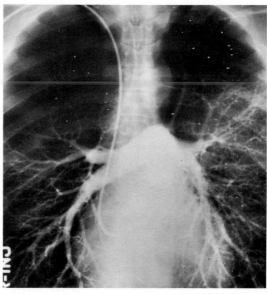

Figure 7–49. PULMONARY ANGIOGRAPHY IN BULLOUS EMPHYSEMA

Upper lobe bullae are outlined by arteriography, and there is increased arterial vascularity in the rest of the lung.

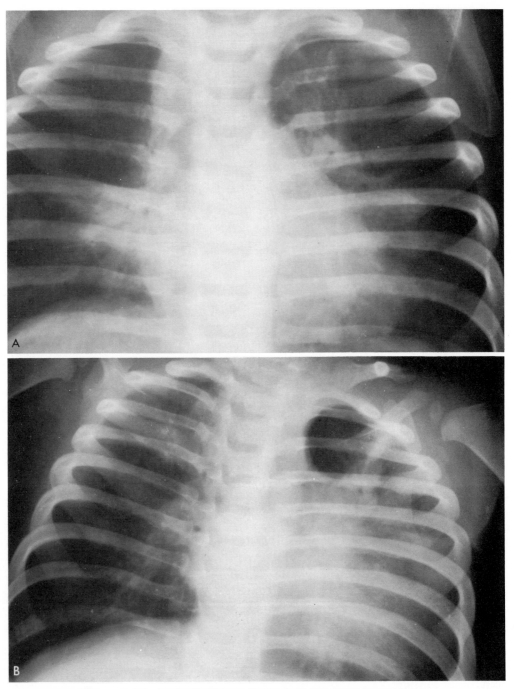

Figure 7–50.   PNEUMATOCELE IN STAPHYLOCOCCAL PNEUMONIA

A, Widespread pneumonia. *B*, 4 days later. A pneumatocele is seen in the left apex.

to a check-valve obstruction. When the bronchus to the affected lobe is normally patent, the mechanism of hyperinflation is unknown.

The pulmonary overdistention that occurs bilaterally with partial tracheal obstruction and unilaterally with malignant tumor also falls into the check-valve group with obstructive overinflation. But in Swyer-James syndrome and in pulmonary bronchogenic cyst, the mechanism of pulmonary overinflation is very likely related to collateral ventilation.[218]

I don't know where honeycomb lung fits into the classification except that it is said to represent dilated respiratory and terminal bronchioles.[941] It is discussed in more detail in the next chapter. The same applies to the bubbly lung pattern associated with oxygen toxicity and the so-called Wilson-Mikity syndrome.[1306]

Pulmonary Cysts

A pulmonary cyst is defined as a sharply outlined lesion containing fluid or air or both. It is round or oval in shape and its wall thickness is no more than a couple of millimeters. It may be lined by flattened or columnar epithelium or have no epithelium at all.

Much has been written about the pathogenesis of pulmonary cysts[44, 132] and conflicting opinions based on meager evidence are dogmatically expressed. I assume this gives me the right to add my own speculations and observations which you may consider or ignore, as you choose.

I doubt if any pulmonary cyst is congenital except for adenomatoid malformation and some bronchogenic cysts, both of which are seen in the newborn. On the contrary, a solitary cyst is extremely unusual in the neonate. It has been observed to develop in an infant after recovery from a severe acute respiratory episode. Cystic bronchiectasis is also acquired, not congenital. I have watched it appear in tuberculosis and histoplasmosis and have never recognized it in a newborn.

As stated earlier in this chapter, pulmonary bronchogenic cyst probably results from a congenital or acquired occlusion of a moderate sized bronchus and can be explained by Culiner's theory. The congenital nature of bronchogenic cyst is supported by its high incidence in pulmonary sequestration.

Whatever a pneumatocele is, its hallmark is an air filled, thin walled cyst that changes in size and appearance from day to day. It may show an air-fluid level. It usually appears during the waning stage of staphylococcal pneumonia in a child and is a favorable prognostic sign (Fig. 7–50). It often disappears in a week or two, but once in a while, like a healed abscess or tuberculous or fungus cavity, it may remain permanently as a stationary bulla-like shadow. I suspect the pneumatocele is caused by a bronchial plug, with inflation of the lung distal to it via the pores of Kohn. The pneumatocele does not fill on bronchography.

Because of their resemblance to cavitary nodules, the roentgen signs of these cystlike lesions will be discussed in the next chapter.

CHAPTER 8

THE INTERSTITIUM

PULMONARY NODULES AND CYSTS

Nodular and cystic lesions are combined in this section because they look alike roentgenographically and have overlapping causes. An air containing cyst is distinguished roentgenologically from an excavated nodule by its smooth inner lining and thinner wall, which measures up to about 2 mm in thickness. To qualify as a nodule or cyst, a pulmonary lesion must present a reasonably sharp outline. Hence, a focal infiltrate with ill-defined borders is excluded. The term *coin lesion* doesn't accurately describe the true shape and is best discarded.

Disseminated nodules less than 1 cm in diameter are considered under interstitial or alveolar lesions and are excluded here. I have set no upper limit of size for a pulmonary nodule, though I usually call the big ones a *mass*.

The Radiopaque Nodule

SOLITARY NODULE

The fluid filled lesion is also included here simply because it cannot be distinguished roentgenographically from a solid one. Table 8–1 is a gamut for the solitary nodule. Before looking at it, close your eyes and try to recall as many causes as you can. Then write in any that were omitted in the table. If you come up with three or more that I don't have, buy yourself a trophy.

Most of the conditions listed present an identical roentgen appearance but certain features may at times help distinguish them.

Although lobulation or lumpiness of the circumference of a nodule favors primary carcinoma, it is certainly not a reliable criterion. The notch or umbilication sometimes seen along the outer surface, especially on tomography, was once considered a clue to malignancy,[275, 1002, 1006] but it is also commonly encountered in granuloma (Fig. 8–1) and other lesions and is therefore not a valid sign.

At one time, I considered strandlike or "sunburst" pseudopodal projections from the margins of a pulmonary nodule an indication that the lesion had contracted and was therefore not a neoplasm but rather a granuloma, mineral oil paraffinoma, or conglomerate mass of pneumoconiosis (Fig. 8–2). This opinion came back to haunt me in two patients eventually shown to have bronchogenic carcinoma (Figs. 8–3 and 8–6D). Shapiro et al. recently found a "tail" or "rabbit ears" extending peripherally from a nodular alveolar cell carcinoma in a number of patients.[1107] I now consider linear projections a sign of benignancy only if there are several such nodules or if the history supports the diagnosis of pneumoconiosis or paraffinoma.

On the contrary, an unusually sharp border—as if delineated with a pencil—speaks against an infiltrating or retracting lesions, such as carcinoma or granuloma, and in favor of an expanding lesion which compresses but does not infiltrate the adjacent lung, such as bronchial adenoma, benign tumor, xanthoma, or hamartoma (Fig. 8–4). Once more though, it's too subtle a point on which to gamble for such high stakes. If a nodule has tapered margins and moves synchronously with the chest wall on respiration, a pleural or extrapleural location is assured (Fig. 10–9).

TABLE 8–1.   Causes of the Radiopaque Pulmonary Nodule

	GROWTH*	SOLITARY	MULTIPLE
Common			
Bronchial adenoma	↑	x	
Carcinoma, primary[54, 152, 712, 898]	↑	x	x
Granuloma—tuberculosis, histoplasmosis, coccidioidomycosis, brucella,[17, 1263] idiopathic	0	x	x
Hamartoma[487, 635, 759, 946, 1064]	0	x	x
Neoplasm, metastatic[32]	↑	x	x
Simulated pulmonary nodule: skin tumor, nipple shadow, rib lesion, foreign body, artifact	0	x	x
Rare			
Abscess, sepsis	↓	x	x
Amyloid[769, 1089]	0	x	x
Arteriovenous fistula, hemangioma, sclerosing hemangioma,[739] varix, anomalous pulmonary vein	0		
Bulla, infected; bronchiectatic cyst	0	x	x
Echinococcus disease[817]	↑	x	x
Heartworm[73, 1231]	↓	x	x
Hematoma	↓	x	
Hernia of spleen, liver, or fluid filled gut	0	x	
Infarct	↓	x	x
Lymph node, intrapulmonary[476, 1034]	0	x	
Mast cell disease[178]	0	x	
Mucoid impaction[1307]	↓	x	x
Neoplasm, benign:[932] leiomyoma, fibroma, chemodectoma, neurofibroma,[40] lipoma, myoblastoma, hemangiopericytoma, plasmacytoma,[1202] endometrioma, papilloma	↑	x	x
Neoplasm, malignant, other than carcinoma: lymphoma (pseudolymphoma), sarcoma,[533] pleural mesothelioma	↑	x	x
Paraffinoma (mineral oil granuloma)	0	x	x
Paragonimiasis	↓	x	x
Pleural fibrin ball	0	x	
Pleural fluid, encapsulated	↓	x	x
Pneumonia, organized	0	x	x
Pneumoconiosis, conglomerate mass	0	x	x
Pseudotumor, xanthoma[1215]	0	x	
Rheumatoid arthritis[147, 961, 1117, 1180]	↓		x
Sarcoid	↓		x
Sequestration (fluid filled cyst)	0	x	
Splenosis	0	x	x
Tracheopathia osteoplastica	0		x
Wegener's granuloma[402]	↑		x

*Usual short term growth potential
↑ = growth,   ↓ = regression,   0 = constant size
x = yes

A well-defined branching or a linear component relates the nodule to the pulmonary vasculature or bronchial tree. Arteriovenous fistula, hemangioma, varix, and anomalous pulmonary vein are readily distinguished from bronchial mucoid impaction by the demonstration on tomography of central feeding or draining vessels or air bubbles (Figs. 5–31 and 7–17).

The importance of looking for calcium in the pulmonary nodule is well known (Fig. 8–5). For this reason as well as for improved visualization and localization of the nodule, tomography is invaluable. Cavitation, perceptible on plain or tomographic films, is also important and is discussed below.

The rate of growth, sometimes measured by the doubling time of a lesion,[202, 866] has been emphasized in the distinction between a benign and malignant lesion. Although this may have some general application to the problem, there is so much

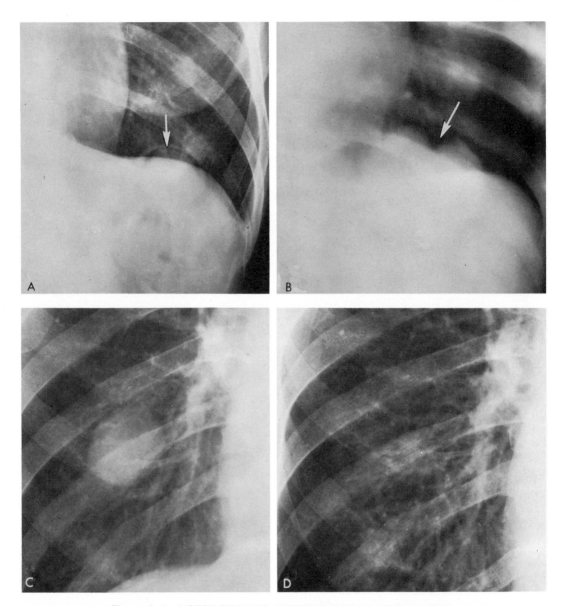

Figure 8–1. NOTCH SIGN AND MENISCUS SIGN IN A GRANULOMA

A, Upright teleroentgenogram reveals a nodule in the LLL capped by a thin rim of air (arrow). *B,* Laminagram 2 years later. The meniscus has disappeared. The nodule is larger and now presents a notch in its superior margin (arrow). Other films showed an annular calcification in its center. *C,* New nodule in the right lung on the same day as *B.* The nodule on the left was resected and found to be a granuloma of unknown etiology. *D,* A year later. The right nodule has almost completely disappeared without treatment.[155] (From Felson, B.[326]; reproduced with permission of Charles C Thomas, Publ.)

overlap in the rate of enlargement of a malignant and a benign lesion that their differentiation on this basis is unreliable. A malignant tumor may grow at a tortoise pace[1003] or spread like a conflagration.

A solitary peripheral carcinoma, if untreated, may show an interesting course. It either arises in or invades a small bronchus, then extends proximally within the bronchus, the line of least resistance. It may then successively cut off a subsegmental, segmental, and eventually a lobar or even the main stem bronchus, producing collapse of a progressively increasing volume of lung

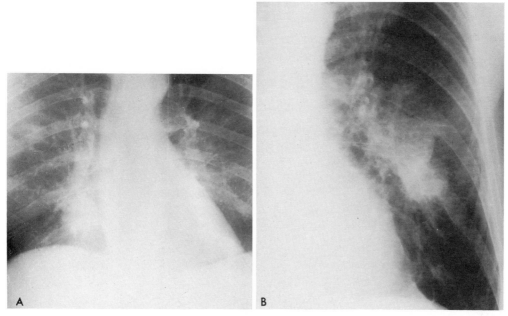

Figure 8–2. STRANDLIKE MARGINS

A, Mineral oil paraffinoma. *B*, Silicotic conglomerate mass.

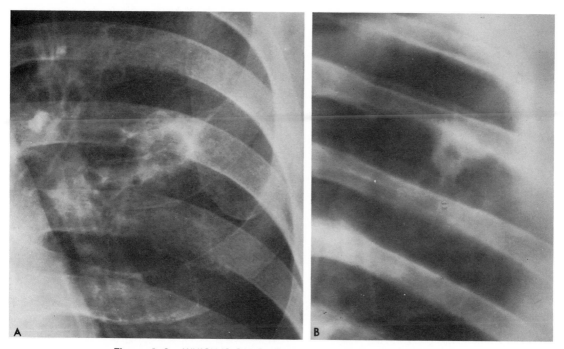

Figure 8–3. WHICH IS CARCINOMA AND WHICH IS GRANULOMA?

Each lesion shows strandlike margins and central cavitation. Both underwent surgery. *A* is a carcinoma, *B* a histoplasmoma . . . I think.

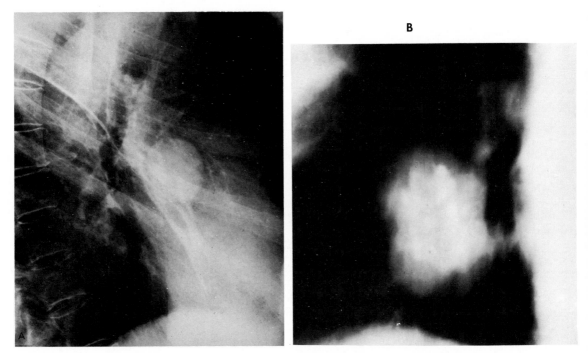

Figure 8–4. PENCIL-SHARP NODULES OF BRONCHIAL ADENOMA

A, The tumor has caused subsegmental collapse. B, Another patient. Partly calcified bronchial adenoma. This was a functioning tumor—the patient had Cushing's syndrome. (Courtesy of Dr. Manuel Viamonte, Jr.).

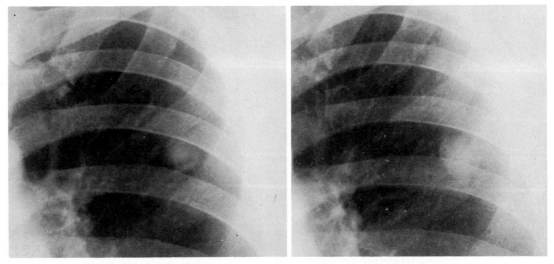

Figure 8–5. GROWTH OF A PARTLY CALCIFIED HISTOPLASMOMA

The films were made 2½ years apart. Note the large central calcification in both films. The resected lesion showed no active inflammation. (Courtesy of Drs. Lee S. Rosenberg and Henry Felson.)

supplied by these units.[424, 1003] The hamartoma, despite its implication of inborn malformation, is seldom seen in children. It may slowly enlarge as may the "quiescent" granuloma (Fig. 8–5).

Table 8–1 includes a column indicating the *usual* short term growth potential of each condition; some variation in behavior is to be expected. Spontaneous diminution of a pulmonary nodule, of course, excludes a malignant process (Fig. 8–1C and D). The rate of change is widely variable. Rapid clearing of a rounded, well-defined pneumonia, contusion, infarct, or abscess is well known, and mucoid impactions may be coughed up. Slow enlargement of a benign tumor is expected. Improvement after introduction of therapy is a modifying factor. Clearing of pulmonary rheumatoid nodules, sarcoid, and Wegener's granuloma with cortisone may be striking.

MULTIPLE NODULES

The list of causes of multiple pulmonary nodules is surprisingly long (Table 8–1). Admittedly, many of the items are museum material (Fig. 8–6). Metastatic malignancy outnumbers all the others put together. A cautious note of optimism is permissible if multiple nodules fail to enlarge over a period of several months in the absence of a known primary neoplasm. Incidentally, patients with metastatic neoplasm need not be symptomatic. It is common experience to hear the clinician protest, "But he's not sick!"

Air Containing Nodules and Cysts

SINGLE CAVITARY LESION

A sharply outlined air containing lesion may represent a bulla, a fluid filled cyst with bronchial communication, or a solid nodule that has become excavated. There are many such lesions (Table 8–2).

It is surprising how frequently the cavitary nodule turns out to be malignant.[42] A variety of mechanisms account for this. Perhaps the most common is neoplastic obstruction of an artery supplying the nodule, resulting in central infarction. Infection of a neoplastic nodule may occur, probably be-

cause of stasis in the adjacent obstructed bronchus. Necrosis may result from toxic drugs, steroids, or even an autophagic enzyme liberated by the tumor itself. Some of these cavitated carcinomas do not show necrosis histologically. This raises other theoretical explanations for its gas content: obstructive emphysema; collateral air drift;[973] sebaceous or serous secretions by a highly differentiated squamous or glandular carcinoma finding their way into a nearby bronchus and permitting air to enter the nodule; and finally, carcinoma developing within a cyst or bulla[61, 452, 928, 1067] (Fig. 8–7). A cavitary carcinoma which seems to defy explanation is illustrated in Figure 8–8.

Certain roentgen features of a cavitated nodule suggest malignant tumor. These include multiple holes, nodular inner or outer wall, and eccentric excavation[345] (Fig. 8–9). However, none of these signs of malignancy is consistently reliable (Fig. 8–10).

A solitary cyst may contain air, fluid, or both. When the cyst is filled with air the wall is seen to be only a few millimeters thick and a small demilune of fluid is present in its base (Fig. 8–11). The fluid filled cyst looks almost exactly like a solid mass, perhaps a little sharper in outline and a little more spherical (Fig. 8–12). The features of bronchogenic cyst (Figs. 4–26 and 7–16), cystic bronchiectasis (Figs. 1–7, 7–3, and 7–20), and pneumatocele (Fig. 7–50) have already been discussed.

MULTIPLE CAVITARY LESIONS

Bullae are by far the most common type of air containing, multicystic lesions involving the lung. When infected, they partly or completely fill with fluid (Fig. 1–16). Cystic bronchiectasis can produce a similar appearance. Otherwise, multiple thin walled cysts are uncommon (Table 8–2).

Multiple, thick walled, cavitated nodules most frequently occur in metastatic neoplasm and granulomas (Table 8–2). Cavitary metastases, attributable to one or another of the mechanisms already described for cavitation in bronchogenic carcinoma, are not at all uncommon (Fig. 8–13).

THE PULMONARY MENISCUS SIGN

As is already apparent, the content of a cavitary lesion has a major bearing on its
(*Text continued on page 327.*)

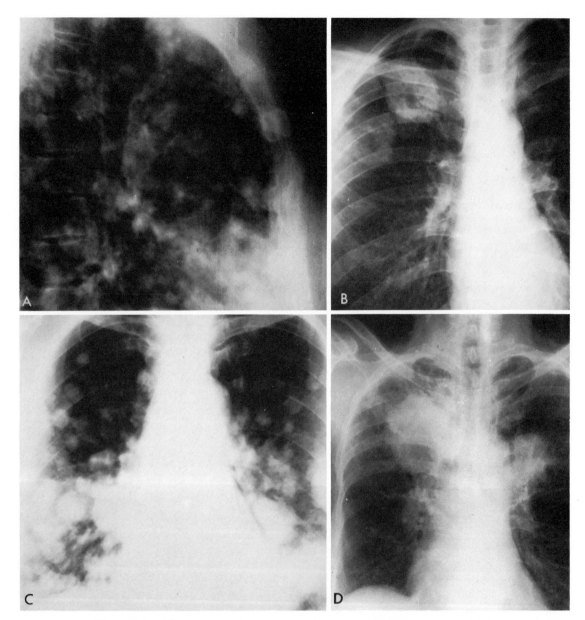

Figure 8–6. SOME UNUSUAL CAUSES OF MULTIPLE PULMONARY NODULES

A, Pulmonary amyloidosis. (Courtesy of Dr. Frederick J. Bonte.) *B,* Multinodular cavitary tuberculosis. The lesions had grown concentrically. *C,* Multiple leiomyomas. (Courtesy of Dr. Henry I. Goldberg.) *D,* Simultaneous primary carcinomas of the lung. The lesion on the right was a squamous carcinoma, that on the left an undifferentiated carcinoma. Note the stranded margins on both lesions. (From Caceres, J., and Felson, B.[152]; reproduced with permission of Radiology.)

TABLE 8-2. Cavitary Nodules and Cysts

	Type of Lesion	Thin Walled	Thick Walled
Common			
Carcinoma, primary	S	x	x
Granuloma—tuberculosis, fungus, idiopathic	SM	x	x
Neoplasm, metastatic[259, 261, 717]	SM	x	x
Rare			
Abscess	SM	0	x
Cyst, bronchiectatic	M	x	x
Echinococcus cyst[817]	SM	x	0
Hematoma, laceration of lung	S	x	x
Hernia	S	x	0
Histiocytosis X[196, 393, 620]	M	x	0
Hydropneumothorax, encapsulated	SM	x	0
Infarct	SM	x	x
Lymphoma[1163]	SM	0	x
Noninfected or infected bulla;[51] other cysts[132, 775]	SM	x	0
Paragonimiasis	SM	x	x
Pneumatocele[31, 151, 256, 272]	SM	x	0
Pneumoconiosis, conglomerate mass	S	0	x
Rheumatoid nodule (ankylosing spondylitis)[147, 961, 1117, 1180]	M	x	x
Sarcoid, cystic[462, 504]	M	x	0
Sarcoma	S	0	x
Sequestration	S	x	0
Wegener's granuloma, periarteritis nodosum[402]	SM	0	x

S = Solitary
M = Multiple
x = Yes
0 = No

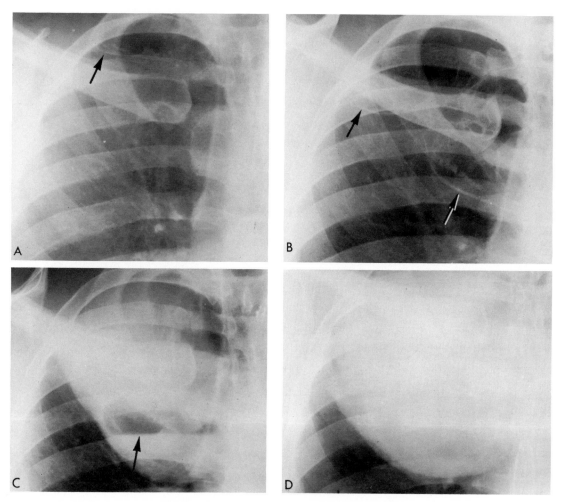

Figure 8–7.   CARCINOMA ARISING IN A BULLA

A, Early bulla formation at extreme right apex (arrow). *B,* 4 years later. The bullae are much larger (arrows). *C,* 2½ years later. Except for an air-fluid level (arrow), the bullae are occupied by a sharply marginated lesion of water density. My diagnosis was infected bulla. (See Fig. 1–16.) *D,* 3 weeks later. There has been considerable enlargement. Exploration revealed a solid inoperable squamous carcinoma!

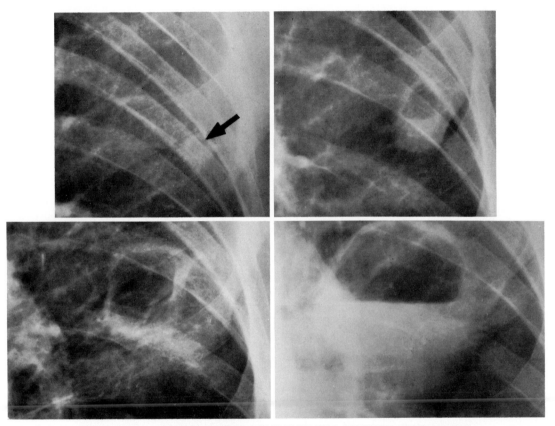

Figure 8–8. SQUAMOUS CARCINOMA THAT WAS CAVITARY THROUGHOUT

A, Tiny circular lesion in left midlung (arrow). *B,* 6 months later. Considerable growth. *C,* 8 months later. The inner wall of the cavitary lesion is irregular. *D,* Another 9 months have passed. Note the large fluid level. Necrosis was absent in the final specimen. The patient had refused operation. (From Felson, B., Fleischner, F. G., McDonald, J. R., and Rabin, C. B.[345]; reproduced with permission of Radiology. Courtesy of Dr. Lee S. Rosenberg.)

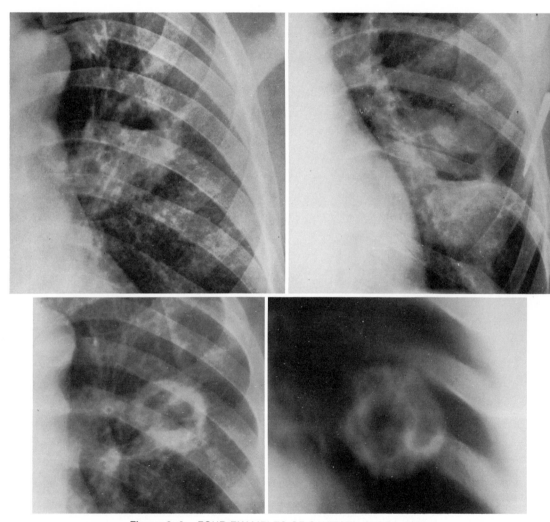

Figure 8–9.   FOUR EXAMPLES OF CAVITARY CARCINOMA

Multiple cavities, nodular inner or outer wall, and excentric excavation are suggestive but not reliable signs of malignancy.

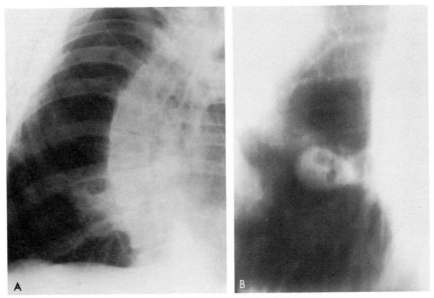

Figure 8–10. PULMONARY LACERATION

A, Film on day of car accident. Note the ill-defined outer margin and central cavity. There is severe scoliosis. *B,* Tomogram 2 weeks later. The lesion now shows a sharp outline and several holes. Operative proof. (Courtesy of Dr. Chapin P. Hawley.)

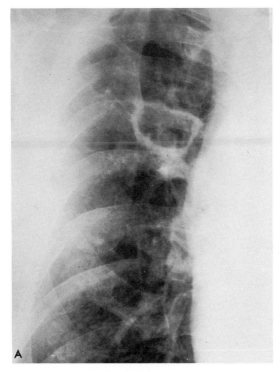
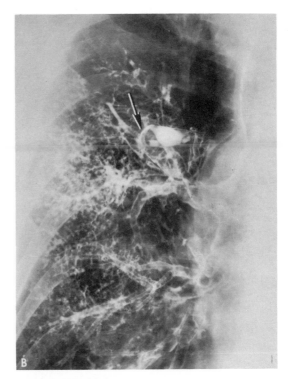

Figure 8–11. CYSTIC BRONCHIECTASIS

A, Note the small demilune of fluid in the floor of the cavity. *B,* A wide bronchus (arrow) leads into the cavity. (From Wisoff, C. P., and Felson, B.[1312a]; reproduced with permission of J. Thorac. Surg.)

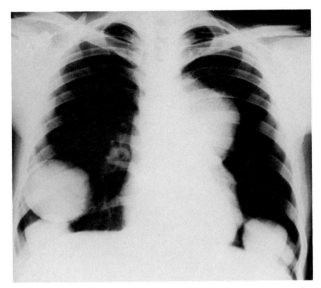

Figure 8–12. ECHINOCOCCUS CYSTS

Note the very sharp margins of the spherical lesions. (Courtesy of Dr. Ali Alizadeh, Meshed, Iran.)

Figure 8–13. CAVITARY METASTASES

The primary was a transitional cell carcinoma of the bladder. Tomogram.

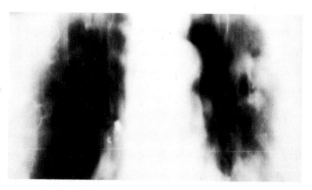

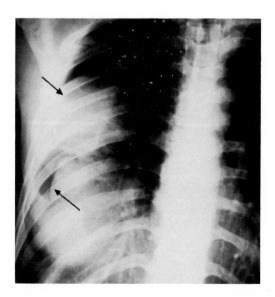

Figure 8–14. MENISCUS SIGN IN HYDATID CYST

The crescent shape gas shadow (lower arrow) outlines the hydatid membrane. A second cyst (upper arrow) is fluid filled. (Courtesy of Dr. Ali Alizadeh, Meshed, Iran.)

roentgen diagnosis. This is most emphatically true in the case of the *pulmonary meniscus sign.* The sign has been described under a variety of other names, including *air cap* and *air crescent.* At one time it was regarded as diagnostic of pulmonary hydatid cyst, the term being applied to the crescentic gas shadow seen along the cyst margin when air enters the space between the hydatid membrane and the host's adventitia, heralding the disintegration of the cyst[250, 636, 700, 826, 1079] (Fig. 8–14). Later, cyst fragments floating in the cavity produce the *lily pad sign.*

TABLE 8–3. Causes of Meniscus Sign

Common
  Fungus ball[447, 732, 843, 1012, 1248, 1267]

Rare
  Blood clot in a tuberculous cavity[121, 297, 355]
  Bronchial adenoma
  Carcinoma,[215] Rasmussen aneurysm[297, 944, 965, 1182]
  Hamartoma
  Hydatid cyst
  Idiopathic
  Lung abscess (inspissated pus)[92, 744]
  Pulmonary gangrene[231]
  Sarcoma
  Tuberculoma[1339]

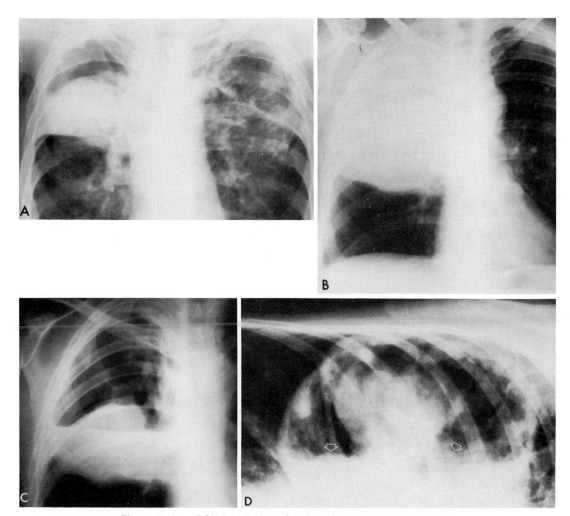

Figure 8–15. SOME UNUSUAL CAUSES OF THE MENISCUS SIGN

A, Blood clot in an active tuberculous cavity. In this patient and another, the mass disappeared a few days after cessation of a severe hemoptysis. *B* and *C,* Gangrene of the lung. Pneumococcic pneumonia with bulging fissure was followed in a few days by disintegration of the lobe within its visceral pleura, with mobile necrotic fragments. (From Danner, P. K., McFarland, D. R., and Felson, B.[231]; reproduced with permission of Charles C Thomas, Publ.) *D,* Bronchogenic carcinoma. Left decubitus view. The huge air containing tumor shows a large attached central mass and loose fragments (arrows) which protrude above the fluid level.

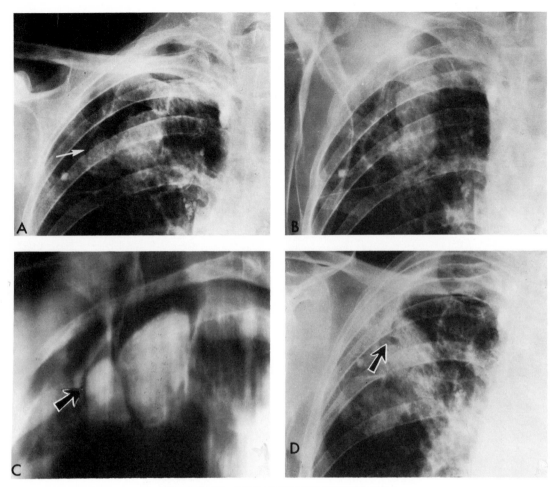

Figure 8–16. INTRACAVITARY FUNGUS BALL

A, Upright teleroentgenogram. The patient was asymptomatic. Note the crescent of air (arrow) around the two large nodules in the RUL. *B,* Left lateral decubitus on same day (printed upright for comparison). The nodules have fallen to the medial side of the cavity. *C,* Laminagram same day. The two fungus balls and the meniscus (arrow) are better seen. Calcification is noted along the superior aspect of the medial fungus ball. *D,* 3 years later. The patient has symptoms and signs of acute pneumonia. Fragments of tissue in the sputum showed mycelia of Aspergillus. A small air-fluid level is present (arrow). Diagnosis was confirmed at operation.

(Figure continued on opposite page.)

The air crescent and lily pad signs are by no means pathognomonic of Ecchinococcus disease, and in nonendemic areas other etiologies are more common. For convenience, I have combined them under the name *meniscus sign* to include either a fixed or mobile mass within a cavity. Table 8–3 lists the conditions in which the meniscus sign occurs (Fig. 8–15). In some instances, only a rim of air may be visible at the periphery of the mass (Fig. 8–1A). In others, the mass may be small and the cavity huge (Fig. 8–15C).

FUNGUS BALL. By far the most frequent cause of the meniscus sign in my own practice has been the intracavitary fungus ball, in which one or more round masses composed of the mycelia of *Aspergillus fumigatus* develops in a preexisting cavity. The cavity is usually a thin walled, air filled structure present for months or years. The background causes of the cystic or cavitary lesion that harbors a fungus ball include bulla, bronchiectasis, active and inactive tuberculosis or histoplasmosis,[1093] lung abscess, cancer, sarcoidosis, and even sequestration.[158, 406, 462, 1335]

The fungus ball may be solitary or multiple and may vary in size from a small pellet to a huge mass. The largest I've seen

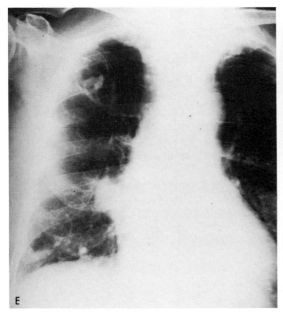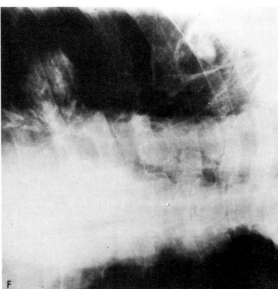

Figure 8–16. *Continued.* *E,* Upright, and *F,* decubitus films of a patient with a renal graft. The mass in the cavity at the right apex did not move. Nocardia was found on brush biopsy of this lesion. Multiple cavitary lesions are common in opportunistic fungus infections.

was at a film reading session in the East. I was told they had bigger balls in Baltimore than anywhere else.

The surface of a fungus ball may be calcified (Fig. 8–16). Perhaps the cavernolith (Fig. 14–28) really represents a completely calcified fungus ball. The ball is generally free within the unilocular or multilocular cavity, but may occasionally be attached to the wall and project into the lumen like a polyp (Fig. 8–16*E* and *F*). The fungus ball is at times soft and may even flatten somewhat in the upright position. It may almost fill the cavity or occupy only a small part of it. A fungus ball has been reported in the pleural cavity.[843]

Although it is generally asymptomatic and indolent, hemoptysis and signs of pneumonia may appear as a result of hemorrhage or from secondary infection of the cyst or the surrounding lung. Very rarely a fungus ball may appear a week or two after the onset of a lung abscess. Disintegration of a fungus ball may occasionally occur, with expectoration of the particles. I have now seen two patients with invasive aspergillosis in which a fungus ball later appeared. A case of coccidioidal fungus ball has recently been reported[53] and I just encountered one caused by an opportunistic infection with Nocardia.

DISSEMINATED INTERSTITIAL DISEASES OF THE LUNG

Many attempts have been made to set down criteria for the roentgenologic recognition of interstitial involvement of the lung. For example a reticulated, short, linear pattern of "dots and dashes" is believed to signify interstitial fibrosis. Similarly, a prominent, longer, branching, linear conformation, so-called "heavy markings," has often been equated with interstitial disease. Although pathologic study in these patients sometimes confirms the presence of interstitial involvement, more often there is another type of lesion or none at all to account for the shadows. Like noses, lung shadows show a wide degree of normal variation.

It is also common experience to encounter a patient with severe respiratory symptoms in whom the chest roentgenogram appears entirely normal, yet autopsy a few days later shows an extensive interstitial disorder, such as miliary tuberculosis or diffuse interstitial fibrosis.[999] Several explanations for this paradox are available. In the first place, the individual nodules or infiltrates may be so small or their edges so ill defined that their detectability falls below the level of resolution of the roentgen method.[1243] Secondly, the interstitial process must encroach extensively upon the alveolar air to become roentgenographically visible (Fig. 8–17A). For Dr. J. Read (and for me), it is hard to conceive of thickened alveolar walls alone ever casting recognizable roentgen shadows.[969] Certainly, if the alveolar lumens retain air, there is less opportunity for coalescence and the individual lesions remain too small to see (Fig. 8–17B). With primary alveolar lesions, on the other hand, the air is quickly replaced, coalescence occurs early, and pulmonary involvement usually becomes visible soon after the onset of symptoms (Fig. 8–17C).

Pathologic Features and Pathogenesis

The interstitium of the lung is comprised of the walls of the alveoli, alveolar sacs and ducts, and the bronchioles as well as the interlobular septa and the tissues that accompany the larger pulmonary vessels and bronchi. Although the vessels and bronchi themselves are interstitial structures, they possess their own normal and abnormal patterns and so I don't include them in the interstitial category. The same applies to interlobular thickening (Kerley's B lines).

Various types of pathologic processes may arise in the interstitial tissues:[609]

(1) Disseminated miliary lesions, espe-

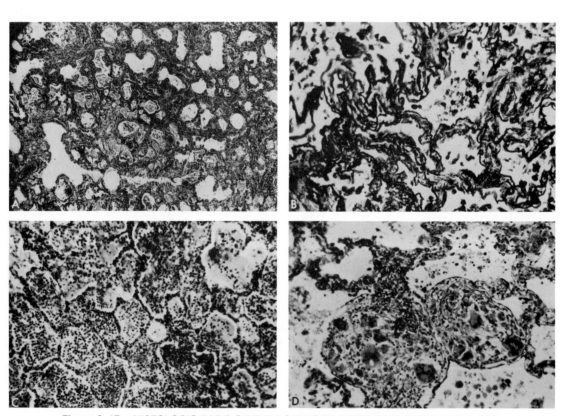

Figure 8–17. HISTOLOGIC BASIS OF THE ROENTGEN FINDINGS IN INTERSTITIAL AND ALVEOLAR INVOLVEMENT

A, Idiopathic diffuse interstitial fibrosis. The greatly thickened alveolar walls encroach strikingly on the air spaces. This degree of involvement is generally visible on the chest roentgenogram. *B,* Severe interstitial amyloidosis. The alveolar walls are only slightly thickened and do not compress the alveolar spaces. Hence there is no coalescence and the roentgenogram will appear normal. The debris in the alveolar lumens is artifactual. *C,* Lobular pneumonia. Contiguous alveolar spaces are filled with exudate. The chest film becomes positive early and shows the alveolar pattern. *D,* Interstitial granulomas caused by histoplasmosis. Coalescence of many such nodules is required for roentgen visualization. (From Felson, B.[331]; reproduced with permission of Ann. Radiol.)

cially those of hematogenous cause such as miliary tuberculosis, originate in the interstitial tissue (Fig. 8–17D). However, by the time the individual nodules become large enough to be seen radiographically, they are no longer confined to the interstitial region, but compress or invade the adjacent alveoli. For want of a better name, I still call these small sharp lesions *interstitial nodules,* but will yield to a better term when it is forthcoming.*

(2) Acute viral pneumonia is believed by many to be an interstitial disease. However, even though it may begin in an interstitial location (and there is some doubt of this), the process rapidly extends into the alveoli.

(3) Similarly, interstitial edema is hardly ever encountered at necropsy without considerable intraalveolar edema.

(4) Diffuse interstitial fibrosis is yet another kind of interstitial lesion. It probably has many causes, but only a few have been identified. Severe respiratory symptoms and signs are often present, usually attributed to the limited pulmonary distensibility and to the separation of the capillaries from the alveolar membranes, both of which impair the gas exchange. In many of these patients, pulmonary emphysema supervenes, often taking the form of myriads of small juxtaposed air cysts (Figs. 8–18 and 8–19) to which the term *honeycombing* has been applied.[532]

The pathogenesis of honeycombing is not yet established. In fact, even the anatomic structures affected were disputed until recently,[682, 827] when Pimentel demonstrated by tridimensional photographic reconstruction that the saccules mainly represented dilated terminal and respiratory bronchioles.[941] The cysts have been attributed to constriction of these bronchioles resulting in small areas of obstructive emphysema. That so many tiny units of lung could simultaneously but independently develop similar amounts of obstructive emphysema stretches credulity. Another possible mechanism is that of coalescence of alveoli consequent to destruction of alveolar walls by the underlying disease. However, histo-

logic evidence of various stages of alveolar wall dissolution has not been reported.

The Culiner theory can also be applied to honeycombing. Obstruction of many small bronchi, bronchioles, and alveolar ducts commonly occurs with interstitial fibrosis. Cough may raise the pressure in the adjacent bronchi sufficiently to overfill, through the pores, the alveoli distal to the occluded bronchi. Overdistended bronchioles and alveoli containing air trapped by the valves might then account for the honeycombing.

It should be emphasized, and this is of considerable importance, that the term *honeycombing* as used here implies a specific pathologic appearance and not merely a radiologic pattern. It is not to be confused with bullae or blebs, in which the air cellules are much larger. Instead, the individual air filled sacs are round, oval, or irregular and have a more or less uniform diameter of 1 to 10 mm (Figs. 8–18 and 8–19). They are usually grouped together in grapelike bunches. The distribution in the lung varies from a single localized area to almost complete involvement of both lungs. A patchy arrangement is common. Heppleston described the histologic appearance.[532] Many air passages, some dilated, are traceable into the cysts through wide or narrow orifices. One cyst often leads into others from which alveolar ducts or sacs arise, so the bunches are often joined to a single stem bronchiole. Thick plugs of mucus are common at the entry of the air passages into the cysts. Irregular strands of fibrous tissue lie between the cysts, with intermingled inflammatory cells and smooth muscle bundles. The fibrotic process also involves the interlobular septa.[969]

Pulmonary fibrosis, of course, need not be confined to the interstitial tissue. It may result from any long-standing inflammatory process, such as tuberculosis, and cut a nondiscriminating path through the parenchyma. The present discussion does not deal with this form of fibrosis.

Roentgen Findings

As previously noted, extensive and clinically serious interstitial involvement may occur in the presence of roentgenologically normal lungs. Unlike alveolar diseases, acute interstitial involvement usually takes

---

*Recently the term *small rounded opacities* has been applied to such lesions in the *UICC/Cincinnati Classification of the Radiographic Appearances of Pneumoconioses.*[1238] Naturally I favor its adoption; I helped select it.

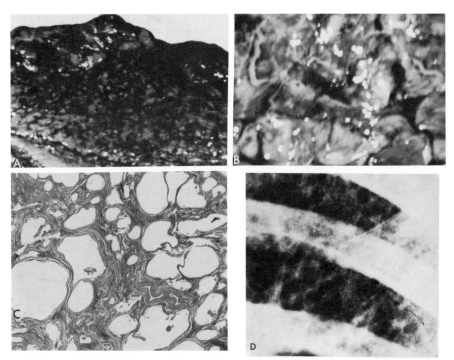

Figure 8–18.   HONEYCOMB LUNG SECONDARY TO IDIOPATHIC INTERSTITIAL FIBROSIS

A, Gross appearance of the external surface of the lung showing innumerable small air saccules. *B,* Enlarge-ment of a section of *A.* The individual sacs (arrows) are round or oval and have a diameter of about 3 mm. *C,* Low power microphotograph of the same lung. The small air cysts are surrounded by fibrous tissue. *D,* Enlargement of a section of the chest roentgenogram, showing honeycombing. (From Felson, B.[331]; reproduced with permission of Ann. Radiol.)

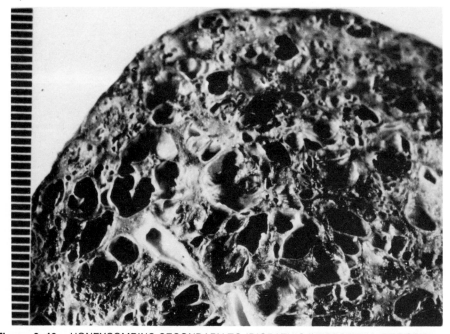

Figure 8–19.   HONEYCOMBING SECONDARY TO IDIOPATHIC INTERSTITIAL FIBROSIS

Each mark on the rule at the left is 1 mm.

about a week from the onset of symptoms to become visible.

INTERSTITIAL NODULATION (SMALL ROUNDED OPACITIES)

The typical roentgen sign of interstitial nodulation is a profusion of discrete round or oval lesions of 1 to 5 mm in diameter (Fig. 8–20). They are usually called *miliary* nodules because they reminded someone of millet seeds. A city dweller all my life, I presume a millet seed looks like a miliary nodule. The individual lesions usually become visible only after they reach 2 to 3 mm in diameter (Fig. 8–20A). Whether these small rounded opacities represent summation images of superimposed nodules[523] or the individual nodules themselves is unsettled. Recent evidence seems to favor the summation theory,[600] but my own inner logician tells me that we are seeing the images of actual nodules, perhaps the ones nearest the film, superimposed on a summation background. My reasons for saying this are several:

1. Experimentally produced summation images are fuzzy, mottled, and irregularly distributed. Small rounded opacities are often sharply defined and uniformly distributed.

2. Individual *calcified* nodules 1.5 mm in diameter and flecks of oily lymphography media are visible without signs of summation. Kerley's lines are only a millimeter or so in width and they are surely not summation images. The same applies to the walls of the cellules of honeycomb lung.

3. How do you explain by summation theory the uniformly punctate nodules in some pneumoconiotics and uniformly larger nodules in others?

4. If summation is the explanation of small rounded shadows, why should the lungs sometimes appear clear in miliary tuberculosis?

The interstitial nodules may enlarge and compress the adjacent alveolar spaces or penetrate them, ultimately coalescing. This late confluence never reaches the degree encountered almost from onset with alveolar lesions. Alveolar nodules (Figs. 7–34 and 7–35) are hardly ever as small or as discrete as interstitial ones; they generally measure over 5 mm in diameter.[333]

Table 8–4 is a gamut of the causes of dis-

seminated interstitial nodulation. The nodules of granulomatous disease are often relatively uniform in size in the individual patient (Fig. 8–20B), whereas those of metastatic neoplasm and alveolar cell carcinoma (Fig. 8–20C, D) usually vary considerably. They are often sharper and more rounded than the granulomatous nodules. Occasionally, neoplastic nodules may be as numerous as those of miliary tuberculosis, but as a rule they are much sparser, appearing in repeated small crops.

INTERSTITIAL EDEMA

Pulmonary edema confined to the interstitial tissue is not common. As Rigler has noted, the chest film may be normal in purely interstitial edema.[999] Generally, however, there are Kerley's lines (page 241) and sometimes perivascular and peribronchial cuffing, hilar blurring, and pleural edema.[444, 516] The Kerley's lines are transient. The B lines, denoting swelling of the interlobular septa, predominate, but A and C lines are not unusual. The other signs of interstitial edema are difficult to elicit and less reliable; when followed to autopsy, alveolar edema is nearly always present.

INTERSTITIAL PNEUMONIA

The same considerations apply to acute interstitial pneumonia, usually (and often falsely) attributed to viral infection. Here again, the alveolar component of the lesion quickly obscures any evidence of interstitial involvement on the roentgenogram.

INTERSTITIAL FIBROSIS

In diffuse interstitial fibrosis, the lungs may also appear entirely normal, even when the disease is incapacitating. In some, the roentgen signs of pulmonary hypertension may be present. Diffuse pulmonary emphysema is sometimes associated with interstitial fibrosis although by no means consistently. In short, some patients with symptomatic, histologically proved generalized interstitial fibrosis present a normal chest roentgenogram, while others show the signs of diffuse emphysema or cor pul-

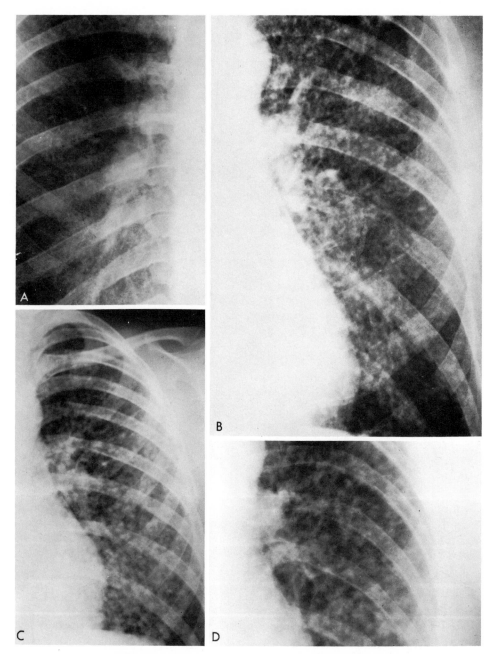

Figure 8–20. INTERSTITIAL (MILIARY) NODULATION IN FOUR DIFFERENT CONDITIONS

A, Berylliosis. The nodules are tiny, only 1 to 2 mm in diameter. (Courtesy of Dr. Oscar Sanders.) *B*, Acute histoplasmosis. The nodules are sharply defined and of uniform size. They average about 3 mm in diameter. *C*, Metastatic thyroid carcinoma. The nodules vary in diameter from 3 to 12 mm. Despite their large size, they have remained discrete. *D*, Alveolar cell carcinoma. The nodules are large and well defined.

**TABLE 8–4. Causes of
Disseminated Interstitial Nodules**

Common
   Tuberculosis
   Fungus diseases (e.g., histoplasmosis)
   Malignancy (metastatic, alveolar cell carcinoma,
    lymphoma)
   Pneumoconiosis
   Sarcoid
   Interstitial fibrosis (subliminal honeycombing)

Rare
   Histiocytosis X
   Amyloidosis
   Rheumatoid arthritis
   Hemosiderosis (mitral stenosis)

monale; yet neither emphysema nor cor pulmonale is reliable evidence of underlying diffuse interstitial fibrosis.

SMALL IRREGULAR OPACITIES I have borrowed this term from the UICC/Cincinnati Classification (see footnote, p. 331) to denote an abnormal degree of shadowing that has been described by such terms as reticular, reticulonodular, network, fibrotic, linear, exaggerated markings, ground glass, and others. This pattern has commonly been assumed to be caused by interstitial fibrosis. At times it is (Fig. 8–21), but don't depend on it. I suspect that the pattern is a summation effect of a combination of different types of lesions, interstitial, lymphangitic, vascular, and yes, even normal lung.

Small irregular shadows are common in pneumoconiosis. They are striking, especially in the lung bases, in asbestosis. They can sometimes be seen in lymphangitic metastasis, scleroderma, chronic inactive tuberculosis, sarcoidosis, lymphoma, sensitivity pneumonitis ("farmer's lung" and bagassosis), and other conditions.

HONEYCOMB LUNG. In my opinion, *the only dependable roentgen sign of interstitial fibrosis is honeycombing.* The air cysts comprising the honeycomb range in size from bare perceptibility to about a centimeter in diameter and are usually fairly uniform in size in a given patient. They are oval or round in shape. The walls are so thin that they are difficult to see, so that the honeycombing may be visible only in scattered areas. One may infer, however, that small ill-defined shadows adjacent to

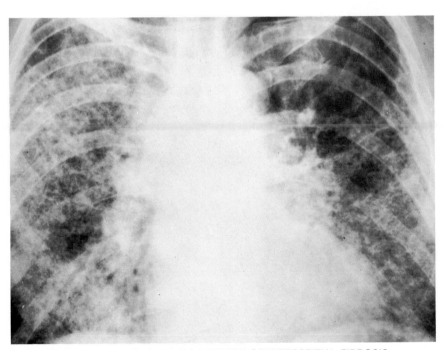

Figure 8–21. NONSPECIFIC PATTERN OF INTERSTITIAL FIBROSIS

This grossly abnormal film shows dots and streaks, short and long linear shadows, and extensive coalescence. Autopsy revealed severe idiopathic interstitial fibrosis with honeycombing and bronchiectasis. (From Felson, B.[331]; reproduced with permission of Ann. Radiol.)

distinct cysts represent similar lesions (Fig. 8–22).

To demonstrate these small, thin walled shadows requires films of good quality and scrutiny of areas of relatively sparse involvement. Bucky films are sometimes helpful, enhancing the contrast and delineating the fine walls of the saccules. Laminagraphy has been disappointing in this respect.

The roentgen differential diagnosis of honeycombing is important but often difficult. Frequently, superimposition and the small size of the innumerable shadows make it impossible to state which are the

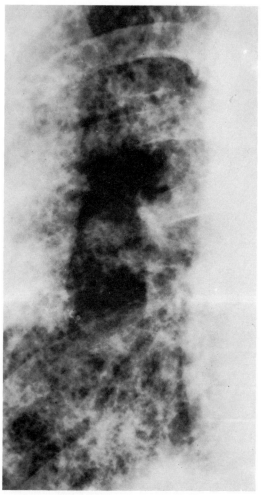

Figure 8–22. IDIOPATHIC INTERSTITIAL FIBROSIS WITH SEVERE DIFFUSE HONEYCOMBING

Confirmed at autopsy. The scapula and adjacent muscles account for the shadow over the upper lateral lung. (From Felson, B.[331]; reproduced with permission of Ann. Radiol.)

lesions—the increased densities or the radiolucencies between them (Fig. 8–21). Thus, the distinction between the honeycombing of interstitial fibrosis and the nodulation of interstitial granulomatosis is often difficult and at times impossible to make.

Similar problems arise in distinguishing the radiolucencies of honeycombing from those seen within alveolar infiltrates (the "air alveologram"). The air alveologram shows more irregularity than the cysts of honeycombing. However, alveolar exudate may be superimposed on honeycombing or emphysema (Fig. 8–38) and the radiolucent cysts shining through will even more closely resemble the alveologram.[1343, 1344]

Cavities within pulmonary lesions (the destructive pattern), as in tuberculosis or fungus disease, give little trouble because their larger size, irregularity, and surrounding infiltrates do not resemble honeycombing. Bullae are usually larger and less uniform than the cellules of honeycombing. On the other hand, cystic bronchiectasis may give indistinguishable shadows (Fig. 8–23A). Usually the bronchiectatic sacs are larger and they often contain tiny meniscus-like fluid levels. Unlike the honeycomb saccules, they distinctly enlarge on inspiration. Bronchography will confirm the diagnosis: the dilated bronchiectatic cavities fill readily (Fig. 8–23B) while the honeycomb cellules do not.

Spontaneous pneumothorax is a common complication of interstitial fibrosis, whatever the cause, particularly when there is associated honeycombing. If pneumothorax occurs during the course of a chronic diffuse pulmonary ailment, interstitial fibrosis should be strongly suspected. Pneumonia, pulmonary hypertension, and respiratory insufficiency may also complicate the clinical and roentgen picture.

CAUSES OF DIFFUSE INTERSTITIAL FIBROSIS AND HONEYCOMBING

Idiopathic Interstitial Fibrosis. In 1944, Hamman and Rich reported four cases of a condition which they called *acute diffuse interstitial fibrosis* of the lungs, characterized by progressive dyspnea, cough, cyanosis, and cardiac decompensation.[498] Death from asphyxia or cor pulmonale resulted within 6 months—the "acute" designation was obviously relative. Autopsy revealed an unusual type of inflam-

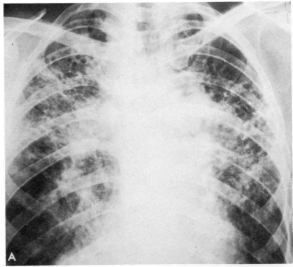

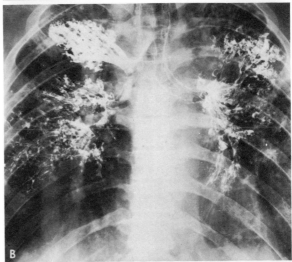

Figure 8–23. CYSTIC BRONCHIECTASIS IN SARCOIDOSIS PRESENTING A HONEYCOMB-LIKE PATTERN

A, Hilar and mediastinal adenopathy are present. There is extensive bullous emphysema at both bases. *B,* Bronchogram shows that cystic bronchiectasis accounts for the cellules in the contracted upper lung fields. (From Felson, B.[327]; reproduced with permission of Dis. Chest.)

mation with (1) enlargement of the epithelial cells lining the alveoli, (2) necrosis of alveolar and bronchial epithelium, (3) formation of hyaline membranes, (4) marked edema and fibrin deposit in the alveolar walls, (5) extensive diffuse interstitial fibrosis, and (6) eosinophilic infiltration. Excessive smooth muscle in the interstitial tissue and emphysema were also noted. The roentgenograms and gross specimens in their reports showed extensive honeycombing in at least two of the four cases. The authors expressed no opinion concerning the etiology of the disease.

Since this report, many cases of interstitial fibrosis of unknown etiology have been labeled *Hamman-Rich syndrome* despite

the fact that the histologic features seldom resemble those described by Hamman and Rich. Diffuse interstitial fibrosis may occur as the end-stage of a variety of pulmonary conditions in which the hallmarks of the original disease are no longer evident. For example, I followed a patient with typical pulmonary sarcoidosis, histologically confirmed. Subsequently, a diffuse honeycomb pattern developed which progressed slowly. The patient eventually died of pulmonary insufficiency about 12 years after his first film. At autopsy, evidence of sarcoidosis was completely lacking. The histologic picture was that of diffuse interstitial fibrosis with honeycombing, and a diagnosis of Hamman-Rich syndrome was made.

I have seen several other examples of sarcoid and one of histiocytosis X with a similar story. I prefer the term *idiopathic interstitial fibrosis* to *Hamman-Rich syndrome* but have no objection to the latter if it is clearly understood that it does not indicate a specific entity but merely the end-result of any one of a number of conditions, known or unknown.

A large number of patients with diffuse interstitial fibrosis fall into this idiopathic group.[127] The condition has been reported in children and a familial distribution has been recorded.[1189] The patient often shows a slowly progressive, irreversible pulmonary condition which generally interferes seriously with pulmonary function, and usually dies of pulmonary insufficiency or cor pulmonale.

On the roentgenogram, ill-defined, small irregular opacities are often seen (Fig. 8–21). Honeycombing is a prominent and common feature (Figs. 8–18*D* and 8–22). There are no roentgen signs that consistently distinguish this condition from other more specific causes of interstitial fibrosis.

Histiocytosis X. Another relatively common cause of interstitial fibrosis is *histiocytosis X*, particularly the eosinophilic granuloma variety. The lungs may be involved alone or in association with lesions in the skin, bone, brain, or other organs.[1300] Mediastinal lymphadenopathy may accompany the lung lesions. Eosinophilic granuloma confined to the lungs has been considered by some to be a separate entity unrelated to histiocytosis X, but the pulmonary abnormality is clinically, radiologically, and histologically identical in the isolated and systemic forms.

The interstitial fibrosis and honeycombing of eosinophilic granuloma (Fig. 8–24) are probably always preceded by disseminated interstitial nodules;[1283] I have observed this transition from nodular to honeycomb pattern over a period of years in two patients. At times, the interstitial nodules and honeycomb lesions may coexist roentgenographically and pathologically. On the other hand, the granulomatous lesions may never progress to honeycombing and instead disappear spontaneously[1300] or after radiation or cortisone.[861]

The honeycombing may appear predominantly in the upper lung fields. Pneumothorax is a fairly frequent complica-

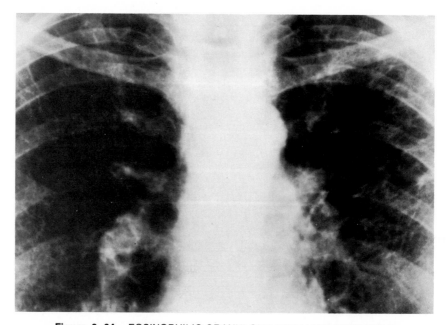

Figure 8–24. EOSINOPHILIC GRANULOMA WITH HONEYCOMBING

For many years, the patient was asymptomatic except for diabetes insipidus. Recently, a mandibular lesion developed. (From Felson, B.[331]; reproduced with permission of Ann. Radiol.)

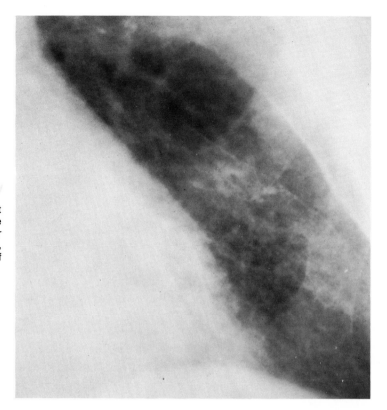

Figure 8–25. SCLERODERMA

Honeycombing is visible in the left lower lung. Similar changes were seen at the right base. The upper lung fields were clear. (From Felson, B.[331]; reproduced with permission of Ann. Radiol.)

tion[1027] but cor pulmonale is quite uncommon. Rarely, the cystic lesions become huge, reaching a diameter of 2 to 6 cm and containing air, fluid, and debris.[620]

Many patients remain essentially asymptomatic despite rather extensive honeycombing.[14, 632, 1300] Two of our patients were asymptomatic except for diabetes insipidus.[814] This symptom may also occur in sarcoidosis.[1152]

Histologically, the pulmonary biopsy may show nonlipid histiocytosis (Letterer-Siwe disease) or cholesterol histiocytosis (Hand-Schüller-Christian disease) instead of eosinophilic granuloma. All three, however, are now considered to be manifestations of histiocytosis X. I have also seen honeycombing with Niemann-Pick and Gaucher's disease.

Scleroderma. Interstitial fibrosis is said to occur in 20 to 25 per cent of all autopsies done on patients with *scleroderma*.[1236] The presence and severity of the pulmonary involvement are unrelated to the extent of the skin lesions; in fact, the skin may occasionally be entirely normal.[19] Esophageal involvement is sometimes, but by no means regularly, associated so that the pulmonary changes cannot be attributed to aspiration. Pathologically, the inferior portion of the lungs is more severely involved than the superior, and honeycombing is common.

The chest roentgenogram may appear normal despite severe respiratory symptoms, significant abnormality in pulmonary function, and frank changes on lung biopsy.[833] As a rule, the roentgen changes are predominantly basilar. Recognizable honeycombing (Fig. 8–25) is a relatively late roentgen manifestation,[1211] generally preceded by inconspicuous, fine, linear, basal streaks. Enlargement of the cardiac outline may occur as a result of either pericardial effusion or sclerodermatous involvement of the myocardium. Cor pulmonale is apparently quite unusual.[1219] A case of dermatomyositis with honeycombing seen at autopsy has been mentioned.[451]

Rheumatoid Arthritis. There are a number of reports of diffuse interstitial fibrosis associated with *rheumatoid arthritis*. An incidence of 1 per cent has been recorded among 700 patients with this disease.[922] I have seen it in a 6 year old child. The pulmonary granulomas that also occur in rheumatoid arthritis may present roentgenologically as diffuse miliary lesions or scattered larger nodules. These often regress,[797] but the interstitial fibrosis is permanent and may be progressive.[1142] Its severity does not parallel that of the joint disease and the pulmonary involvement may occasionally precede the signs and symptoms of arthritis.[122] A relationship between idiopathic chronic interstitial fibrosis and rheumatoid disease has been suggested on the basis of serologic studies,[1259] but clinical evidence does not support this view.[16]

The interstitial fibrosis seen with rheumatoid arthritis has no specific histologic or roentgen features[465, 937, 1044] (Fig. 8–26). Honeycombing is frequent.[258] Pleural effusion or hilar adenopathy may be present.[845] Occasionally the diffuse pulmonary process may be preceded by basilar alveolar infiltrates.[122, 750]

Chronic diffuse interstitial fibrosis associated with systemic lupus erythematosus or periarteritis nodosa is mentioned in the literature.[127, 299, 309, 1068, 1142] Hoffbrand, however, was unable to find a documented case report of interstitial fibrosis in lupus,[555] nor do I know of one in periarteritis.

Sarcoidosis. Pulmonary sarcoidosis may cause diffuse interstitial fibrosis with or without honeycombing. Most if not all of these cases are preceded by the interstitial nodular form of the disease. The nodular granulomas may regress completely, only to be followed later by interstitial fibrosis, or may progress imperceptibly into the fibrotic stage. The interstitial fibrosis is irreversible and may slowly evolve into extensive bullous emphysema. When this occurs the outlook for survival is poor.[327] During the honeycomb phase of the disorder, symptoms and functional impairment may be severe.

In the interstitial fibrosis of sarcoidosis, the lungs may be normal or show changes indistinguishable from those of other causes. However, persistent thoracic lymph node enlargement is common in sarcoid and provides an important diagnostic clue (Fig. 8–27). Residual microscopic sarcoid lesions at the time of the interstitial fibrosis may be lacking. Cor pulmonale is a common complication. As already noted, cystic bronchiectasis may develop and simulate honeycombing (Fig. 8–23).

Pneumoconiosis. Interstitial fibrosis with honeycombing is also commonly present in pneumoconiosis. It is almost always accompanied by other roentgen manifestations, including disseminated nodules, small irregular opacities, and/or conglomerate masses.[877, 1075] Honeycombing is particularly frequent in the advanced stages of asbestosis (Fig. 8–28A) but is not rare in silicosis (Fig. 8–28B), berylliosis, and other reactive dust diseases. There has been no attempt to correlate the honeycombing with the severity of symptoms and prognosis in these conditions, but I suspect that its presence does not bode well for the patient.

Other Causes of Honeycombing. Chronic lipoid pneumonia may also produce interstitial fibrosis with honeycombing. Originally showing an alveolar pattern (Fig. 7–46), the phagocytosed oil is carried

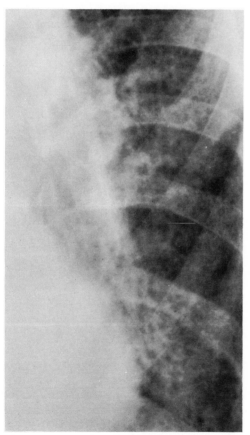

Figure 8–26. HONEYCOMBING IN RHEUMATOID ARTHRITIS

The right lung showed similar changes.

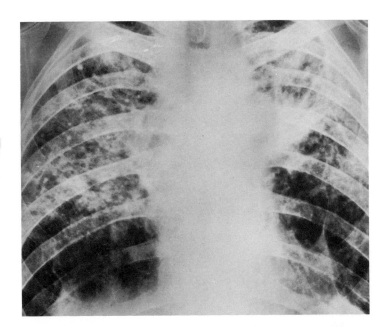

Figure 8–27. SARCOIDOSIS

Honeycombing is seen in the upper portions of the lungs with extensive bullous emphysema in the bases. The mediastinal widening is attributed to lymph node enlargement. Compare with Figure 8–23. (From Felson, B.[328]; reproduced with permission of Amer. J. Roentgen.)

to the interstitial tissue where it incites a fibrotic reaction. The honeycombing is usually confined to the lower lung fields, since the aspirated oil gravitates to these parts. Progression is extremely slow and the condition is seldom accompanied by significant symptoms.

A similar sequence occurs in *desquamative pneumonitis*.[414, 741, 743] In this condition of unknown cause (and it may not be a clinical entity),[682] granular pneumocytes initially slough into the alveoli. This produces an extensive alveolar pattern, usually basilar in location (Fig. 7–45). Eventually interstitial fibrosis with honeycombing ensues. *Idiopathic pulmonary hemosiderosis* is another condition that starts as an alveolar lesion but may terminate in honeycombing.[475]

There are several other conditions in which honeycombing is a feature but these are not, strictly speaking, associated with interstitial fibrosis. One is *tuberous sclerosis*; in this anomaly, the interstitium consists predominantly of smooth muscle, although fibrous tissue is also present.[832] Symptoms, when they occur, usually first appear in adult life. Pneumothorax, pulmonary insufficiency, and cor pulmonale may complicate the syndrome.[245, 1120] The chest roentgenogram shows no features that distinguish this condition from other causes of honeycombing[474] (Fig. 8–29). However, the clinical and

roentgen manifestations of the disease in the brain, bones, kidneys, and skin readily establish the diagnosis.

Similar pulmonary lesions have rarely been recorded in neurofibromatosis[244, 591, 801] and lymphangiomyomatosis.[149, 293, 397] Interstitial *amyloidosis* can also cause honeycombing[200, 1257] (Fig. 8–30). A few years ago, one of my friends (?) showed me a case of pulmonary amyloidosis with honeycombing on three different film reading sessions, and I failed to mention the entity on each occasion. It's now on the list. Amyloidosis may explain the honeycombing I recently saw in a patient with Waldenström's macroglobulinemia.

Muscular cirrhosis of the lungs is believed by some to represent a pathologic concomitant of interstitial fibrosis of any cause, resulting from an excessive proliferation of the smooth muscle component commonly accompanying interstitial fibrosis.[102, 398, 465, 681, 682, 739] Others consider it to be a separate entity, congenital or acquired.[146, 187, 546, 1043, 1109, 1209] Heppleston states that the amount of smooth muscle in these cases far exceeds that seen in other types of honeycomb lung and he therefore places it in a separate category.[532] Whether or not muscular cirrhosis is a separate entity, honeycombing is constantly associated.[103] Bronchography in several patients has shown a diffuse "bronchiolectasis."[187] Although the

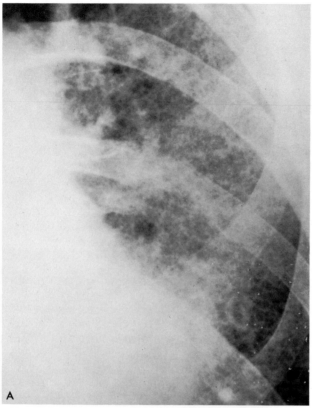

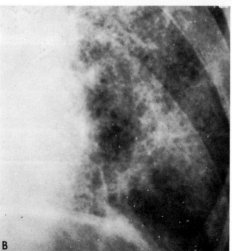

Figure 8–28. HONEYCOMBING IN
PNEUMOCONIOSIS

A, Asbestosis. The honeycombing predomi-
nates in the lower half of the lung fields. Note
the small irregular opacities and the "shaggy
heart." *B,* Silicosis. Interstitial nodulation is
also present. (From Felson, B.[331]; reproduced
with permission of Ann. Radiol.)

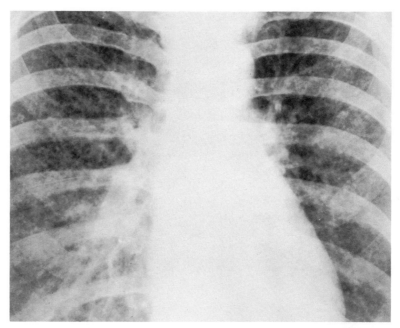

Figure 8–29. TUBEROUS SCLEROSIS WITH HONEYCOMBING

There had been no change in the chest roentgenogram over many years except for one episode of spontaneous pneumothorax. The patient was asymptomatic at the time of this film. The left lung showed similar lesions. Some of the cysts are so small that they look like small rounded nodules.

condition may terminate fatally as a result of right heart failure or pulmonary insufficiency, patients have lived with it for many years with relatively few symptoms.[210]

Congenital *adenomatoid malformation,* considered by some to represent a diffuse hamartomatous anomaly of the lung, is a disease of newborn infants in which the lung contains many small cysts. The process is always unilateral, the affected lung enlarging progressively like a tumor and dis-

placing the mediastinal structures toward the contralateral side. The roentgen signs are diagnostic. The large mass of tissue which replaces the lung usually contains many small cystic air bubbles, resembling honeycombing (Fig. 8–31).

Another cause of honeycombing in the infant is the so-called *Wilson-Mikity syndrome.* Many of these babies have received concentrated oxygen therapy.[865, 890, 950] The cysts are probably not caused by interstitial

Figure 8–30. AMYLOIDOSIS WITH HONEYCOMBING

Close-up of the right lower thorax. Both bases were diffusely involved.

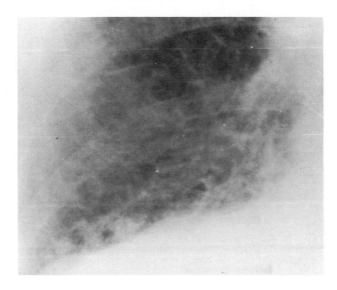

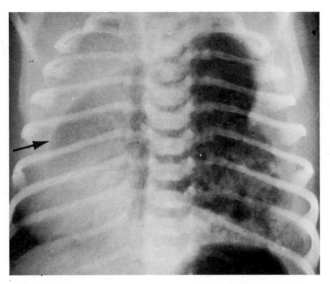

Figure 8–31. ADENOMATOID MALFORMATION OF LEFT LUNG

The bubbly honeycomb pattern is bordered laterally by an irregular vertical strip of solid pulmonary opacity. The enlarged left lung has herniated far into the right thorax (arrow).

fibrosis, since they are disproportionately large for the size of the patient and they may clear spontaneously. At necropsy, there is alveolar overdistention with fibrous pulmonary septa. The roentgen pattern is one of coarse lacelike infiltration surrounding many cystic foci measuring 2 to 10 mm in diameter. The pattern has been described as "bubbly" and is slightly coarser than that of honeycombing, considering the small size of the lungs (Fig. 8–32). Although the mortality is high, complete regression occurred in about half of the reported cases.[30]

Prolonged stay in a respirator is believed to cause a severe interstitial pneumonitis with eventual fibrosis and even honeycombing. The specific cause of "respirator lung" or its relatives "stiff lung"[164a, 1347] or "shock lung" has not been established, although the clinical settings include shock, transfusion reaction, trauma, oxygen therapy, and heart-lung bypass. The mortality is high.[779]

A variety of other conditions have been mentioned as causes of diffuse interstitial fibrosis and sometimes honeycombing. These include farmer's lung,[739] radiation injury, inhalation of cadmium[282, 827] and mercury fumes, streptomycin treated tuberculous bronchopneumonia,[1127] mucoviscidosis,[1127] mesenchymomatosis,[681] xanthomatous biliary cirrhosis,[681] chronic mitral valve disease,[646] and the pneumonitis caused by various drugs, including busulfan,[900] hexamethonium,[263] nitrofurantoin,[1033] and methysergide.[124] However, it is still unsettled whether all of them can produce roentgenographically evident honeycomb-

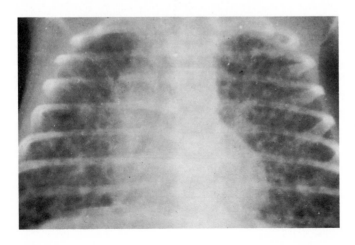

Figure 8–32. WILSON-MIKITY SYNDROME

Newborn infant. The lungs appear bubbly, but it's hard to rule out a nodular pattern. The chest slowly cleared and was normal 4 months later. Oxygen had been administered. (From Felson, B.[331]; reproduced with permission of Ann. Radiol.)

ing. I know farmer's lung and pigeon breeder's lung[1239] can; I've seen it. Until documentation is more definite, I prefer to omit the others from the list of causes of honeycombing (Table 8–5).

DIFFERENTIAL DIAGNOSIS. As stated, honeycombing is easily confused with cystic bronchiectasis, bullous emphysema, air alveologram, fine cavitation, and normal lung intervening between miliary nodules. If the distinction is not clear to you from the film, it is better to say so than to guess; otherwise wrong diagnoses will undermine confidence in this valuable sign.

The differential diagnosis of honeycomb lung cannot be based on the chest roentgenogram alone. All available information must be utilized in each individual case. Severe respiratory symptoms and pronounced alterations in pulmonary function are the rule in idiopathic pulmonary fibrosis but infrequent in other forms of interstitial fibrosis, perhaps because the former represents a later stage of the fibrotic process. The nonpulmonary manifestations of histiocytosis X, scleroderma, and tuberous sclerosis help to establish these diagnoses, whereas a history of exposure to noxious dust or an oily substance lends support to the diagnosis of pneumoconiosis and lipoid pneumonitis, respectively. Age is, of course, the key to the diagnosis of pulmonary dysmaturity and adenomatoid malformation.

TABLE 8–5. Causes of Honeycombing

Common
  Idiopathic interstitial fibrosis
  Histiocytosis X
  Scleroderma
  Rheumatoid arthritis
  Sarcoidosis
  Pneumoconiosis

Rare
  Gaucher's, Niemann-Pick disease
  Lipoid pneumonia
  Desquamative pneumonitis
  Idiopathic pulmonary hemosiderosis
  Tuberous sclerosis, neurofibromatosis, lymphangio-
    myomatosis
  Amyloid
  Recurrent sensitivity pneumonitis: "farmer's lung,"
    "pigeon breeder's lung," bagassosis, etc.
  Muscular cirrhosis (?)
  Adenomatoid malformation
  Wilson-Mikity syndrome, "respirator lung,"
    "shock lung"[4a]

Certain chest roentgen features may also be helpful. Predominance of the lesions in the upper lung fields in eosinophilic granuloma and in the lower fields in scleroderma, oil aspiration, and desquamative pneumonitis are helpful clues. Lymph node enlargement may persist into the fibrotic stage of sarcoidosis, and nodulation and conglomerate shadows aid in establishing the diagnosis of pneumoconiosis. The unilaterality of adenomatoid malformation is diagnostic. In pulmonary dysmaturity, the honeycombing may disappear; this is also said to happen occasionally in eosinophilic granuloma but I have never seen it documented. A previous chest roentgenogram is important to determine the background upon which the honeycombing has been etched. Earlier evidence of diffuse miliary nodulation favors sarcoid, eosinophilic granuloma, and pneumoconiosis.

Honeycombing, then, is an important roentgen finding and its recognition enables us to reduce the ponderous list of diagnostic possibilities of disseminated lesions of the lung. Once identified—and you must be *certain* of it—the differential diagnosis is greatly simplified by consulting a list of the possibilities (Table 8–5).

THE DESTRUCTIVE PATTERN

A variety of diseases destroy pulmonary tissue without regard to histologic boundaries.[688] They cut a swath across the lung, invading or destroying alveoli, bronchi, vessels, and interstitium indiscriminately. However, except for certain of the deep fungi, especially actinomycosis,[391] blastomycosis,[515] and torulosis (Fig. 9–33), they seldom violate the pleural surfaces. Their roentgen hallmark is the cavity (Fig. 8–33).

Table 8–6 lists as many of the causes of the destructive pattern as I could think of. If you can recall others, write them in. Pneumoconiosis is included because bland necrosis may occur within a conglomerate mass. These diseases often closely resemble each other roentgenologically, so that differentiation usually depends upon clinical, bacteriologic, and histopathologic findings.

The lesions are ill defined on their pe-

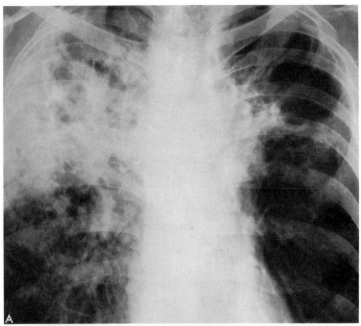

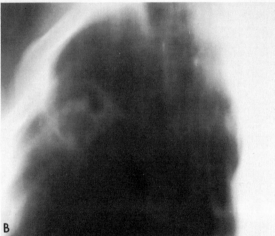

Figure 8–33. DESTRUCTIVE PAT-
TERN: THE CAVITY

A, Chronic fibrocavitary histoplasmosis. Small cavities in the right
apex and a large one in the left. *B, M.
kansasii* tuberculosis. Tomogram.

TABLE 8–6. Causes of Destructive Pattern

Common
  Bronchogenic carcinoma
  Tuberculosis
  Fungus diseases[46, 391, 515, 1095]
  Lung abscess,[38] sepsis[597]
  Laceration, missile wound[310, 584, 697, 733, 914, 1146, 1214]

Rare
  Pneumoconiosis[169]
  Infarct[889, 1071]
  Wegener's granuloma[342]
  Chronic granulomatous disease of childhood[125, 662]
  Parasitic or tropical diseases (e.g., amebic abscess,
    paragonimiasis, melioidosis[719, 764]
  Lymphoma[1163]

riphery, where they often show an alveolar
pattern (Fig. 8–34). One or more cavities are
usually visible within the infiltrate as variable sized irregular pockets of air (Fig. 8–
35), sometimes containing an air-fluid level
(Figs. 8–36 and 8–37). What I call an *up-
stairs-downstairs distribution,* i.e., apical
involvement on one side and basal involvement on the same or opposite side, is common, especially in tuberculosis.

Spontaneous or therapeutic regression of
the exudates surrounding a cavity may
leave a residual thin walled, bulla-like structure, often with open bronchial communication.[38, 46] Long linear fibrous strands

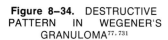
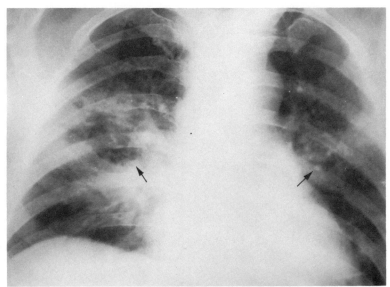

Figure 8–34. DESTRUCTIVE PATTERN IN WEGENER'S GRANULOMA[77, 731]

The peripheral margins of the bilateral infiltrates present an alveolar pattern. Note the cavities (arrows). (From Felson, B., and Braunstein, H.[342]; reproduced with permission of Charles C Thomas, Publ.)

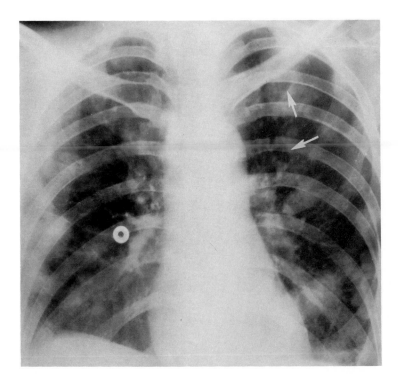

Figure 8–35. DESTRUCTIVE PATTERN IN SEPTICEMIA

The ill-defined infiltrates represent infected infarcts. Central breakdown (arrows) was eventually seen in most of the lesions. Autopsy proof.

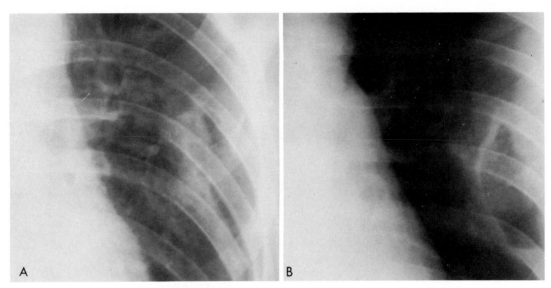

Figure 8–36. DESTRUCTIVE PATTERN IN PULMONARY LACERATION

A, This film was obtained on the day of a blunt chest injury. Note the cavity. *B,* The next day an air-fluid level is present in it. Early cavity formation is common.

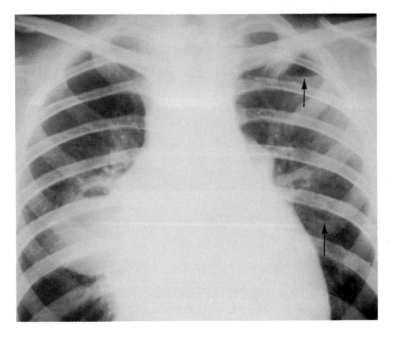

Figure 8–37. DESTRUCTIVE PATTERN IN HODGKIN'S DISEASE

Fluid levels are present (arrows).

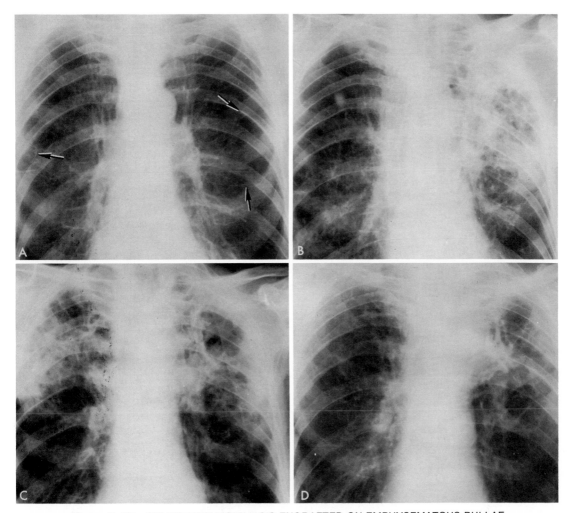

Figure 8–38. PULMONARY MONILIASIS ENGRAFTED ON EMPHYSEMATOUS BULLAE

A, Chest normal except for bullae (arrows). *B*, 7 months later. Chronic respiratory symptoms. The bullae show through the left-sided infiltrate. A destructive pattern is suggested. *C*, 4 months later. The infiltrate now involves the RUL. *D*, 1½ years later. Scar formation with hilar retraction remains. Repeated cultures at the time of *B* and *C* were positive for *Candida albicans.*

with retraction of mediastinum, hilum, or interlobar septum also indicate past or recent efforts at healing. The fibrotic scars do not regress. Lobar collapse of either contractive or obstructive type is a common sequela, especially in healed tuberculosis.

Pneumonia engrafted upon preexisting bullous emphysema gives difficulty in differential diagnosis. The bullae show through the alveolar exudate as air or air-fluid pockets and are impossible to distinguish from true lung destruction without preexisting or early follow-up films showing the bullae without the infiltrate.[1343, 1344]

The superimposition of an indolent infiltrate on existing bullae suggests particularly the possibility of Monilia infection (Fig. 8–38). Once in a while histoplasmosis[962] or tuberculosis[597, 1036] may behave in a similar manner. Cystic bronchiectasis surrounded by pneumonia may also simulate the destructive pattern.

In the absence of bronchial communication, the cavities of destructive lung disease may be filled with fluid and the resemblance to alveolar disease is then striking. Pneumonia with pneumatocele may present an appearance identical to the destructive pattern, but the day-to-day change identifies the pneumatocele (Fig. 7–50).

CHAPTER 9

THE PLEURA

ANATOMIC CONSIDERATIONS

The parietal and visceral layers of the pleura are not visible on the normal chest film because their shadows blend with the water density of the chest wall, mediastinum, and diaphragm. Where the pleura is outlined on both sides by air density, as in the interlobar planes, it can often be seen. Even under these circumstances, visibility depends on the central beam striking the interlobar surface tangentially. This has been discussed in greater detail at the beginning of Chapter 3.

The mediastinal surfaces of the pleura can occasionally be demonstrated at or near the midline where the right and left pleurae come in contact.[443] They are best seen on Bucky, lordotic, or high kilovoltage films that adequately penetrate the mediastinal and spinal shadows.[68, 686] The chief zones of junction of the two pleural surfaces are three in number and are located anterior to the ascending aorta, immediately behind the heart, and under the aortic arch. In the presence of unilateral emphysema or collapse, the lung may herniate through one or more of these areas into the opposite thorax (Fig. 3–51). The mediastinal pleural reflections are discussed further in Chapter 11.

Another anatomic consideration that bears emphasis is the surprising depth of the posterior component of the costophrenic sulcus. The posterior reflections of the pleura onto the diaphragm are often visible

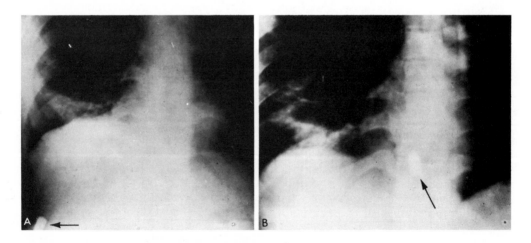

Figure 9–1. BULLET IN THE PLEURAL CAVITY

This Lothario slammed the back door behind him as the husband fired. The bullet that struck the fleeing lover was almost as spent as he, barely penetrating the chest and dropping free into the pleural cavity. *A*, Upright. *B*, Recumbent. The shifting bullet (arrows) illustrates the depth of the posterior costophrenic sinus and one of the hazards of clandestine sex in Cincinnati.

on a well-penetrated abdominal or chest film as a horizontal line with medial ascent or slight upward concavity on each side, a considerable distance below the dome.[686] Relatively large amounts of pleural fluid may accumulate here without being apparent on the upright PA teleroentgenogram. A pulmonary lesion or foreign body located within or adjacent to it is often projected well down into the abdomen on conventional films. It may, in fact, appear virtually certain that such a density lies within the abdomen (Fig. 9–1). Fluoroscopy and spot films with oblique positioning will often clarify the location.

FREE FLUID

The configuration of free pleural fluid does not appear to be related to the nature of the fluid or to its etiology[279, 649] (Table 9–1). Such fluid often presents the familiar appearance of a homogeneous opacity with a concave upper border, higher laterally than medially, the so-called *pleural meniscus* (Fig. 9–2). Actually, there is nothing in the pleural sac of this shape; were it possible to quick-freeze the upright patient, there would be no ice wedge to cast this meniscus shadow. Instead, a hollow cup of ice much taller than its roentgen shadow, thicker at the base and tapering to a fine edge at the top, would be found encasing the lower lung. Although the only thing I've ever frozen is an ice cube, the evidence for this configuration of pleural effusion is well supported.[242, 376] Simply stated, the meniscus is a tangential projection of the lateral side of the cup. There is also a meniscus shadow medially and anteriorly and posteriorly, but an upright film of adequate penetration and appropriate projection is required to show it. In fact, if you turn the upright patient as on a spit during fluoroscopy there will always be a meniscus at the outer margin.

Free pleural fluid may show a variety of other patterns on the upright film. One of these, the subpulmonary, occurs with such frequency that Hessen[538] considered it to be the normal distribution, and I am inclined to agree. Rigler first called attention to this collection of fluid apparently trapped between the diaphragm and the undersurface of the lung on the upright film.[995]

TABLE 9–1. Causes of Pleural Fluid

Common
  Acute pancreatitis
  Cirrhosis
  Collagen disease
  Congestive heart failure
  Idiopathic
  Infection (bacterial, fungus, parasitic, tuberculous, viral)[1140]
  Malignancy
  Postmyocardial infarction syndrome
  Pulmonary infarction
  Renal disease
  Subphrenic abscess[1059]
  Trauma to lung, mediastinum, spine[988]

Rare
  Amebiasis[723]
  Asbestosis
  Coagulation defect
  Hydrocarbon ingestion
  Hypoproteinemia
  Iatrogenic (surgery, instillation of drugs)
  Infectious mononucleosis
  Löffler's syndrome
  Mediterranean fever
  Meigs' syndrome
  Methysergide therapy[543]
  Myxedema
  Nephrosis and other renal disease
  Niemann-Pick disease
  Obstructed superior vena cava or azygos vein
  Radiation therapy[1290]
  Rheumatoid disease[60]
  Ruptured aneurysm
  Ruptured dermoid cyst
  Ruptured esophagus
  Sarcoid
  Spontaneous chylothorax
  Waldenström's macroglobulinemia
  Wegener's granulomatosis
  Whipple's disease

Roentgenologically, it presents as an opaque shadow with upward convexity, parallel to the hemidiaphragm in both frontal and lateral projections. The appearance closely simulates that of an elevated diaphragm (Figs. 9–3 to 9–5) and, on this account, is commonly ignored or misinterpreted. Certain recognizable differences suggest the true diagnosis. The "costophrenic" and "cardiophrenic" angles are often shallow or obliterated. The fluid density is generally greater than that of the diaphragm, since the aerated lung in the posterior costophrenic sinus, which normally reduces diaphragmatic opacity, has been replaced by fluid. There may be evidence of pleural disease elsewhere in the affected hemithorax, e.g., in the interlobar

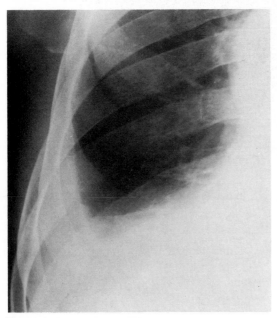

Figure 9–2. FREE PLEURAL FLUID, MENISCUS
PATTERN

planes. The crest of the shadow of the sub-pulmonary fluid often lies more lateral than that of an elevated hemidiaphragm. On the left side, the gas bubble in the fundus of the stomach lies some distance below the dome

of the "diaphragm," but this finding is sometimes seen normally (Chap. 12). On the right side, the lower margin of the liver is usually at its normal level and the minor fissure lies closer to the "diaphragm" than normal. In the lateral upright view, the posterior costophrenic angle usually shows a small meniscus while anteriorly the shadow appears to flatten against the major fissure.[376, 934]

Any of these signs should lead you to suspect free pleural fluid. Confirmation is readily obtained with recumbent or decubitus views or with fluoroscopy.[994] In the supine view, the true diaphragm is now seen at its normal level and there is a haze over the affected thorax caused by the layer of pleural fluid which has gravitated posteriorly (Fig. 9–4B). In the decubitus view with the involved side dependent, the fluid will, of course, accumulate along its lateral wall. This is demonstrated better with the table in slight Trendelenburg position to empty the costophrenic angle. It should be noted that in some normal individuals a small amount of free pleural fluid, as little as 5 to 10 cc, can be demonstrated by this maneuver, and even aspirated.[848a, 851, 1332] The incidence is higher after exercise and during pregnancy.

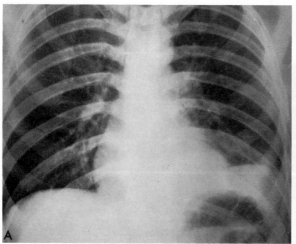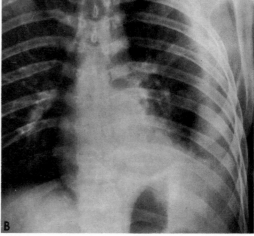

Figure 9–3. SUBPULMONARY FLUID, LEFT

A, Upright film. The crest of the fluid lies slightly more lateral than that of an elevated diaphragm. There is considerable distance between the gas bubble of the stomach and the top of the "diaphragm." The left side of the heart is denser than the right. The "cardiophrenic" and "costophrenic" angles are shallow. *B,* Left lateral decubitus view (printed upright for comparison). The fluid extends along the dependent left lateral chest wall. Note the elevated left hemidiaphragm.

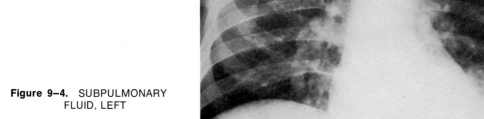

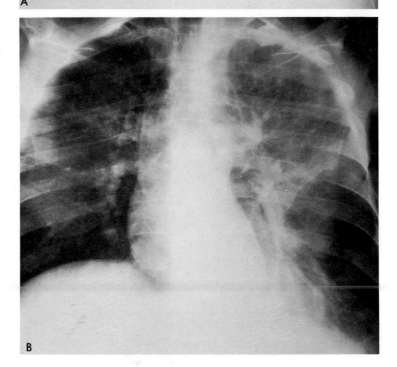

Figure 9–4. SUBPULMONARY FLUID, LEFT

A, Upright teleroentgenogram. The left hemidiaphragm appears elevated. The left lower portion of the cardiac density is increased because of fluid behind it. So is the left diaphragm. The left costophrenic angle is shallow. The gastric bubble is not seen. *B,* Patient supine. The left pleural fluid has shifted upward, causing a difference in radiolucency of the two sides of the thorax. The left hemidiaphragm is now seen to be in normal position. Note the normal vasculature in the left lung, indicating that the underlying pulmonary tissue is well aerated.

I prefer the decubitus position for small effusions, since the eye may fail to detect the slight unilateral increase in density on the supine film. The lateral decubitus film has one disadvantage: the elevated hemidiaphragm that normally occurs in this position (Fig. 9–3*B*) may hide a good part of the underlying lower lobe.

On fluoroscopy, the shadow of the subpulmonary effusion may move well with respiration, but on deep expiration the fluid often shifts into a meniscus pattern.[701] This will also occur on inspiration if the patient is tilted laterally[538] or if the table is lowered partially from the upright position. Ripples synchronous with cardiac pulsation may be seen. The high frequency of subpulmonary distribution of free pleural fluid and the difficulties in its recognition have led us to adopt the policy of recommending recum-

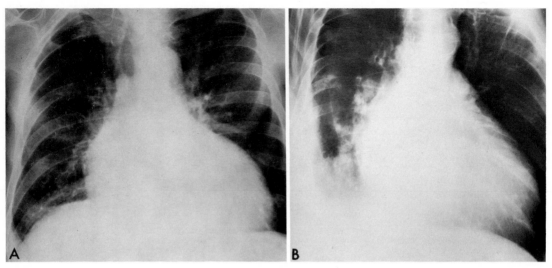

Figure 9–5. SUBPULMONARY FLUID, RIGHT

A, Teleroentgenogram. The right "hemidiaphragm" appears slightly elevated and a little more radiopaque than normal. The costophrenic sinus shows a small meniscus. *B,* Right lateral decubitus (printed upright). A large effusion is revealed. The patient was in congestive failure.

bent or decubitus films whenever one or both hemidiaphragms appear to be elevated.[345, 409, 613, 1037]

Other patterns of free fluid on the PA and lateral teleroentgenogram are much less common.[995, 1011] Occasionally, free fluid may arrange itself about an individual lobe and simulate lobar consolidation or collapse (Fig. 9–6). Rarely, it may present a fairly straight upper border (Fig. 9–7). Not infrequently it appears to rise higher on the mediastinal than on the lateral side. Free fluid may parallel the heart border so closely that cardiac enlargement is simulated (Fig. 9–8). Fluid may collect along the lateral thoracic wall on the upright film. Occasionally some of the fluid is trapped in an interlobar fissure, causing a step-off. More often the fluid collects in the minor fissure[376]; major fissure accumulation may result in a visible vertical fissure line on the frontal projection[1222] (Fig. 3–3). A paraspinal pleural fluid collection is often recognizable on the supine abdominal film, obliterating or overlapping the shadow of the descending aorta (Fig. 9–9). An interesting challenge is presented in Figure 9–10.

Several theories have been propounded to explain the inconsistencies in fluid distribution. The most versatile of these is that of Fleischner, who postulated an increased tendency of portions of the lung underlying the fluid to collapse because of multifocal bronchial obstructions.[376] The negative pressure thus created attracts the fluid as in a pocket. Since the relative retractility of the individual lobes can vary from patient to patient, a variety of roentgen patterns of free fluid may occur.

It is generally assumed that a large amount of fluid will displace the heart and other mediastinal structures to the contralateral side, but it is surprising how much fluid can sometimes be present without such displacement. On a number of occasions I have seen free fluid extending almost to the first rib without detectable shift of the midline structures. However, when the *entire* thorax is opacified by free fluid, mediastinal displacement is nearly always seen and occasionally even mediastinal herniation (Fig. 9–11). In fact, if the entire thorax is filled with fluid without mediastinal displacement, or if there is a shift toward the side of the fluid, one should strongly suspect collapse in the underlying lung, antedating the development of the fluid. Bronchogenic carcinoma is by far the most frequent cause of this sign[735] (Fig. 3–53). It is better to rely on tracheal rather than on cardiac displacement, since only one heart border is visible in these patients.

(*Text continued on page 359.*)

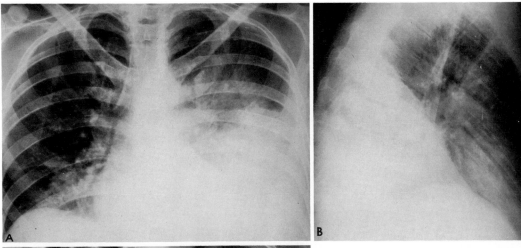

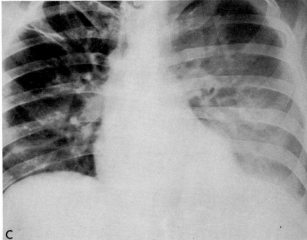

Figure 9–6. FREE FLUID SIMULATING LOBAR CONSOLIDATION

A and *B*, PA and left lateral upright teleroentgenograms. On the lateral view, the anterior margin of the density seems to outline the left major fissure. The appearance is easily mistaken for LLL pneumonia. *C*, Recumbent film made the same day. The fluid has now shifted to the posterior portion of the thorax. Biliary cirrhosis with ascites. Incidentally, compare the azygos vein in *A* and *C*. (From Felson, B., Fleischner, F. G., McDonald, J. R., and Rabin, C. B.[345]; reproduced with permission of Radiology.)

Figure 9–7. FREE PLEURAL FLUID, RIGHT, WITH AN ALMOST HORIZONTAL UPPER BORDER

The fluid may be contained in the subpulmonary pleural space. The upper margin of the fluid is not as sharply defined as an air-fluid level and is not parallel to the bottom of the film. Congestive failure.

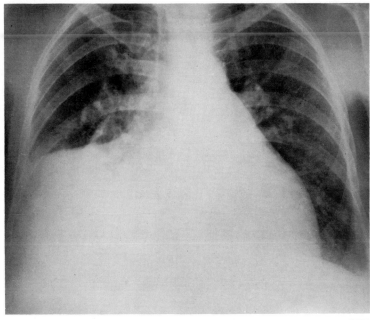

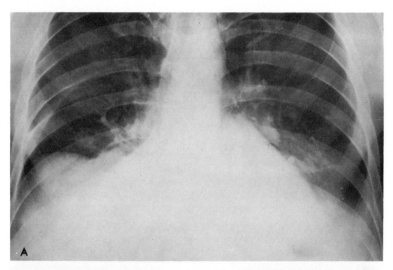

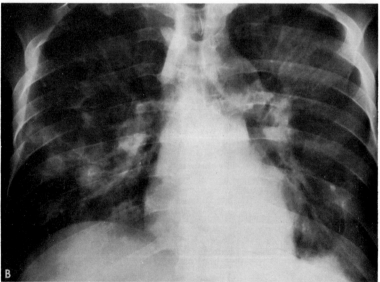

Figure 9–8. FREE PLEURAL FLUID SIMULATING CARDIAC ENLARGEMENT

A, The heart appears extremely enlarged and a diagnosis of congestive failure was made despite absent clinical signs of heart disease. *B,* Recumbent film, made the same day, reveals a normal heart. The free fluid has been displaced into the posterior portion of each pleural cavity. A ductus node is shown on the left. Hodgkin's disease. (From Felson, B., Fleischner, F. G., McDonald, J. R., and Rabin, C. B.[345]; reproduced with permission of Radiology.)

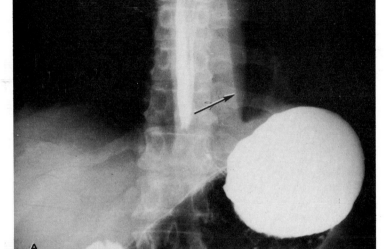

Figure 9–9. NOW YOU SEE IT,
        NOW YOU DON'T

A, Supine film shows a left jux-
tamediastinal collection of fluid
(arrow) medial to the lateral
border of the descending aorta. B,
Prone film a few moments later.
The fluid has gravitated out of the
medial gutter.

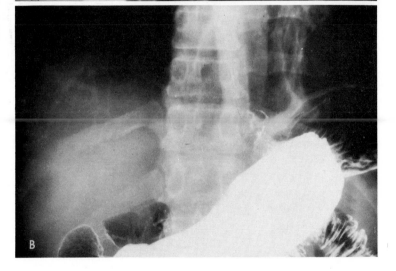

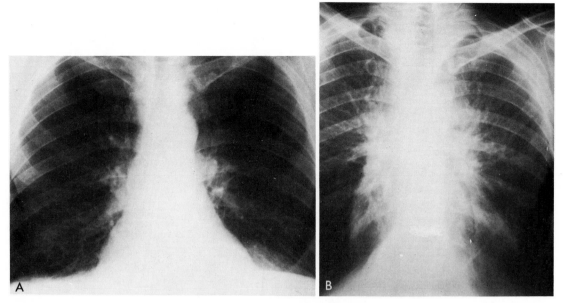

Figure 9–10.   UPRIGHT AND BUCKY RECUMBENT CHEST FILMS

The heart borders are obliterated only on the recumbent film *(B)*. Can you figure it out? The answer is in the legend of Figure 9–12.

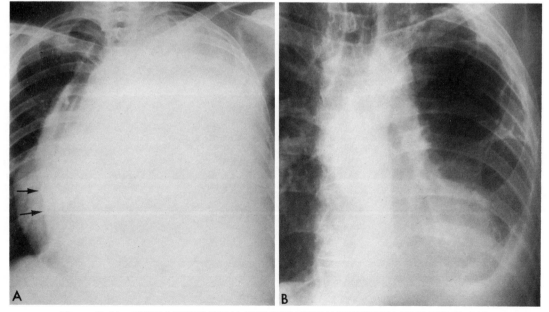

Figure 9–11.   HUGE LEFT PLEURAL EFFUSION WITH HERNIATION OF PLEURAL SAC

A, The trachea is grossly displaced but the mediastinal herniation (arrows) extends beyond it. *B,* After treatment. The trachea is now midline and the heart is deviated to the left. Tuberculous pleural effusion.

A large left effusion or lower intrathoracic mass will frequently invert the left leaf of the diaphragm. This results in a smooth hemispherical opacity in the left upper quadrant of the abdomen that impinges on and displaces the fundus of the stomach. Phrenic inversion is discussed in detail in Chapter 12.

It is often desirable to see the lung underneath a pleural effusion. Although Bucky recumbent films are useful for this purpose, a decubitus view with the affected side uppermost will often prove more helpful, since free fluid will gravitate along the mediastinum and the unobscured lung will rise toward the lateral chest wall. Better yet is filming immediately after a pleural tap. Pleural injection of gas at the time of the tap will reveal the thickness of the pleura and sometimes even show the nodules of pleural metastases (Fig. 9–12).

In uncomplicated congestive failure, the pleural fluid accumulation is often greater on the right than on the left for some unexplained reason. The reverse is hardly ever true.[816, 1291] Therefore, if one demonstrates distinctly more fluid in the left pleural space than in the right, or if the fluid is present only on the left side, causes of pleural effusion other than heart failure *per se* should receive first consideration. I have seen but one proved instance of unilateral left effusion from cardiac failure. By far the commonest cause of predominantly left-sided effusion associated with enlargement of the heart is pulmonary infarction.[958] However, what's to prevent a cardiac patient from having a left tuberculous, pancreatitic, cirrhotic, or neoplastic effusion (Fig. 9–13)?

A partial exception to this rule occurs when the right pleural cavity is totally obliterated or almost so, as it is in a small percentage of all individuals. But these cases can be recognized by the obvious pleural thickening and encapsulation of fluid that occurs on the right side with pleural symphysis (Fig. 9–15C). Although there are some dissenting opinions, in my experience the sign has held up well and has enabled us to suspect and later confirm the presence of some other disease in many cardiac patients.

A discussion of the relationship of pleural fluid to abdominal disease will be found in Chapter 12. At this time, I would merely

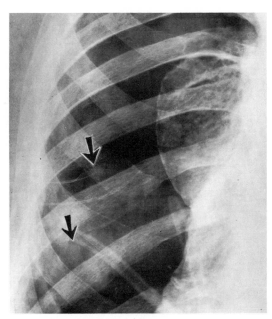

Figure 9–12. PLEURAL METASTASES DEMONSTRATED BY DIAGNOSTIC PNEUMOTHORAX

Upright film following pleural tap and injection of air. In addition to the nodular thickening of the pleura seen laterally, many individual nodules are visible (arrows).

Answer to Figure 9–10: *B* is a *prone* film of a patient with bilateral free subpulmonary pleural fluid (*A*) which has gravitated forward alongside the heart, obliterating its borders. (Courtesy of Dr. Richard C. Cavanagh.)

like to note that the diaphragm under certain circumstances is leaky.

Encapsulated Fluid

Pleural fluid encapsulation is the result of obliteration of the pleural space by fusion of the parietal and visceral layers. Extensive unilateral pleural symphysis, encountered in 5 per cent of autopsies, may be developmental or acquired from past or current pleural disease. Some portion of the pleural cavity remains patent in nearly every instance, and here fluid can still accumulate.

As already noted, the distribution of free fluid seen on the upright film may at times resemble that of encapsulated fluid. Gravitational methods will readily distinguish the two. Differentiation between en-

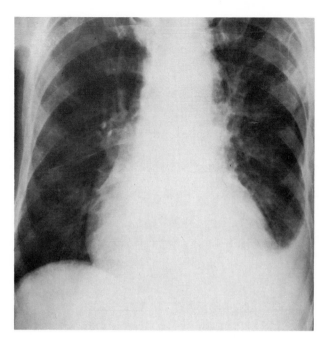

Figure 9–13.   LEFT PLEURAL EFFUSION IN A
CARDIAC PATIENT

The cause of the fluid was metastatic malignancy.

capsulated pleural fluid and extrapleural lesions will be discussed in the next chapter.

At times, pleural encapsulation may closely simulate pulmonary consolidation or collapse or mediastinal tumor.[1185] For example, encapsulated fluid in the posteromedial portion of the lower pleural cavity is sometimes mistaken for lower lobe pneumonia. The borders of an encapsulation are generally more convex than those outlining a collapsed or consolidated lobe. In the lateral view, the major septum is usually visible anterior to the encapsulated fluid. Pleural thickening elsewhere in the thorax generally accompanies loculated fluid. Demonstration of an air bronchogram within the shadow in question has helped us on a number of occasions to recognize that it is pulmonary rather than pleural in location. Bronchography, by delineating the lobar margins, serves admirably to distinguish the two conditions (Fig. 9–14).

Interlobar effusion is encountered most commonly in heart failure. The interlobar fluid may cast a sharply marginated elliptical or circular shadow which, on the frontal roentgenogram, may closely resemble a solid tumor. As the cardiac status improves,

the rapid regression of such densities has led to the terms *pseudo-* or *vanishing tumor.*[317, 320, 823, 919, 1272] Vanishing tumor is most often encountered with minor fissure encapsulation. A tendency for the shadow to recur in the same area with subsequent bouts of heart failure has been noted (Fig. 9–15).

The diagnosis of interlobar fluid can be suspected or made on the frontal roentgenogram from the location of the opacity at the site of projection of an interlobar septum; the slight tapering of the medial and lateral margins in the case of minor fissure encapsulation; the broad, ill-defined, medially concave, kidney shaped density with major fissure involvement (Fig. 9–16); the double bubble shadow of minor and superior major fissure loculation (Fig. 9–17); and the detection of pleural involvement elsewhere in the hemithorax.[368, 996] Confirmation is obtained from the lateral view, in which the long axis of the opacity conforms to the position of the distended fissure and the tapering extremities are more clearly depicted (Figs. 9–17*B* and 9–18). A large effusion may cause the fissure to sag (Fig. 9–19).

The distinction between RML collapse and fluid encapsulated in the lower part of the right major fissure or in the minor fissure may be difficult[604] (Fig. 9–20). Many cases diagnosed as interlobar encapsulation in the past were, in fact, instances of middle lobe collapse. I found a number of such errors on reviewing some of my own material of 20 years ago.

In the frontal view interlobar fluid, unlike RML collapse, rarely causes the silhouette sign. However, the two conditions are better differentiated on the lateral roentgenogram. In RML collapse, at least one border of the density is concave or straight, whereas in interlobar effusion the margins are generally convex, so that the opacity appears spindle shaped or cigar shaped. The collapsed middle lobe nearly always makes contact with the caudal portion of the anterior chest wall, too low for the position of the minor fissure and too high for the major fissure, which intersects the diaphragm, not the chest wall. Both extremities of the en-

capsulation are usually tapered, whereas in collapse the anterior end is broad. In the lateral view, the minor and lower half of the major septa are not visible as separate linear shadows in RML collapse, since they form the margins of the pulmonary density. But in interlobar encapsulation, one or the other fissure is usually seen, especially since appreciable thickening of the pleura elsewhere in the hemithorax often accompanies fluid encapsulation. If an air bronchogram is demonstrated within the opaque shadow, interlobar effusion can, of course, be excluded.

Localized pleural mesothelioma may also closely simulate encapsulated effusion (Fig. 10–4). Lobulation of the roentgen shadow favors tumor. In the lateral film, interlobar encapsulation may be simulated by the *overlap shadow* of RLL collapse or consolidation. Differentiation is easily made by identifying the back of the heart (Fig. 2–9).

(*Text continued on page 366.*)

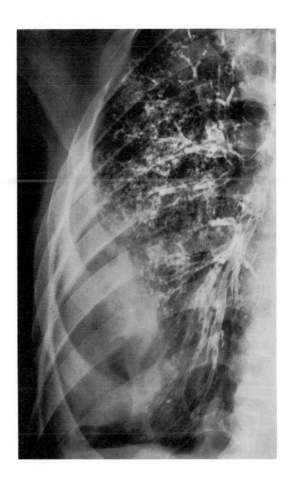

Figure 9–14. PLEURAL ENCAPSULATION RESEMBLING PULMONARY DISEASE

The bronchogram delineates the entire right lung and reveals extrinsic compression. On the plain film, differentiation between encapsulated pyopneumothorax and lung abscess could not be made with certainty.

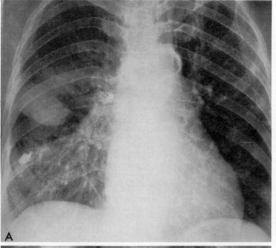

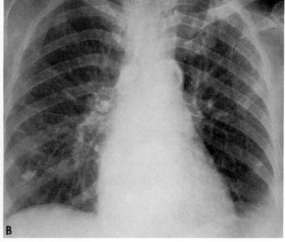

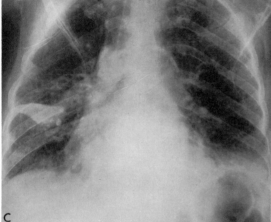

Figure 9–15. "VANISHING TUMOR"

A, The encapsulated fluid in the minor fissure simulates a tumor. The patient is in congestive failure. *B,* 1 week later the interlobar effusion has cleared. The minor fissure is thickened. The cardiac status has improved. *C,* 9 days later the interlobar fluid has recurred coincident with another episode of congestive failure. There is now also free fluid in the left pleural cavity. (From Felson, B.[326]; reproduced with permission of Charles C Thomas, Publisher.)

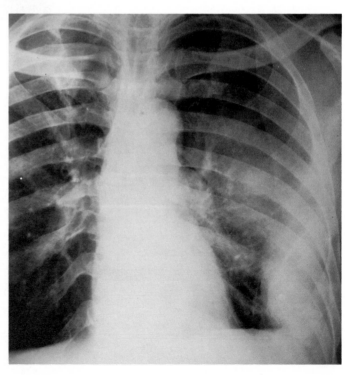

Figure 9–16. FLUID ENCAPSULATED IN LEFT MAJOR FISSURE

The ill-defined reniform density is characteristic of oblique fissure loculation. Postpneumonic empyema.

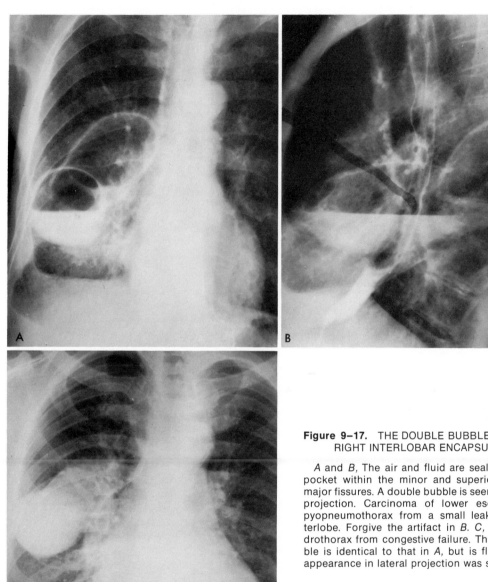

Figure 9–17. THE DOUBLE BUBBLE SHADOW OF RIGHT INTERLOBAR ENCAPSULATION

A and *B*, The air and fluid are sealed in a single pocket within the minor and superior half of the major fissures. A double bubble is seen in the frontal projection. Carcinoma of lower esophagus with pyopneumothorax from a small leak into the interlobe. Forgive the artifact in *B*. *C*, Interlobar hydrothorax from congestive failure. The double bubble is identical to that in *A*, but is fluid filled. The appearance in lateral projection was similar to *B*.

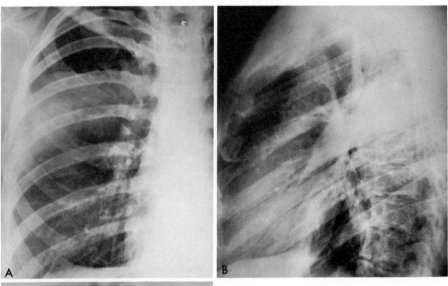

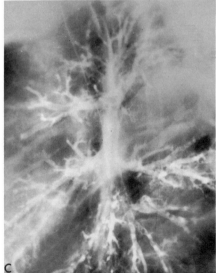

Figure 9–18. ENCAPSULATED FLUID IN SUPERIOR HALF OF RIGHT MAJOR FISSURE

A, The lower border of the opacity is not sharply defined, as by the minor fissure (see Fig. 9–15). *B,* The right lateral view shows tapering inferiorly and convexity of the anterior and posterior margins. *C,* Right lateral bronchogram performed at the insistence of a disbeliever. The fluid separates the posterior segment of the RUL from the superior segment of the RLL. (Courtesy of Dr. Lee S. Rosenberg.)

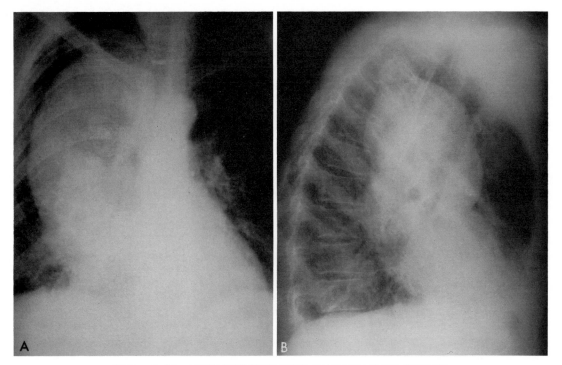

Figure 9–19. HUGE ENCAPSULATION IN RIGHT MAJOR FISSURE

The large major interlobar effusion has a reniform configuration in *A* and shows a lobulated or buckled outline in *B.* Inflammatory etiology.

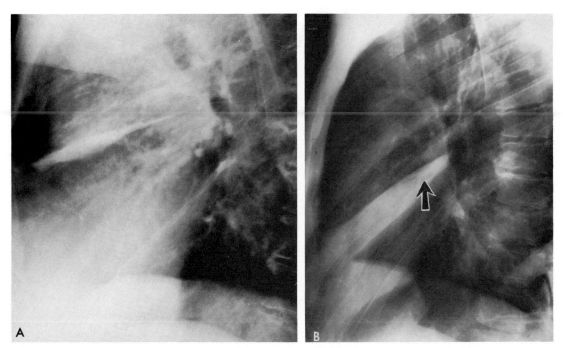

Figure 9–20. DIFFERENTIAL DIAGNOSIS BETWEEN INTERLOBAR EFFUSION AND RML COLLAPSE

A, Cigar shaped encapsulation in the minor fissure. Note visibility of the thickened major fissure. *B,* Triangular shaped RML collapse. The arrow points to several air filled bronchi.

PNEUMOTHORAX

The demonstration of a small pneumothorax is facilitated by expiration (Fig. 1–15). In a previous book, I attributed the expiratory enlargement of a pneumothorax to expansion of the pleural air because of the lowered pressure within the lung. Fleischner, among others, tactfully chided me, noting that intrapulmonary pressure is *higher* during expiration. He further stated, "The slight changes during the respiratory phases by 2 to 4 cm water, as compared with atmospheric pressure of about 100 cm water, have very little influence upon the pneumothorax air in the way of compression or expansion. The explanation is quite simple. In maximal inspiration and expiration we change the lung not only in volume by the vital capacity, we increase and decrease also correspondingly the surface of the lung or the inner surface of the chest. Let us assume that we have two equal squares of butter, and a big and small slice of bread. We cover these slices each with one pat of butter. On the small slice the butter forms a thick layer, on the big slice we have to spread it thin. Thus the pleural air forms a thin layer about the lung in inspiratory standstill; in expiration, covering only a small surface, it is arranged in a thick layer. The compression occurs, of course, but I am sure that it contributes to our visible change not more than 5 per cent."

Dr. David Gelfand, one of our residents at the time, spelled it out with films (Fig. 9–21), less tasty than bread and butter but more edible than crow. Occasionally the effect of expiration may be quite striking (Fig. 9–22).

A lateral decubitus film with the affected side uppermost is just as useful in the diagnosis of pneumothorax as the expiration film, since it allows all the pleural air to collect along the lateral chest wall where even minute amounts can be visualized. This position also serves to distinguish pneumothorax from other intrathoracic collections of air, such as extensive bullous emphysema ("vanishing lung"), pneumomediastinum, and pneumopericardium (Fig. 11–8). This view, or a cross-table lateral,[279, 773] is important in infants in whom the recumbent AP film often fails to show a small amount of pleural air collected near the sternum, the highest point in the thorax in this position.

A word of caution concerning the interpretation of shadows within lung tissue partially compressed by pneumothorax is indicated. Not infrequently, a spurious shadow that simulates a cavitary or pulmonary consolidation results from the irregular compression collapse of segments in the underlying lung. However, it is occasionally possible to see interstitial air bubbles in the lung compressed by pneumothorax secondary to spontaneous pneumomediastinum, indicating the track of the air leak.[388, 907]

It is extremely important to recognize tension pneumothorax because it requires emergency thoracentesis. Generally this is easy because of the marked compression of the lung. The lung tends to retain its shape in pneumothorax due to its elastic recoil[376] (Fig. 9–22) and to traction by the pulmonary ligament[957] (Fig. 9–25). High pressure pneumothorax secondary to valvelike communication with the lung or through the chest wall often overcomes this tendency, squeezing the lung into a formless shadow along the spine and often displacing it across the midline (Fig. 9–23). The high pressure sometimes even inverts the diaphragm (Fig. 12–14). Acquired communication between the two pleural cavities may occur.[1262] If the lung is splinted from within by air bubbles in the interstitial tissue or extensive disease in the parenchyma, a deceptive situation arises: the lung cannot collapse completely[197] (Fig. 9–24). However, in this event pleural tension is still recognizable by the displacement of the mediastinal structures, though the lung itself shows only mild compression collapse. Remember, though, some degree of contralateral mediastinal shift occurs on expiration in every pneumothorax, so only inspiratory displacement counts.

Oh, Fleischner, and Wyman have called attention to a sign in traumatic pneumothorax that implies a fractured main stem bronchus.[897] The entire mediastinal surface of the lung, including the hilar region, is outlined by the mediastinal air. It worked in one instance (Fig. 9–24), but it shouldn't. The medial edge of a lung is often outlined by pleural or mediastinal air, even with an intact bronchus.

(Text continued on page 370.)

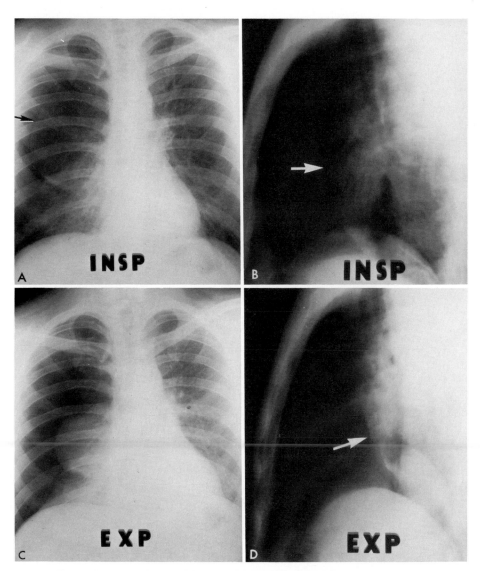

Figure 9–21. RESPIRATORY EFFECT ON THE SIZE OF A PNEUMOTHORAX

The volume of pleural air is the same on inspiration as on expiration; the lung (arrows) and thorax are smaller on expiration. Confirmed by volumetry. The lateral views were made with the patient supine; the frontal views are PA teleroentgenograms.

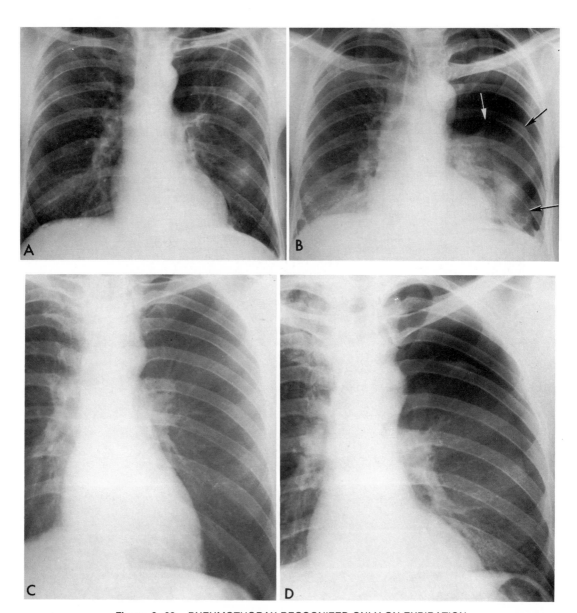

Figure 9–22. PNEUMOTHORAX RECOGNIZED ONLY ON EXPIRATION

A, Inspiratory film. There is a small radiolucency along the lower left heart border and adjacent to the aortic knob. *B,* Expiratory film made immediately after *A.* The pneumothorax appears much larger. Arrows outline the compressed lung. Note that the compressed lung has retained its normal configuration. (Courtesy of Dr. Samuel H. Fisher.) *C* and *D,* Another patient. The pneumothorax is invisible on the inspiration film. Note the shift of the heart to the right on expiration (*B* and *D*).

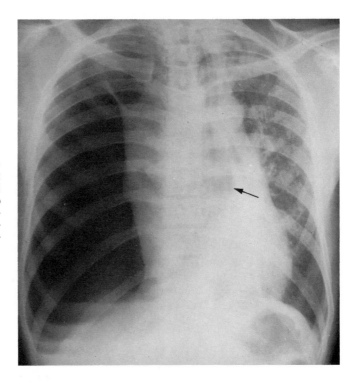

Figure 9–23. TENSION
PNEUMOTHORAX

An adhesion has prevented complete
collapse of the apex but the rest of the right
lung is compressed medially (arrow), and
the air filled right pleural sac extends into
the left thorax (arrow) along with the mediastinal structures. The costal attachments of the right hemidiaphragm are visible because the dome is depressed.

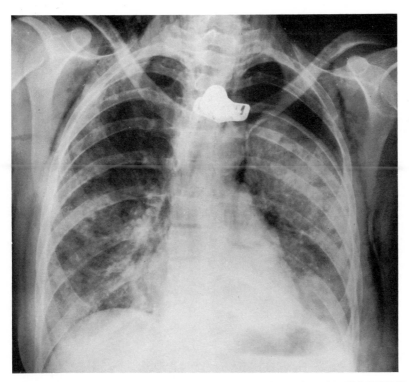

Figure 9–24. PNEUMOMEDIASTINUM AND PNEUMOTHORAX CAUSED BY FRACTURED LEFT MAIN
BRONCHUS

The medial surface of the lung is clearly visible along the hilum, indicating discontinuity. Contusion and interstitial air have splinted the left lung from within so that it cannot collapse completely. Tension pneumothorax is difficult to recognize in this situation. The roentgen findings were present before the tracheotomy.

369

Deep in the lateral costophrenic angle in pneumothorax one commonly sees two intersecting lines forming a V, with the apex pointing laterally (Fig. 9–25).* For some time I thought this represented the parietal pleural reflection. However, a skeptical resident proved to me, by tilting the patient, that the V represents a small amount of free fluid. The roentgen beam, striking the peripheral portion of the thorax obliquely rather than tangentially, projects the anterior and posterior surfaces of the air-fluid level into different planes, neither of which is quite parallel to the floor.

Air loculated under the left lung has been called *subpulmonary pneumothorax*.[683] In reality, it represents extrapleural extension from a pneumomediastinum. Recently, it has been shown that Hamman's sign ("mediastinal crunch") is not diagnostic of pneumomediastinum but is commonly

---

*Not to be confused with the V sign of Naclerio seen with pneumomediastinum in the left mediastinophrenic angle, resulting from ruptured esophagus.[860]

also caused by a small left pneumothorax (Chap. 11).

When pneumomediastinum and pneumothorax coexist, as they often do in infants,[1048] one may safely assume that the pneumomediastinum developed first.[179] Macklin and Macklin showed experimentally that air in the pleural space cannot be forced through the intact visceral or mediastinal pleura but that, conversely, air in the mediastinum readily perforates the pleura to enter the pleural cavity.[778] Occasionally, the lower end of the esophagus will perforate into the left pleural sac directly instead of via the mediastinum, resulting in a large hydropneumothorax.[860]

Spontaneous pneumothorax, probably the result of a ruptured bulla, generally clears in 2 to 4 weeks, but lasts longer if complicated by pleural infection or bleeding, as occurs once in a while. Recurrent pneumothorax is seen in about one fourth of these patients.[585]

Table 9–2 lists the causes of pneumothorax. Curiously, osteogenic and other sarcomas account for many of the cases of

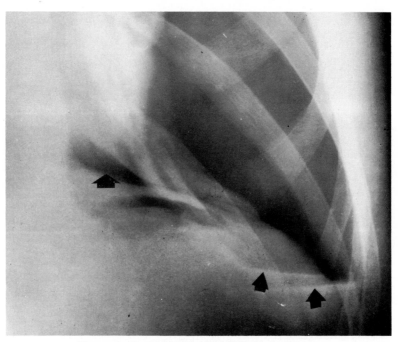

Figure 9–25. THE *V* LINE IN PNEUMOTHORAX

On the upright teleroentgenogram, the two intersecting lines (lower arrows) form a *V* with its apex directed laterally. This represents an air-fluid level in which the roentgen beam strikes the surface of the fluid obliquely. The triangular inferior pulmonary ligament (upper arrow) preserves the shape of the base of the collapsed lung.

TABLE 9-2. Causes of Pneumothorax

Common
  Iatrogenic
  Mediastinal emphysema
  Spontaneous (ruptured bulla)
  Trauma

Rare
  Bronchopleural fistula from lung abscess or
    granuloma (tuberculosis)
  Fibrocystic disease of the pancreas
  Honeycomb lung (Table 8-5)
  Hyaline membrane disease
  Oxygen toxicity; Wilson-Mikity syndrome
  Pneumonia
  Pneumoperitoneum with passage through
    diaphragm
  Primary or metastatic neoplasm
  Pulmonary infarction
  Ruptured esophagus

metastatic neoplasm[230] (Fig. 9-26). Infarct causing pneumothorax need not be of the infected variety.[91]

The differential diagnosis between a large bulla or lung abscess and encapsulated pneumothorax or hydropneumothorax is at times difficult (Figs. 1-11,

2-14, and 9-27). If the fissures are visible on the frontal or lateral projection, the location of the air or air-fluid pocket is facilitated, since pneumothorax, of course, does not conform to lobar boundaries. Roentgenograms of excellent detail in various projections may be helpful in demonstrating the very thin walls of bullae, although strandlike pleural adhesions extending across a pneumothorax may resemble them (Fig. 9-23). An expiratory film will generally show "enlargement" of the pneumothorax but not of the bulla or lung abscess. One may have to resort to bronchography to distinguish between these conditions (Fig. 9-14).

PLEURAL THICKENING

Obliteration of a lateral costophrenic angle, generally attributed to past inflammatory disease, is a common finding in the normal patient. It was encountered in 1.2 per cent of 600 Army inductees (Chap. 15). It is occasionally bilateral. Thickening of the apical pleura—the *apical cap* described by early writers—was visible to an appreciable degree in about 1 per cent of a similar group

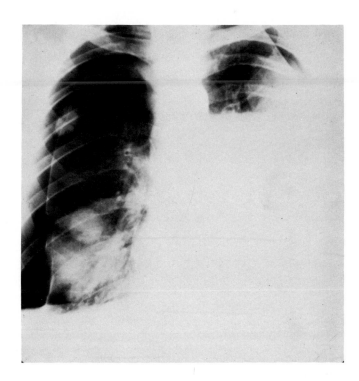

Figure 9-26. BILATERAL PNEUMOTHORAX FROM METASTATIC OSTEOGENIC SARCOMA

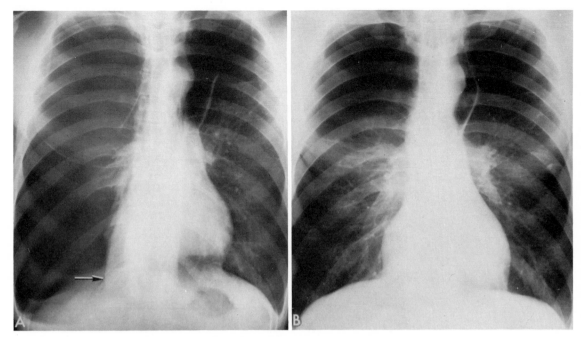

Figure 9–27. BULLOUS EMPHYSEMA VS. PNEUMOTHORAX

A, Obvious bullae are seen in both upper lung fields. What about the right lower lung? Note the collapsed RLL (arrow). Its triangular shape speaks for pneumothorax. An expiration or decubitus film would have established the diagnosis. *B*, Several weeks later. The pneumothorax has cleared and the RLL has expanded.

of inductees. It was bilateral in about one third and occurred more frequently on the left than on the right for no apparent reason. Small bullae often are seen adjacent to the thickened apical pleura. The etiology of apical cap has been attributed to the effects of past tuberculosis, but Pernice et al. found no evidence of tuberculosis in their carefully studied autopsy series.[933a] In about half of the 57 patients, they found no lesion to explain the roentgen sign. In the remainder, nonspecific fibrotic thickening of the visceral pleura and subpleural pulmonary tissue was apparent. Apical cap was visible roentgenographically in 11 per cent of their patients, who were considerably older than my Army inductees.

The "companion" shadow of the upper ribs, a much more common normal finding, may be mistaken for it. More important is the simulation of unilateral apical cap by superior sulcus carcinoma, sometimes referred to as *Pancoast's tumor*. When the tumor is advanced, there is no problem: its shadow is thick and lumpy, rib destruction is evident (Fig. 1–17), and Horner's syn-

drome and severe pain are usually present; but early, the tumor may present merely as a slight apical thickening. These tumors often break through the visceral and parietal pleura to extend into the neck. At one time they were even considered a special type of tumor that arose in a branchial arch.

Differentiation between pleural thickening and free fluid is readily made by utilizing gravitational techniques. A small encapsulation, however, may closely simulate old pleural thickening. Convexity toward the lung generally indicates encapsulated fluid, but exceptions are not uncommon and the distinction may be impossible to make. The normal internal thoracic shadow[1073,1113] often seen along the sternum in the lateral view should not be mistaken for pleural thickening or encapsulation (Chap. 13).

A pulmonary infarct in the costophrenic angle, a favored site, may also give difficulty. Hampton and Castleman pointed out that pleural thickening and free fluid are generally concave toward the hilum, whereas infarct is usually convex.[499] Their Boston colleagues euphonically dubbed

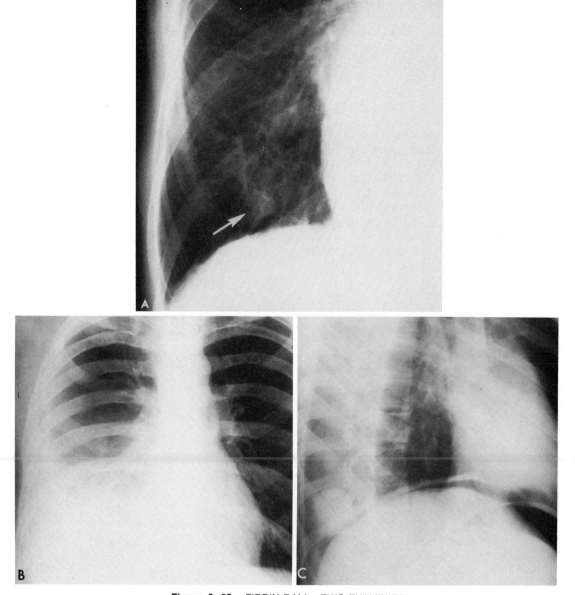

Figure 9–28.   FIBRIN BALL—TWO EXAMPLES

A, The pleural nodule (arrow) developed after a pleural effusion complicating right thoracotomy for mitral stenosis. Tomography showed ill-defined margins. At autopsy, the mass was found attached to the visceral pleura. *B,* Pleural effusion in another patient. *C,* Several months later. Right oblique view after diagnostic pneumoperitoneum. The large nodule and thickened pleura are residua of the effusion. (Courtesy of Dr. Henry I. Goldberg.)

this convexity "Hampton's hump" (Figs. 3–1 and 5–39). The proximal margin of an infarct is usually less sharp than pleural disease.

A fibrin ball, probably resulting from defibrination of blood or pus or effusion by cardiac pulsations, occasionally may form within pleural fluid. Pneumothorax is not essential for its development. As the effusion regresses, the fibrin ball becomes visible as a small pleural mass (Fig. 9–28). The condition should be suspected whenever a nodular lesion appears after a pleural effusion or thoracotomy.

Pleural mesothelioma may also resemble nonspecific pleural thickening or effusion (Fig. 10–4). The tumor may be diffuse or localized. The diffuse form, often related to asbestos exposure[1096] and generally highly malignant, is usually accompanied and obscured by pleural fluid. After tap, the lung is still compressed by an irregular vise of tumor (Fig. 9–29). Pulmonary and pericardial invasion and lymph node metastases are frequent.[984]

Circumscribed mesothelioma, accompanied in a high percentage of patients by pulmonary osteoarthropathy, may be benign or malignant.[664, 1091, 1186] It can arise from the external or the internal surface of the parietal or visceral layer of pleura.[985] So can other tumors, especially of the mesenchymal or spindle cell type. The location can sometimes be determined roentgenologically. An external parietal pleural lesion may be dumbbell shaped, since it commonly extends into the chest wall. It sometimes involves a rib. An internal parietal tumor, if unattached to the visceral pleura, moves with the rib cage and independently of the lung on respiration. The reverse is true for the visceral pleural tumor. External and internal visceral pleural tumors are generally indistinguishable on the plain film, although they may project into the lung differently, the latter with a narrower base against the pleura than the former. An analogy can be made with gastrointestinal lesions. The internal visceral pleural tumor is like a sessile polyp, whereas the external is similar to an intramural extramucosal lesion. Interlobar pleural tumor is not rare[150]

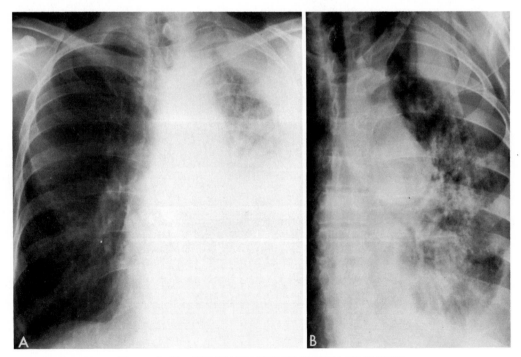

Figure 9–29. MALIGNANT MESOTHELIOMA OF PLEURA

A, Teleroentgenogram showing signs of a large pleural effusion. *B,* Bucky recumbent film after thoracentesis. The lung is encased in tumor. The patient had been exposed to asbestos many years ago.

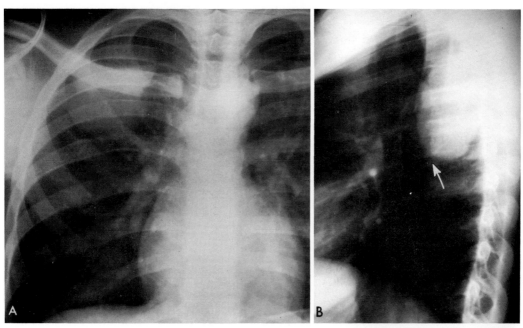

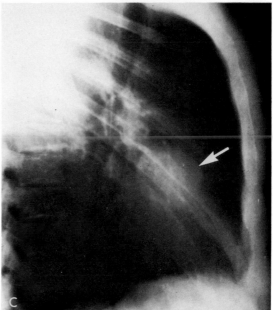

Figure 9–30. INTERLOBAR PLEURAL
MESOTHELIOMAS

A and *B,* A 16 year old boy with a fibrous mesothelioma in the upper portion of the right major
fissure. Note tapering border in *B* (arrow). *C,* An
adult with benign mesothelioma (arrow) in major
fissure.

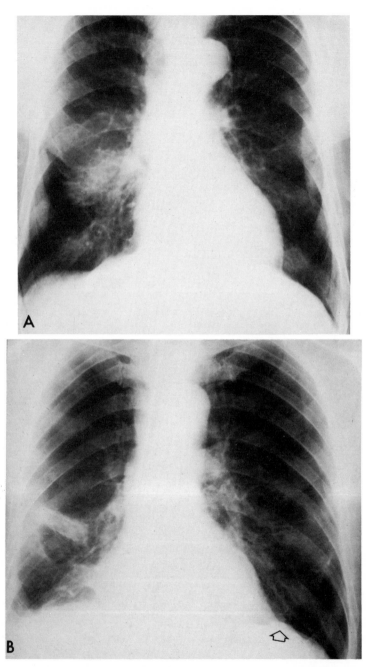

Figure 9-31.   NONCALCIFIED PLEURAL PLAQUES IN ASBESTOSIS

A, The lateral wall of each thorax shows a large plaque. There is also a conglomerate mass adjacent to the right hilum. *B,* A low flat plaque is seen on the left leaf of the diaphragm (arrow). Diffuse right pleural thickening and a broad calcific pleural band are also present.

(Fig. 9–30) and may be indistinguishable from interlobar fluid encapsulation (Fig. 9–18).

A pedunculated tumor in the pleural sac may arise in the pleura, lung, or mediastinum. It can sometimes be recognized by its mobility on respiration and with change in patient position.[69] The roentgen diagnosis of a tumor localized to or pedunculated into the pleural sac is greatly simplified by induced pneumothorax (Figs. 11–4 and 11–14).

Pleural calcification is discussed in Chapter 14. Generally attributed to organization of past pleural effusion or hemothorax, it is a fairly common finding. Plaque-like deposits of calcium in the pleura, often bilateral and best seen in the diaphragm (Fig. 14–27), occur with great frequency in asbestosis,[12, 380, 390, 593, 614, 659] occasionally in talcosis,[1115, 1137] and other silicate pneumoconioses.

Similar but *noncalcified* pleural plaques are also common in asbestosis[12, 389, 390, 418, 777] (Fig. 9–31). They vary in number, size, and location. They are found on the parietal surface, the lung moving freely over them.

Diagnostic pneumothorax has confirmed their parietal location.[660]

Similar plaques have been reported in lymphoma and other tumors. The pads of parietal pleural fat so commonly seen along the lateral costal surfaces at autopsy sometimes show as multiple, faint, ill-defined shadows, often parallel to the ribs and symmetrical[306] (Fig. 13–2). Their incidence is tabulated in Chapter 15. They do not resemble asbestotic plaques at all.

THE DISRUPTED PLEURA

As a rule, the interlobar pleura presents an effective barrier to the spread of a disease process from one lobe to another. However, disruption of the septum does occasionally occur and is indicated roentgenographically by evidence of extension of a lesion across a fissure. Since certain pathologic conditions (especially neoplasm) arising in the region of the hilum may spread simultaneously into several lobes, the assumption that a lesion has violated the rules should be

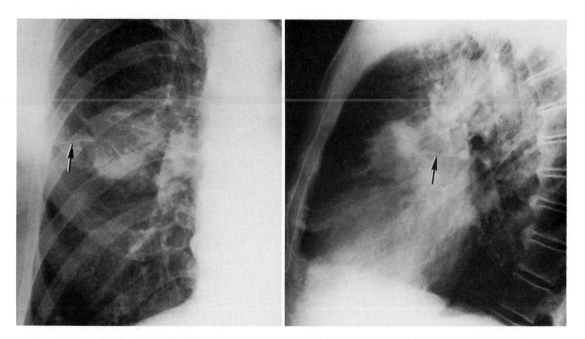

Figure 9–32. BRONCHOGENIC CARCINOMA EXTENDING THROUGH THE MINOR FISSURE

The intact portion of the minor fissure is well delineated (arrows). At operation, the tumor straddled the fissure and destroyed the central portion of the contiguous pleural surfaces.

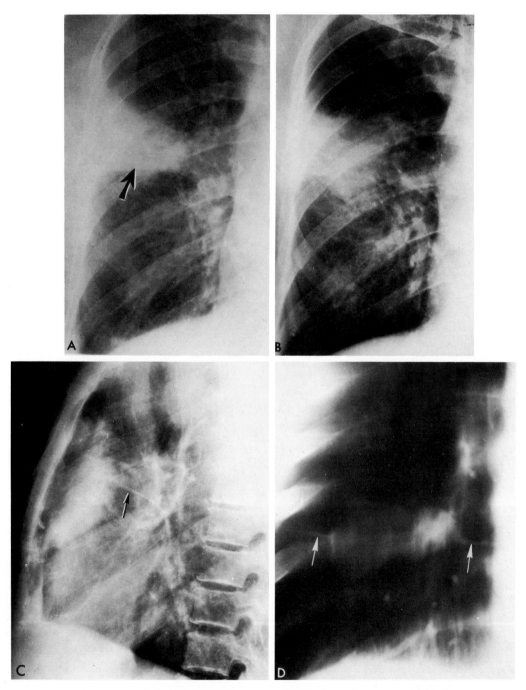

Figure 9–33.   DISRUPTION OF INTERLOBAR SEPTUM IN FUNGUS DISEASES

A and *B*, Blastomycosis. At first restricted to the RUL by the minor septum (arrow), after several months *(B)* the lesion extended across the fissure into the RML. *C*, Actinomycosis crossing minor fissure (arrow). *D*, Torulosis penetrating minor fissure (arrows). Tomogram.

made only when it lies well away from the hilum. The lesion itself should present unsharp margins to distinguish it from interlobar pleural fluid. In some instances, serial films may demonstrate the actual penetration of the fissure.

Bronchogenic carcinoma, tuberculosis, and lung abscess are sometimes found to trespass an interlobar septum at autopsy,[1297] but this is seldom detected radiographically (Fig. 9–32). Roentgen evidence of a disrupted septum should suggest all the above possibilities, but on the basis of incidence, mycotic infection should be given prime consideration. We have encountered the sign in blastomycosis,[325, 515] actinomycosis,[391] and torulosis[1145] (Fig. 9–33). Penetration of the parietal pleura has a similar connotation. It is discussed in Chapter 10.

CHAPTER 10

THE EXTRAPLEURAL SPACE

The extrapleural space is represented in the normal individual by a potential line of cleavage in the loose connective tissue comprising the endothoracic fascia. It lies between the parietal pleura and the thoracic cage. The structures within and adjacent to this region include connective tissue, nerves, vessels, muscles, and ribs.

Lesions involving the extrapleural region usually produce a characteristic shadow on the roentgenogram. Because of the intact parietal and visceral pleura overlying it, a tumefaction in this space will present an extremely sharp convex contour facing the lung.[923] The pleural cover smoothes out the minor surface irregularities of the mass so that it has better definition than a pulmonary lesion.

Since the parietal pleura is adherent to the internal surface of the thoracic wall and is not readily stripped away, the horizontal diameter of an extrapleural lesion is often almost as great as the vertical. For the same reason the superior and inferior edges are usually tapered and may even be slightly concave toward the lung (Fig. 10–1). The widest part is usually opposite the center of attachment.[1040] The pleura is thus displaced toward the lung by the thrust of the central part of the extrapleural mass, like a well-filled maternity dress whose profile closely simulates that of an extrapleural lesion (Fig. 10–2).

In most instances the pleural cavity itself is uninvolved. Because extrapleural lesions usually arise in or near a rib, periostitis and even frank bone destruction are commonly present (Fig. 10–3). The soft tissues external to the ribs may also be involved, clinically and radiographically, depending on the nature of the disease process.[410] On respiration, the shadow of the extrapleural lesion

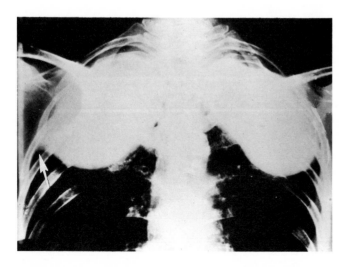

Figure 10–1. BILATERAL EXTRAPLEURAL OLEOTHORAX

Oil was introduced extrapleurally years ago as collapse therapy for bilateral apical pulmonary tuberculosis. Note the extremely sharp convex margin and the tapering lower lateral edges (arrow) characteristic of extrapleural lesions. (From Felson, B.[326]; reproduced with permission of Charles C Thomas, Publ.)

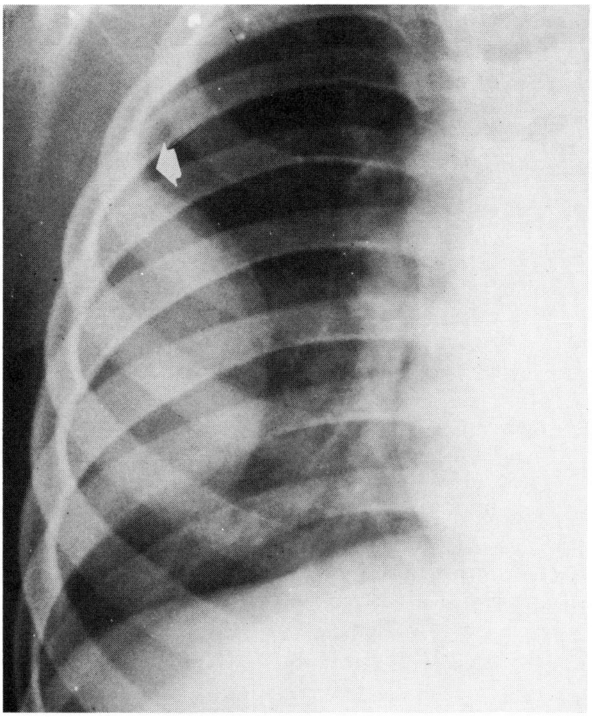

Figure 10–2. EXTRAPLEURAL LIPOMA

The sharp convex border, tapered upper margin (arrow), and wide transverse diameter are characteristic of the profile of an extrapleural lesion—and of a pregnant woman.

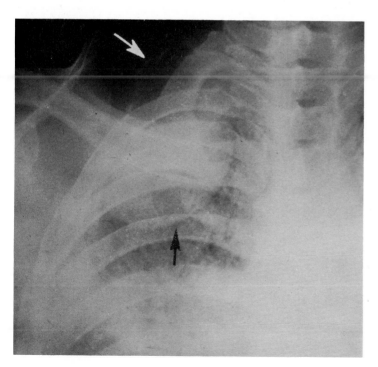

Figure 10–3. RIB INVOLVEMENT IN EXTRAPLEURAL BLASTOMYCOSIS

Note the destruction of the right second rib (upper arrow) and the sharp margin of the localized opacity in the upper thorax (lower arrow). Extensive pulmonary involvement is also present. An extrapleural abscess involving the rib was found at autopsy.

moves with the overlying rib and independently of the lung. I apply the term *extrapleural sign* to the combination of a pencil sharp convex outline and tapering margins, with or without the other findings. Not all extrapleural lesions exhibit these changes, nor can they be considered pathognomonic of disease in this location unless rib involvement is demonstrated.

Encapsulated effusion in the pleural space, especially when long-standing, may produce similar roentgen findings (Fig. 2–14). However, in effusion the margins are seldom quite so well defined, there are pleural changes elsewhere in the thorax, and, of course, rib involvement does not occur. Interlobar pleural fluid presents an identical sharply defined shadow with tapering ends but is readily distinguished by its anatomic location (Fig. 9–18). Free pleural fluid is easily identified by its shift with change in position. A pulmonary tumor rarely shows the degree of sharpness in outline or the flattening against the chest wall exhibited by the extrapleural mass. In addition, such a tumor generally moves independently of the ribs on respiration. A localized primary tumor of the pleura may, on occasion, give roentgen signs identical to those of an extrapleural lesion except for the tapering margins[56, 90, 664] (Fig. 9–30). Malignant mesothelioma shows a smaller transverse diameter, thickening in other pleural areas, and often pleural effusion (Fig. 10–4). Rarely, a mesothelioma may arise from the external surface of the parietal pleura and, in truth, be entirely extrapleural.[580]

If the roentgen beam strikes an extrapleural lesion perpendicular to its presenting surface, the typical findings will not be observed. In order to bring out all the extrapleural characteristics, it is necessary to bring the lesion into profile. Fluoroscopy with spot films is ideal for this purpose. Bucky films are important for the demonstration of the rib changes.

The fact that the mediastinum and diaphragm are also, in essence, extrapleural in location gives the extrapleural sign added significance.[229, 338] Mediastinal tumor (Figs. 10–5 and 10–6*) and diaphragmatic hernia (Fig. 12–9) can usually be distinguished

---

*See also Figures 1–3 and 11–3.

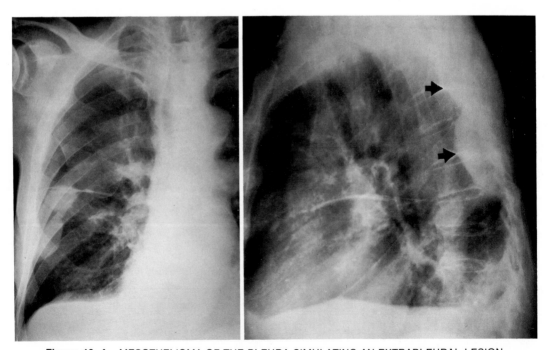

Figure 10–4. MESOTHELIOMA OF THE PLEURA SIMULATING AN EXTRAPLEURAL LESION

The margins are sharp (arrows) and the borders tapered. However, there is lobulation, the transverse diameter of the opacity is small in relation to its height, and extensive pleural thickening is seen throughout the right thorax.

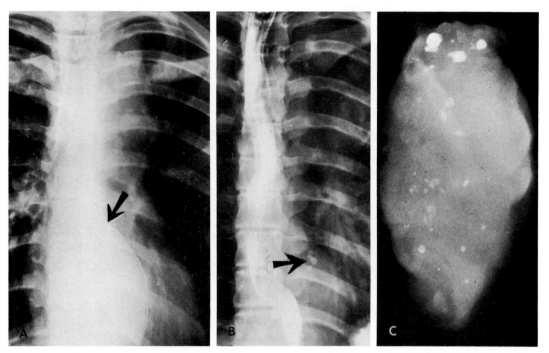

Figure 10-5. THE EXTRAPLEURAL SIGN IN MEDIASTINAL HEMANGIOMA[726, 1103]

A, Teleroentgenogram. Two masses: one in the posterior inferior mediastinum (retouched), the other blending with the shadow of the aortic knob. Note the sharp lateral border and tapering superior edge of each mass (arrow). *B,* Bucky film reveals phleboliths (arrow) in the lower mass, permitting a correct preoperative diagnosis. *C,* Roentgenogram of the resected owlish lower hemangioma.

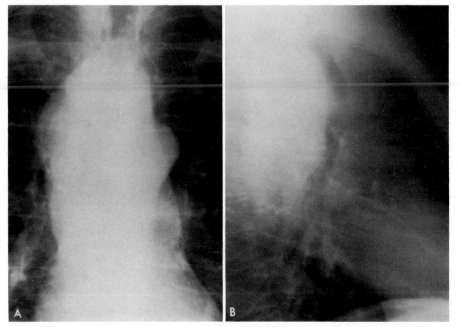

Figure 10-6. THE EXTRAPLEURAL SIGN IN LEIOMYOMA OF ESOPHAGUS

The tapered upper right margin and sharp lateral borders of the mass indicate its mediastinal location. The trachea is bowed forward in the lateral view. (From Felson, B.[338]; reproduced with permission of Seminars in Roentgenology.)

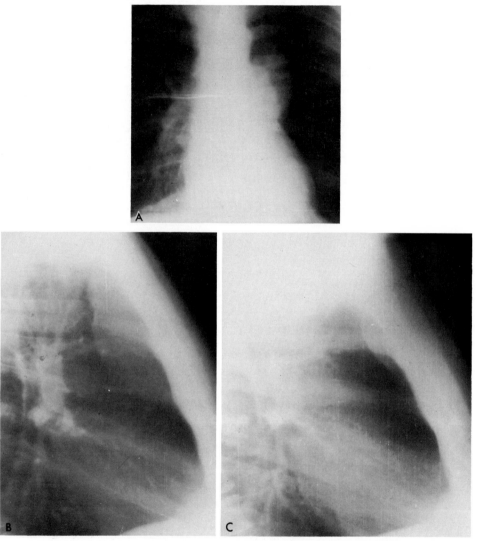

Figure 10–7.   STERNAL HEMATOMA WITH EXTRAPLEURAL SIGN

A and *B* were obtained soon after the injury, and *C* is 9 weeks later. The discrete posterior margin and the anterior tapering edges exclude a mass arising in the mediastinum. Not proved. (Courtesy of Dr. Chapin P. Hawley.)

from pulmonary or pleural lesions by the presence of this sign. The paraaortic line is commonly elevated by a posterior mediastinal lesion (Fig. 1–2).

A sternal lesion that extends or protrudes intrathoracically usually shows the extrapleural sign in the lateral projection (Fig. 10–7). Visibility of the posterior margin of such a mass distinguishes it from an anterior mediastinal tumor, which generally blends with the anterior cardiac silhouette (Fig. 11–3).

A pathologic process arising in any of the extrapleural structures may produce the sign, but by far the commonest cause is metastatic tumor in a rib. On the PA teleroentgenogram, we often see a sharp shadow far peripherally which we have learned from experience usually indicates rib metastasis, even though the rib destruction itself is not apparent (Fig. 10–8). Actually, this shadow represents, in part, the extrapleural sign.

Extrapleural involvement may also occur with myeloma, lymphoma,[927] primary neoplasm,[79, 470, 923, 1097] and inflammatory pro-

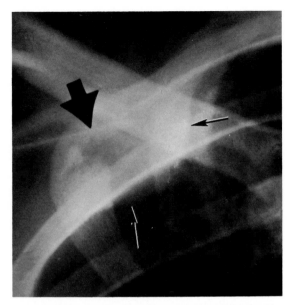

Figure 10–9. EXTRAPLEURAL INVOLVEMENT IN RIB TUBERCULOSIS

The large arrow points to the rib destruction, the smaller arrows delineate the extrapleural mass. The tapered margins are well depicted.

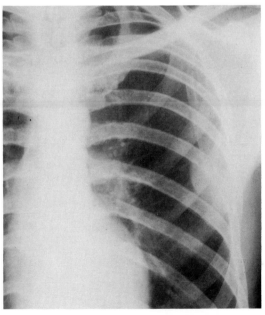

Figure 10–8. THE EXTRAPLEURAL SIGN IN RIB METASTASES

Although bone destruction is not evident, the typical density adjacent to the axillary segment of the left 7th rib indicates extrapleural disease.

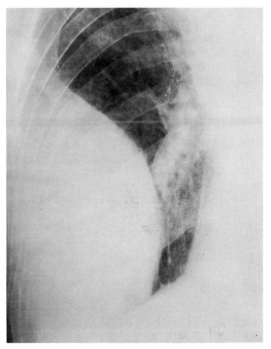

Figure 10–10. EXTRAPLEURAL HEMATOMA

Chest trauma had occurred 2 days earlier. The hematoma spontaneously drained via the skin a week later.

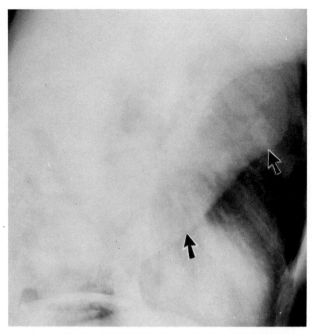

Figure 10–11.   HUGE EXTRAPLEURAL HEMATOMA

Lateral view. Note the sharp anterior margin (arrows) and the otherwise normal pleural sac. Autopsy confirmation. No cause was demonstrated, but a ruptured intercostal artery was suspected. There was no history of trauma.

cesses of tuberculous, mycotic, or pyogenic etiology[1133] arising in a rib or in the soft tissues (Figs. 10–3 and 10–9). Extrapleural lipoma[1097] (Fig. 10–2) and fat pad are particularly frequent causes. The now abandoned procedure of extrapleural injection of mineral oil or other substances in the treatment of tuberculosis produced the extrapleural sign in its classic form[908] (Fig. 10–1). Accumulation of blood or serous fluid in the extrapleural space may occur following external thoracic trauma (Fig. 10–10), ruptured aneurysm (Fig. 10–11), parietal pleurectomy, and sympathectomy.[933, 1072, 1136] A similar appearance is seen with congenital lobar agenesis, in which the missing lobe is often replaced by a chunk of extrapleural areolar tissue.[243] This causes a loss of the right heart border in the frontal view and an anterior shadow in the lateral view that parallels the sternum (Figs. 3–12 and 3–19). Table 10–1 is a list of extrapleural lesions.

Direct extension of a pulmonary or pleural lesion into the extrapleural space, or vice versa, does occasionally occur. This is most frequently encountered in patients with malignant tumor, especially in the superior sulcus of the lung. I have also seen such extensions in rib metastasis, empyema necessitatis, lung abscess, tuberculosis, blastomycosis,[515] and actinomycosis.[902] In these conditions, however, the pulmonary and pleural changes overshadow the ex-

TABLE 10–1.   Extrapleural Lesions

Common
Metastasis to rib or extrapleural soft tissues
Rib fracture
Other bone mass (myeloma, fibrous dysplasia, histiocytosis X, etc.)
Mediastinal mass
Subphrenic mass

Rare
Hematoma
Lipoma, neurofibroma, or other soft tissue mass
Postsympathectomy, plombage, or other operation
Chest wall infection
Lobar agenesis

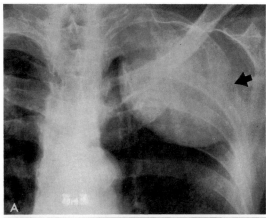

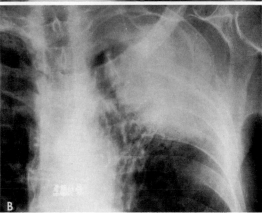

Figure 10–12. THE EXTRAPLEURAL SIGN IN RIB METASTASIS

A, The left 3rd rib is destroyed (arrow). *B,* 6 months later the extrapleural sign has disappeared. There is now obvious pleural and pulmonary invasion. At autopsy the tumor had broken through the pleura into the lung. Adenocarcinoma of the stomach.

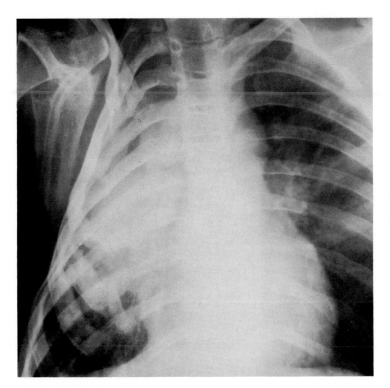

Figure 10–13. ACTINOMYCOSIS WITH CHEST WALL INVOLVEMENT

Right pulmonary involvement with bone sclerosis and periostitis is present. (Courtesy of Dr. William A. Altemeier.)

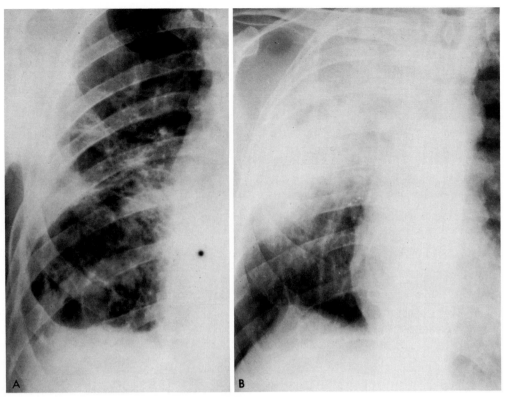

Figure 10–14. ACTINOMYCOSIS WITH INVOLVEMENT OF LUNG, PLEURA, AND EXTRAPLEURAL STRUC-
TURES

Two different patients. Each had a draining cutaneous fistula in the right axilla. Note the "parachute string" stranding in the lower thorax.

trapleural manifestations, except for the bone and soft tissue involvement (Fig. 10–12). Bronchography may help in delineating the extrapleural component (Fig. 7–2). The *en bloc* involvement of lung, pleura, and ribs, except in the superior sulcus, is most commonly encountered in actinomycosis (Figs. 10–13 and 10–14). In this condition, a characteristic stranding of the pleura, like the strings of a parachute, and a peculiar wavy costal periostitis may occur[391] (Fig. 13–9).

CHAPTER 11

THE MEDIASTINUM

The diagnosis of a mediastinal lesion is far from an accurate science and many physicians, like horsebettors, play it by hunch. Dr. Jan Schwarz once told me, "Any fool can make the right diagnosis for the right reasons. It takes a genius to make the right diagnosis for the wrong reasons." There aren't many geniuses around.

My own approach is to play the percentages. But just to determine the odds for or against a disease requires some knowledge of basic principles of anatomy, pathology, clinical medicine, and roentgenology. The roentgen principles, many of which have already been discussed, present special features in the mediastinum and some of them are worth reviewing here.

There is little to add to the discussion of techniques and methods in Chapter 1 in regard to the study of mediastinal lesions. A high kilovoltage film offers little advantage over a well-exposed Bucky film, and tomography is superior to both. Angiography is important in distinguishing cardiovascular from other conditions, and bronchography will exclude a pulmonary lesion. Artificial pneumothorax, pneumoperitoneum, or pneumomediastinum is only occasionally useful, as is myelography.[70] Fluoroscopy is ideal for the study of mediastinal lesions and should *never* be omitted.

MEDIASTINAL VS. PULMONARY AND PLEURAL LESIONS

We're frequently confronted with the problem of differentiating a mediastinal lesion from one arising in adjacent lung or pleura. Since the mediastinum lies outside the pleural sac, the extrapleural signs used to identify chest wall lesions are, with certain limitations, also applicable to mediastinal tumors (Figs. 10–5 and 10–6), including the sharply penciled margin and the tapering upper and lower borders. The paravertebral shadow is elevated in a similar manner by a posterior mediastinal mass (Fig. 11–1). Involvement of the spine or adjacent ribs, or even the sternum, is a clear-cut indication that a central mass is extrapleural (and therefore mediastinal) in location.* Bilaterality of a mass excludes a pulmonary location (Fig. 2–16).

Mediastinal and pulmonary lesions can also be differentiated by their respiratory motion. Intrapulmonary shadows move synchronously with the adjacent lung markings, whereas mediastinal lesions do not.[141] Instead, their respiratory excursion varies with their location in the mediastinum: those in the posterior gutter (i.e., involving the nerves or spine) seldom move at all (Fig. 1–3); anterior tumors (e.g., thymoma and dermoid) move more or less in conjunction with the heart; lesions attached to the esophagus or trachea move with these organs; masses elsewhere in the mediastinum move independently of all these structures (Fig. 1–2).

The presence of an air bronchogram within the lesion indicates that it lies in the lung rather than in the mediastinum (Fig. 2–48). Bronchography or diagnostic pneumothorax may occasionally be necessary to exclude a pulmonary or pleural localization (Fig. 11–4).

---

*For present purposes, we include the paravertebral region with the posterior mediastinum.

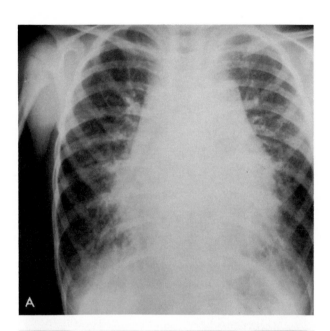

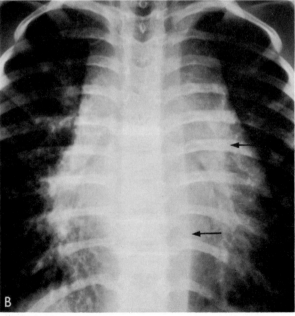

Figure 11–1. HILUM OVERLAY SIGN IN AN ANTERIOR MEDIASTINAL TUMOR

The initial film *(A)* was thought to indicate congestive failure. *B,* Bucky film. The left pulmonary artery lies well within the cardiac silhouette (upper arrow). The left paraspinal line is displaced laterally (lower arrow). At autopsy, this child had lymphangiomatosis involving the mediastinum, lung, and bone. Pericardial effusion was also present. (Courtesy of Dr. Patrick Lynch.)

MEDIASTINAL VS. CARDIAC AND PERICARDIAL DISEASE

Surprisingly, an anterior mediastinal mass may closely resemble a dilated heart or pericardial effusion. The clinical findings will usually resolve the dilemma but are not infallible. The *hilum overlay* and *convergence* signs (Figs. 2–18, 2–19, and 11–1), are helpful in making this distinction.

However, certain types of congenital heart disease, especially among infants, may result in a lateral bulge anterior to the pulmonary trunk, causing the left pulmonary artery to appear well within the left border of the cardiac silhouette. Examples of this are shown in Figures 11–2 and 14–12. Collapse of the LLL may also displace the first left pulmonary bifurcation posteromedial to its normal position. Rarely, a pericardial effusion may bulge anterolaterally in front of the right and left main pulmonary arteries and overlap them for several centimeters on the frontal projection. These are uncommon exceptions, particularly in the adult, but they make the hilum overlay sign less secure.

The absence of pulsation signifies a non-cardiac origin. However, more often than not, pericardial effusion and tumor pulsate (transmitted) and can't be distinguished from an enlarged heart or from each other on this basis alone. Angiocardiography will solve the problem.

CONTENT OF MEDIASTINAL LESIONS

The specific diagnosis of a mediastinal lesion can sometimes be suggested by studying its contents. Surprisingly, it is not always an easy matter to recognize gas, fat, or calcium on plain films, and Bucky films or laminagrams are often required.*

Fat

Even with these methods, the distinction between fat and water density in the thorax

---

*Supervoltage technique has been advocated for visualization of gas in the trachea, central bronchi, and mediastinal soft tissues. It will, however, tend to "burn out" calcium density.

Figure 11–2. FAILURE OF HILUM OVERLAY SIGN

Atrial septal defect. The left main pulmonary artery (arrowhead) is projected well inside the shadow of the left cardiopericardial border.

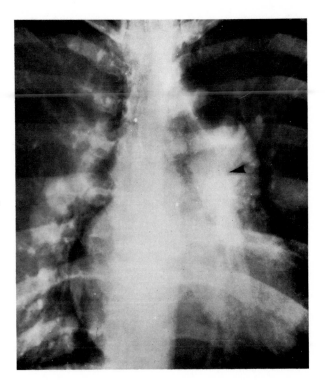

is sometimes difficult.[549] For reasons that escape me, fat is easier to identify in an ovarian than in a mediastinal dermoid, and the cardiac fat pad usually obliterates the heart border. More simply stated, fat on the chest film often looks like water density (Figs. 10–2 and 11–3). I can understand this when fat is inflamed (Fig. 2–15) or involved with malignant tumor—cellular infiltrate has water density—but not otherwise. Does the adjacent gas play some trick on the eye of the X-ray tube or radiologist?

When fat is identified in a thoracic lesion, the diagnosis rests between mediastinal teratoma, lipoma,[213] thymolipoma[57] (Fig. 11–4), fat pad, omental hernia, excess fat subsequent to steroid therapy,[667] and possibly hibernoma. Occasionally, a lipoma may lie entirely within the pericardial sac and fat density completely surrounds the heart.[802] In the one case I have seen, the fat density was not evident but, on fluoroscopy, pulsations were absent at the edge of the cardiopericardial shadow and visible along the margins of the heart itself. A fatty (chylous?) pericardial effusion can be detected (Fig. 11–5), but is about as rare as sunburn in a convent. It may resemble epicardial fatty tissue.[674]

Calcium

Calcium in mediastinal lesions will be discussed in Chapter 14.

Pneumomediastinum

Gas within a mediastinal mass generally indicates a hernia, esophageal diverticulum, locally or diffusely dilated esophagus,[88] mediastinal abscess, or communicating duplication cyst (Fig. 11–6).

Diffuse pneumomediastinum has many sources (Table 11–1), including the esophagus, trachea, or bronchus, from perforation or operation; the retroperitoneal space, after diagnostic pneumoretroperitoneum or perforation of the duodenum or colon; the neck, following trauma, a surgical procedure (such as dental drilling),[577] or a perforating cervical lesion; and the lung itself, from

a tear in the parenchyma that permits air to leak into the interstitial tissue and dissect to the hilum and into the mediastinum.

The latter, the so-called *spontaneous pneumomediastinum*, usually appears suddenly without obvious cause, although it may at times occur during respiratory therapy, anesthesia, labor, diabetic acidosis,[1050] resuscitative attempts on the newborn, from other injuries, from straining, and from cough associated with pulmonary disease.[50, 126, 206, 472, 715, 856, 896, 1094] Measles has been listed as a common cause in Africa.[963] The bubbles of air in the interstices of the lung are sometimes visible as they track along the walls of the vessels and bronchi toward the hilum and mediastinum[158a, 388, 907] (Fig. 11–8E).

Air in the mediastinum is visible as streaklike shadows or bubbles located centrally or in small collections along the margins. These are often especially well seen between the sternum and the heart and aorta on the lateral view. Larger collections may displace the mediastinal pleura far laterally on frontal projection. In the infant, the thymus is often dissected from the rest of the mediastinal structures and elevated by the gas, producing the spinnaker sail sign[770, 896, 1131] (Fig. 11–7).

Since all connective tissue planes in the body intercommunicate, the gas may spread far from the mediastinum. Dissection into the neck is common, less so in children, whereas extension into the retroperitoneum is unusual. Spread to the shoulder, chest wall, and even the head and extremities may occur. Sometimes the gas dissects under the parietal pleura in the diaphragm, causing a loculated collection resembling pneumothorax, except that it does not shift with change in position.[745, 896] Dr. Bertram Levin recently called my attention to the fact that in pneumomediastinum the central tendon of the diaphragm is sometimes visible along the caudal surface of the cardiopericardial shadow.

With spontaneous rupture of the esophagus, gas may extend into adjacent fascial planes of the mediastinum and diaphragm, forming a V in the left phrenovertebral angle.[860] Rupture into the pleural space results in pneumothorax. It has been said to be more frequent on the left,[988, 1038] but

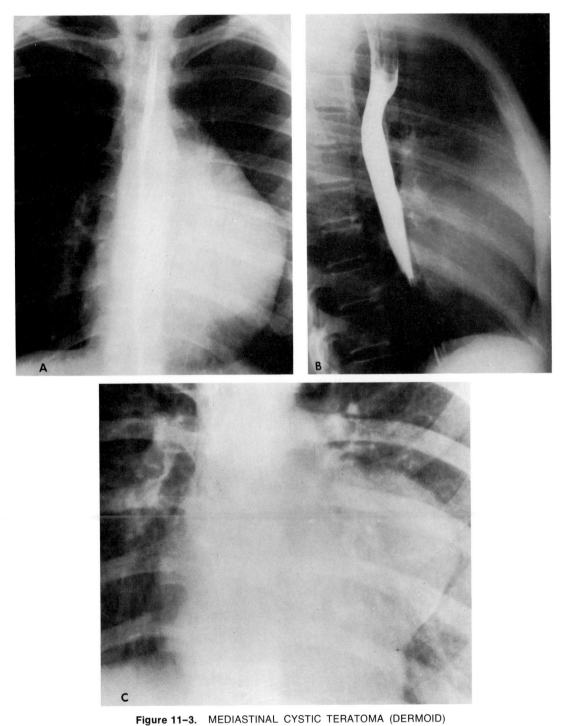

Figure 11-3.   MEDIASTINAL CYSTIC TERATOMA (DERMOID)

A and *B*, The fat content is not recognizable. Note the hilum overlay sign. *C*, Another patient.

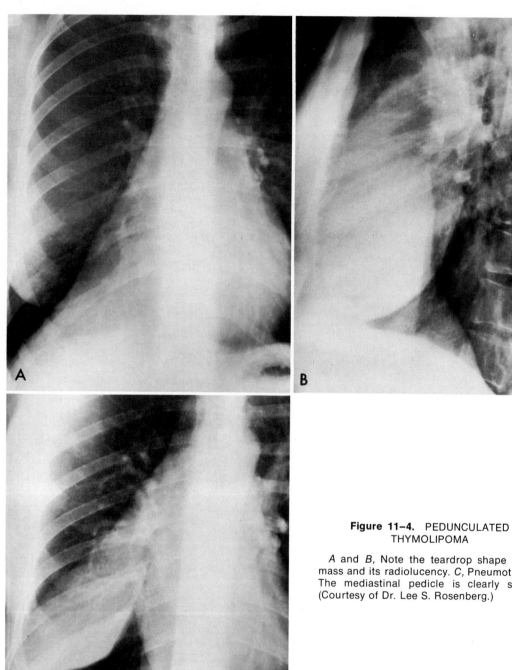

Figure 11–4. PEDUNCULATED
THYMOLIPOMA

A and *B*, Note the teardrop shape of the
mass and its radiolucency. *C*, Pneumothorax.
The mediastinal pedicle is clearly shown.
(Courtesy of Dr. Lee S. Rosenberg.)

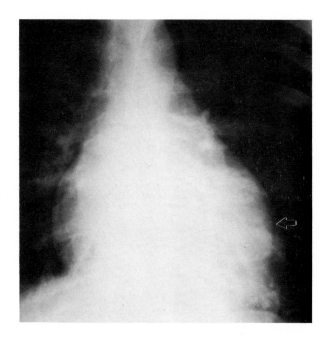

Figure 11–5. PROBABLE FAT CONTAINING PERICARDIAL EFFUSION

The heart (arrow) is visible inside the cardio-pericardial shadow in a patient with proved pericardial effusion. Nine days later the heart appeared normal. (Courtesy of Dr. Herbert S. Francis.)

Macklin and Macklin found no such predilection in their experiments on cats.[778] The reverse, pleural air causing pneumomediastinum, does not occur.[778, 1094]

Pneumomediastinum is at times difficult to distinguish from pneumopericardium and pneumothorax on routine roentgenograms. The problem is settled by simply obtaining frontal views with the patient in right and left decubitus positions (Fig. 11–8). Here are some other obvious points of differentiation: (1) An air-fluid level in the lung or pleura stops at the midline; a mediastinal air-fluid level often crosses it. (2) Pneumopericardium seldom rises to the level of the aortic knob which, of course, is outside the pericardial sac. (3) The main pulmonary artery is often clearly outlined by pericardial air (Fig. 11–9).

Incidentally, pneumopericardium is rare and is generally the result of trauma, a surgical procedure, perforation of the esophagus or stomach (Fig. 11–10), carcinoma of the lung, or inflammatory disease caused by gas producing organisms.[757, 920, 1016, 1029] Figures 11–11 to 11–13 illustrate still another cause of pneumopericardium — congenital pericardial defect.[295, 351, 445]

It is now known that Hamman's sign ("mediastinal crunch")[497] is *not* pathognomonic of pneumomediastinum; as noted first by McGuire and Bean in 1939, it may be caused by a small left pneumothorax, and just about as frequently.[811] In pneumothorax, the sound is produced by the touching of the two pleural surfaces with each heart beat and respiratory excursion.[1325] The crunch usually disappears in the right lateral decubitus position[177] or when more air is injected into the pleural sac.[1070, 1094, 1099] A small pneumothorax may not show on an inspiratory film, so that a patient with a mediastinal crunch and negative roentgenogram should have an expiratory film and perhaps a decubitus view as well.

CONFIGURATION

The shape of a mediastinal lesion seldom offers much assistance in its diagnosis. True, lymph node enlargement is often lobulated and a dilated esophagus has a long vertical diameter and sometimes broad undulated margins. So has aortic disease (e.g., dissecting aneurysm), azygos vein enlargement[168, 269] (Fig. 2–25), and mediastinal hematoma[964] (Fig. 11–22). A teardrop shaped shadow, broad along the diaphragm and narrower above, generally signifies a soft pedunculated mass such as a pericardial cyst (Fig. 11–14) or thymolipoma[69, 549, 1047] (Fig. 11–4). But these are infrequent shapes.

(*Text continued on page 399.*)

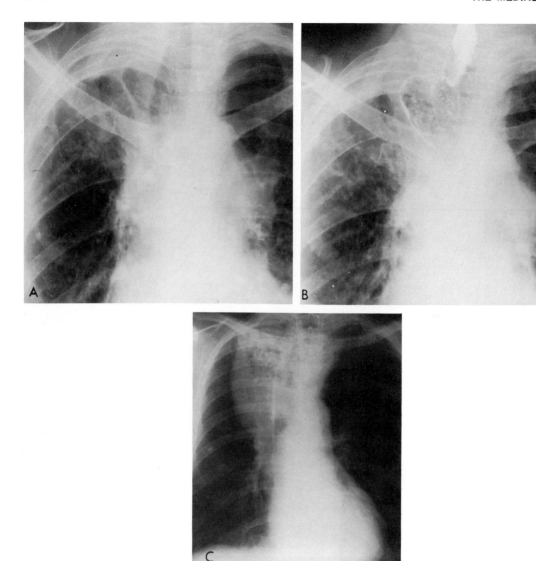

Figure 11–6. GAS IN A MEDIASTINAL "MASS"

A, Several years after RUL resection for tuberculosis, a cavity is seen in the right apex or superior mediastinum. *B,* Barium swallow. Localized dilatation of the esophagus explains the gas shadow.[88] *C,* Another patient. Cardiospasm. Note the gas bubbles trapped within food in dilated esophagus.

TABLE 11–1. Causes of Gas in the Mediastinum (Pneumomediastinum)

Common	*Rare*
Esophageal dilatation or diverticulum	Belch
Hiatal hernia	Communicating duplication cyst
Respiratory distress, birth trauma	Diagnostic pneumoretroperitoneum
Rib fracture	Mediastinal abscess
"Spontaneous" pneumomediastinum	Perforation of trachea or bronchus
Surgical procedure (tracheostomy, mediastinotomy,	Retroperitoneal perforation of GI tract
dental drilling, etc.)	Ruptured esophagus

Figure 11–7. SPINNAKER SAIL SIGN
IN PNEUMOMEDIASTINUM

A, Newborn with respiratory distress. The lungs appear emphysematous. *B,* A few hours later a peculiar
shadow has appeared along the left
upper and lateral thoracic wall. This
was initially interpreted as encapsulated fluid. The midline structures have
shifted to the right. *C,* Pneumothorax
(arrows) has resulted from an unsuc-
cessful attempt to tap the "fluid." It is
obvious that pneumomediastinum outlines the left lobe of the thymus. The
midline structures are deviated farther
to the right. Returning to *B,* it is now
apparent that the sail-like shadow is
the thymic gland, displaced far laterally by a large left-sided pneumomediastinum. The chest appeared normal
a few days later. (From Felson, B.[338];
reproduced with permission of Seminars in Roentgenology.)

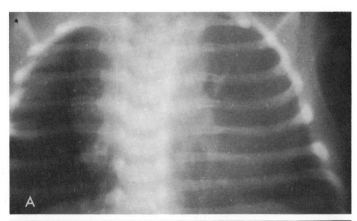

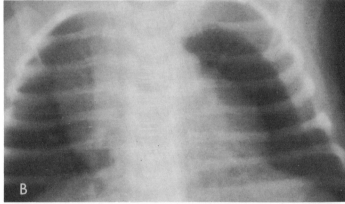

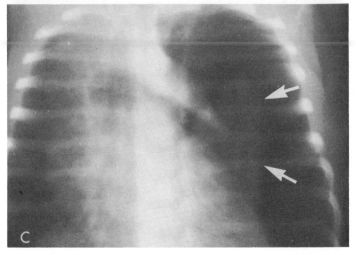

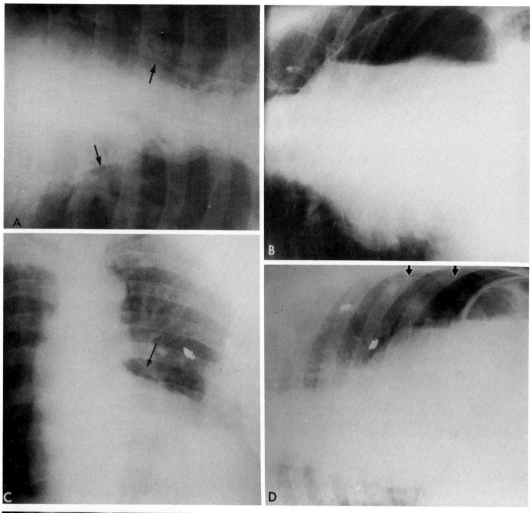

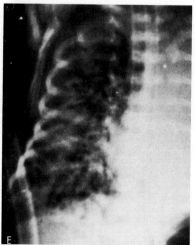

Figure 11–8. DECUBITUS VIEWS FOR DIFFERENTIATING PNEUMOMEDIASTINUM, PNEUMOPERICARDIUM, AND PNEUMOTHORAX

A, Pneumomediastinum. The air streaks (arrows) did not rise in the left decubitus position. The air distribution was identical to that in the upright and right decubitus views. There is a suggestion of interstitial air tracking in the juxta-hilar region of the left lung. *B,* Pneumopericardium. The left side of the heart and pericardium are clearly delineated in this right decubitus view. The opposite decubitus film depicted the right pericardium. *C,* Right pneumothorax secondary to bullet wound. Recumbent view. A small air shadow is seen alongside the heart. *D,* Right decubitus view. The air has risen to the left lateral thoracic wall (arrows). I guess this point is pretty obvious. My apologies. *E,* Intrapulmonary air tracking in right lung in the late stages with hyaline membrane disease.

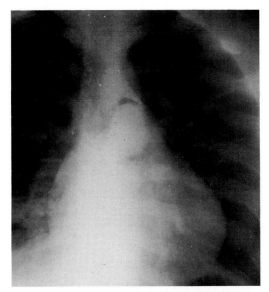

Figure 11–9. PNEUMOPERICARDIUM

A small amount of air outlines the main pulmonary artery. Right pleuropericardial stab wound.

A more common problem arises in relation to various bumps on the abnormal heart which simulate anterior mediastinal tumor. Awareness of their usual locations and etiologies is helpful in their recognition. One of these, "the third mogul," was named and popularized by Daves.[234] It lies just below

the pulmonary arc on the left border (Fig. 11–15) and has a variety of causes (Table 11–2).

The Thymic Signs

Differentiation of the normal thymus gland from mediastinal tumor in children can usually be made on the basis of its configuration. Because of its far anterior location, the thymus often spreads out laterally in front of the lung and mediastinal pleura. Hence, it may not show the typical extrapleural signs, but instead may produce a triangular sail shadow, unilateral or bilateral, projecting from the upper mediastinum on the frontal film (Fig. 11–16). Kemp et al., in a roentgen survey of 498 healthy children, observed the sail shadow in 8.8 per cent; 6.2 per cent on the right, 2.4 per cent on the left, and 0.2 per cent bilaterally.[638] Postmortem studies have demonstrated conclusively that the normal thymus gland is responsible for this shadow.

The sail shadow is readily differentiated from RUL consolidation by its well-defined vertical lateral border, and from encapsulated fluid by its sharp inferior angle, which forms a notch with the heart border.[512] It usually shrinks considerably on deep inspiration.

(*Text continued on page 403.*)

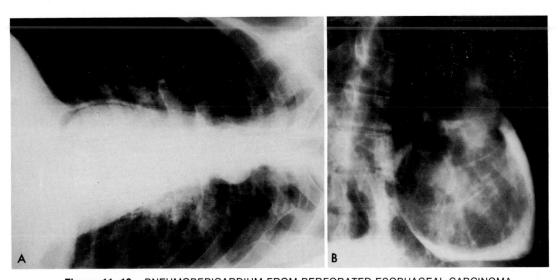

Figure 11–10. PNEUMOPERICARDIUM FROM PERFORATED ESOPHAGEAL CARCINOMA

A, Left decubitus. *B,* Ingested barium has entered the pericardium. (Courtesy of Dr. Harold G. Margolin.)

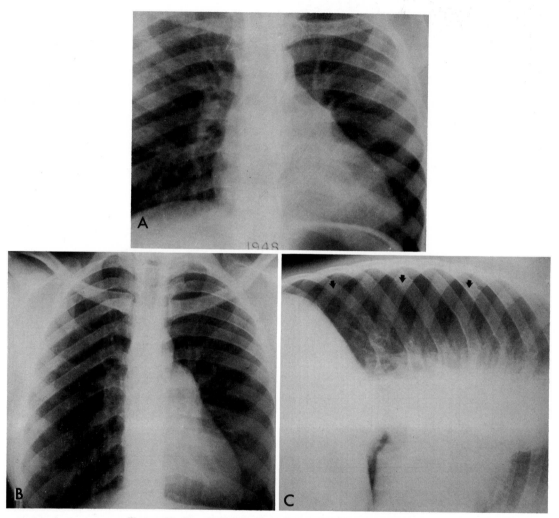

Figure 11-11.   CONGENITAL LEFT PERICARDIAL DEFECT

A, Age 4. *B,* Age 17. Note extension of the heart to the left and the prominent pulmonary arc. *C,* Left decubitus film after induced left pneumothorax. Air outlines the undersurface of the heart. A small *right* pneumothorax (arrows) has occurred, probably as a result of an associated defect in the mediastinal pleura. (From Felson, B., and Wiot, J. F.[351]; reproduced with permission of Charles C Thomas, Publ.)

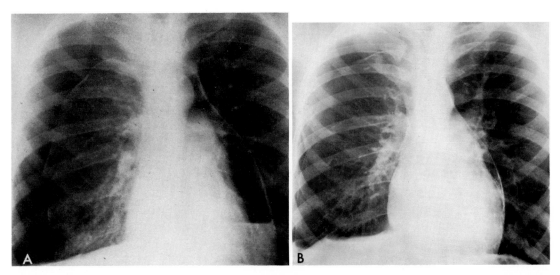

Figure 11–12. SPONTANEOUS PNEUMOTHORAX IN A PATIENT WITH CONGENITAL RIGHT PERICARDIAL
DEFECT

A, Note that air extends from the right pleural cavity into the left side of the pericardial sac. *B,* Lipiodol instilled in
the right lateral pleural cavity outlines the left surface of the heart! The patient had Marfan's syndrome.

Figure 11–13. PERICARDIAL HERNIA

Congenital absence of the transverse septum of
the diaphragm and caudal segment of the pericardium with intrapericardial small intestine. Chief
complaint: barking cough. (Courtesy of William J.
Roenigk, D.V.M.)

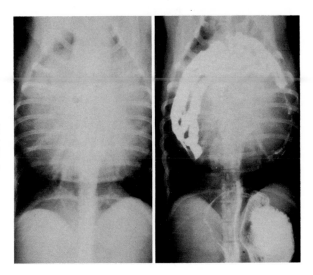

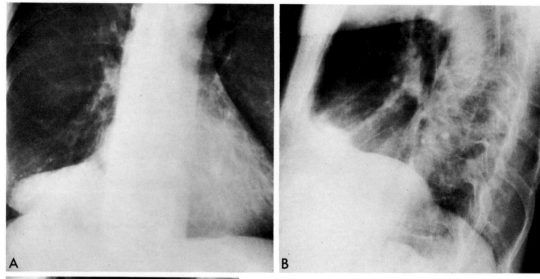

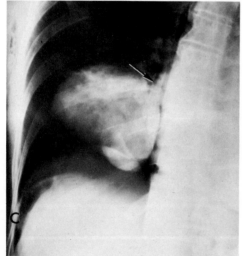

Figure 11–14. PEDUNCULATED PERICARDIAL CYST

Note obliteration of the anterior silhouette of the diaphragm in *A* and *B. C*, Pneumothorax and pneumoperitoneum reveal the pedicle attached to the pericardium
(arrow). (Courtesy of Dr. Lee S. Rosenberg.)

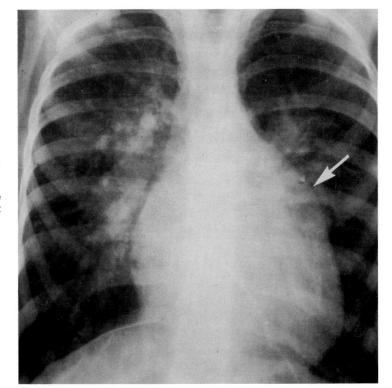

Figure 11–15. THE "THIRD MOGUL" IN CORRECTED TRANS-POSITION

The bump (arrow) represents the ascending aorta. Note that the left pulmonary artery shadow lies well within the cardiac silhouette, a false hilum overlay sign.

The normal thymus lies so far forward that its soft lateral borders are often slightly indented by the internal protrusion of the osteocartilaginous junctions of the adjacent ribs. This produces a subtle wavy margin on frontal projection, first described by Mulvey as the *thymic wave sign*[853] (Figs. 11–16 and 11–17). Thymic tumor and other anterior mediastinal masses do not show this sign.

TABLE 11–2.   Causes of the "Third Mogul"

Cardiac aneurysm
Cardiac or pericardial tumor or cyst
Coronary artery aneurysm or fistula
Corrected transposition
Ebstein's malformation
Left atrial appendage enlargement, double
   atrial appendage
Mediastinal tumor
Myocardial hypertrophy, severe
Pericardial defect
Sinus of Valsalva aneurysm
Thymus gland, normal
"Wooden-shoe" configuration in Fallot's tetrad, etc.

They are firmer and less subject to indentation by the anterior thoracic cage.[294]

As already noted, the spinnaker sail sign indicates pneumomediastinum. Ignoring the two sail signs and the wave sign may shipwreck patient and radiologist together.

The involution of the thymic shadow usually begins at the end of the first year of life and is generally complete by the age of three.[294] The persistent thymus and the large normal gland frequently plague the radiologist.[292] Could it be a tumor? Steroid is said to shrink the normal gland,[153] but in two of our three patients who were tested with it, the thymic shadow remained unchanged. Both patients proved to have a normal thymus.

Absent thymic shadow is seen in DiGeorge syndrome (aplasia of thymus and parathyroid glands)[656] and certain other immunoglobulin anomalies (Fig. 11–18). However, following extensive burns and other severely stressful conditions, the normal infant thymus may shrink. As recovery occurs, the thrust of thymic regeneration may simulate a growing mediastinal mass.[433]

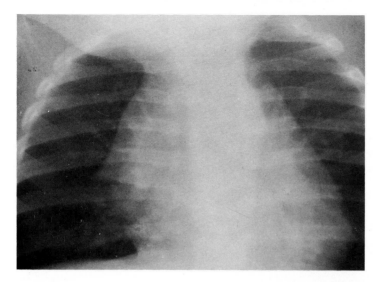

Figure 11–16. THE SAIL SHADOW OF THE NORMAL THYMUS GLAND

Note also the thymic wave sign, not exactly of seasick propensity.

Figure 11–17. THYMIC WAVE SIGN

The wavy right border is caused by indentation of the soft normal thymic tissue by each of the adjacent costochondral junctions. There is also a hilum overlay sign bilaterally. (From Felson, B.[338]; reproduced with permission of Seminars in Roentgenology.)

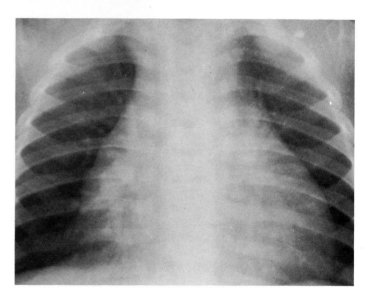

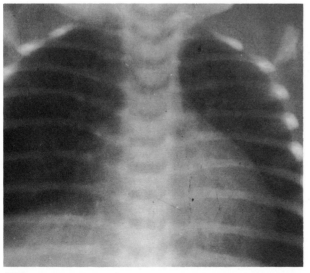

Figure 11–18. ABSENT THYMUS GLAND IN DI GEORGE SYNDROME

OTHER SIGNS

There is great variation in the size of mediastinal tumors, from the small thymoma often associated with myasthenia gravis to the huge mass of lymph nodes in Hodgkin's disease. But size alone is of limited value as a parameter for diagnosis. Unilaterality is sometimes helpful. For example, neurogenic tumor, pericardial cyst,[658] and persistent left cardinal vein (left superior cava) are almost always unilateral.

Change in size is not as reliable an indicator of the benign or malignant nature of a mediastinal mass as you might expect. A pericardial cyst or dermoid may expand fairly rapidly, whereas a malignant tumor may enlarge slowly. Decrease in size of lymphoma after radiation or chemotherapy and regression of tuberculosis after antibiotics and of sarcoidosis after steroids are well known. But these modalities are no longer used as therapeutic tests, since a surgical approach is quicker, more reliable, and almost as safe.

The presence of a localized pulmonary lesion provides an important roentgen clue to the nature of a mediastinal mass (e.g., malignancy, primary tuberculosis, or histoplasmosis). Basal infiltrates may result from aspiration secondary to an esophageal lesion. Poor definition of a margin of a mediastinal mass may indicate *en bloc* pulmonary-mediastinal involvement, and therefore malignant disease.

Abdominal involvement may also hold the key to the diagnosis of a mediastinal lesion and vice versa. An inflammatory lesion in the pancreas may "migrate" into the mediastinum; hepatosplenomegaly supports the diagnosis of lymphoma of the mediastinal nodes; a too small liver may signify hepatic herniation; spread from an abdominal neuroblastoma may explain a widened thoracic paravertebral shadow or *iceberg sign* (page 41.)[289]

ANATOMIC LOCATION

One of the most important roentgen aids in diagnosing a mediastinal mass is its location on the AP axis of the thorax, i.e., in the coronal plane. Often the lesion is not visible in the lateral projection because its margins are in contact with other structures of water density or because it doesn't present a border tangential to the X-ray beam. Occasionally, the lesion is poorly delineated in the frontal view for similar reasons. In these cases, fluoroscopy is essential for accurately localizing the mass. Oblique roentgenograms are a poor substitute.

The various ramifications of the silhouette sign are invaluable in determining the position and extent of a mediastinal lesion. The sign can be applied in all projections, not only to the heart but also to the aorta and other structures in the mediastinum as well as to the mass itself.

As stated earlier, bone erosion or destruction is helpful in locating and diagnosing a mediastinal mass. A lesion that involves the spine, sternum, or a rib is readily localized and its nature often histologically predicted. Even if the bone adjacent to a lesion is not visibly involved, attachment can be suspected on the basis of synchronous movement of the bone and the lesion with respiration. This is especially true of lesions in the retrosternal space.[938] Bucky films and laminagrams are often helpful in demonstrating the bone involvement and occasionally even myelography may add important information (Fig. 11-31).

Neurenteric Lesions

An interesting relationship exists between congenital hemivertebra and mediastinal cyst. This has to do with the neurenteric canal, a rudimentary linkage between the gut and spinal canal. The subject is best understood by considering the tracheoesophageal tube as an offshoot of the neural canal.[302, 867, 1243] As with any such embryonic separation, there are six possibilities of retained connections (Fig. 11-19). Each has a clinical counterpart (Table 11-3 and Figs. 11-20 and 11-21) except perhaps type 5, but I'll bet this exists too because it does at other similar embryologic junction sites.

Occasionally the type 1 anomaly arises from an intestinal loop and meanders through the diaphragm and mediastinum.[483] I am not certain that all esophageal and bronchogenic duplication cysts have a neurenteric origin. At any rate, relatively few of them show a spinal anomaly.

(*Text continued on page 409.*)

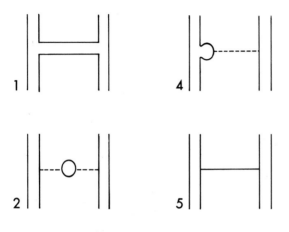

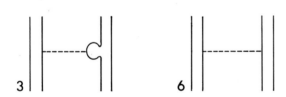

Figure 11-19. RETAINED CONNECTIONS AT EM-BRYONIC POINTS OF SEPARATION

Type 1, Patent all the way. *Type 2*, Closed at both ends, patent in center. *Type 3*, Open at one end. *Type 4*, Open at other end. *Type 5*, Obliterated all the way. *Type 6*, Totally absorbed.

TABLE 11-3. *Embryonic Connections (See Figure 11-19)*

TYPE	*Pulmonary Artery to Aorta*	*Umbilical Cord to Intestine*	*Umbilical Cord to Urinary Bladder*	*Neural Canal to Tracheoesophagus*
1	Patent ductus	Patent vitelline duct	Patent urachus	Neurenteric canal
2	Isolated ductus (from left subclavian artery)	Vitelline cyst	Urachal cyst	Duplication cyst (enteric, bronchogenic)
3	Aortic diverticulum	Umbilical sinus	Umbilical sinus	Congenital esophageal or tracheal diverticulum
4	Pulmonary artery diverticulum	Meckel's diverticulum	Congenital fundal diverticulum of bladder	Anterior meningocele
5	Ligamentum arteriosum	Umbilical ligament	Urachal ligament	?
6	Absent ligamentum arteriosum	Normal	Normal	Normal

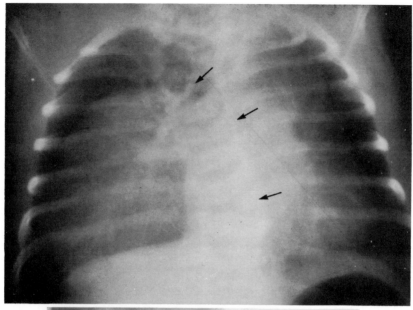

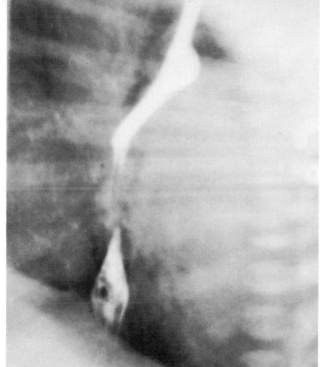

Figure 11–20.   NEURENTERIC ANOMALY: DUPLICATION CYST OF ESOPHAGUS (Type 2)

Multiple hemivertebrae (arrows). The large mediastinal mass lies between the esophagus and the spine. This proved to be a gastric lined cyst attached to the spine. We have a similar case in which the cyst was lined by bronchial mucosa.

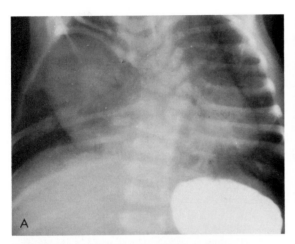

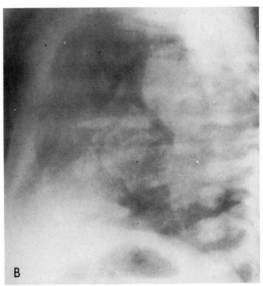

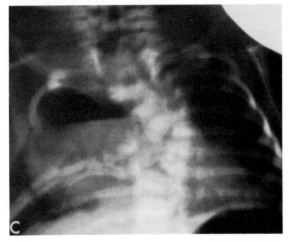

Figure 11–21. NEURENTERIC ANOMALY: AN-
TERIOR MENINGOCELE (Type 4)

A, PA teleroentgenogram. Note the severe vertebral and rib anomalies. Even a mild dorsal spine
anomaly has a similar connotation. B, In the lateral
view, the cyst lies between the spine and esophagus.
At operation, a nodule of gastrointestinal tissue was
found in the wall of the meningocele. (Courtesy of
Dr. William H. McAlister.)

The Mediastinal Lines

A variety of vertical lines are visible in the mediastinum on the frontal view of the chest. These lines represent pleural reflections delineated by air in the adjacent lungs. The chest film must be well penetrated and the pleural lines optimally oriented for their demonstration, i.e., with an edge tangential to the beam. It is difficult to differentiate one normal pleural line from another, or even to distinguish the anterior ones from the posterior. But knowledge of their anatomy often provides information concerning the presence and localization of an adjacent lesion. I have borrowed freely from many others[68, 359, 443, 686] under the supposition that if you steal from one it is called plagiarism, but if you steal from many it is called research. I forget from whom I plagiarized that statement.

The *right paraspinal line* runs from the thoracic inlet to the diaphragm, a millimeter or two from the right border of the thoracic spine. It is produced by the normal soft tissues covering the bone. It is displaced laterally by osteophytes (Fig. 11–30B); an expanding lesion of the vertebrae; a paravertebral mass such as a neurogenic tumor, abscess, or lymphoma;[831, 1314] azygos vein enlargement (Fig. 5–50); and hematoma (Fig. 11–22).

The *left paraspinal line* lies medial to the lateral border of the descending aorta and is seldom seen above the aortic knob[745] (Figs. 11–23 and 11–26). When it is pulled to the left by aortic dilatation a juxtavertebral lesion is simulated. Osteophytes are less frequently present on this side, presumably because pulsation of the aorta interferes with their formation. Otherwise, the left paraspinal line is displaced by similar conditions as the right (Figs. 2–25, 11–1, and 11–24). Free pleural fluid in the phrenicovertebral angle in the supine position may simulate displacement[229] (Fig. 9–9).

Dr. J. J. Crittenden, when he was a member of our staff, examined 100 consecutive normal supine Bucky AP films of the chest and noted that the left paraspinal line lay up to 1 cm from the spine when the aorta was of approximately normal size and contour, and 2 to 3 cm when the aorta was tortuous.

The *right paraesophageal* line (Figs. 11–25, 11–26, and 11–30B) is concave to the right in the upper thorax. It extends from the pulmonary apex down to about the level of the right main stem bronchus. Here it appears to deviate to the right over the azygos vein and sometimes also over the confluence of the right pulmonary veins, except when the esophagus is pulled to the left by the elongated tortuous aorta. Below the azygos vein, the line deviates toward the left, forming the azygoesophageal recess.[526, 527]

The upper segment of the right paraesophageal line is visible through the trachea in about 10 per cent of adults and 50 per cent of children.[192] The width, as visualized with barium in the esophagus, measures from 3 to 7 mm.[905] In peptic esophagitis, cardiospasm, and esophageal varices (Fig. 5–51), it may increase to 20 mm in width.[905, 1281] Enlargement of the heart, especially of the left atrium, may displace the right paraesophageal line.

The *left paraesophageal line* is less often seen because the adjacent descending aorta obliterates it. This line is normally indented from the left by the aortic knob and left main stem bronchus. Its lower end at the diaphragm is often visible. Any mass that displaces the esophagus will, of course, alter the paraesophageal lines. The barium esophagram is helpful in identifying them.

The *left paraaortic line* lies parallel to the left paraspinal line but alongside the lateral border of the aorta (Fig. 11–26). The lower end of the *right paraaortic line* may sometimes be seen just above the diaphragm on a well-penetrated film but is difficult to disassociate from the right paraesophageal line (Fig. 1–2). A right paraaortic line is seen with right-sided descending aorta (Fig. 11–27).

There is a *posterior junction line* between the two lungs behind the esophagus. It is difficult or impossible to distinguish from the paraesophageal lines without barium, although it is thinner and extends from the thoracic inlet to the diaphragm. On the right it becomes confluent with the azygos vein.[526]

The *anterior junction line* between the lungs usually lies near the midline and is never visible above the sternal notch. It is seen in about 20 per cent of chests as a V shaped structure only 2 to 3 inches in length,[194] extending downward from the level of the angle of Louis (Figs. 11–28 and

(*Text continued on page 416.*)

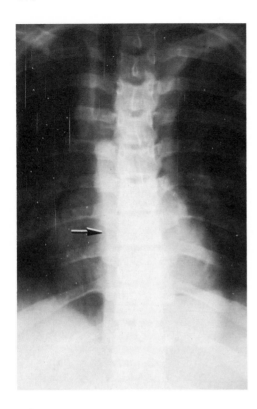

Figure 11–22. DISPLACED RIGHT PARASPINAL LINE
(arrow)

Hematoma from aortic laceration.

Figure 11–23. TOMOGRAM SHOWING NORMAL
LEFT PARAVERTEBRAL LINE

It is not visible above the aortic knob.

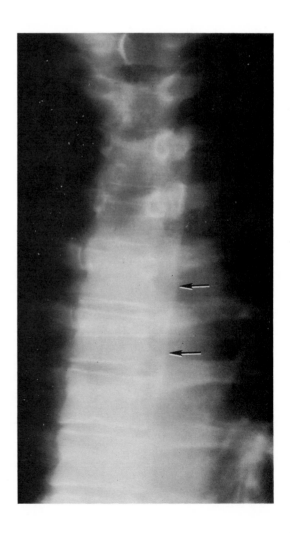

Figure 11-24. DEVIATION OF LEFT PARA-
SPINAL LINE

Intrathoracic extension of an abdominal
neuroblastoma (arrow) in a child.

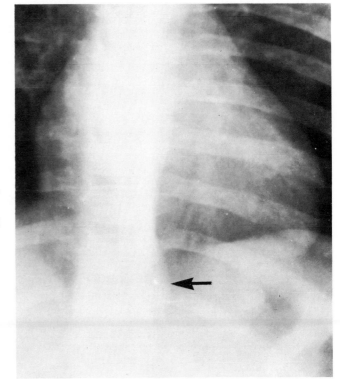

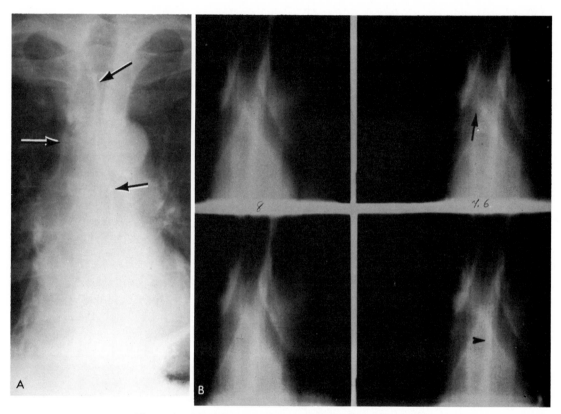

Figure 11–25.   NORMAL RIGHT PARAESOPHAGEAL LINE

A, The upper segment (top arrow) is seen through the trachea. In this elderly man, the aorta has pulled the lower part of the line to the left (bottom arrow). An esophagram clearly identified the line as the right wall of the esophagus. The right paratracheal line is also well shown (middle arrow). *B,* Tomograms and *C,* barium swallow of a young patient. The supra- and infra-azygos segments of the paraesophageal line are denoted by arrowheads, the azygos segment by arrows.

(Figure continued on opposite page.)

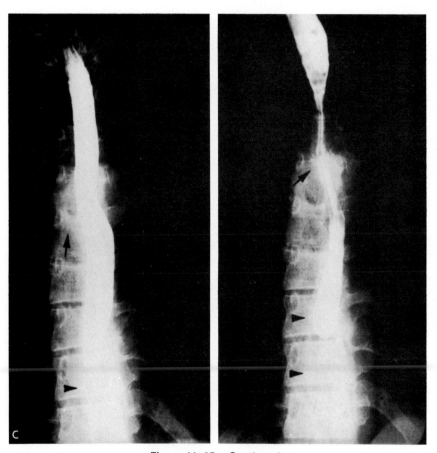

Figure 11–25. *Continued.*

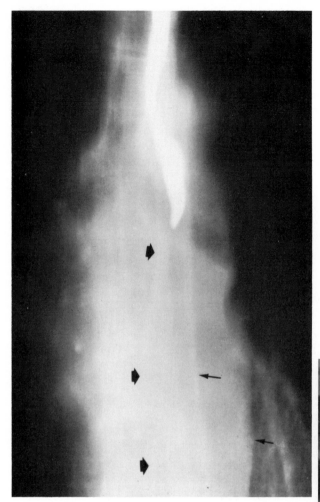

Figure 11–26. NORMAL MEDIASTINAL PARA
LINES ON TOMOGRAPHY

The right paraesophageal (thick arrows), left
paraspinal (upper thin arrow), and left paraaortic (lower thin arrow) lines are shown.

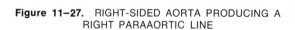

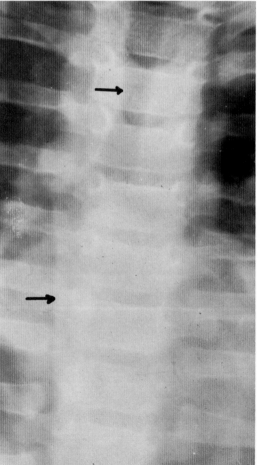

Figure 11–27. RIGHT-SIDED AORTA PRODUCING A
RIGHT PARAAORTIC LINE

The right paratracheal line is indented by the right arch
(upper arrow) and ends below in the azygos arch. The aorta
descends on the right (lower arrow), as it usually does in
these patients. The azygos arch has produced a silhouette
sign on the right descending aorta. Supine film. (From
Felson, B., and Palayew, M. J.[348]; reproduced with permission of Radiology.)

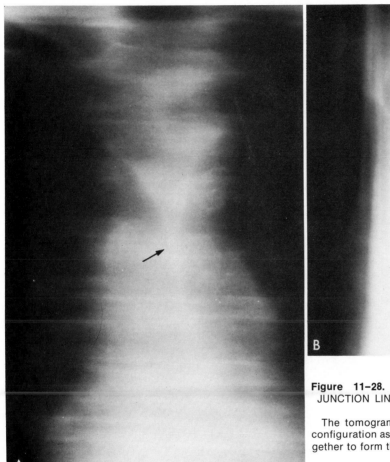

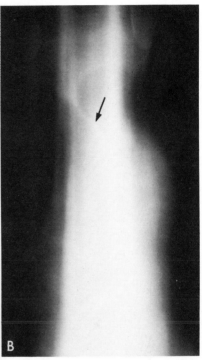

Figure 11–28. NORMAL ANTERIOR JUNCTION LINE IN TWO PATIENTS

The tomograms show the V shaped configuration as the two lungs come together to form the line (arrow).

11–29). This line is seldom apparent in infants because of the thymus.

The *right paratracheal line* is visible in 63 per cent of normal adult chest films (Figs. 11–25A and 11–30A). The azygos vein shadow is always seen at its lower end on the recumbent film but not so often in the upright (Fig. 11–27). Carcinoma of the tracheal wall,[603] lymph node enlargement, and other mediastinal masses and nearby lung lesions may efface its border. The left paratracheal line is seldom seen because the adjacent great vessels generally obliterate it.

A *left pericardial line* (Fig. 11–30C) is sometimes demonstrated as it obliquely crosses the aortic knob. It is, of course, continuous with the left heart border. Enlarged anterior mediastinal nodes may elevate this line.[83] Keats calls it the aortic-pulmonary mediastinal stripe.[631a]

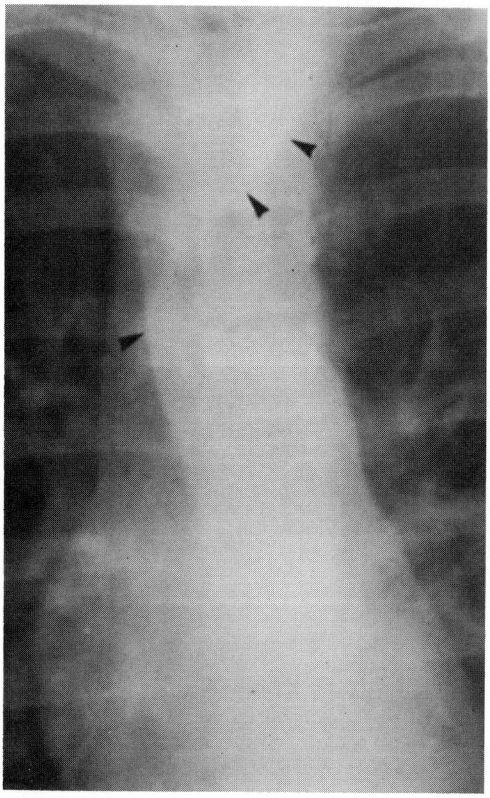

The soft tissues of the extrapleural space are continuous with those of the mediastinum superiorly, perhaps along the subclavian arteries.[453] Pneumomediastinum seldom extends into this space but seems to prefer the easier pathway into the neck, even in children. However, blood or spinal fluid in the mediastinum may spread extrapleurally over one or both pulmonary apices (Fig. 11–31). I have seen it most often in traumatic laceration of the aorta.

Don't be too meticulous in trying to demonstrate the mediastinal lines, nor too glib about naming them. They can confuse you, too. Like the fable of the grasshopper and the centipede: The grasshopper asked the centipede, "Do you move all your right legs, then all your left, or do you move them one pair at a time?" The centipede thought and thought about it—and hasn't walked since.

The Mediastinal Compartments

The divisions of the mediastinum defined by the great anatomists are not suitable for the roentgen diagnosis of mediastinal lesions. A mass anterior to the heart (anterior mediastinum) usually blends with the heart shadow (middle mediastinum) so that its compartment of origin is uncertain. Lesions found between the heart and the spine are different from those in the vertebral gutter, although both lie in the posterior mediastinum. The same histologic lesion may occur in either the superior division or lower down in the mediastinum. Indeed, mediastinal masses seem to extend more readily in a craniocaudal direction than anteroposteriorly.[563, 715] With *chuzpah** born of desperation, I have ignored the great teachings of the past and use an anatomic classification based on roentgen projection rather than anatomic dissection. It has proved eminently practical for me and I hope it will for you.

The radiologic subdivisions of the mediastinum are ascertained from the lateral roentgenogram (Fig. 11–32) as follows: An

Figure 11–29. SEPARATION OF THE TWO LUNGS ANTERIORLY BY A HEMATOMA (arrowheads)

Widening of the V is indicative of an anterior mediastinal abnormality except in infants (thymus).

---

*When your brother-in-law comes in wearing your suit, it's nerve. When he smiles at you through your own false teeth, that's *chuzpah*.

(Text continued on page 420.)

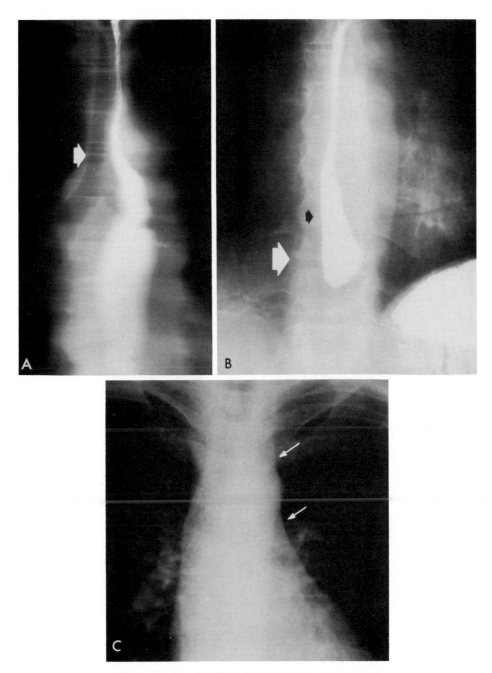

Figure 11–30. NORMAL MEDIASTINAL PARA LINES

A, Tomogram showing right paratracheal line (arrow), ending below in the azygos vein. *B*, The right paraeso-phageal (small arrow) and right paraspinal (large arrow) lines are shown. *C*, The left pericardial line (arrows) ex-tends across the upper descending knob.

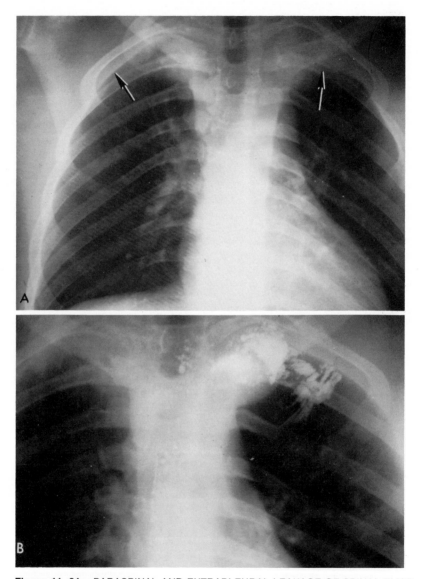

Figure 11–31. PARASPINAL AND EXTRAPLEURAL LEAKAGE OF SPINAL FLUID

   A, The paraspinal lines are displaced laterally and are contiguous with the extrapleural extension over both pulmonary apices (arrows). Neurologic signs after severe trauma led to myelography, which showed the extraspinal seepage of contrast medium shown in *B.*

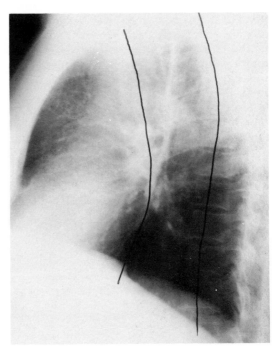

Figure 11–32. THE MEDIASTINAL COMPARTMENTS

The "anterior" and "middle" mediastinum are divided by the line extending along the back of the heart and front of the trachea. The "middle" and "posterior" mediastinal compartments are separated by the line connecting a point on each thoracic vertebra about a centimeter behind its anterior margin.

TABLE 11–4.   *Conditions Found in Each of the Roentgen Compartments of the Mediastinum*[338, 520, 521, 615, 715, 716, 771, 872, 1025]

"Anterior"	"Middle"	"Posterior"
Anomalous or dilated superior vena cava[335]		
Parathyroid tumor[715, 912]	Thyroid tumor	Neurogenic tumor, benign or malignant
Thyroid, ectopic	Parathyroid tumor[715]	Glomus tumor[715]
Thymic lesion[57, 285, 335, 492, 507, 549, 673, 1098, 1102]	Vagus or phrenic neurinoma[430]	Pheochromocytoma[217]
Chemodectoma[492, 939]	Chemodectoma[492, 939]	Chemodectoma[492, 939]
Mediastinitis,[715] abscess, fibrosis[271, 762, 765]	Mediastinitis,[715] abscess, fibrosis[271, 765]	Mediastinitis,[715] abscess, fibrosis[271, 765]
Mesenchymal tumor°[191, 213, 715, 788, 911]	Mesenchymal tumor°[191, 213, 715, 788, 911]	Mesenchymal tumor°[191, 213, 715, 788, 911]
Teratoma, choriocarcinoma[913, 1275]	Tracheal tumor[603, 715, 716]	Extramedullary hematopoiesis[209, 549, 765]
Aneurysm of aorta or sinus of Valsalva; buckled innominate artery[1081]	Aneurysm of aorta or major arteries or veins; right aortic arch; kinked aorta[249, 348, 859]	Aneurysm, descending aorta
Lymphoma°°[549]	Lymph node disease[357, 549, 1251]	Lymphoma°°
Pericardial tumor, cyst, or diverticulum[746, 768, 836]	Bronchogenic, enteric, or neurenteric cyst[58, 867, 910, 1026]	Neurenteric cyst[58, 867]
Pericardial tumor[802]	Esophageal lesion	Lateral meningocele[141, 189]
Cardiac tumor or aneurysm	Azygos vein enlargement	Cyst of thoracic duct
Hematoma[964]	Hematoma[964]	Hematoma[358, 964]
Hernia, Morgagni or hepatic[23, 58]	Hernia, hiatal, hepatic	Hernia, Bochdalek, kidney, spleen
Pericardial fat pad or fat pad necrosis[49, 184, 684]	Pancreatic pseudocyst[715]	Spinal disease
		Pancreatic pseudocyst

°Mesenchymal tumor includes lipoma, fibroma, myoma, hemangioma, lymphangioma, chondroma, xanthofibroma, mixtures of these, and their malignant counterparts.

°°Lymphoma includes lymphosarcoma, leukemia, reticulum cell sarcoma, Hodgkin's disease, and the like.

imaginary line is traced upward from the diaphragm along the back of the heart and front of the trachea to the neck. This divides the "anterior" from the "middle" mediastinum.* A second imaginary vertical line connects a point on each of the thoracic vertebrae 1 cm behind its anterior margin. This divides the "middle" from the "posterior" mediastinum. The position of the posterior line is not critical, since a lesion in the "posterior" mediastinum must make contact with the posteromedial thoracic wall, i.e., it must involve the paravertebral gutter. Thus,

---

*Quotation marks are used to distinguish the roentgen from the anatomic subdivisions.

if the posterior surface of a mass is outlined by air, it is still considered to lie in the "middle" mediastinum.

Table 11–4 lists the various conditions found in each of these compartments. Note that certain lesions may occur in any of the three compartments. An effort was made to group the lesions in the table according to their vertical level in the patient, but this was only partly successful. A lesion may, of course, extend from its compartment of origin to the next one or arise along the border between them, so that it is sometimes difficult to determine roentgenographically the original site. Nonetheless, we have found this chart of considerable value in the differential diagnosis of mediastinal masses.

CHAPTER 12

THE DIAPHRAGM

THE HIGH DIAPHRAGM

As is well known, diaphragm levels vary considerably from patient to patient. The average level of the right cupola is at the anterior end of the sixth rib.[720] The right hemidiaphragm is usually about half an interspace higher than the left, but appreciable unilateral elevation is not uncommon.[1334a] I noted a raised diaphragm in 11 per cent of a series of 500 normal chests; in 9 per cent it occurred on the left and in 2 per cent on the right. In half of the 9 per cent, the two domes were at the same level; in the other half the left was actually higher than the right. Fifty per cent of those with left-sided elevation showed gaseous distention of the stomach, splenic flexure, or both (Chap. 15).

I have encountered a number of healthy individuals who have had left-sided elevation for prolonged periods (up to 15 years), and have been struck by the frequent persistence of the finding—even including the associated distention of the gut. I refuse to believe that each of the many chest films was made after a heavy meal or that every patient had constipation all those years. I think the excess gas represents "filler," i.e., expansion of gut to fill in the increased space in the left upper quadrant created by the high diaphragm. Pain and dyspnea have been attributed to this form of meteorism ("splenic flexure syndrome"), but I wonder. . . .

The normally higher position of the right hemidiaphragm is generally attributed to the bulk of the underlying liver, but the fact is, the left hemidiaphragm is depressed by the heart. In partial situs inversus with liver and heart on the same side, the diaphragm leaflet on that side is the one that is *lower*[1315]

(Fig. 3–19). Put this in your drawer of useless information.

A moderately high hemidiaphragm may result from a number of pathologic processes. It is common in such thoracic conditions as pulmonary collapse, pneumonia, infarction, rib fracture, and pleurisy. The raised hemidiaphragm in most of these situations is attributed to "splinting" from the chest pain. More striking elevation of a leaf of the diaphragm follows damage to the phrenic nerve by tumor, trauma, or surgical procedures. Table 12–1 is a list of the causes of phrenic paralysis. In eventration, the affected hemidiaphragm (generally the left) also shows marked elevation,[1210] but because of the absence or sparsity of muscle fibers (Fig. 12–22).

Upper abdominal conditions also frequently cause unilateral elevation. Enlargement of the liver or spleen (Figs. 12–1 and 12–2), pancreatitis, and subphrenic abscess are the commonest of these, but any lesion that produces inflammation or pain in the

TABLE 12–1. Causes of Paralyzed Hemidiaphragm

Common
    Thoracic tumor (phrenic nerve involvement)
    Operation (phrenic nerve injury or resection)
    Subphrenic abscess

Rare
    Trauma; Erb's palsy
    Neurologic disease (stroke, poliomyelitis)
    Tumor or infection of the neck or cervical spine
    Pneumonia[416, 948]
    Radiation therapy
    Muscular disease (myotonia)
    Eventration
    Idiopathic[1174]

421

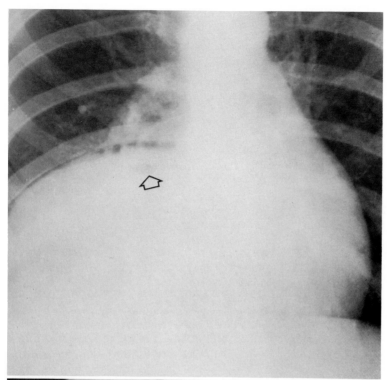

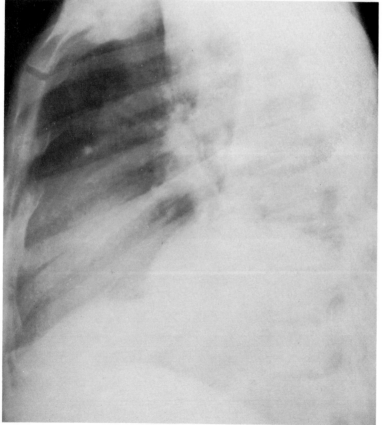

Figure 12–1. AMEBIC ABSCESS OF THE LIVER

The right hemidiaphragm shows a rounded posterior elevation. The small gas bubble (arrow) is attributed to incipient perforation into the lung.

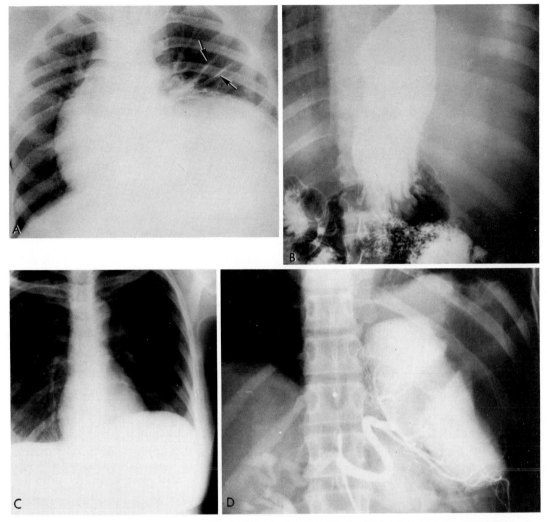

Figure 12–2. ENLARGED SPLEEN CAUSING ELEVATION OF THE LEFT HEMIDIAPHRAGM

A, The heart is displaced to the right. There are two oblique disks of atelectasis above the left hemidiaphragm (arrows). *B,* Upper GI series shows medial displacement of the stomach by the huge spleen. *C* and *D,* Another patient. Recent trauma. The selective splenic arteriogram shows a large subcapsular hematoma.

vicinity of its undersurface may raise the diaphragm.

In *subphrenic abscess,* the hemidiaphragm is elevated and often loses its normal convexity as its posterior segment is lifted. Its respiratory movement is absent or greatly limited. Gas may be present in the abscess and, on the left, the gastric bubble may be displaced. The recognition of gas within a left subphrenic abscess depends on visualization of the normal confines of the gastric fundus and splenic flexure. Pleural

fluid and disk atelectasis are common thoracic manifestations.[1059] The roentgen signs may be minimal or absent if antibiotic therapy has been administered.[193] *Hepatic abscess,* including the amebic variety, may give identical signs (Fig. 12–1).

There are, in addition, several entities that closely resemble a high hemidiaphragm but in which the diaphragm itself is actually in normal position. One of these, free pleural fluid trapped between the lung and diaphragm, has already been discussed in Chapter 9. The other, traumatic diaphragmatic hernia, will be described below.

Germane to the problem of the elevated diaphragm are the position and contour of the stomach and colon as seen on plain films or with contrast medium. In about 500 normal chests with gas outlined fundus, the distance between the top of the gastric bubble and the left cupola was less than 1 cm in about 88 per cent; 1 to 2 cm in about 11 per cent; and over 2 cm in less than 1 per cent. A surprising number of films had to be discarded (over 200) because no gas bubble was visible at all (Chap. 15). Underexposure accounted for some of these. Perhaps in others, the fundus-cupola distance was so great that the gas bubble was not on the film. Remember though, the gas bubble does not necessarily lie under the *highest* portion of the left hemidiaphragm. When it doesn't, even though the stomach rests against the undersurface of a segment of diaphragm, the dome may project considerably above the gas bubble on the frontal view.

Downward displacement of the stomach and/or colon occurs in a number of normal and abnormal situations. Most of these are included in Table 12–2. Inversion of the diaphragm will also depress these structures. Left subpulmonary pleural effusion often

TABLE 12–2. Causes of Increased Space Between Gastric Fundus and Diaphragm[761, 1318]

Normal variation
Left lobe of liver, normal or enlarged
Spleen, normal or enlarged
Ascites
Subphrenic abscess
Tumor of fundus of stomach
Tumor of kidney, adrenal, pancreas, or diaphragm

appears to increase the fundus-diaphragm distance (Fig. 9–3).

The key to the diagnosis of the underlying cause of apparent elevation of the *right* hemidiaphragm is the position of the lower border of the liver shadow. In the high diaphragm caused by paralysis, eventration, or intrapulmonary lesion, and in hepatic herniation,[930] the lower border of the liver is elevated (Figs. 3–15, 12–3, and 12–28C). When there is subpulmonary fluid, the normal position of the lower border of the liver is not altered. In subphrenic abscess or enlarged liver, the inferior edge of the liver will either be in a normal or low position, but never elevated (Fig. 12–4). The position of the spleen, when visible, can be utilized in similar fashion on the left side (Fig. 12–2).

Transient or persistent hepatodiaphrag-

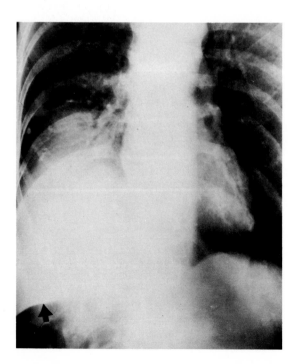

Figure 12–3. ELEVATED RIGHT DIAPHRAGM FROM COLLAPSED RLL

The lower border of the liver (arrow) is also elevated.

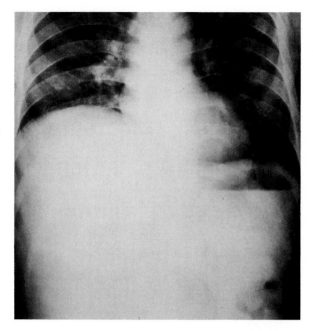

Figure 12–4. ELEVATION OF DIAPHRAGM BY ENLARGED LIVER

The liver also shows marked downward enlargement. Hepatoma.

matic interposition of the colon or small intestine (Chilaiditi's syndrome) is a frequent and generally asymptomatic condition.[48] However, I have seen a patient with acute small bowel obstruction from herniation through the falciform ligament, and another with recurrent, temporary, alternating volvulus of the sigmoid and stomach into the right subphrenic space. Interposition of the large or small bowel between the spleen or stomach and the left hemidiaphragm is not uncommon.

Bilateral elevation of the diaphragm may be seen with ascites, pregnancy, hepatosplenomegaly, and large abdominal neoplasm or cyst. It may also be encountered in association with bilateral intrathoracic or subphrenic disease. We have seen a few examples in lupus erythematosus, presumably the result of the pleural involvement so frequently encountered in this disease.

Examination in the lateral projection is indispensable to the study of lesions in the vicinity of the diaphragm. For example, the lateral view may show that the elevation of a hemidiaphragm is predominantly anterior or posterior. On the right side, liver enlargement is, of course, the most likely cause of anterior elevation, and subphrenic abscess most often produces posterior elevation. However, I have seen a number of examples of subphrenic abscess with anterior elevation and several of hepatic enlargement with posterior elevation.

ABNORMAL DIAPHRAGM CONTOUR

Alterations in the shape of the diaphragm are common. *Scalloping*, a polyarcuate appearance, results from the visibility of small muscle fascicles near their individual insertions on each of the lower ribs. Among 540 normal chest films, scalloping was found in 30 instances, or 5.5 per cent. It was seen with much less frequency on the left side than on the right, probably because of obscuration by the heart. It was sometimes bilateral, and was commoner among asthenic individuals (Chap. 15). The incidence is greater in patients with pulmonary emphysema or pneumothorax. In these cases, the dome of the diaphragm is so depressed that the attachments are silhouetted against the air containing lung (Fig. 12–5).

Localized Bumps on the Diaphragm

Elevation of a *segment* of diaphragm is a fairly frequent roentgen finding. Since the localized hump must contain subjacent tis-

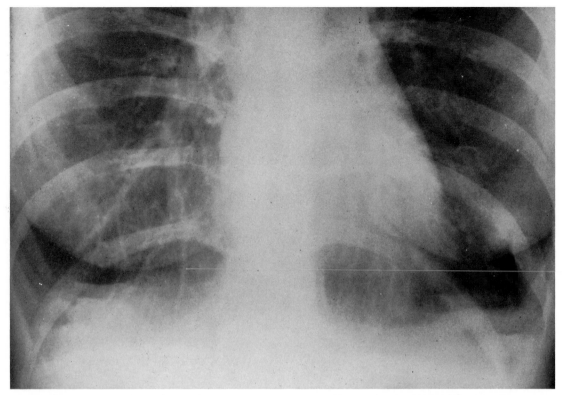

Figure 12–5. SCALLOPING OF THE DIAPHRAGM DURING AN ACUTE ASTHMATIC ATTACK

A chest film 1 month earlier was normal. The diffuse emphysema has so depressed the dome of the diaphragm that its costal attachments are uncovered.

sue, usually liver—a vacuum is impossible—some difficulty is encountered in its classification. Is it a hernia or a localized eventration? Since muscle fibers may be meager or absent in eventration, differentiation from a hernial sac cannot even be resolved pathologically. The commonest site of this bump is along the anteromedial portion of the right hemidiaphragm adjacent to the heart. A lump of liver generally extends into it. The condition has been variously reported as localized eventration, hepatic herniation, and ectopic lobe of the liver.[23, 408, 924] It is usually congenital and may be associated with other anomalies. Diagnostic pneumoperitoneum may show a hump, bump, or lump on the liver, with a membrane, the thinned diaphragm or hernial sac, above it (Fig. 12–6). However, the peritoneal air may fail to enter the sac. Anyway, a liver scan is a simpler and safer way of establishing the diagnosis (Fig. 12–

7). Figure 12–8 illustrates a fascinating example of a similar localized bump which appeared shortly after a major surgical procedure on the neck. This suggests that segmental paralysis from injury to fibrils of the phrenic nerve may at times cause localized "eventration."

Localized diaphragmatic hernia with other viscera in the chest can produce a similar shadow. A tumor or cyst of the diaphragm or liver may also cause a solitary upward convexity[1, 1054, 1244] (Fig. 12–9), as can accessory diaphragm.

ACCESSORY DIAPHRAGM

Accessory diaphragm is a partial duplication of a hemidiaphragm, nearly always the right, that extends obliquely upward and backward to join the posterior thoracic wall. Part or all of the lower lobe is contained

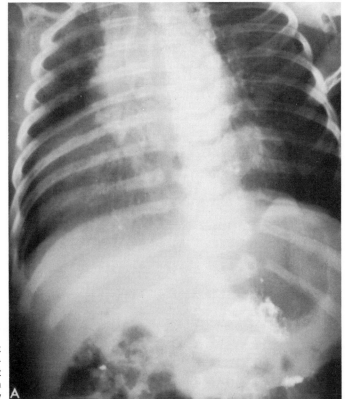

Figure 12–6. CONGENITAL IN-
TRATHORACIC HERNIATION OF LIVER

A, The large mass in the lower thorax
simulates a greatly enlarged heart of bi-
zarre configuration. However, the amount
of liver substance visible in the abdomen
is abnormally small, and the pulmonary
arteries converge on the heart high in the
thorax. *B,* Diagnostic pneumoperitoneum. The hernial sac is outlined with
air (arrows). More than half of the liver
lies in the lower thorax. A normal heart
lies above the hernia. A liver scan would
have been just as diagnostic but hadn't
been invented when this patient was seen.

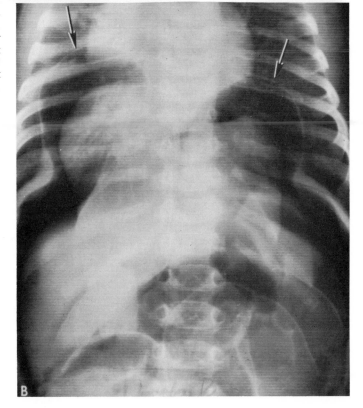

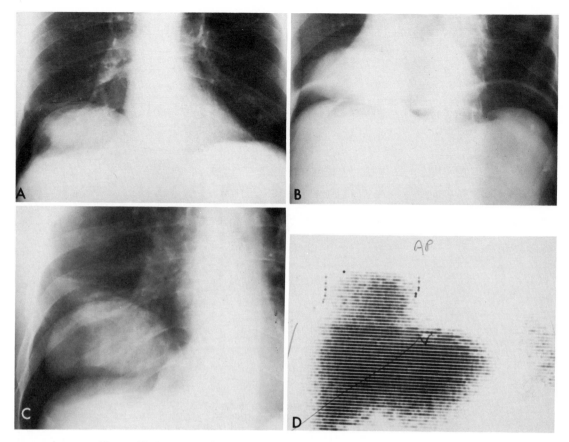

Figure 12–7. HEPATIC HERNIA, PROBABLY CONGENITAL, IN AN ADULT

A, PA teleroentgenogram. *B,* Diagnostic pneumoperitoneum. No air enters the thorax. *C,* Diagnostic pneumo-thorax. The mass is outlined by air. *B* and *C* need not have been done because *D,* the liver scan, proved diagnostic. No operative confirmation.

between it and the true hemidiaphragm. It is commonly associated with scimitar syndrome (Chap. 3).

On the frontal view of the chest, the entire hemidiaphragm may be elevated or show a flat prominence (Fig. 3–18). In the lateral view, the extra diaphragm may appear as an oblique shadow, lower anteriorly. The heart is generally deviated toward the right.[243, 273, 340, 881, 1061]

Inversion of the Diaphragm

Have you ever wondered why, after removal of 500 cc or so of pleural fluid, the chest film sometimes still looks the same as before the tap? Or why a patient may be very short of breath when one pleural cavity is only half filled with fluid? The explanation for these seeming inconsistencies rests with the subject of inversion of the diaphragm.

A large collection of pleural fluid or an intrathoracic mass may invert the left hemidiaphragm so that its convexity is directed downward. The liver ordinarily prevents the right hemidiaphragm from inverting under similar circumstances. I have long been aware of this condition and even illustrated it in an earlier publication,[330] but considered it extremely rare and generally unimportant. It remained for one of our former residents, Dr. Richard B. Mulvey, to demonstrate that inversion is common and has considerable clinical significance.[854]

He pointed out in the first place that, since the diaphragm itself is invisible under

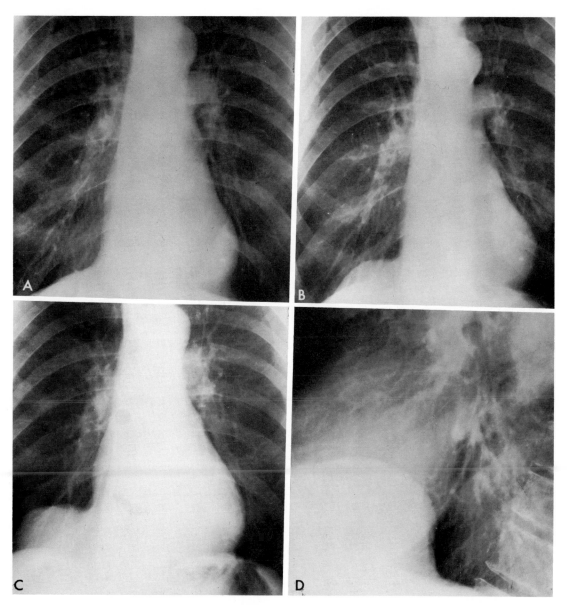

Figure 12–8. ACQUIRED LOCALIZED "EVENTRATION"

A, Normal chest 4 days prior to laryngectomy and tracheotomy for carcinoma. *B*, 6 days after operation. The medial segment of the right leaf of the diaphragm is moderately elevated. *C* and *D*, A year later. The anteromedial bulge on the right is now more prominent. Fluoroscopy showed limitation of motion of the abnormal segment. The findings were unchanged 4 years later.

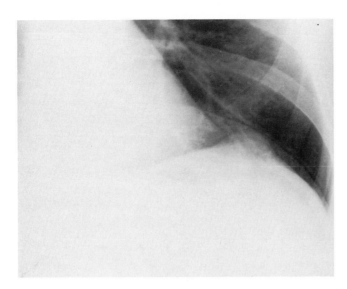

Figure 12–9. SIMPLE CYST OF LEFT DIA-
PHRAGM

(Courtesy of Dr. Roland G. Wintzinger.)

these circumstances, the gastric fundus can readily serve as its marker. And obviously, if you can't make out the gas bubble on the chest film, give barium. With diaphragm inversion, the fundus is displaced downward and medially and its lateral contour is often deformed as by an extrinsic mass (Fig. 12–10). The spleen and splenic flexure are also depressed, and sometimes even the kidney. Occasionally the outline of the inverted diaphragm may be visible as a smooth margined left upper quadrant mass (Fig.

12–11). Pneumoperitoneum should be diagnostic but is hardly necessary.

The trough formed by the inverted diaphragm can hold a lot of fluid. The first result of thoracentesis in these patients is return of the diaphragm to its normal upright position. Thus, the crest of the fluid doesn't fall after chest tap; the bottom simply rises (Fig. 12–12).

Now, why the shortness of breath? After all, pneumonectomy isn't usually followed by dyspnea, so why should half a chest full

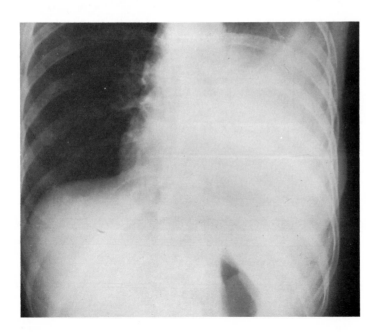

Figure 12–10. INVERSION OF LEFT HEMIDIAPHRAGM BY PLEURAL EF-
FUSION

The gastric bubble is depressed and flattened on its outer contour. The heart is shifted only slightly to the right. Upright film. (Courtesy of Dr. Richard B. Mulvey.)

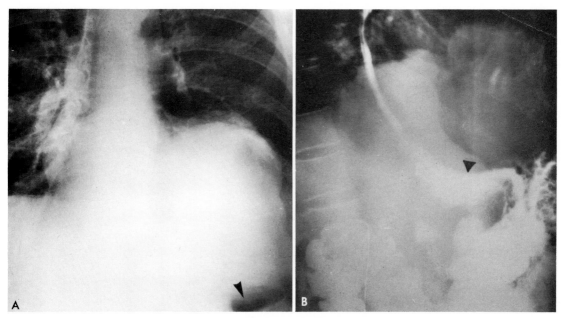

Figure 12–11. INVERSION OF LEFT HEMIDIAPHRAGM

A, Large lobulated opacity in the left lower thorax. A sharply outlined mass is also seen in the left upper abdomen (arrowhead), depressing the gastric air bubble. *B,* There is extrinsic pressure on the fundus of the stomach by the soft tissue mass (arrowhead). A chest film made several years earlier was normal except for a hump at the cardiac apex. At operation an enormous pericardial coelomic cyst was found resting against the intact inverted diaphragm. (Courtesy of Dr. William R. Dickens.)

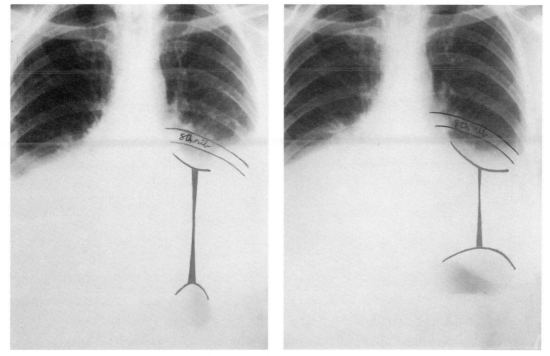

Figure 12–12. WHY PLEURAL EFFUSION MAY LOOK THE SAME BEFORE AND AFTER THORACENTESIS

A, Congestive failure with bilateral pleural effusion before pleural tap. Note the low position of the gastric bubble and the height of the fluid, which extends to the level of the 8th rib posteriorly. *B,* After removal of over 500 cc of fluid from the left thorax. The height of the fluid is considerably reduced as the gas bubble (retouched) rises; the crest of the fluid shows little change. (Courtesy of Dr. Richard B. Mulvey.)

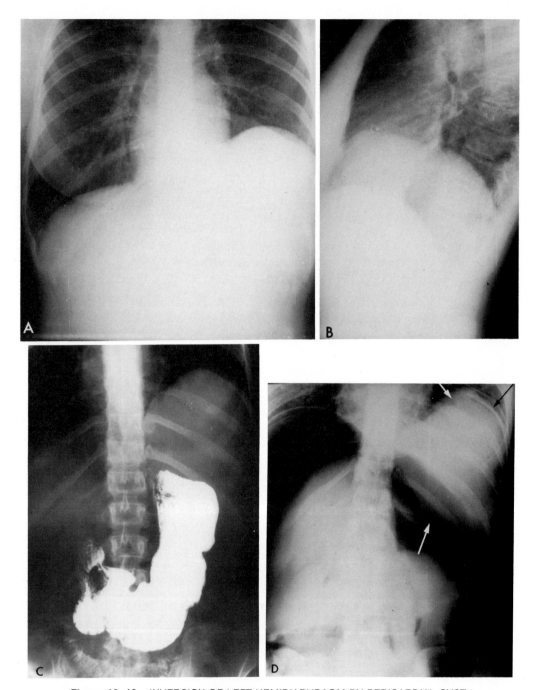

Figure 12–13. INVERSION OF LEFT HEMIDIAPHRAGM BY PERICARDIAL CYST

A and *B*, Apparent elevation of left hemidiaphragm by a large left upper quadrant mass. *C*, The mass depresses and flattens the gastric fundus. The splenic flexure and left kidney were also depressed. *D*, Diagnostic pneumo-peritoneum. The downward convexity (lower arrow) is the inverted diaphragm. The cyst (upper arrows) is connected by a pedicle to the lower border of the pericardium. I called it a large spleen! (Courtesy of Dr. Richard Ashcom.)

of fluid cause it? To begin with, an inverted diaphragm behaves inversely: it rises actively on inspiration and falls on expiration, just as you might expect if you think about it. This can be clearly observed during fluoroscopy by watching the gastric bubble. If you remove just enough fluid to leave the diaphragm flat (flat-topped gas bubble), little or no respiratory excursion is visible. Remove still more fluid and the now-upright diaphragm is seen to move in normal direction.

For years, chest physicians and surgeons have invoked a condition known as pendulum respiration or *pendelluft* to explain the respiratory malfunction that occurs after thoracoplasty or chest wall injury. Air was believed to pass back and forth between the two lungs during breathing.[22, 123, 747] More recently the theory has been discarded.[415, 789, 1162, 1323] Mulvey has applied the pendulum theory to inversion of the diaphragm by pleural fluid. What happens when the two hemidiaphragms move in opposite directions? On inspiration, as the inverted left hemidiaphragm rises and the right descends, some air goes from the left lung into

the right. The converse occurs during expiration. Of course, some air must come from the outside or this would be incompatible with life. Removal of enough fluid to bring the diaphragm upright corrects the *pendelluft* and often the dyspnea. So pendulum respiration may account for the dyspnea in patients with inverted diaphragm. As A. D. Steinfeld* remarked, "The theory is dead though not yet buried." Perhaps Mulvey has resurrected it.

As I stated earlier, inversion of the diaphragm is a frequent event. Swingle et al. encountered 11 cases in a year.[1191] I have observed inversion in a number of patients with left pleural effusion: in two instances of pericardial cyst (Figs. 12–11 and 12–13), in two cases of huge myocardial aneurysm at the undersurface of the left ventricle, and in a child with left tension pneumothorax. I have also seen one patient with inversion of the *right* hemidiaphragm, a child with severe tension pneumothorax (Fig. 12–14),

*A medical student who reviewed the literature on *pendelluft* for me.

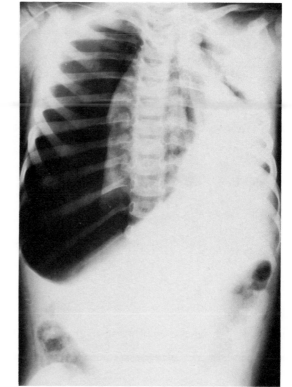

Figure 12–14. INVERTED RIGHT HEMIDIAPHRAGM BY TENSION PNEUMOTHORAX

The right pleural sac is greatly enlarged by the traumatic pneumothorax. Postmortem film.

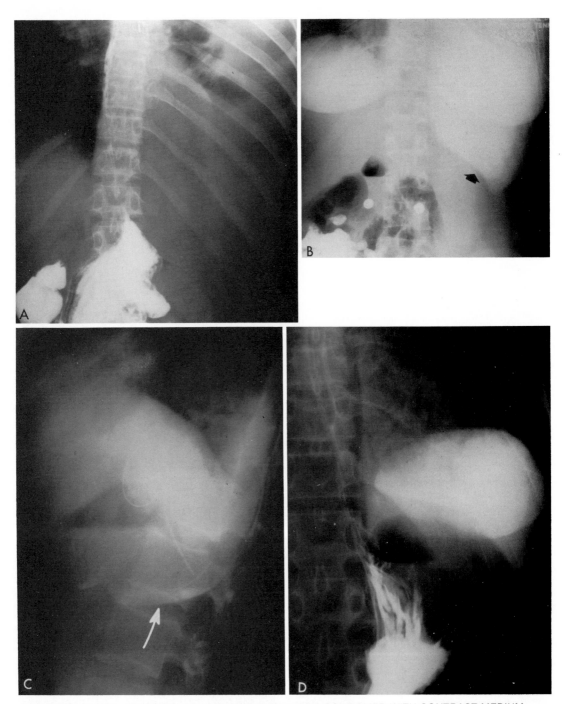

Figure 12–15. INVERSION OF LEFT HEMIDIAPHRAGM CONFIRMED WITH CONTRAST MEDIUM

A, Recumbent film shows depression, displacement, and distortion of the barium filled gastric fundus and low position of the left kidney. *B,* Upright film. Hypaque has been injected into the left pleural cavity. Note low position of left posterior costophrenic recess (arrow). *C,* Upright lateral film 1 month later. Recurrence of fluid. More Hypaque has been injected via catheter. The inverted diaphragm is beautifully shown (arrow). *D,* Same day, after tap. Note the upward convex diaphragm and the opacified subpulmonary fluid. The gas bubble is now normal. The overlying breast shadow obscures some of the detail. (Courtesy of Dr. Elizabeth Ann Rush and Medical Division, Oak Ridge Institute of Nuclear Studies, Inc.)

and one with bilateral inversion caused by congenital lobar emphysema (Fig. 3–70).

Why inversion develops in some patients with left pleural effusion and not in others, I have no idea. It is certainly not related to the nature of the pleural fluid. The inverted left diaphragm might be expected to "pop" upright when the patient assumes a recumbent position, since the fluid should leave the trough, but this doesn't seem to happen. That inversion is not merely a theoretical consideration is illustrated in Figure 12–15.

DIAPHRAGMATIC MOTION

Normal Motion

Normal diaphragm movement during respiration is not always smooth and even. Asymmetrical motion occurred in 77 per cent of normal patients in one series, although the difference in excursion was usually less than 1 cm.[6, 402] The left leaf is more often the one with greater mobility.[6, 699] The excursion in one group of normals ranged from 3 to 6 cm in 75 per cent, with 23 per cent less than 3 cm and 2 per cent more than 6 cm.[1128] In another series, the mean motion was 5 to 7 cm, with less than 3 cm excursion in 14 per cent.[1334a] Minor asynchronous motion of the two hemidiaphragms and even momentary minimal paradoxical movement are also common. The dome may also move differently from the rest of the diaphragm.

Quiet inspiration is usually performed by contraction of the diaphragm and external intercostal muscles.[699] Quiet expiration does not involve muscular action, but deep expiration requires active contraction of the abdominal and thoracic expiratory muscles. Hitzenberger's sniff test is made by inhaling suddenly through the nose with the mouth closed. Normally, the rapid increase of intrathoracic pressure is associated with a downward movement of both hemidiaphragms. Unilateral passive upward movement is seen with paralysis, eventration, and other conditions involving the diaphragm.[1346]

In lateral recumbency, the dependent leaf of the diaphragm rises high and its respiratory excursion is greatly exaggerated.

Incidentally, the lateral recumbent view is useful for demonstrating paradoxical motion, especially since the small screen in modern fluoroscopic equipment prevents adequate comparison of the two sides in the frontal position.

Occasionally, unusual diaphragmatic movements are seen. Hiccups are produced by sudden diaphragm contraction with abrupt inspiration through a partly closed glottis.[544] Diaphragm flutter consists of uni- or bilateral fibrillary contractions, 60 to 300 per minute, and is of unknown etiology.[274] Diaphragm contraction synchronous with each cardiac systole has also been recorded.[411]

I once had the unusual opportunity of examining fluoroscopically a young woman who had pseudocyesis. The lower abdomen was protuberant and there was moderate intestinal gaseous distention. Both leaves of the diaphragm were remarkably low and showed essentially no respiratory movement; the patient utilized costal breathing. She was then hypnotized by a psychiatrist and was told that she was in labor and would shortly give birth to a baby. Rapid contractions of her abdominal muscles followed, punctuated by a few screams, and the patient promptly delivered—a large amount of audible gas. Her abdomen became flat. Fluoroscopy now showed normal position and excursion of the diaphragm. Nevertheless, when she was released from hypnosis all the original findings promptly recurred. Paternity of the new false pregnancy was never established.

Abnormal Motion

Altered mobility of the diaphragm on respiration is an important roentgen sign of phrenic or juxtaphrenic disease. All the conditions mentioned in connection with elevation of the diaphragm may also be associated with distinct limitation in its excursion. *Complete* fixation is encountered with subphrenic abscess and other suppurative processes in contact with the diaphragm. It also occurs in some cases of paralysis, eventration, traumatic hernia, unilateral obstructive hyperaeration, and pneumothorax.[624, 1207] In many of these con-

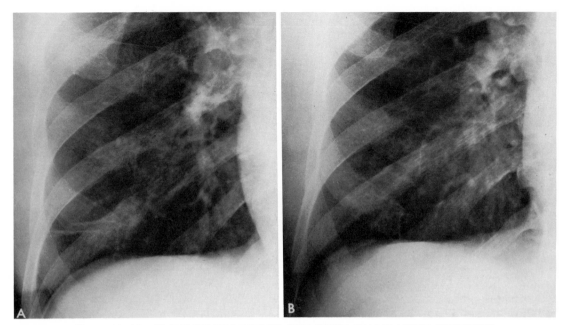

Figure 12–16. PLATELIKE ATELECTASIS FOLLOWING GALLBLADDER OPERATION

A, Several disks of atelectasis are seen above the right hemidiaphragm several days postoperatively. *B,* 1 week later the Fleischner lines have cleared.

ditions, paradoxical movement, i.e., upward displacement of the affected side on inspiration, is also common.[101] This type of paradoxical motion, unlike the active movement of diaphragmatic inversion, is passive and results from the increased intraabdominal pressure that occurs during inspiration as well as from the sucking effect of expansion of the normal hemithorax.[624] Fluoroscopic differentiation between complete fixation and impaired or paradoxical motion is facilitated by the use of sniffing[1346] and snorting maneuvers. It requires at least a 2 cm difference in movement on the two sides to be significant.[6]

Greatly limited or absent mobility is the rule in subphrenic abscess, but in two proved cases that I observed, a normal excursion was demonstrated. Needless to say, in both instances I missed the diagnosis. As noted earlier, normal excursion in subphrenic abscess is more common after antibiotic therapy.[193] The limitation of movement caused by nonsuppurative processes in the chest or abdomen is seldom striking.[301] The differential diagnosis between paralysis or eventration and traumatic diaphragmatic hernia cannot be made on the basis of paradoxical or absent move-

ment, despite oft-repeated statements to the contrary. A simple and reliable method of distinguishing them will be discussed later.

DISK ATELECTASIS

Impaired diaphragmatic motion is often associated with Fleischner's lines, or platelike atelectasis.[370, 381, 784] At this point a brief digression to consider the nature and recognition of these lines seems in order. They are several millimeters in width and 2 to 5 cm in length, and usually lie transversely in the base of one or both lungs (Fig. 12–16). At times they take an oblique or even vertical course (Fig. 12–2A).

They are readily distinguished from septal or Kerley's B lines (Figs. 5–54 and 5–58) in that they are fewer in number (usually only one or two), are spaced more irregularly, are located more deeply within the lung, and are often thicker. On rotating the patient, an atelectatic disk becomes foreshortened or may disappear,[1194] whereas a septal line, which is really a circle outlining the periphery of a lobule, does not change. Differentiation of a disk from the linear scar of a healed infarct or an inflammatory lesion is more difficult.[1139] The linear scar may show fine strands emanating from its borders and is often associated with pleural thickening; it is also permanent, whereas the Fleischner line is often evanescent. At times, however, it is impossible to distinguish between the two.

Fleischner proved that the discoid lines were the result of collapse of small pulmonary subdivisions. They may occasionally be seen in the normal hypersthenic individual with a high diaphragm and are commonly present following thoracic trauma, with subphrenic disease, or with pathologic elevation of the diaphragm from any cause.[796] The lines may also be seen in bronchopneumonia and were particularly frequent in the World War II epidemic of so-called primary atypical pneumonia. They are relatively common in cardiac patients,[514] but here the distinction from infarction is practically impossible; the two often coexist.[1126] To me, disk atelectasis usually signifies that the mobility of the underlying hemidiaphragm is, for one reason or another, impaired.

DIAPHRAGMATIC HERNIA

Traumatic Type

The roentgen distinction between eventration, elevation, or paralysis of the diaphragm on the one hand and traumatic diaphragmatic hernia on the other, is an extremely important one from the standpoint of the patient's survival.[166] Traumatic hernia, of increasing incidence in this era of violent injury, is preponderantly a left-sided lesion. Either blunt or penetrating trauma may be responsible. The herniated viscus — usually the colon or stomach, sometimes accompanied by the spleen or left kidney[251] — often parallels the superior contour of the diaphragm in both frontal and lateral projections. Obstruction is frequent, probably because of the angular margins of the

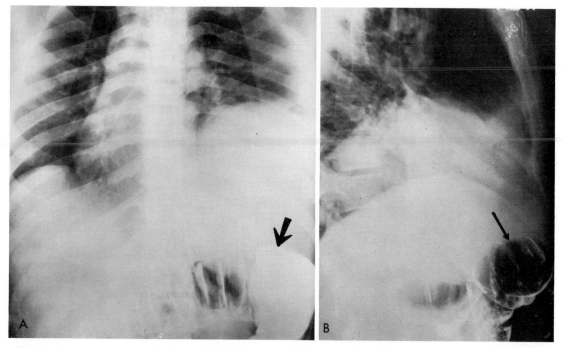

Figure 12–17. OBSTRUCTED TRAUMATIC DIAPHRAGMATIC HERNIA SIMULATING A HIGH DIAPHRAGM

The patient had received a severe blow to the left upper abdomen several months previously. The barium filled splenic flexure (arrow) appears depressed. Barium swallow was not performed. A diagnosis of late rupture of the spleen was made and surgery delayed. At operation, the stomach was found to be strangulated in the left thorax. The patient died. (From Carter, B. N., Giusseffi, J., and Felson, B.[166]; reproduced with permission of Charles C Thomas, Publ.)

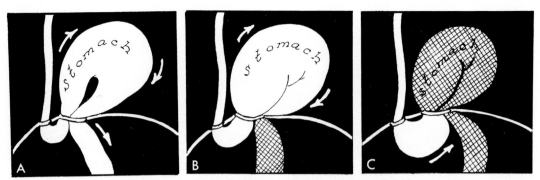

Figure 12–18. DIAGRAM OF BARIUM MEAL FINDINGS IN HERNIATION OF THE STOMACH THROUGH A DIAPHRAGMATIC TEAR (BARIUM IS INDICATED IN WHITE)

A, No obstruction. *B*, Obstruction of efferent segment. *C*, Obstruction of afferent segment. (From Carter, B. N., Giusseffi, J., and Felson, B.[166]; reproduced with permission of Charles C Thomas, Publ.)

phrenic defect, but it is often delayed for several years after the injury.[84] If incarcerated or strangulated, the herniated gut may fill with fluid and the resulting roentgen appearance closely resembles that of subphrenic abscess or ruptured spleen (Fig. 12–17).

The nature of the diaphragmatic excursion is not helpful in differentiating traumatic hernia from the various causes of elevated diaphragm, and the plain film findings often appear identical. However, the administration of radiopaque medium by mouth or rectum provides information that is essentially infallible in this differential diagnosis. In left-sided traumatic hernia, either the colon or, less commonly, the stomach extends through the rent in the dia-

phragm. Whichever of these organs is herniated, its entry and exit through the torn diaphragm obviously must occur through the single defect. Furthermore, the edges of the phrenic laceration are closely applied to the herniated viscus. Consequently, the points of entry and exit of the gut lie in close apposition and their margins are constricted like a funnel by the edges of the diaphragm. This side by side, beaklike narrowing reminds me of two pairs of lovebirds on a perch (Fig. 12–20A).

Should the herniated gut become obstructed, either as it enters or as it leaves the thorax, the number of beaks will be reduced accordingly, and dilatation proximal to the constriction will occur (Figs. 12–18 to 12–20). The obstruction is often of the closed

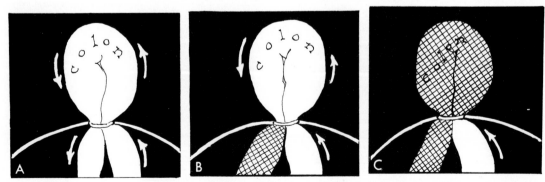

Figure 12–19. DIAGRAM OF BARIUM ENEMA FINDINGS IN HERNIATION OF THE COLON THROUGH A DIAPHRAGMATIC TEAR (BARIUM IS INDICATED IN WHITE)

A, No obstruction. *B*, Obstruction of proximal segment. *C*, Obstruction of distal segment. (From Carter, B. N., Giusseffi, J., and Felson, B.[166]; reproduced with permission of Charles C Thomas, Publ.)

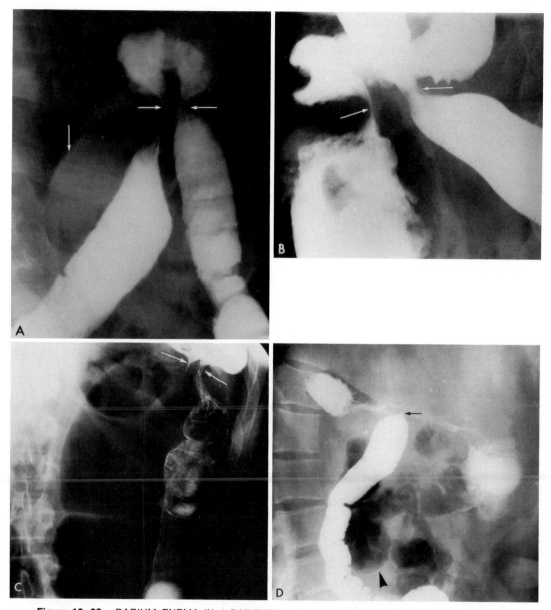

Figure 12–20. BARIUM ENEMA IN 4 PATIENTS WITH TRAUMATIC DIAPHRAGMATIC HERNIA

The horizontal arrows indicate the approximate position of the rent in the diaphragm in each patient. *A,* Counter-incision breakdown after hiatal hernia repair. Nonobstructive hernia. The medial portion of the diaphragm is visible (vertical arrow). The lovebird sign is well shown. *B,* A rare example involving the right hemidiaphragm. Nonobstructive. (Courtesy of Dr. Richard H. Greenspan.) *C,* Obstruction of the proximal segment. There is marked distention of the ascending and transverse colon. Three beaks are seen. *D,* Obstruction of the distal segment. Lateral view. Note the single beak (arrow). The stomach, outlined with barium, is not herniated. The proximal colon shows moderate gaseous distention (arrowhead).

loop or strangulation variety, so distention may be striking. The combination of splenic flexure obstruction and a high "left hemidiaphragm" is almost diagnostic of traumatic hernia (Fig. 12–21).

Curiously, these signs of traumatic hernia, which were first set down in 1951[166] and have never failed me in dozens of instances, have been ignored in nearly every article on the subject since. Pneumoperitoneum, pneumothorax, and even angiography have been attempted to establish the diagnosis, but are neither as simple nor as safe and reliable as barium studies.

In eventration or phrenic paralysis, the colon or stomach drapes itself beneath the elevated diaphragm and the proximal and distal limbs neither lie alongside each other nor show narrowing (Fig. 12–22).

Bochdalek and Morgagni Hernias

Roentgen findings similar to those of traumatic diaphragmatic hernia occur in any form of herniation of the colon or stomach through the diaphragm or elsewhere (Fig. 12–23). However, hernia through a foramen of Bochdalek[534, 1295] or through the central tendon into the pericardial sac (Fig. 11–13) has a large orifice and usually contains small intestine, so that the lovebird sign is seldom well shown. The beaks are more difficult to detect in hernia of the small bowel because of the multiple overlapping loops, small caliber of the intestine, and peristaltic contractions.

The diagnosis of hernia through the foramen of Morgagni is usually obvious if gut lies within the hernial sac.[655, 924] If, however, only the omentum or transverse mesocolon is herniated, the absence of gas in the sac makes the problem more difficult. A barium enema, especially when filmed in the upright position, will usually show elevation of the anchored transverse colon in contrast to the gravitational descent of the remainder of the colon[1025] (Fig. 12–24). A cane shaped contour of the properitoneal fat line at the anterior inferior margin of the thorax in the lateral view has recently been described as a sign of small Morgagni hernia.[696]

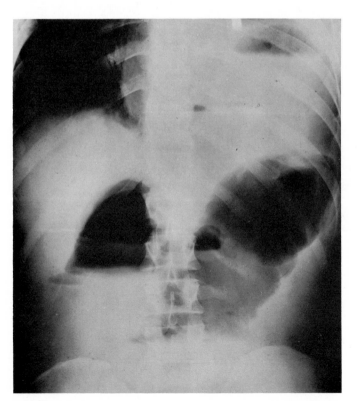

Figure 12–21. STRANGULATION OBSTRUCTION OF THE COLON IN TRAUMATIC DIAPHRAGMATIC HERNIA

The colon is obstructed at the splenic flexure, and what appears to be the left hemidiaphragm is elevated. However, the fluid level lies in the thorax within a distended herniated segment of colon proximal to an efferent obstruction.

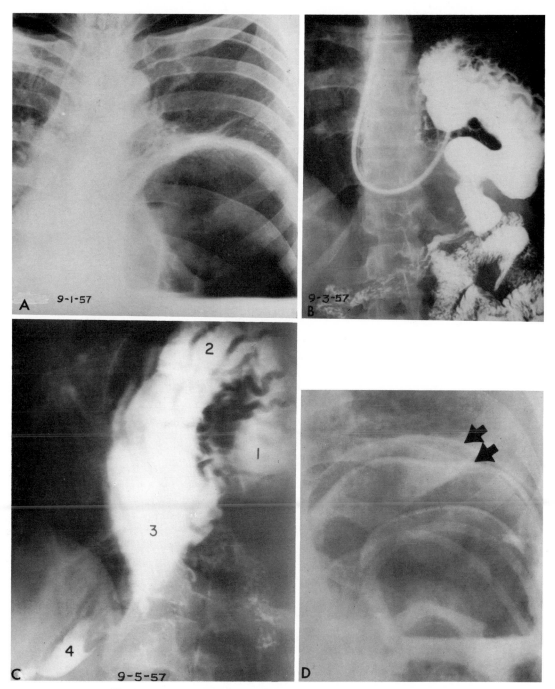

Figure 12–22. EVENTRATION WITH ACUTE GASTRIC VOLVULUS

A, The upright chest film shows a tremendously distended stomach. *B*, Upper GI series after tube decompression; the lovebird sign is absent. *C*, Barium study after recurrence of acute volvulus. *(1)* Fundus. *(2)* Body. *(3)* Antrum. *(4)* Bulb. *D*, Diagnostic pneumoperitoneum verifies the positions of the diaphragm (upper arrow) and stomach (lower arrow). Operative confirmation.

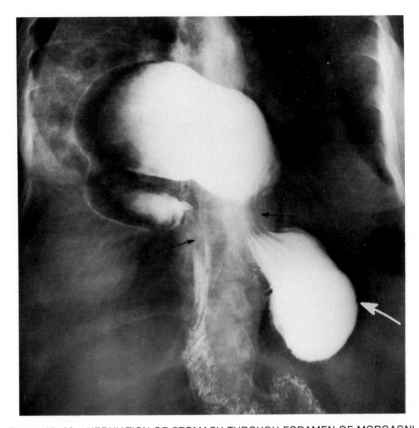

Figure 12–23. HERNIATION OF STOMACH THROUGH FORAMEN OF MORGAGNI

The fundus of the stomach (lower arrow) lies below the diaphragm. Note the lovebird sign (upper arrows).

Obstructed Hiatal Hernia

Acute obstruction of a hiatal hernia presents a fascinating roentgen picture. It is not an uncommon event—I have seen about a dozen patients with 20 episodes.[84, 698] The pattern is remarkably consistent. The obstruction nearly always results from volvulus of a large sliding hernia. Before the acute episode, the esophagogastric junction, fundus, and a variable segment of the body of the stomach are in the thorax. After the twist, the distal and proximal segments of the stomach change places, the esophagogastric junction and fundus now lying below the diaphragm and the antrum above (Fig. 12–25). The segment of the stomach proximal to the twist—the fundus beneath the diaphragm—becomes tensely distended. The distal stomach within the mediastinum may also distend if the obstruction is at its efferent segment. Thus, the

Figure 12–25. OBSTRUCTED HIATAL HERNIA

(1) Proximal stomach. *(2)* Distal stomach. *A,* On admission, the esophagogastric junction lies below the diaphragm. *B,* Intubation. There is less gastric distention. Note beak shaped constriction and twisted mucosa at the hiatus. *C,* Reduction of volvulus. The esophagogastric junction is now in the thorax. (From Blatt, E. S., Schneider, H. J., Wiot, J. F., and Felson, B.[84]; reproduced with permission of Radiology.)

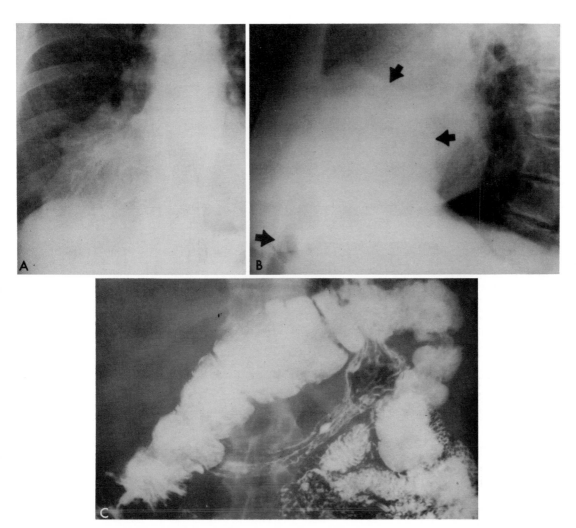

Figure 12–24. OMENTAL HERNIA THROUGH THE RIGHT FORAMEN OF MORGAGNI

A, Upright teleroentgenogram. The large lobulated mass blends with the right heart border and diaphragm. No gas shadows are seen within it. *B*, Right lateral teleroentgenogram. The mass (upper arrows) lies anteriorly. The colon (lower arrow) rises rather high anteriorly but does not enter the thorax. *C*, Prone film with barium in the stomach, small bowel, and colon. The midtransverse colon is elevated. An upright film would have been preferable. (From Carter, B. N., Giusseffi, J., and Felson, B.[166]; reproduced with permission of Charles C Thomas, Publ.)

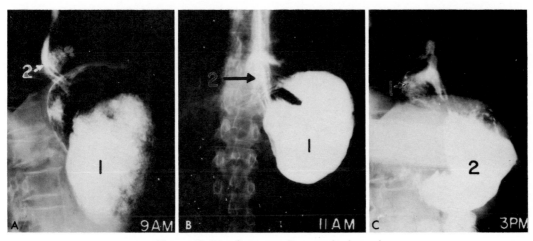

Figure 12–25. See opposite page for legend.

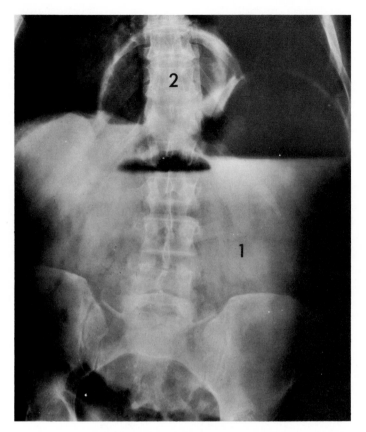

Figure 12–26. OBSTRUCTED HIATAL HERNIA

Upright film. Tremendous dilatation of the proximal stomach *(1)* which fills most of abdomen and shows two gas-fluid levels. The mediastinal locule *(2)* is the distended distal stomach. Removal of two liters of fluid by intubation resulted in reduction of the volvulus. (From Blatt, E. S., Schneider, H. J., Wiot, J. F., and Felson, B.[84]; reproduced with permission of Radiology.)

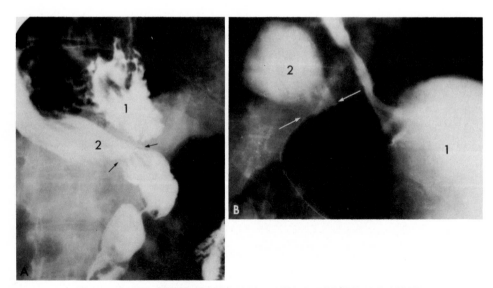

Figure 12–27. OBSTRUCTED HIATAL HERNIA, BEFORE AND AFTER

90 year old man with 3 prior documented bouts, each relieved by intubation. *(1)* Proximal stomach. *(2)* Distal stomach. The hiatus region is marked with arrows. *A,* Patient asymptomatic. *B,* The obstruction was at the distal end of the antrum. (From Blatt, E. S., Schneider, H. J., Wiot, J. F., and Felson, B.[84]; reproduced with permission of Radiology.)

plain films are usually diagnostic, showing two balloon-like, gas-fluid pockets, one in the mediastinum and the other beneath the left hemidiaphragm (Figs. 12–26 and 12–27).

Confirmation is readily obtained by barium swallow. Barium freely enters the overdistended subphrenic fundus; a beak and sometimes a twist are seen as the column extends toward the esophageal hiatus. A little barium may enter the thoracic locule.

Tube decompression of the gastric fundus usually results in quick recovery, with untwisting of the volvulus and return of the prevolvulus relationships. But recurrence is so frequent that surgical correction of the hernia is indicated as soon as feasible after gastric deflation.

Hepatic Hernia

Intrathoracic herniation of the liver may be congenital or acquired. The latter results from severe abdominal trauma. It is a com-

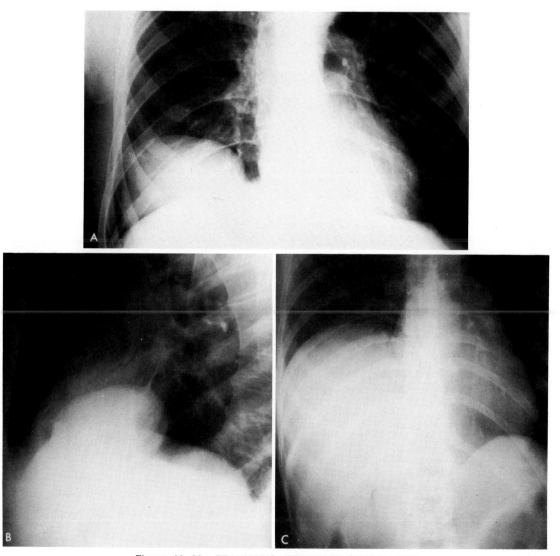

Figure 12–28. TRAUMATIC HERNIATION OF THE LIVER

A and *B,* Localized intrathoracic hepatic mass. (Courtesy of Dr. Warner A. Peck, Jr.) *C,* Another patient. Large phrenic tear with the entire liver displaced upward. Note elevation of liver edge in abdomen.

mon autopsy finding after fatal accidents, especially airplane crashes. A deceleration injury followed by a chest film showing local or generalized bulging in the region of the right hemidiaphragm is usually enough for the diagnosis (Fig. 12–28). A liver scan is helpful; induced pneumoperitoneum will likely demonstrate the phrenic tear but the resulting pneumothorax may aggravate the patient's condition.

Congenital hernia of the liver is more common on the right (Fig. 12–7) but may be bilateral (Fig. 12–6) or, occasionally, confined to the left thorax. Unlike the traumatic variety, it has a hernial sac.

The spleen is rarely involved in congenital diaphragmatic hernia. Renal herniation occasionally occurs posteriorly, more commonly on the left side.[66]

pleura to such an extent that the fibers pull apart. The widened interstices permit the diaphragm to become microscopically and even grossly permeable to air or fluid. Lieberman and his co-workers[737, 738] have convincingly established this hypothesis with the following evidence, based on an ingenious study of a group of cirrhotics:

1. [131]I injected into the ascites appeared in higher concentration in the pleural fluid than in the blood plasma or lymph.
2. Thoracentesis reduced the volume of the ascites.
3. Air (500–1000 cc) injected into the peritoneal sac of the sitting patient appeared in the pleural fluid within 1 to 48 hours.
4. A small opening or leaking blister in the diaphragm was identified at thoracoscopy or autopsy in several of these patients.

THE LEAKY DIAPHRAGM

A small pleural effusion is commonly observed in subphrenic inflammatory processes such as subphrenic abscess, pancreatitis,[484] and liver abscess. This has been termed *sympathetic pleurisy,* but the pleura is about as sympathetic as Lady Macbeth. The effusion is doubtless an extension of the inflammatory process through the interstices of the parietal peritoneum, diaphragm, and parietal pleura. Involvement of the mediastinum may also occur secondary to penetrating inflammation, particularly from pancreatitis.

This mechanism of pleural or mediastinal involvement from subphrenic inflammation is easy to understand. But what about cirrhosis and Meigs' syndrome (Fig. 12–29), in which the pleural effusion is constantly associated with ascites and is noninflammatory? Along with others, I have long suspected that the diaphragm was sometimes pervious to fluid.[612, 1167, 1324] In this connection, it is interesting that in the dim past, when therapeutic pneumoperitoneum for pulmonary tuberculosis was widely used, air occasionally appeared in the pleural cavity.[489]

The *leaky diaphragm* concept clearly explains these mysteries. Severe and prolonged distention of the peritoneal sac by fluid or air stretches the diaphragm and its closely attached parietal peritoneum and

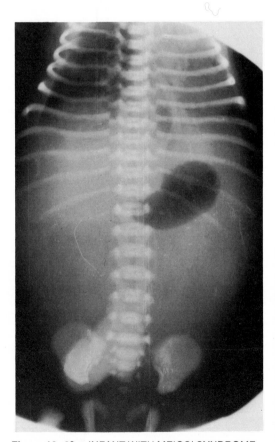

Figure 12–29.   INFANT WITH MEIGS' SYNDROME

Recumbent film showing bilateral pleural effusion and segmental collapse in LLL. Ovarian fibroma. (Courtesy of Drs. Richard B. Mulvey and Nicholas M. Katona.)

5. Separation of collagenous bundles in the tendinous portion of the diaphragm was demonstrated at autopsy in each of the patients.

PNEUMOPERITONEUM

Since pneumoperitoneum is so commonly detected on a chest film, I have included it in this chapter. The demonstration of free peritoneal gas on the chest film is not as simple as it sounds. With appropriate technique, the great majority of patients with pneumoperitoneum can be recognized even with amounts of gas as small as 1 cc. The best method is to keep the patient on his left side for 10 minutes and then take a decubitus film in this position, centering over the dome of the liver. This is followed immediately by an upright chest film, care being taken to keep the liver uppermost during the change in position, so that the air doesn't escape from the phrenic region.[137, 834]

It may sound pedantic, but don't mistake a subphrenic fat deposit,[1288] basal lung disease, or an overlapping costal edge for free gas. They can fool the expert. When in doubt, always change the position and centering a little, and take another film.

Postoperative Pneumoperitoneum

Free peritoneal gas is a common finding following laparotomy. How, then, does one detect perforation or anastomotic disruption in a recently operated patient? In other words, how long does gas remain in the peritoneal sac following an uncomplicated operation?

A study of 200 consecutive patients who underwent laparotomy at the Cincinnati General Hospital was made by Bryant, Wiot, and Kloecker in 1963.[137] Upright or decubitus films were made on the day of operation and every day or two thereafter, until all the gas had disappeared. Postoperative pneumoperitoneum was demonstrated in 58 per cent of the cases. The amount of gas appeared greater on the upright than on the decubitus film. The time required for absorption of the pneumoperitoneum varied from 1 to 24 days and appeared to depend only on the volume originally trapped, as seen on the first film.

Surprisingly, peritonitis seemed to be without influence so far as the presence and rate of absorption of the gas were concerned. The body habitus of the patient, however, appeared to play a major role. Over 80 per cent of the asthenic patients showed pneumoperitoneum, while only 25 per cent of the obese showed it. The thin patients also showed larger amounts of gas, and consequently it persisted longer. In the obese patients, the gas was nearly always gone by the third postoperative day.

In another study at this center, Wiot, Benton, and McAlister obtained early postoperative roentgenograms on about 100 infants and children from newborn to age sixteen.[1311] About 30 per cent showed free air on the first postoperative day. Each day thereafter, for the next three days, the number of cases decreased by about one half, so that at four days free gas was still present in four patients, and at six days gas was still seen in two, in one of whom it remained for 38 days. Essentially, all the findings in the first study were corroborated. It was concluded that children were similar to obese adults in that they tended to trap less air initially and therefore to retain it only briefly.

To sum up, in the event of postoperative abdominal symptoms, the roentgen demonstration of free gas should not enter into decisions of diagnosis or management, with the important exception that in obese patients and children more than three days postoperative, free peritoneal gas suggests perforation. Increase in postoperative pneumoperitoneum has significance only if the films were made with the patient in the same position for the same length of time and in the absence of abdominal drains.

Spontaneous Pneumoperitoneum Without Peritonitis

Spontaneous pneumoperitoneum is generally considered pathognomonic of ruptured hollow viscus. However, occasional instances of free peritoneal gas without perforation have been reported. Although asymptomatic or only mildly ill, many of these patients have been subjected to immediate laparotomy, with puzzling results: no perforation, no peritonitis, and no explanation for the presence of the peritoneal gas. Although only 30 cases were found in a review of the literature, we encountered 10 cases at the University of Cincinnati Medical Center in 10 years.

I believe that a variety of mechanisms accounts for these cases of pneumoperitoneum without peritonitis. In young females, the genital system appears to be the commonest site of entry of the air, a spontaneous Rubin's test, as it were, that probably occurred during douching. In other groups, intraperitoneal rupture of an intestinal gas cyst is probably a fairly common cause, and downward dissection from a pneumomediastinum an occasional one. The high incidence of peptic ulcer and other gastro-

intestinal diseases, especially those associated with distention of the stomach or intestine, cannot be ignored, although the actual route of entry of gas into the peritoneum is speculative. I'm pretty sure that distended gut is not always air-tight and may leak gas through a normal but thinned wall.

It is important that the surgeon and the roentgenologist realize that pneumoperitoneum does not invariably mean visceral perforation and therefore does not always require operation. Spontaneous pneumoperitoneum without peritonitis can be recognized by the trivial or absent clinical and laboratory signs. Obviously, patients on steroid therapy and those in whom the level of consciousness is impaired may have frank perforation of the gut with few symp-

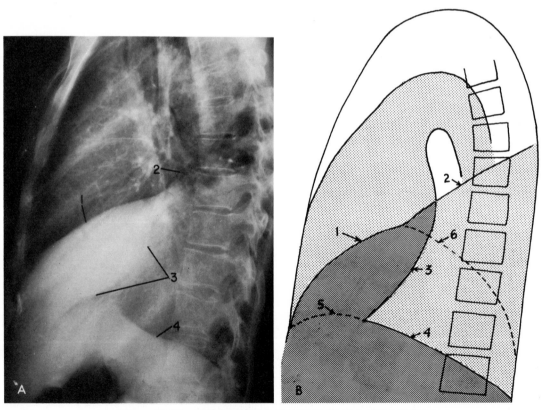

Figure 12–30. THE OVERLAP SHADOW IN RLL COLLAPSE

A, Interlobar effusion is simulated by overlapping of the left-sided heart shadow by the collapsed RLL and elevated right hemidiaphragm. The lower border of the liver is also elevated. *B,* Diagrammatic representation. *(1)* Anterior portion of elevated right leaf of diaphragm; *(2)* right major septum; *(3)* posterior surface of heart (in left thorax); *(4)* posterior segment of left hemidiaphragm; *(5)* approximate position of the anterior segment of the left hemidiaphragm, obliterated by the bottom of the heart; *(6)* approximate position of the posterior portion of the right hemidiaphragm, obliterated by the airless RLL.

toms and signs. Prudent judgment and meticulous observation are, of course, always required.[334]

THE OVERLAP SHADOW

On the lateral chest film, a composite shadow that can be mistaken for interlobar effusion is frequently seen. Usually the right hemidiaphragm is elevated and the RLL is consolidated or collapsed. One or both of these structures make up the anterior aspect of this spindle shaped, overlapping shadow. Its posterior margin is formed by the posterior border of the heart, which lies in the *left* thorax (Figs. 2–9, 2–28, and 12–30). Sometimes the shadow is seen in the normal subject, especially in right lateral recumbency, the high riding right hemidiaphragm overlapping the left-sided heart. Lesions in the left lower thorax don't produce this false shadow because they obliterate the back of the heart shadow. On occasion, thoracentesis of this spurious opacity, aptly named the *overlap shadow*, has been attempted. The resulting reddish aspirate which quickly clots is called blood, and it comes from the liver.

CHAPTER 13

THE THORACIC WALL

THE RIBS

Normal and Variations

One of the many fascinations of radiology is illustrated in Figure 13–1. SEX! Equal rights, similar attire and hairdo, transves- tism, and iatrogenic genital reversal make the usual visual hallmarks of the sexes less reliable. Actually, the film illustrated is that of a man with gynecomastia from estrogen therapy for carcinoma of the prostate. And you can suspect this from the pattern of cal- cification in the lower costal cartilages!

When the Lord created Eve, He shaped the calcium in her lower costal cartilages

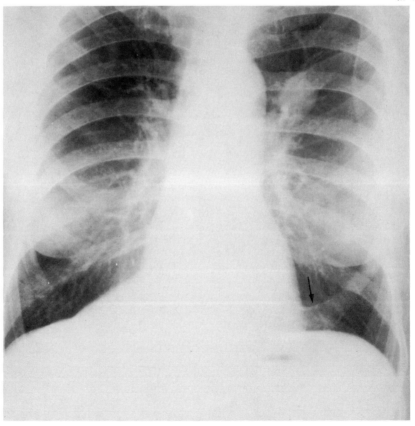

Figure 13–1. SEX AND THE COSTAL CARTILAGES

Man or woman? The calcification of the margins of the lower costal cartilages (arrow) is of the male type. This man was receiving estrogen therapy for carcinoma of the prostate with pulmonary metastases.

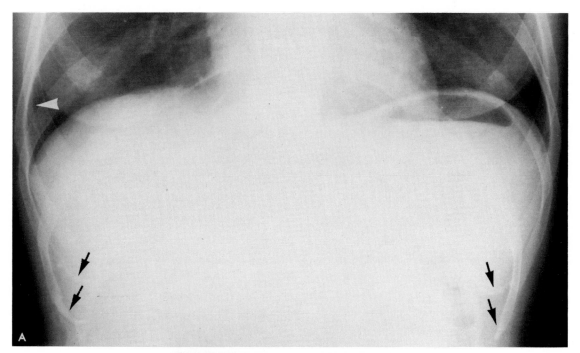

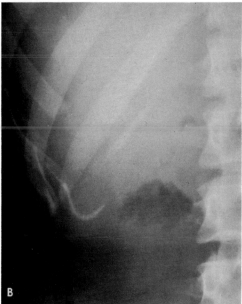

Figure 13–2. FEMALE TYPE OF CARTILAGE OSSIFICATION

A, Note that the center of the cartilages is opacified (arrows). A subpleural fat deposit is visible on the right (arrowhead). *B,* Another patient.

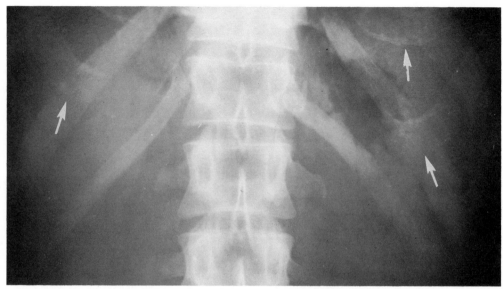

Figure 13–3. MALE TYPE OF CARTILAGE OSSIFICATION

Note that the calcification is confined to the edges of the cartilages (arrows).

(and in those of many women since) in the form of a penis, perhaps in memory of the donor (Fig. 13–2). He also formed the lower costal cartilage calcifications in man to resemble a vagina[362, 869, 1057] (Fig. 13–3). This was first called to my attention by one of our Fellows, Dr. Richard D. Gerle. My own experience with sexing of patients is based on a study of the lower costochondral patterns in over 700 individuals. The female *central* calcification is usually solid but occasionally takes the form of a row of small circles or solid nodules. The male *marginal* calcification is sometimes confined to one side of the cartilage.

From Table 13–1, it is apparent that the calcification pattern will indicate the sex more than 95 per cent of the time. I have no knowledge of the incidence of homosexuality among the exceptions nor of hermaphroditism in the few patients who have

both male and female types of calcification on different ribs (Fig. 13–4). But weird as it sounds, the five women with male calcification configuration in Sanders' series had each had a pelvic operation some years earlier—oophorectomy in three and unknown type in two.[1057]

These normal costal cartilages really contain bone rather than amorphous calcium.[654] Once adulthood is reached, there seems to be no clear-cut increase in the incidence of ossification with advancing age.[869] Identical twins have an identical pattern of calcification.[1242] Except for the first rib, the lower cartilages are involved more often than the upper.[312] The costal cartilage of the first rib is ossified much more often and more extensively than the others.[654] The pattern varies greatly from one patient to the next, with symmetry the rule (Chap. 15). Early extensive costal cartilage ossification has

TABLE 13–1. *Calcification of Lower Costal Cartilages**

	NUMBER OF PATIENTS*	NONE	CENTRAL	MARGINAL	BOTH
Females	323	122 (38%)	199 (61%)	1 (0.3%)	1 (0.3%)
Males	418	250 (60%)	9 (2%)	156 (37%)	3 (0.7%)

*An additional 250 films were discarded because the lower ribs were not well shown.

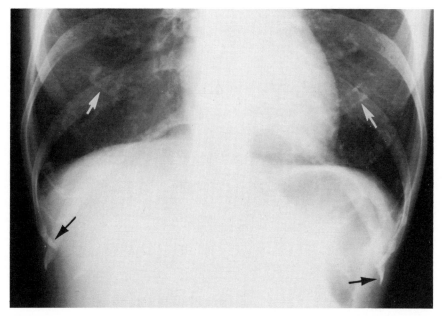

Figure 13–4. MALE AND FEMALE TYPE OF CARTILAGE CALCIFICATION IN A WOMAN

The lower arrows denote central calcifications, the upper ones marginal calcifications.

been related to the adrenogenital syndrome[362] and to psychoneurosis,[437, 564] but I'm skeptical.

The so-called *cervical rib* is seen about once in every 75 individuals; it is usually bilateral but often asymmetrical. It is sometimes really an underdeveloped first thoracic rib, as determined by the number of cervical vertebrae above it. Although it may occasionally cause symptoms by compressing the subclavian artery or brachial plexus, the vast majority are asymptomatic. Eleven pairs of ribs are found about three times as often in girls as in boys, and are about six times as common among mongoloids as among normal children.[47] Intrathoracic rib is discussed in Chapter 14.

A congenitally bifid, spurred, or widened rib is also a common variant,[1060] more so among Samoans than Cincinnatians.[798] It is one of the manifestations of the basal cell nevus syndrome.[461]

The *companion shadow* is a faint soft tissue density that parallels a segment of rib (Fig. 13–5) and sometimes the clavicles. If you look closely, you'll see it on at least one rib in about three of every four chest films.

One third have it on the first rib, often bilaterally. A similar incidence is found on the second rib (Chap. 15). It represents an internal bulge of intercostal tissues.[1104] If you look inside the chest of a cadaver, you can see that the soft parts over the inner rib surfaces are not in the same plane as the soft tissue strips between the ribs; the ribs jut into the thorax more than the intercostal soft tissues. This is also the case during life, though probably to a lesser degree. If the central ray strikes tangentially a part of the step-off between these two levels of soft tissue, the soft tissue-lung interface will become apparent as a companion shadow.[1013, 1336] A similar arrangement of the supraclavicular cutaneous tissues explains the clavicular companion shadow.[80]

A wavy, flaring rib border, a normal variant, may simulate a companion shadow.[80] Pleural thickening may present one or more arcs, but does not parallel individual ribs. It is generally wider inferiorly and is seldom bilateral. The common subpleural fat or muscle collections along the lower lateral thoracic wall (Fig. 13–2) are usually thicker than a companion shadow and con-

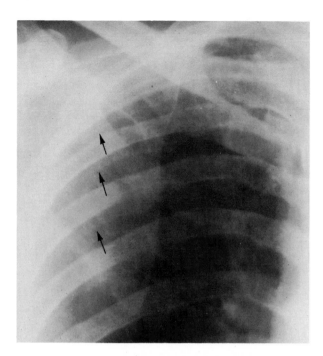

Figure 13–5. COMPANION SHADOWS ALONG THE POSTERIOR SEGMENT OF THE RIGHT 3RD TO 5TH RIBS (arrows)

vex toward the lung (Chap. 15). Similar shadows are very common along the upper thorax in oblique roentgenograms.

Rib Notching

Once thought to be pathognomonic of coarctation of the aorta, notching of the ribs is now known to occur in a variety of other conditions as well, for the most part related to components of the intercostal space, especially the intercostal artery, vein, and nerve. Enlargement of any of these structures from whatever cause may result in erosion of the inferior border of one or more ribs (Fig. 13–6). Table 13–2 lists 16 causes of rib notching and Figures 5–6 and 5–52 illustrate some of them.[97, 350]

Of course, far and away the most common is coarctation of the aorta. The collateral flow bypassing the aortic constriction to get to the abdomen and lower extremities comes almost entirely from the two subclavian arteries. It passes via the thyrocervical, costocervical, and internal mammary arteries and their subdivisions to the posterior intercostals and thence into the descending aorta. The large volume of blood traversing this route causes dilatation, tortuosity, and increased pulsation of the intercostal arte-

ries, which result in gradual erosion of the adjacent bone.

Unilateral notching in coarctation occasionally occurs on the left side when the constriction is located proximal to an anomalous right subclavian artery (Fig. 13–7A), and on the right side when the coarctation occurs proximal to the left subclavian (Fig. 13–7B). Only the subclavian artery that arises proximal to the aortic obstruction transmits the collateral blood to the intercostals. Rarely, unilateral notching occurs in conventional coarctation, without explanation.

Rib notching in coarctation is seen fairly often in children under 12 but is quite rare in infants. Duration is not the only factor influencing the presence of notching; the severity of the coarctation also plays a role. Notching is not seen in so-called *pseudocoarctation* of the aorta, which I consider to be a mild form of congenital coarctation with buckling of the aortic arch but little actual constriction or collateral circulation.

Notching of the first two ribs doesn't happen because the first two intercostal arteries, arising from the supreme intercostal, do not convey blood directly to the postcoarctation segment of the aorta. The last three intercostal arteries conduct blood away from the postcoarctation aortic seg-

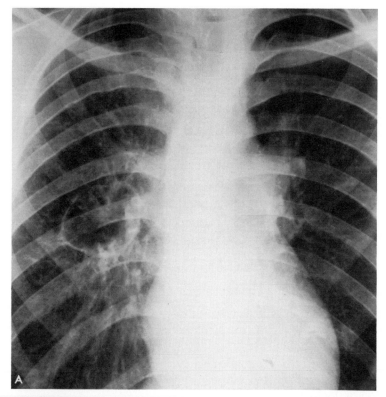

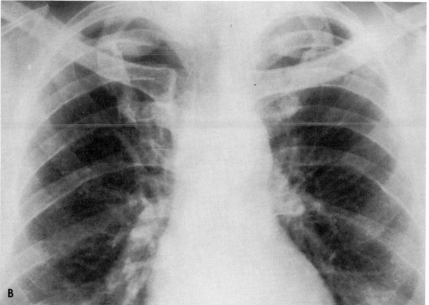

Figure 13–6. TWO UNUSUAL CAUSES OF RIB NOTCHING

A, Valvular pulmonary stenosis. The right 4th, 5th, and 6th ribs show scalloping. There is poststenotic dilatation of the left pulmonary artery and a cyst in the right midlung. *B,* Neurofibromatosis. The 7th right and 7th and 8th left ribs are scalloped. The bilateral apical masses represent neurinomas of the 3rd intercostal nerves. (From Boone, M. L., Swenson, B. E., and Felson, B.[97]; reproduced with permission of Charles C Thomas, Publ.)

TABLE 13–2. *Sixteen Causes of Rib Notching*

I. Arterial
   A. Aortic obstruction
      1. Coarctation of the aorta
      2. Thrombosis of the abdominal aorta
   B. Subclavian artery obstruction
      3. Blalock-Taussig operation
      4. "Pulseless disease": Takayasu's arteritis, arteriosclerosis obliterans
   C. Decreased pulmonary arterial blood flow
      5. Tetralogy of Fallot
      6. Pseudotruncus
      7. Pulmonary valve stenosis
      8. Unilateral absence of the pulmonary artery
      9. Pulmonary emphysema
II. Venous
      10. Superior vena cava obstruction
III. Vascular shunt
      11. Pulmonary arteriovenous fistula
      12. Intercostal arteriovenous fistula
      13. Intercostal to pulmonary artery fistula[239]
IV. Neurogenic
      14. Intercostal neurinoma
V. Osseous
      15. Hyperparathyroidism
      16. Idiopathic, normal variant

ment and are therefore not significantly enlarged, so notching doesn't occur at this level. In the other arterial causes for notching listed in Table 13–2, the flow in the dilated intercostals is from the aorta, the reverse of that in coarctation.

Occasional examples of unequivocal rib notching have been encountered in which thorough investigation has failed to reveal a cause. I have seen this with surprising frequency, minor in degree, in a survey of healthy chests (Chap. 15). For this I have been accused of having a notched retina. The location of the indentation on the ribs

may be helpful in differentiating the normal from the abnormal. Significant notching is seldom limited to the rib segment adjacent to the spine but is often confined to the midthird of the posterior rib. Shallow, wavy, elongated scalloping is just as meaningful as deeper, narrower, solitary notching.

Other Rib Lesions

It is not my intention here to discuss rib abnormalities as such, but only as they relate to intrathoracic disease.

A rib lesion *en face* may closely simulate a lung mass (Fig. 13–8), so before embarking on tomography you should fluoroscope every thoracic nodule that does not clearly lie in the lung on both frontal and lateral views. Once in a while a healed rib fracture will be indicated and embarrassment averted. Even if the lesion does lie in the lung, fluoroscopy will often save you time, films, and tomographic radiation by providing an estimate of the depth of the lesion and demonstrating its attachment.

Tietze's syndrome, painful nonsuppurative swelling of one or more costal cartilages and adjacent bone of unknown etiology, is a self-limited condition. It most often involves the second costal cartilage. Usually the roentgenogram appears normal, but sometimes enlargement of the rib end occurs, with faint mottled sclerosis that simulates pulmonary infiltration. The differentiation can be made by tomography or by tangential projection, the position predetermined by image amplified fluoroscopy.[161, 1135, 1256]

Cough fracture is an extremely common event, though often missed because dis-

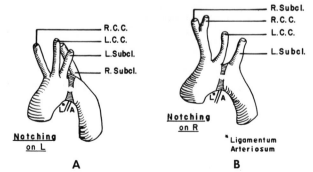

Figure 13–7. EXPLANATION OF UNILATERAL RIB NOTCHING IN AORTIC COARCTATION

The subclavian artery on the side of notching must arise from the precoarctation segment of the aorta. (From Boone, M. L., Swenson, B. E., and Felson, B.[97]; reproduced with permission of Charles C Thomas, Publ.)

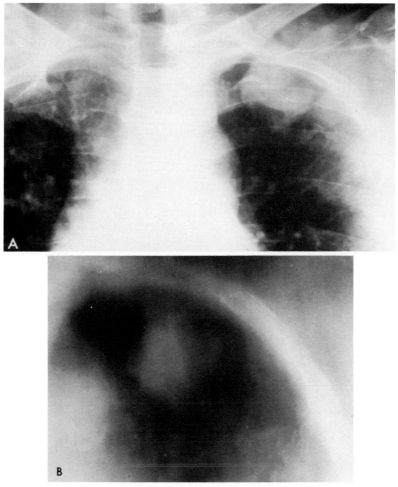

Figure 13–8. CHONDROMA OF FIRST RIB SIMULATING A LUNG NODULE

Fluoroscopy revealed that the lesion moved with the rib. *A,* Bucky film. *B,* Tomogram certainly suggests a pulmonary nodule, doesn't it?

placement is seldom a feature. Frequently bilateral, it usually involves the axillary segment of the sixth to ninth ribs.[402] The first rib may also fracture once in a while from the stress of severe dyspnea or cough.[86, 278]

Rib and soft tissue involvement in continuity with a lung and/or pleural lesion is highly suggestive of *actinomycosis,* particularly if there is a wavy periostitis[391] (Figs. 10–13 and 13–9). However, this does not apply to the superior sulcus of the lung, where rib destruction associated with pulmonary disease nearly always turns out to be carcinoma (Fig. 1–17).

Posterior rib expansion of striking proportion associated with posterior mediastinal masses of extramedullary hematopoiesis is seen in *thalassemia*[669] (Fig. 13–10). Rib lesions may relate to intrathoracic involvement in other ways, including the pneumonia and emphysema of asphyxiating thoracic dystrophy of the newborn,[942] the aspiration pneumonia of costovertebral rheumatoid arthritis, and, of course, the combination of rib and lung nodules in metastatic neoplasm. A large rib mass, e.g., in myeloma,[1320] may intrude intrathoracically, producing an extrapleural sign.

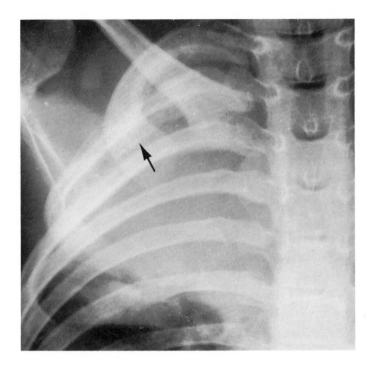

Figure 13–9. ACTINOMYCOSIS WITH RIB INVOLVEMENT

The wavy periostitis on the right second rib (arrow) is almost diagnostic. (Courtesy of Dr. William A. Altemeier.)

Figure 13–10. THALASSEMIA WITH EXPANDED RIBS

The transverse processes of the vertebrae are also involved. Intrathoracic juxtaspinal soft tissue masses of hematopoietic tissue are also present (arrows).

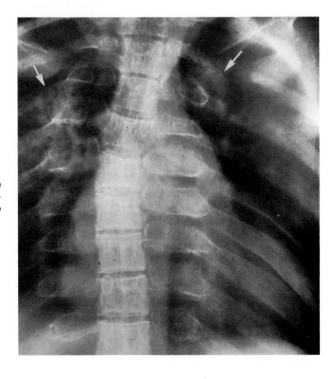

THE STERNUM

Funnel breast of more than minimal degree can usually be recognized on the PA teleroentgenogram.[286, 413, 1221] The heart usually shifts to the left, its left border is straightened, and the pulmonary arc is prominent because of slight cardiac rotation toward the right oblique. Increased transverse diameter and a subtle central radiolucency of the heart may be present, attributable to the thinner anteroposterior diameter secondary to intrusion by the depressed sternum. This also explains the unusual clarity of the spine and of the right cardiophrenic angle vasculature. The ribs are often asymmetrical and take an abnormal course. The lower right heart border is commonly obliterated by the soft tissues of the chest wall (Fig. 2–32). The end-on shadow of the depressed sternum may exaggerate the right cardiophrenic radiopacity. In severe funnel breast, the upper segment of the sternum is said to move outward with inspiration while the lower third moves inward.[548]

Pigeon breast (pectus carinatum) also deforms the chest but is more difficult to detect in frontal view than is funnel breast.[1060] Premature obliteration of the sternal sutures, seen in the lateral film of newborn infants, is associated with a high incidence of congenital heart disease.[225] Eventually pigeon breast deformity may occur. Atrial septal defect is commonly associated with thoracic deformity, especially pigeon breast.[1153]

The presence of double ossification centers in the manubrium, an unusual finding in normal children, is encountered in about 90 per cent of mongoloids.[675] Cretinism and other endocrine conditions may cause delayed fusion of the sternal segments.

A sternal mass caused by plasmacytoma, chondrosarcoma, lymphoma, fracture, or other lesions is easily confused with an anterior mediastinal tumor. The distinction can usually be made in the lateral view by recognizing the extrapleural signs along the posterior border of the mass, outlined by the lung intervening between the mass and the mediastinal soft tissues (Fig. 10–7).

THE SPINE

The *straight back syndrome* refers to thoracic compression symptoms secondary to straightening of the normal dorsal kyphosis. This results in narrowing of the space between the vertebral column and the sternum. The heart is often displaced to the left, as in funnel breast (Fig. 13–11). A systolic

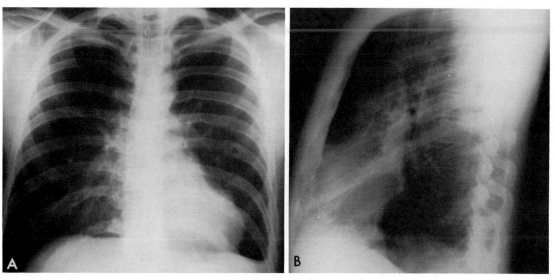

Figure 13–11. STRAIGHT BACK SYNDROME

A, In the PA view funnel breast is closely simulated. *B*, The lateral view shows loss of the normal dorsal kyphosis.

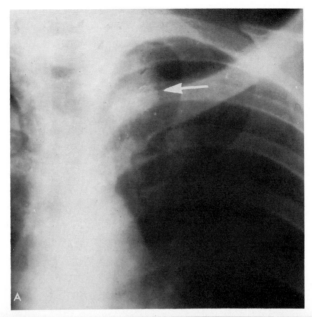

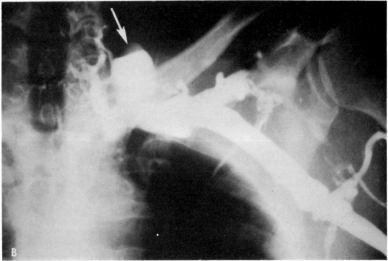

Figure 13–12. JUGULAR LYMPH SAC

This rare anomalous vessel lies at the junction of the thoracic duct and left jugular vein.[471, 1177] *A*, Plain film. A soft tissue mass (arrow) bulges from the left supraclavicular region. *B*, Brachial venogram. Retrograde filling of the sac is shown (arrow).

murmur is common.[966, 1237] As with funnel breast, symptom production has been questioned.

The relationship of spinal anomalies to mediastinal lesions has already been discussed (Chap. 11).

THE SOFT TISSUES

A soft tissue lesion superimposed over the lung can often be suspected by its unusually sharp outline produced by the room air.[95, 270] It is seen only when elevated above the skin surface and at least one edge profiled by the X-ray beam (Figs. 2–38 and 13–12). If the margins are diffuse or the lesion lies on the skin surface nearest the tube, it is less apt to be shown. Artifacts are frequently troublesome but can often be recognized by their too white appearance for the quality of grayness elsewhere on the film.

Outward bulging of the intercostal spaces in a child or adult has long been assumed to indicate pulmonary emphysema. Kattan, Spitz, and Moskowitz of our department have shown that this finding has no real significance since it is also seen in skinny and cachectic individuals[627] (Fig. 13–13).

True pulmonary herniation between the ribs or into the neck may occasionally occur. Intercostal hernia is usually the result of trauma or surgical incision. In cervical hernia, a tear in Sibson's fascia from coughing or emphysema is generally responsible. The pulmonary hernia is elicited by in-

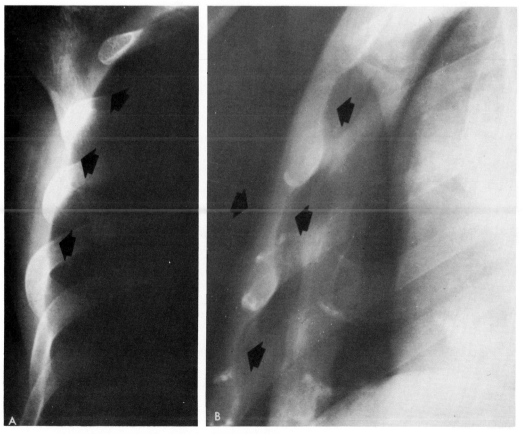

Figure 13–13. BULGING OF THE INTERCOSTAL SPACES (arrows)

A, AP film of an emaciated alcoholic woman, age 60, with no clinical signs of emphysema. *B*, Off-lateral view of a 60 year old emaciated man. No emphysema was apparent clinically or fluoroscopically. (Courtesy of Kattan, K., Spitz, H. B., and Moskowitz, M.[627]; reproduced with permission of Radiology.)

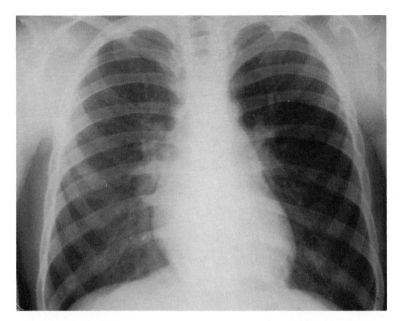

Figure 13–14. ABSENT PEC-
TORAL MUSCLE

Though the left thorax is radiolucent, the vasculature in the left
lung is normal. Note the difference in the lateral soft tissues
on the two sides.

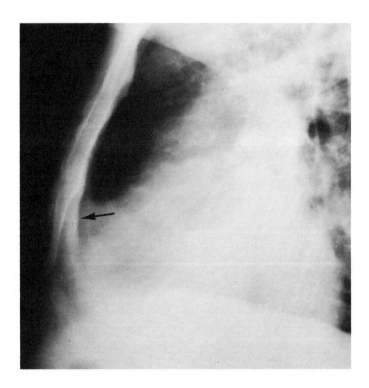

Figure 13–15. ANTERIOR SOFT
TISSUE SHADOW (arrow)

Internal thoracis muscle? Anterior
surface of lingula? This is not quite a
true lateral projection.

creasing the intrathoracic pressure. It is best demonstrated by fluoroscopy.[75, 402, 531, 578, 916, 1116, 1201]

Congenital absence of the pectoral muscle results in greater radiolucency of the lung on that side (Fig. 13–14). It is distinguished on the frontal projection by the altered position of the axillary skin folds and by the normal number and distribution of the pulmonary vessels.[450, 1166, 1255] A similar appearance is seen after mastectomy and other surgical procedures on the chest wall.

The retrosternal soft tissues (premediastinal space) may not be part of the chest wall but I can't find a more suitable cubbyhole for it, so here it stays. The space in front of and between the anterior pleural reflections contains muscles, nerves, vessels, lymphatics, and connective tissue.

On a not quite lateral view of the chest, an irregular or triangular shadow based on the anterior costophrenic angle is often seen (Fig. 13–15). It has sometimes been misinterpreted as a pleural, mediastinal, or chest wall lesion. Shopfner[1113] and Scheff[1073] be-

lieve it represents the internal thoracis muscle, which originates from the back of the lower sternum and inserts on the adjacent costal cartilages. But Whalen et al. are sure it represents the mediastinal areolar tissue in front of the anterior pleural reflection of the left lung.[1287] They point out that in the lateral view the anterior surface of the lingula is not projected as far forward as that of the middle lobe, so that the soft tissues show through.

Since the retrosternal region is poorly visualized in frontal projection, it should be carefully scrutinized on all lateral films. Sternal tumor, dilated internal mammary arteries in coarctation, hematoma from fractured sternum, lymphoma,[379] and other tumors of the soft tissues—all may involve this area.[675, 938] In pericardial effusion, the epicardial and retrosternal fat can sometimes be distinguished in the lower anterior thorax on the lateral view, separated by a broad band of pericardial fluid.[691] Epicardial fat necrosis is a rare but interesting cause of a mediastinal mass[49, 184, 684] (Fig. 2–15).

CHAPTER 14

THORACIC CALCIFICATIONS

When interpreting chest roentgenograms, short shrift is usually given to the ubiquitous thoracic calcifications. In fact, so accustomed do we become to seeing them that we're seldom even aware of their presence. Yet they are, at times, as important to man as the oosik is to the walrus, and just as opaque (Fig. 14–1). There can be no alternative but to consciously examine every chest film closely for the presence of calcium and then attempt to appraise its significance.

In the early 1940s, I recorded the calcifications seen on routine chest teleroentgenograms of more than a thousand inductees in an Army reception center in Indiana. Calcification was seen in the hila, mediastinum, or lungs in 63 per cent. The films were taken without a grid and at low kilovoltage so I probably missed a number of calcifications, especially among the heavier men. For the skeptic, I would point out that any shadow that looked like it might possibly be an end-on vessel was scrupulously excluded.* Many of the calcifications were 5 mm or more in greatest diameter. There appeared to be no difference in prevalence or average size among men under and over 40.

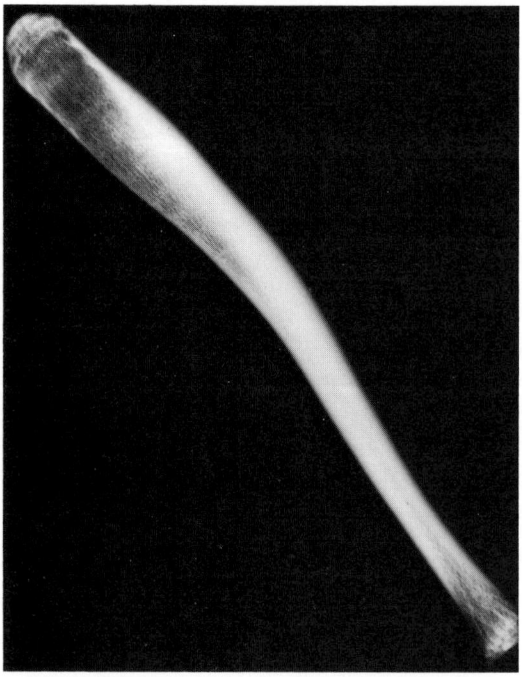

Most of these thoracic calcifications, lymph node and parenchymal, are the result of a "burned out" granulomatous infection by a fungus or by the tubercle bacillus. *Histoplasma capsulatum* is generally the culprit in the midwestern U.S.A., the "histoplasmosis belt," where most of the soldiers in the study came from.[185, 1187] *Coccidioides immitis* has been incriminated in the southwest.[544, 1063] Other fungi, as yet unidentified, may be a cause elsewhere in this country and in other parts of the world.

These static rocks of healed granuloma may become stumbling blocks along the respiratory pathways. Further, there are also many noninfectious lesions that calcify and these, too, require recognition. So let's now examine the lowly calcification critically to see if we can determine its true role in chest roentgenology.

Figure 14–1. OOSIK OF A WALRUS

*Dr. Robert Stadalnik of Sacramento has written me about his spectacle sign. If you look carefully, adjacent to a normal vessel on end you will see a bronchus on end. The two shadows appear thus: ● ○ . In my own perverse way, I have renamed it the *seminoma sign*.

LYMPH NODE CALCIFICATION

Calcified granulomatous infection in the hilar and mediastinal nodes practically never becomes reactivated. The calcium may enlarge as healing continues. Over the years it may even ossify. Conversely, a calcification occasionally seems to melt or even disappear (Fig. 14–2). Most unusually, a carcinoma or other destructive process is responsible for its dissolution; a far more frequent cause is broncholithiasis.

Broncholithiasis

This condition is the result of erosion of a calcified lymph node or parenchymal focus into a bronchus, where the fragments may lodge and cause obstruction or be expectorated.[43, 198, 405, 442, 1266] It is often associated with hemoptysis or pulmonary infection. A broncholith should be suspected if calcium is identified close to the proximal margin of an area of pulmonary collapse (Figs. 14–3 and 14–4). Occasionally, a thin rim of air surrounding the intrabronchial calcification gives it an unusual degree of sharpness. Laminagraphy, bronchography, or bronchoscopy will demonstrate that part or all of the calcific shadow lies within the bronchial lumen.

Expectoration of broncholiths is not unusual. The patient may bring them to his physician, but more often takes a surprisingly casual attitude toward this event. While performing a GI series on a young man, I noted many calcifications in his thorax and asked him if he ever spit up stones. "Sure I do," he answered, in a tone that implied, "Doesn't everyone?" There is even a report, which I won't vouch for, of a troubadour in medieval times who, as part of his act, spat up broncholiths ringingly into a spittoon to the accompaniment of his lyre (probably spelled incorrectly!).

Chronic Pulmonary Collapse

Closely related but not identical to broncholithiasis is the chronic collapse that occurs secondary to the pressure of a granulomatous lymph node on a segmental or lobar bronchus (Fig. 6–18). The lymph node often contains calcium and this can be demonstrated near the obstructed bronchus. Of course, the presence and location of the calcium may be purely fortuitous, so before one assumes a cause-and-effect relationship, a bronchogram or laminagram should clearly indicate that the bronchial obstruction is of the extrinsic type.

Vascular Compression

Granulomatous mediastinal nodes, often calcified, may directly compress the superior vena cava or obstruct it indirectly by inciting fibrosis in the mediastinum. The diagnosis rests in part on pinpointing the location of the calcium with Bucky films, laminagrams, or angiograms. Rib notching[97] or "downhill" varices[347] may ensue (Figs. 5–51 and 5–52). Pulmonary veins may be obstructed in a similar manner (Fig. 5–59).

Esophageal Involvement

A mass of inflammatory mediastinal nodes, usually histoplasmic, may indent or displace the esophagus, or even attach to its wall, sometimes causing dysphagia. This intimate relationship commonly results in a traction diverticulum of the esophagus (Fig. 6–7). I have observed this sequence in four patients, 6 to 12 months elapsing between indentation and diverticulum. In two, calcium could be seen at the apex of the diverticulum.

An unusual case of "milk of calcium" within an intramural mass in the lower end of the esophagus is illustrated in Figure 14–5.[545] Similar granules or fragments of calcium suspended in fluid are seen once in a while in mediastinal lymph nodes and in pulmonary and pleural lesions.

Eggshell Calcification

In the granulomatous conditions, the calcium is ordinarily distributed throughout the involved nodes or scattered indiscriminately within them. Occasionally, the calcium assumes an annular arrangement at the periphery of the node, the so-called *eggshell calcification*. These are most com-

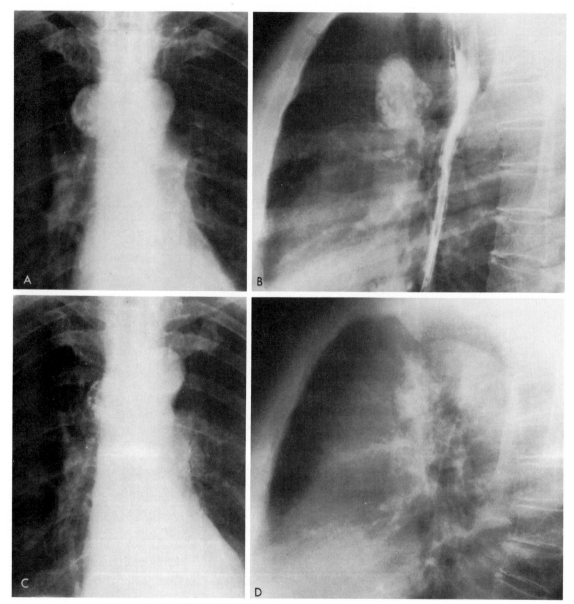

Figure 14–2. "MELTING" OF CALCIFICATION IN RIGHT TRACHEAL NODE
A and *B*, 1953. *C* and *D*, 1971. The patient recalled no expectoration of calcium.

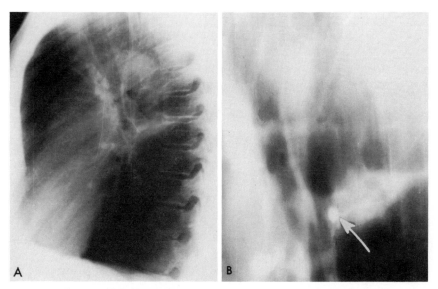

Figure 14–3. BRONCHOLITH WITH PULMONARY INFECTION

A, Right lateral view. Collapse of superior segment of RLL. *B,* Lateral tomogram. The calcified nodule (arrow) lay partly in the lumen of the bronchus to the superior segment.

monly seen in silicosis[55, 417, 473, 1190] (Fig. 14–6). They have also been found in the abdominal, axillary, and cervical lymph nodes of silicotics, but always accompanied by similar intrathoracic node calcifications.[351, 947] No explanation for the unusual peripheral deposits of the calcium in this disease has been forthcoming. In one instance in which we studied several such nodes pathologically, the calcium was in truth circumferentially located, but the silica was evenly distributed throughout the nodes (Fig. 14–7).

In a survey conducted by the Radiology Panel on Pneumoconiosis of the U. S. Public Health Service Occupational Health Division, eggshell calcification in lymph nodes was observed in 0.4 per cent of 16,000 miners. Of 724 miners with definite roentgen evidence of pneumoconiosis, 6.3 per cent showed eggshell calcification.[595] The percentage was the same in soft coal miners as in hard rock metal miners. The rate was much higher in "complicated" pneumoconiosis (progressive massive fibrosis) than in "simple" nodular silicosis. No relationship to a specific type of industrial exposure to silica has been demonstrated.

Identical calcification may occur in the absence of industrial dust exposure.[34, 287, 587] I have seen about six examples (Fig. 14–8). In one a meticulous search at autopsy failed to reveal evidence of silicosis; two others had sarcoidosis.[1160] One had blastomycosis. Nonetheless, when eggshell calcifications are accompanied by small pulmonary. nodules or conglomerate areas of fibrosis, or even only by a positive occupational history, the diagnosis of silicosis is virtually certain. The sign is not encountered after exposure to other types of dust, except for soft coal. This lends support to my own view that coalworkers' pneumoconiosis may merely be a form of silicosis and not a separate entity.[332]

VASCULAR CALCIFICATION

Long-standing organized thromboemboli often calcify in the vessels of the legs and even in the abdomen, so why not in the thorax? Actually this does occur and probably much more frequently than we realize. However, it is difficult to identify a calcified clot on the chest film because it usually resembles the far more common lymph node calcification. It can be recognized only when it assumes the cylindrical or branch-

(Text continued on page 474.)

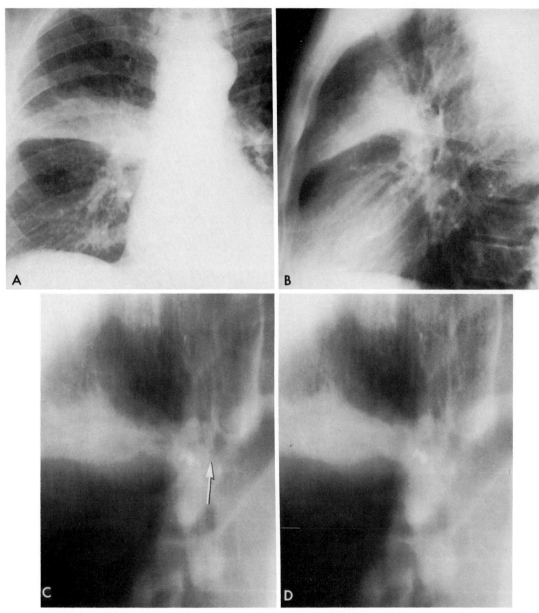

Figure 14–4. BRONCHOLITHIASIS WITH RECURRENT PNEUMONIA

A and *B,* Anterior segment collapse of RUL. One year before, the same segment was similarly involved but cleared completely in about 2 months. *C* and *D,* Tomographic cuts showing occluded anterior segment bronchus (arrow) and adjacent calcifications.

(*Figure continued on opposite page.*)

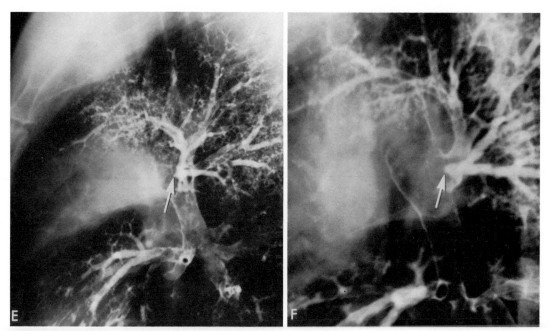

Figure 14–4. *Continued. E,* The occluded bronchus is also seen on lateral bronchography (arrow). *F,* The "wrong" obliquity shows it better (arrow). Broncholiths were found at operation. (Courtesy of Dr. Charles M. Barrett.)

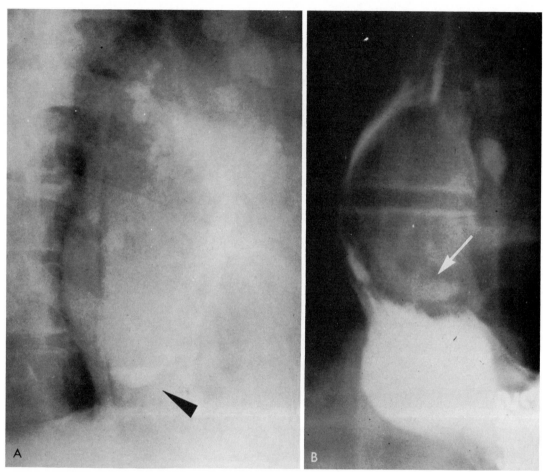

Figure 14–5.   LIQUEFIED CALCIFIC MASS IN WALL OF THE LOWER ESOPHAGUS

A 41 year old man with occasional epigastric distress for 2 years. *A,* Upright film reveals a calcium-water level (arrowhead). *B,* Barium esophagram shows an intramural mass containing calcium (arrow). The "milk of calcium" shifted about with gravity. A cystic intramural mass containing flakes of calcium was excised at operation. There were no periesophageal adhesions. Special stains revealed *H. capsulatum.* It is probable that the histoplasmosis involved the esophageal lymphatic tissue. (Courtesy of Hinshaw, R. J., and Guilfoil, P. H.[545]; reproduced with permission of Dis. Chest.)

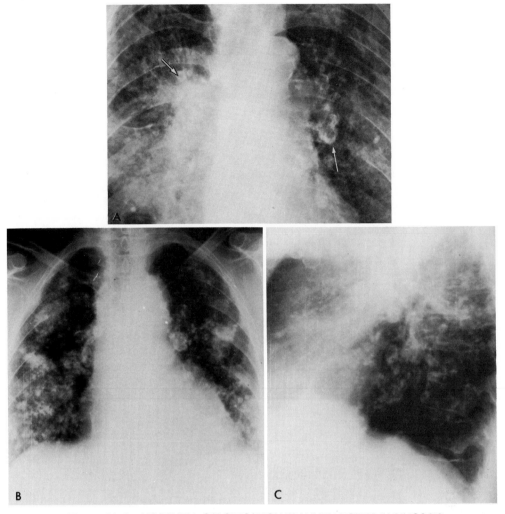

Figure 14–6. EGGSHELL CALCIFICATION IN LYMPH NODES IN SILICOSIS

A, The hilar nodes are affected (arrows). A large conglomerate mass is present at the right base. *B* and *C,* Another patient. Many of the small pulmonary lesions also contain calcium.

Figure 14–7. EGGSHELL CALCIFICATION IN LYMPH NODES

Autopsy specimen. The calcium was also confined to the periphery of the nodes on gross examination. Silica deposits, however, were evenly scattered throughout the nodes.

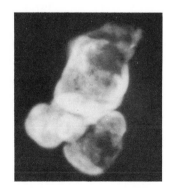

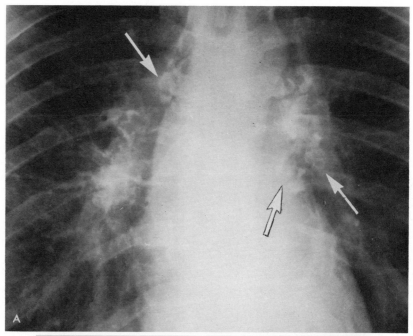

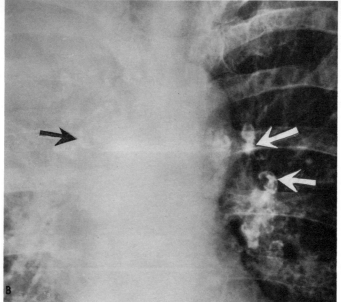

Figure 14–8. NONSILICOTIC EGGSHELL CALCIFICATION (arrows)

A, Sarcoidosis. Chest film 5 years earlier was normal. *B,* Another patient. Thorough autopsy study revealed no evidence of silicosis. The patient died of carcinoma of the right lung.

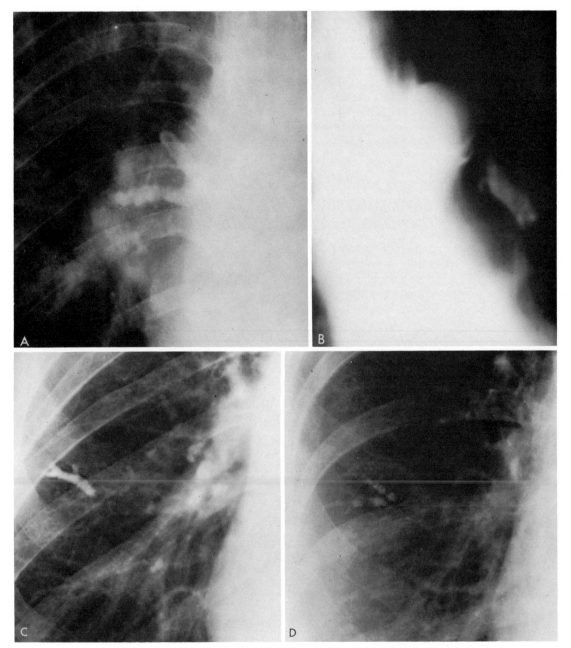

Figure 14–9. CALCIFIED PULMONARY ARTERY THROMBOEMBOLI

A, Proved at autopsy. *B*, Present for at least 10 years, but unproved. *C*, Past history suggested postoperative pulmonary embolism. (Courtesy of Dr. Warner A. Peck, Jr.) *D*, Unproved case. (From Felson, B.[339]; permission of Chest.)

ing configuration of a vessel or is obviously located at a vascular site. The calcified clot may occur in a central or peripheral branch of a pulmonary artery[806] (Fig. 14–9) or vein, in the superior or inferior vena cava[1118] (Fig. 14–10), or even in the aorta[81, 351, 1197] (Fig. 14–11).

Calcification in the *walls* of central pulmonary arteries usually signifies severe pulmonary hypertension superimposed either on lung disease or on a left to right congenital cardiac shunt (Fig. 14–12). Aneurysm of the pulmonary artery or of the aorta or its branches may, of course, also show calcification in its margins.

WIDESPREAD PARENCHYMAL CALCIFICATIONS

Infection

The disseminated miliary lesions of active histoplasmosis usually disappear one to six months after onset.[346] However, many tiny calcific nodules often appear several years later.[1092] In two of our 12 cases of epidemic miliary histoplasmosis, calcium ultimately appeared, but only after about 15 years.[346] The disease is common in dogs, in which the calcium deposits are often more flocculent (Fig. 14–13).

Miliary calcification also occurs in coccidioidomycosis, but is extremely rare in miliary tuberculosis.[442, 1052] Figure 14–14 illustrates the difficulties of documenting such a case.

Indigenous cases of disseminated miliary calcifications are encountered in many lands. Histoplasmosis has been recorded in a number of countries and undoubtedly accounts for many of these cases. Identical calcifications have been reported in a number of patients in Australia, New Zealand, England, and the U.S. many years after an episode of widespread chickenpox pneumonia incurred during adulthood.[233, 666, 776, 1052] Recently I obtained chest films on three of my friends who had had documented episodes of this serious adult disease about 15 years ago. One now showed many small nodular calcifications. Schistosoma,[830] *Armillifer armillatus*,[1168] and Paragonimus[1188] may also give rise to multiple small pulmonary calcifications.

Silicosis

Parenchymal calcifications are frequently seen in the small pulmonary nodules of silicotics (Figs. 14–6 and 14–15). In fact, the ILO/UICC/Cincinnati Radiological Classification of the Pneumoconioses has a specific designation *(cn)* for this finding.[332, 1238] It was encountered in slightly over 1 per cent of the 16,000 miners mentioned earlier (about 20 per cent of those showing roentgen signs of pneumoconiosis), occurring with about the same frequency among the soft coalworkers as among the hard rock metal miners. It is by no means always associated with eggshell calcification in the nodes.

This type of calcification has been de-

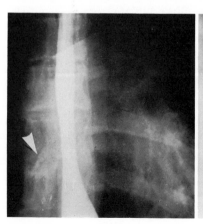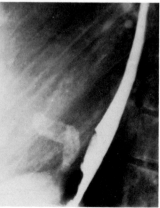

Figure 14–10. CALCIFIED THROMBUS IN THE INFERIOR VENA CAVA

The anterior segment of the boomerang shaped calcification (arrowhead) protruded into the right atrium. *A*, AP view. *B*, Lateral view. Surgically confirmed.

A   B

edge, it is not encountered from exposure to other types of dust. The metallic densities of baritosis and stannosis are much more opaque (Figs. 14–16 and 14–17). Post-lymphangiography and postbronchography deposition of contrast medium also presents as a fine metallic density in the lungs.

Pulmonary Ossification

A rare condition, *idiopathic pulmonary ossification,* (synonyms: pulmonary osteopathia, ossifying pneumonitis, and bony metaplasia of the lung) is associated with fine, branching linear shadows, usually involving a limited area of the lung. The dendritic shadows represent trabeculated bone in the interstitial pulmonary tissue. The calcium density may be difficult to appreciate on the chest film, since the shadows are very thin, and hence the lesion is generally discovered incidentally at autopsy. The condition, most often seen in elderly men, is slowly progressive but seldom gives rise to symptoms.[535, 572, 929, 981, 1076, 1149] The four patients I have seen were all elderly men and showed a strikingly similar roentgen pattern (Fig. 14–18).

Bony nodules in the lungs are sometimes associated with rheumatic mitral stenosis.[422, 482, 1076] These osseous nodules are fairly large and more prominent in the lung bases. Their ossific nature is generally not apparent radiographically, although the calcium content is obvious. The pathogenesis is not established; pulmonary hemorrhage and hemosiderosis have been implicated.

A note of caution, however, is in order: the widespread nodular pulmonary calcification of histoplasmosis, with or without ossification, is so common that coincidence may account for coexistence with mitral stenosis. For years we carried a case in our teaching file as rheumatic mitral valve disease with pulmonary ossification. Pathologically the nodules consisted of trabeculated bone which contained marrow. One day our mycologist reviewed the case and demonstrated *Histoplasma capsulatum* in the bony nodules in the preserved autopsy specimen.*

(*Text continued on page 479.*)

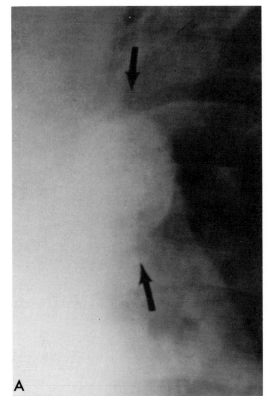

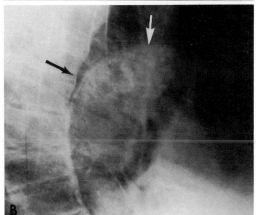

Figure 14–11. CALCIFIED THROMBUS OBSTRUCTING THE LUMEN OF THE AORTIC ARCH (arrows)

AP and lateral views. The patient had absent pulses in the lower extremities and left arm. Autopsy proved. (Courtesy of Taguchi, J. T.[1197]; reproduced with permission of Amer. J. Cardiol.)

scribed in South African gold miners, in sandstone masons, and in Sheffield cutlery grinders, and has been called "Liverpool silicosis."[643] It is also seen among the coal-workers of Great Britain.[772] To my knowl-

---

H. capsulatum is one of the few organisms that retains its morphology long after it dies.[1187]

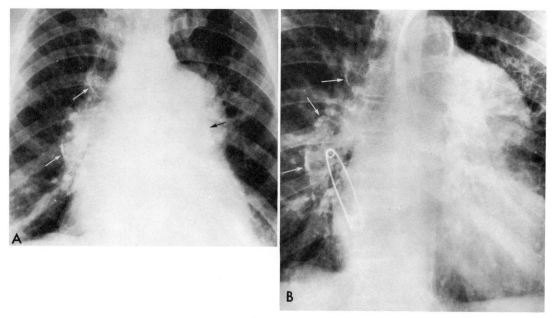

Figure 14–12. PULMONARY HYPERTENSION WITH CALCIFIED WALLS OF CENTRAL PULMONARY
ARTERIES (arrows)

Which patient has the atrial septal defect and which the diffuse pulmonary emphysema? The answer is in the
legend of Figure 14–13.

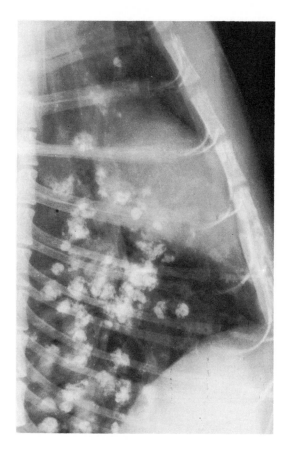

Figure 14–13. HEALED HISTOPLASMOSIS IN A
DOG

Answer to Figure 14–12: *A*, Emphysema. *B*, Atrial
septal defect. (Courtesy of William J. Roenigk, D.V.M.)

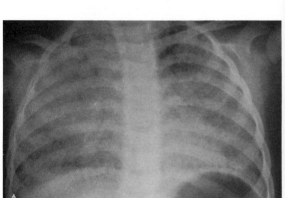
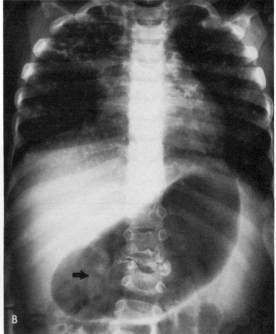

Figure 14–14. SPONTANEOUS HEALING OF MILIARY TUBERCULOSIS WITH DISSEMINATED
CALCIFICATIONS?

In October, 1944, this child had an acute febrile illness with intense miliary nodulation in the lungs *(A)* and enlarged liver and spleen. He was transferred to a tuberculosis sanatorium, although bacteriologic proof was lacking.
His lungs cleared with bed rest. *B*, 3 years later he had Pott's disease of the lumbar spine with calcified paravertebral abscess (arrow) from which tubercle bacilli were isolated. Meanwhile, disseminated punctate calcifications appeared in the lungs. Histoplasmin and tuberculin skin tests were positive 7 years later. Was this
histoplasmosis with superimposed spinal tuberculosis contracted in the sanatorium, or was it spontaneous
healing of miliary tuberculosis with subsequent calcification?

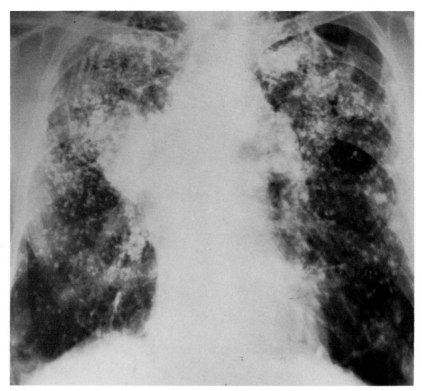

Figure 14–15. PARENCHYMAL CALCIFICATIONS IN SILICOSIS

Even the conglomerate masses are studded with calcium. Eggshell calcification is present in the left hilar nodes.

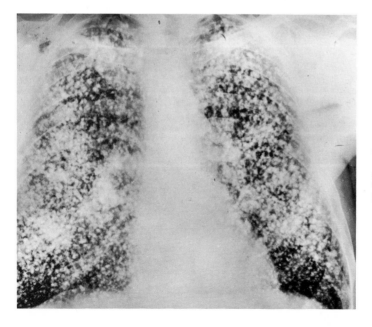

Figure 14–16. BARITOSIS

Pneumoconiosis from packaging barium. The chest was greatly improved 15 years later, after dust control was instituted. The patient was always asymptomatic. (Courtesy of Dr. James Hughes.)

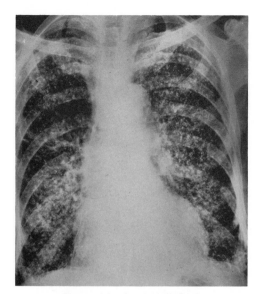

Figure 14–17. STANNOSIS

(Courtesy of Dr. James Hughes.)

Alveolar Microlithiasis

Among the rarer causes of widespread parenchymal calcification is alveolar microlithiasis, a condition in which myriad alveoli and alveolar sacs contain tiny spherules of calcium phosphate.[29, 640, 1108] The disease is often familial.[154, 1147] Its cause remains unknown, but for those who need a conversation piece, the condition has been encountered among snuff-dippers in Thailand.[183]

Roentgenographically, there is diffuse alveolar infiltrate, often of dramatic extent and opacity (Fig. 14–19). Amazingly, these patients are seldom clinically ill. The infiltrate is of calcium density, although not always easily recognizable as such. Tiny dense stippling can usually be seen on close scrutiny.

I have noted a roentgen sign that I believe is diagnostic of extensive alveolar calcification, as seen in microlithiasis.[333] The pleura appears as a *negative* shadow, i.e., a black line instead of a white one, because it lies between the bony rib cage and the calcified pulmonary infiltrate. The water density of the pleura appears black by comparison with the adjacent calcium. I have personally observed the sign in five patients (Fig. 14–19) and have noted it in a number

of illustrations in the literature as well. It has since been confirmed by others.[35, 1208] I have also recognized the sign in a case of hyperparathyroidism (Fig. 14–20). Of course, the pulmonary involvement must be extensive and extend to the periphery of the lung. A well-penetrated film is required, preferably a Bucky. In fact, on an overexposed Bucky film, even the heart, thoracic aorta, diaphragm, and solid abdominal viscera may appear black instead of white. Figure 14–19C illustrates this weird phenomenon.

Metabolic Calcification

Histologically, widespread pulmonary calcification secondary to altered calcium and phosphorous metabolism is not rare. However, detection of the calcium on the chest radiograph is extremely unusual. In sarcoidosis, it is occasionally visible in the small pulmonary nodules.[665] In the two examples I have seen, the serum calcium was not elevated,[140] at least not at the time the films were obtained. Scadding encountered six instances among 136 sarcoid patients in England.[1069]

Calcium is also rarely seen in the lungs in hyperparathyroidism (primary or secondary),[619] renal failure,[813] milk-alkali syndrome, hypervitaminosis D, and after intravenous calcium administration.[205, 1052] Since the calcium is finely divided, differentiation from alveolar disease of water density may be difficult. As stated above, the black pleura sign may be helpful (Fig. 14–20).

CALCIFICATION IN THE SOLITARY PULMONARY NODULE

Identification of calcium in a solitary pulmonary nodule is of great consequence in its diagnosis and management.[2, 1001] A calcium nidus of about 1 mm in diameter and containing as little as 0.1 mg of elemental calcium has been visualized experimentally.[201a] Central calcification (annular, stippled, or solid) is a reliable sign that the lesion is benign and almost always indicates a granuloma or hamartoma (Fig.

(Text continued on page 484.)

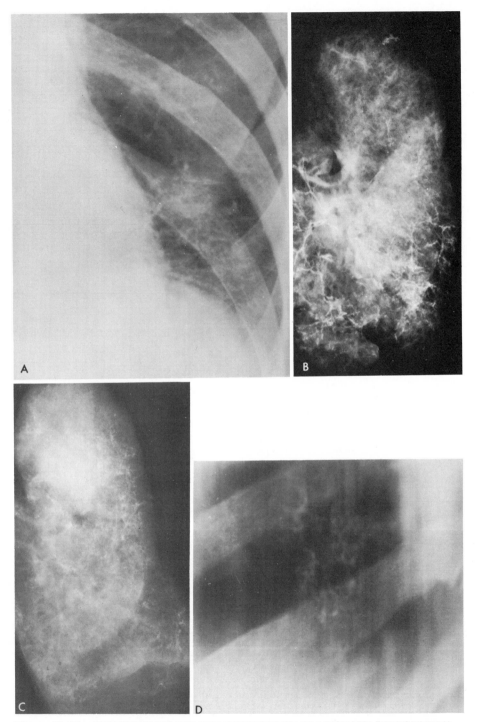

Figure 14–18. IDIOPATHIC PULMONARY OSSIFICATION (PULMONARY OSTEOPATHIA)

A, The lesion had spread slowly during the 6 years prior to this film. *B,* Roentgenogram of postmortem specimen. The patient died of unrelated disease. (Courtesy of Dr. Hans Plaut.) *C,* Another postmortem specimen. The lesions were bilateral. They were barely perceptible on chest films during life, but the calcium content was recognizable. (Courtesy of Dr. Stephen Kieffer.) *D,* Another patient, unproved.

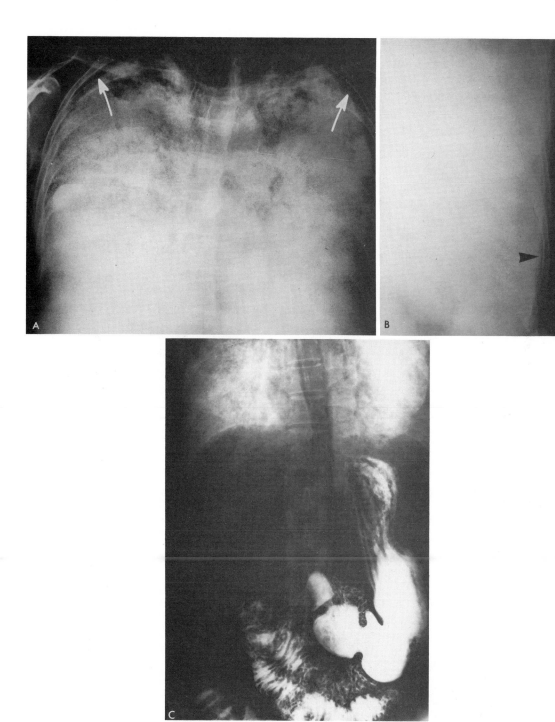

Figure 14–19. THREE PATIENTS WITH ALVEOLAR MICROLITHIASIS

A, Extensive disease in an asymptomatic woman. The ''black pleura'' is best seen at the lateral apices (arrows). (Courtesy of Dr. Charles V. Mooers.) *B,* A fine black pleural line is seen in the left lower thorax between the ribs and the calcified alveolar infiltrate (arrowhead). *C,* A black-hearted patient. Note that the heart, descending thoracic aorta, liver, and spleen appear radiolucent, while the calcium laden lungs and the barium filled stomach are radiopaque. This is an overexposed Bucky film of the abdomen made during a GI series. (Courtesy of Dr. Burke Winget, Travis Air Force Base.)

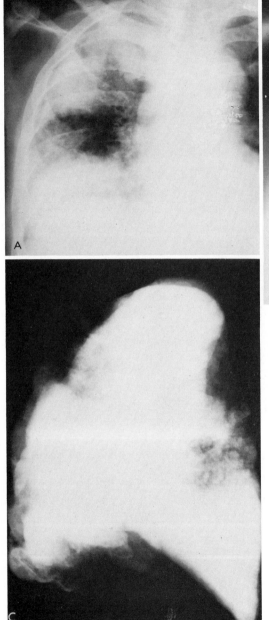

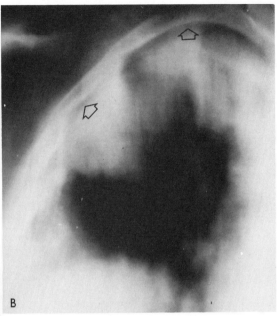

Figure 14–20. PULMONARY CALCINOSIS IN PRIMARY HYPERPARATHYROIDISM

The patient had a greatly elevated serum calcium and phosphorus. *A,* The chest roentgenogram reveals extensive alveolar involvement confined to the right lung. A chest film 3 months earlier had been normal. *B,* Laminagram shows a black pleural line (arrows) overlying the infiltrate, indicating that the alveolar disease is extensively calcified. *C,* Postmortem roentgenogram of the right lung. Histologically, the alveolar calcinosis was limited to areas of organized pneumonia. A parathyroid adenoma was found. Apparently, the pneumonic exudate contained considerable calcium, which precipitated.

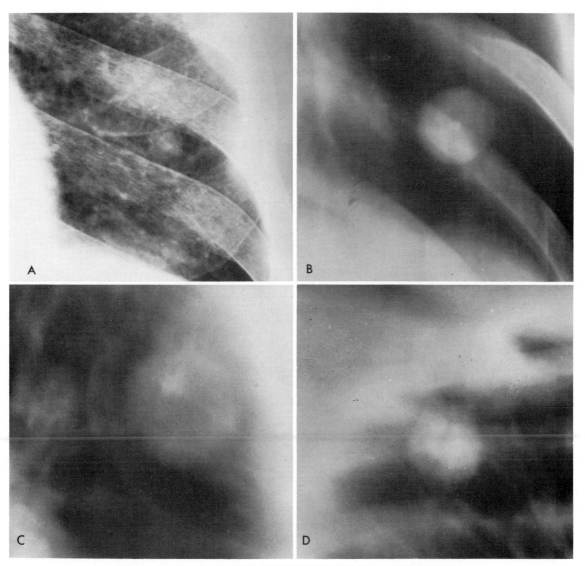

Figure 14–21. PATTERNS OF CALCIFICATION IN HISTOPLASMOMA

Four different patients. *A*, Laminated rings. *B*, Central solid sphere. *C*, Excentric irregular nodule. *D*, Central ring.

14-21). A solid calcification nearer the margin of the lesion usually indicates benignity, but in rare instances may represent a preexisting granuloma engulfed by a neoplasm (Fig. 14-22) or even a cancer arising in a scar.[442] True neoplastic calcification, though frequently identified histologically, is hardly ever seen on chest films, even on laminagrams.[899]

What approach, then, should we take to the solitary, partly calcified nodule in the lung? I believe that the statistics dictate conservative management whenever there is *any* type of calcium in *any* part of the lesion. Given 100 such cases, perhaps one or two will prove to be malignant; for the argument's sake, let's say two. The remainder are not only benign but innocuous, since breakdown or extension of such lesions is exceedingly rare. Thus, 98 healthy individuals would have to be operated on to pick up these two carcinomas — and there is no guarantee that both would be cured. And maybe one or two would die of operative complications.

Considering surgical mortality and morbidity and cancer cure rate, close roentgen observation seems to me to be the wiser choice for these calcium-containing lesions.

If growth of the nodule occurs, prompt surgery is recommended, though the lesion may still prove to be a granuloma.[1092] Delay in operation of a malignant lesion does not imply certain doom, since the outcome often rests more on the biological nature of the tumor than on its duration.

Other types of solitary pulmonary nodule may also calcify or ossify. Pulmonary hamartoma (hamartochondroma) may show various types of calcification, including an irregular dense opacity that has been likened to a popped kernel of corn (Fig. 14-23). The carcinoid type of bronchial adenoma may now and then show extensive ossification[1230] (Fig. 8-4B), as may an occasional arteriovenous malformation, the rare pulmonary plasmocytoma,[652] amyloidoma, and primary pulmonary osteosarcoma.[982]

CALCIFICATION IN MULTIPLE LARGE PULMONARY NODULES

Benign Lesions

Tuberculosis, histoplasmosis, coccidioidomycosis,[545, 1063] and perhaps other fungus

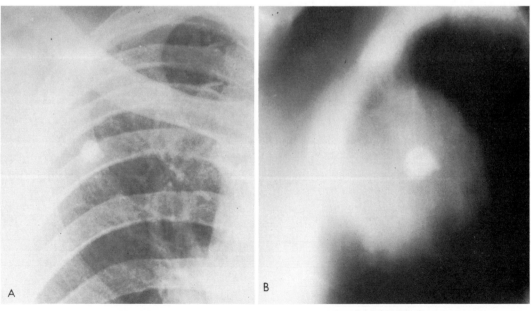

Figure 14-22.   GRANULOMA ENGULFED BY A CARCINOMA

A, 1960. Calcified nodule. *B,* Tomogram of a tumor that appeared in 1967. Squamous carcinoma.

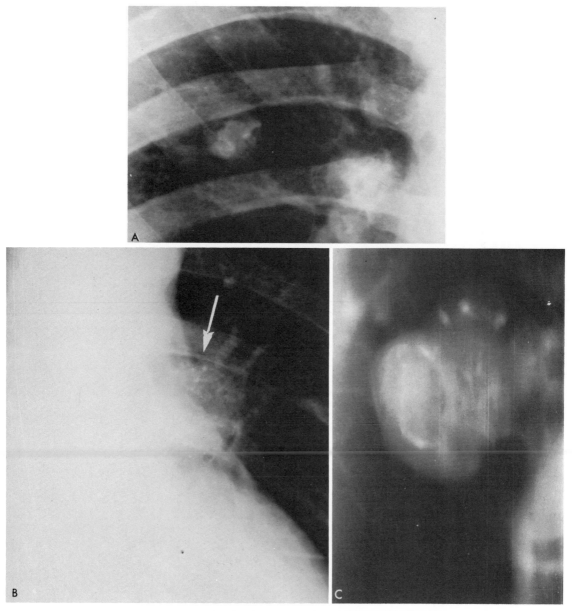

Figure 14–23. CALCIFICATION IN PULMONARY HAMARTOMA

Three cases. *A*, Popcorn type. *B*, Stippled. *C*, Annular and stippled.

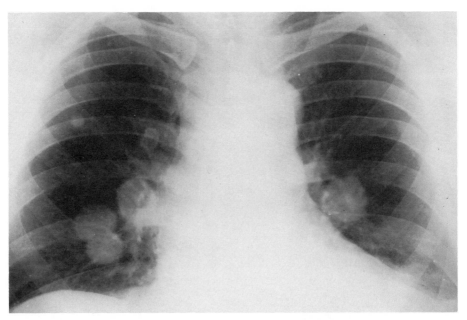

Figure 14–24. CALCIFIED HISTOPLASMOMAS

The lesions did not change over many years. Note the central calcification in some of the nodules.

diseases may present with multiple large nodules of various sizes, some containing calcification (Fig. 14–24). Although usually stable, the nodules may change in size. In one of our patients, they enlarged and several eventually cavitated, at which time the sputum became positive for tubercle bacilli. In another, three nodules were present, one of which was calcified. A few months after this one was resected, the other two nodules spontaneously disappeared. The resected lesion was a granuloma in which no organisms were demonstrated. Palayew recently presented five cases of progressive growth in large multinodular histoplasmosis.[915a]

Rarely, similar partly calcified nodules are seen in the lungs in rheumatoid arthritis and multiple hamartochondromas and in the trachea, bronchi, and lungs in *amyloid disease*[769, 1052] (Fig. 14–25) and *tracheopathia osteoplastica*. The latter is a rare condition, usually asymptomatic but occasionally causing cough and hemoptysis, in

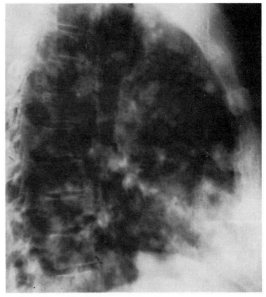

Figure 14–25. CALCIFIED AMYLOID NODULES IN THE LUNG

Lateral view. Chronic cough for 12 years with intermittent sputum. (Courtesy of Dr. Frederick J. Bonte.)

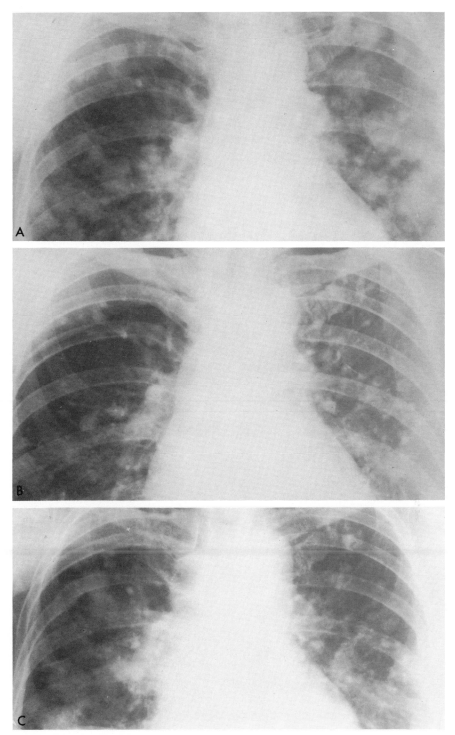

Figure 14–26. CALCIFICATION IN METASTATIC CARCINOMA FROM THE BREAST

The right breast was removed in 1937. *A*, 1946. These pulmonary nodules appeared in 1939 and slowly enlarged despite radiotherapy. *B*, 1951. Spontaneous regression has occurred and the nodules are small and calcified. *C*, By 1958, 20 years after they appeared, the nodules have again enlarged. The patient died a few months later. Autopsy showed partially calcified metastatic nodules histologically identical to the original breast lesion. There was no inflammatory component.

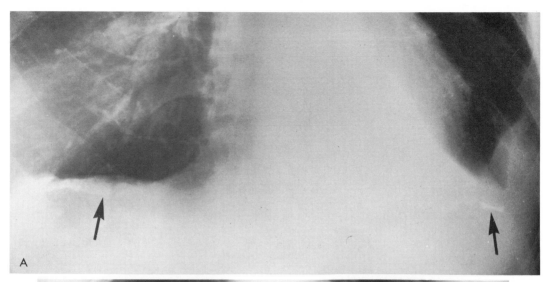

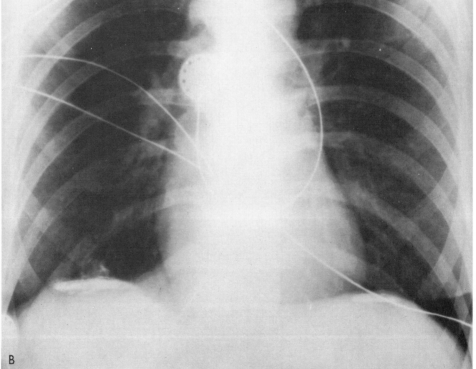

Figure 14–27. PNEUMOCONIOSIS WITH CALCIFIED PLEURAL PLAQUES (arrows)

A, This patient was exposed for many years to talc, silica, and asbestos. The opacity in the LLL followed trauma and later cleared. (Courtesy of Dr. Sanford Blank.) *B,* This 41 year old woman factory worker was exposed to asbestos. She was admitted in status epilepticus, which explains the use of monitoring equipment. The plaques in *A* and *B* are confined to the diaphragmatic pleura.

(*Figure continued on opposite page.*)

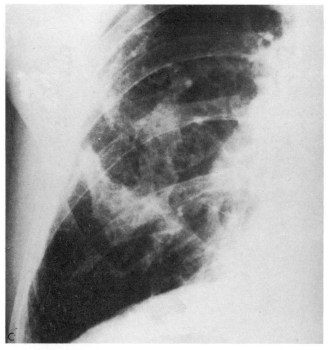

Figure 14–27. *Continued.   C, En face* calcification in another patient with asbestosis.

which cartilaginous masses, often calcified or ossified, are found in the trachea and large bronchi.[164, 208, 567] The nodules are irregular in outline and unevenly distributed so they are readily distinguished from calcification of the tracheal and bronchial rings (Fig. 5–34). They may contain amyloid.[8a]

Multiple Malignant Tumors

Three principal mechanisms account for calcification in malignant tumors in the lungs: (1) *bone formation,* seen with primary[981] and metastatic osteogenic sarcoma and multiple primary chondrosarcomas of the lung; (2) *psammoma formation,* as in metastases from thyroid tumor and papillary cystadenocarcinoma of the ovary and in some bronchogenic carcinomas;[740] and (3) *mucoid calcification,* seen in metastatic colloid carcinoma from the breast[921] (Fig. 14–26) and gastrointestinal tract. *Engulfment* of preexisting calcium by bronchogenic carcinoma, already discussed (Fig. 14–22), might properly be considered a fourth mechanism. Lymphoma, especially Hodgkin's disease, may show calcification,

usually but not invariably after radiation therapy.[366] Presumably, the calcium is the result of necrosis or fibrosis with healing. Encrustation, as seen in the urinary tract, does not seem to occur with bronchial tumors. Differentiation of the nature of the calcification on the basis of its roentgen appearance is not reliable.

PLEURAL CALCIFICATION

Pleural calcification, generally attributable to organized pleural effusion, empyema, or hemothorax,[442] is a fairly common finding. A well-penetrated Bucky film is ideal for its demonstration. The calcium is deposited near the inner surface of the greatly thickened pleura. This results in a clear space of water density interposed between the calcification and the bony thorax on tangential projection.[380]

Small plaques of calcium in the pleura, often multiple and bilateral, occur frequently in asbestosis and in tremolite talc,[326] mica, Bakelite, and calcimine pneumoconiosis.[579, 659, 660, 708, 1028, 1083, 1115, 1137] The calcifications are especially well seen at the domes of the diaphragm (Fig. 14–27) but may also be visible in profile along the lateral chest wall and pericardium. They are more difficult to detect face-on, since they then resemble pulmonary infiltrate; however, the margins of the plaques appear sharper and more angular (Fig. 14–27C).

When two or more of these calcific plaques are seen, the diagnosis of asbestosis (or talc pneumoconiosis, a close relative) can be made with reasonable assurance, even when the lungs are clear. However, I have seen two examples of multiple plaque-like calcifications in the diaphragm associated with chronic pneumonitis secondary to mineral oil aspiration. The calcifications of asbestosis are confined to the parietal pleura. They are probably the result of mechanical irritation by the ragged

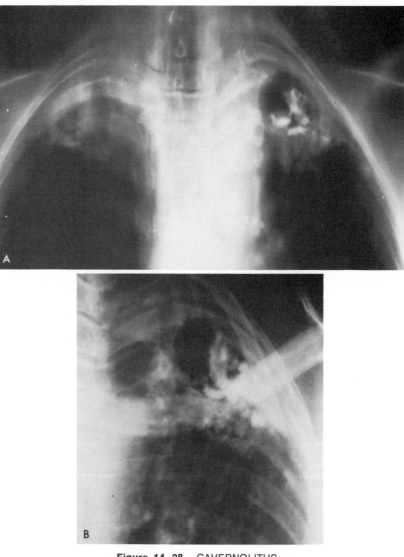

Figure 14–28. CAVERNOLITHS

A, Recumbent AP tomogram shows bilateral apical cavities containing calcified masses. The lesion on the right is not in focus on this cut. *B,* Cross-table AP view with left side dependent (but printed upright) shows that the calcified mass on the left has shifted to the dependent portion of the cavity. There was similar mobility of the mass in the right cavity. Although the patient had been treated many years earlier for tuberculosis, sputum cultures were now negative.

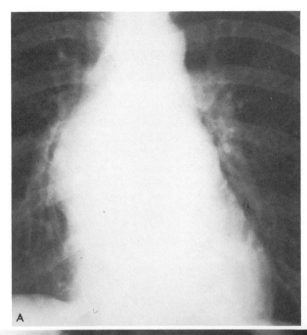

Figure 14–29. CALCIFICATION IN AN INTRAPERICARDIAL CYST

A calcium fluid level is shown on the lateral view. The pathologist thought the cyst was probably post-traumatic, but intrapericardial bronchogenic cyst can also produce this sign.[227] (Courtesy of Drs. Howard Franz and John B. Hearn.)

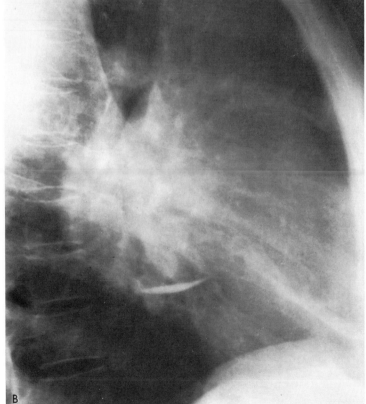

asbestos fragments that have migrated along the bronchi to the periphery of the lungs and protrude into the pleural space.[659]

OTHER THORACIC CALCIFICATIONS

A cavernolith is a calcified mass freely movable in a pulmonary cavity[956, 1052, 1127] (Fig. 14–28). This rare condition has been attributed to tuberculosis, but I have seen several proved fungus balls with surface calcification, so I suspect that the cavernolith is also a fungus ball that has become extensively calcified.[1249]

Calcium is commonly present in mediastinal lesions. If it lies within the substance of a mass and doesn't shift with gravity, a solid tumor is indicated. Layering indicates a cystic lesion (Fig. 14–29). Similar "milk of calcium" may occur in a pulmonary bronchogenic cyst.[214] Calcium in the margin of a mediastinal mass does not necessarily signify a cyst, thymic or otherwise.[1098] A solid thymoma or substernal thyroid may show rim calcification and, of course, so will an aneurysm. Calcification within a tumor does not exclude malignant neoplasm. Annular or stippled calcification may be present in thyroid carcinoma and neurosarcoma.[715] When a thymoma shows calcification, myasthenia gravis is usually associated. A

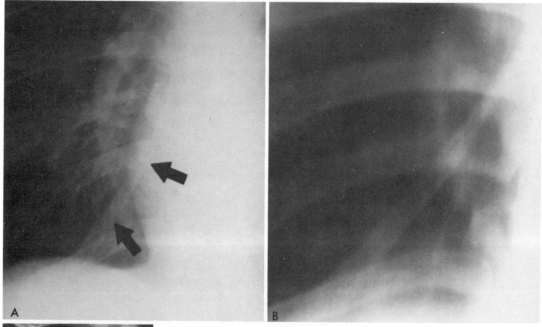

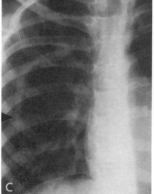

Figure 14–30. INTRATHORACIC RIB

A, The rib extends from the middorsal spine to the base of the lung (arrows). *B,* Tomogram showing typical cortex and medulla. (Courtesy of Weinstein, A. S., and Mueller, C. F.[1271]; reproduced with permission of Charles C Thomas, Publ.) *C,* Another patient.

tooth or bone is diagnostic of teratoma, and phleboliths indicate a hemangioma (Fig. 10–5). The significance of eggshell calcification has already been discussed. Otherwise, there is little specificity of the calcium pattern.

Occasionally the wall of a bulla appears calcified. It is presumed that the bulla developed as a result of a fibrocalcific tuberculous lesion and that the preexisting calcification became incorporated in the bulla wall. Curiously, hydatid cyst in the lung, unlike that in other areas of the body, seldom shows calcification.

An intrathoracic rib, a congenital anomaly, may produce a confusing ribbon-like roentgen shadow near the spine, attached at one end or both to a posterior rib. The diagnosis is easy if you're aware of the condition. It looks like a rib[945, 1271] (Fig. 14–30).

Calcified lesions of the chest wall are often mistaken for intrathoracic shadows. The extrapleural signs are helpful in localizing such lesions. Of course, fluoroscopy with tangential views will settle the issue. Multiple chest wall calcifications may be caused by parasites (*Armillifer ar-* *millatus*,[1168] Cysticercus, Trichinella, etc.), Ehlers-Danlos disease, myositis ossificans progressiva,[351] and scleroderma. Solitary calcification occurs in breast lesions, enchondroma, chondrosarcoma of the bony structures, and other soft tissue or rib tumors.

It is obvious from the foregoing that the presence of calcium in a thoracic lesion is often of considerable importance. Logically, steps should be taken to demonstrate calcium when it is not seen within a lesion on conventional films. However, irrelevant calcification is frequent in significant lesions. Clearly, we cannot study every lesion or every calcification thoroughly. How then should we approach this problem?

My own compromise is to obtain a slightly overexposed Bucky film in every thoracic lesion in which the diagnosis is uncertain. Laminagraphy is reserved for those lesions in which calcification is suspected from the Bucky films, in which visible calcium needs to be accurately localized, or in which the presence of calcium might alter the therapy. The diagnosis may rest on that piece of calcium. Watch for it.

CHAPTER 15

A REVIEW OF OVER 30,000 NORMAL CHEST ROENTGENOGRAMS

Anyone who has participated in extensive chest roentgen surveys will, I believe, agree with me that it is painfully dull work. During the Second World War, I received an "In-Addition-to-Your-Other-Duties" notice assigning me the daily task of interpreting several hundred routine 14×17 chest roentgenograms. To combat the boredom, and at the same time to convince myself that these hours were not a total loss, I tabulated the incidence of certain "normal" roentgen findings. Soon I had accumulated reams of useless information. One day I ran across my notes and decided to include some of the hard-won figures for those readers who, like myself, take pleasure in confirming what they already know or enjoy the acquisition of bits of impractical knowledge. I am reminded of the advertisement, "Used tombstone for sale. Wonderful bargain for anyone named Burdzynski."

Most of the first group of roentgenograms were obtained in connection with a routine physical examination made on Army recruits, officer candidates, etc. About 80 per cent of these individuals were between 17 and 40 years of age, the remainder ranging from 40 to 55 years; about 90 per cent were men. More recently, many films came from a survey by the United States Public Health Service of mine workers. Most of these subjects were adult men over 40, and no parameter was applied to these films that might be influenced by age or dust exposure. For example, I did not use these particular films to study Kerley's lines or aortic disease.

All of the films were PA teleroentgenograms; all interpretations were my own.

One parameter at a time was studied for several hundred to a thousand consecutive films. Each film was first interpreted and reported. If there were no significant abnormalities, the finding being tabulated was then recorded on a chart prepared after a trial run of about 100 cases. On the following pages, my experience with these groups of apparently normal individuals is summarized.

I. THE BONY STRUCTURES
   A. Cervical rib and related anomalies – 350 cases*
      1. Cervical rib was present in 1.5%. Nearly all were bilateral, but half differed distinctly in size on the two sides. They were often well developed.
      2. In 1.2%, underdeveloped first rib was present.** In about half of these individuals the changes were bilateral.
      3. 2.4% showed an unusually long transverse process of the seventh cervical vertebra with no evidence of an articulated cervical rib. Of these, one fourth were unilateral and three fourths were bilateral.
   B. Companion shadows on the ribs – 1350 cases
      1. 35% of 300 cases showed a companion shadow along the first rib. In

---

*The number of cases listed here and on the following pages represents the total number of films reviewed, not the number of variations or abnormalities observed.

**Back in the 1940s, I could tell the difference between a cervical rib and an underdeveloped first rib on the PA chest teleroentgenogram. Now I seem to have forgotten how.

494

almost half it was bilateral. When unilateral, it was about three times as common on the right as on the left.

2. In 31% of the same 300 cases there was a companion shadow along the second rib. In two fifths it was bilateral. Again, it was more common on the right side in the unilateral cases. About 10% showed unilateral or bilateral companion shadows on *both* the first and second ribs. In 56%, there was a unilateral or bilateral companion shadow on *either* the first or second rib.

3. Companion shadows on the lower ribs were seen in about 75% of 700 cases. In 4% they were striking. There did not appear to be any correlation between the presence of companion shadows and body habitus.

4. The incidence of shadows consistent with subpleural fat deposition was recorded in 350 subjects. The internal surface of the lower right thoracic wall was closely scrutinized for these faint shadows, convex toward the lung (Fig. 13–2). In 31%, the films did not show the area adequately. In 29%, no shadow was visible despite adequate penetration, in 18% there was a small shadow, in 17% a moderate sized one, and in 5% the shadow was about 1 cm thick. Often several of these shadows were present.

C. Rib notching — 1500 cases
A localized indentation along the undersurface of the medial half of one or more ribs was seen in about 21% (mild in 19% and moderate in 2%), in the lateral half in 6.5% (5% mild and 1.5% moderate). These notches were seldom of a degree to suggest aortic coarctation. In most, only one or two ribs were affected.

D. Calcification of the lower costal cartilages — 1000 cases*
1. About 250 cases were discarded because the lower ribs were poorly shown.
2. Of about 300 women, 38% showed no calcium, 61% had the central ("female") type, 0.3% had the marginal ("male") type, and 0.3% had both.
3. Of approximately 400 men, 60% showed no calcium, 37% had the marginal ("male") type, 2% had the central ("female") type, and 0.7% had both.
4. When calcium was visible in the

lower ribs, the patient's sex could be predicted with 96% accuracy.

II. THE AORTA
A. Width of the aortic knob — 500 cases
The aortic knob was measured transversely from the left border of the trachea to the left lateral margin of the aorta (A in Fig. 15–1). As expected, the width increased with age. Of those under 30, 95% measured less than 3 cm. Between ages 30 and 40, 91% measured less than 3 cm; over 40, 69% measured less than 3 cm. In no case did the aortic knob measure more than 4 cm in width. One third of this particular group of cases were women.

B. Length of ascending aorta — 1350 cases
1. In 350 cases, the length of the ascending aorta was measured perpendicularly from the level of the lower end of its visible takeoff from the right heart border to the level of the highest point of the arch. It was compared with the length of the right heart border measured perpendicularly from the level of its junction with the diaphragm to the level of the aortic takeoff (B and C in Fig. 15–1). In only 0.3% of those under the age of 30 was the aorta longer than the right heart border. This figure rose to 26% between the ages of 30 and 40, and to 27% over the age of 40.
2. The proximity of the top of the aortic arch to the clavicles was studied in 1000 cases (D in Fig. 15–1). In about 10%, the aorta reached the level of the lower border of the clavicles. There appeared to be no significant rise in incidence with increasing age. It was concluded that this sign was of little value in determining aortic elongation and was probably a function of individual variation or of centering the roentgen beam.

C. Atherosclerosis — 500 cases
Roentgen evidence of definite aortic atherosclerosis, such as calcification in the knob, increase in width, and unusual tortuosity or "uncoiling," was not seen in those under the age of 30, and was encountered in only 2.5% of individuals under 40.

D. Visibility of the top of the aortic knob — 800 cases
The cephalic margin of the aortic knob was observed through the mediastinal tissues. In about 77%, it could be followed to the spine (G in Fig. 15–2). In 23%, it stopped short of the spine, i.e., its silhouette was obliterated before it

*See Table 13–1.

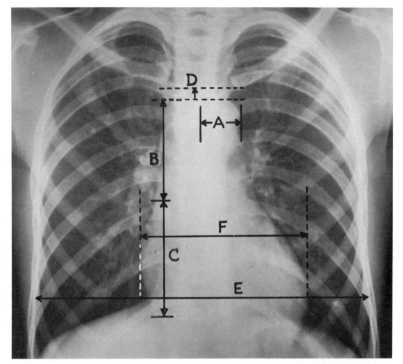

Figure 15–1. SITES OF MEASUREMENT OF NORMAL VARIATIONS

A, Width of aortic knob. *B*, Length of ascending aorta. *C*, Length of right heart border. *D*, Distance from top of aortic arch to clavicles. *E*, Internal diameter of chest. *F*, Transverse diameter of heart.

reached the spine. About 100 cases had to be discarded because the aortic knob wasn't adequately penetrated.

III. THE HEART SHADOW

A. The cardiothoracic ratio—1125 cases
The internal diameter of the chest was measured at the level of the highest point on the right hemidiaphragm (E in Figure 15–1). The transverse diameter of the heart was measured as the sum of the widest portions of the heart to the right and to the left of the midline of the spine, exclusive of the fat pad (F in Fig. 15–1). There were 2.1% with a cardiothoracic ratio greater than 0.5. Surprisingly, the incidence of increased cardiothoracic ratio did not appear to be significantly different among the thin, average, and heavy subjects. However, there were many more cases with a low ratio in the asthenic group. The conclusion was drawn that many adult hearts showing a ratio above 0.5 are enlarged but some are not, so in the individual patient you should not rely on car-

diothoracic ratio alone for the diagnosis of cardiomegaly. And, of course, enlargement may be present despite a normal cardiothoracic ratio.

B. Configuration—1625 cases
1. Some degree of straightening of the left border of the heart was observed in 19%. A distinct rounded prominence of the main pulmonary artery segment was seen in about one sixth of these. Straightening or convexity of the pulmonary arc was frequent among the thin subjects and uncommon among the heavy ones. A fairly deep concavity in the region of the main pulmonary artery segment was seen in 12% of the cases. This occurred more frequently in the hypersthenic individual but was not rare in the hyposthenic. In 68%, the cardiac "waistline" was considered to be midway between the mitral and aortic configuration, i.e., there was a mild concavity of the pulmonary artery segment.

2. Daves has noted an abnormal prominence along the left heart border in a variety of pathologic conditions.[234] He calls it the *third mogul*, after the small hillock on a ski slope that is designed to separate the men from the boys and send the boys to the cast room. I have scanned the left border of the normal heart for such moguls and have found, along the left border somewhere below the pulmonary artery, a small bump (H in Fig. 15–2) in 5%, and one of moderate size in 1%. They were more common along the lower segment of the left ventricle.

C. Position of the right heart border—500 cases

In 87.5%, a small to moderate segment of the heart lay to the right of the spine (J in Fig. 15–2). In 7%, the heart extended to the right almost as far as to the left of the spine. In 0.2% (1 case), it extended even more to the right than to the left. In 3.3%, the right border of the heart and spine coincided, and in about 2%, this heart border lay even more to the left. In half of these, the rib configuration suggested funnel breast, but lateral views were not available.

D. The fat pad—600 cases

60% of the cases showed a distinct pad along the left lower cardiac border. In about a third of these, it appeared to be of fat density. A fat pad was more common in heavy people, but not strikingly so.

E. Visibility of the hepatic vein or inferior vena cava—500 cases

Attention was centered on the broad vascular shadow often superimposed upon the inferior right heart border and usually attributed to the inferior vena cava or one of the hepatic veins. This shadow was visible in 13% of the cases. It was rarely seen in heavy patients.

F. Double shadow visible through the right side of the heart—500 cases

This shadow (Fig. 5–15) simulates the one sometimes seen with enlargement of the left atrium and is produced by con-

Figure 15–2. SITES OF MEASUREMENT OF NORMAL VARIATIONS (continued)

G, Visibility of the top of the aortic knob. *H,* The "third mogul." *J,* Position of the right heart border. *K,* Visibility of the subcardiac segment of the left hemidiaphragm. *L,* Obliteration of the cardiac silhouette by the left hilum. *M,* Obliteration of the ascending aorta by the right hilum.

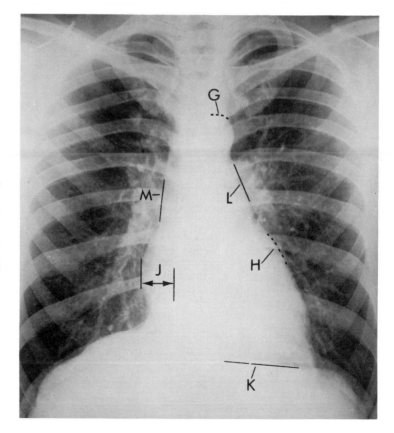

fluence of the right pulmonary veins. Many cases were discarded because the film was too light to visualize the area or because the spine overlapped it. Of the remainder, 68% showed no such shadow, 27% showed a questionable one, while in 5% a definite double shadow could be seen.

IV. THE TRACHEA

A. Tracheal deviation on "true" films—500 cases

The position of the trachea in relation to the midline of the spine just above the clavicles was recorded. Only true PA roentgenograms, as determined by a symmetrical relationship between the inner ends of the two clavicles and the lateral borders of the upper thoracic spine, were utilized. In 2%, a definite although not striking deviation of the trachea from the midline was encountered. The displacement was of about equal frequency toward the left and right. There was no apparent cause for this deviation.

B. Tracheal deviation in rotated patients—100 cases

This study was confined to films showing a mild degree of patient rotation to learn whether the position of the trachea was predictable on the rotated film, information that might occasionally prove useful in the recognition of pulmonary collapse. The presence of rotation was determined from the relation of the inner ends of the clavicles to the spine. A midline vertical interspinous line was used as the reference point for the tracheal deviation. The trachea appeared to deviate in the expected manner or remained in the midline in 98% of the cases. In 2%, however, it appeared to be displaced the wrong way, i.e., the reverse of the expected manner. For example, with the patient rotated into a slight right anterior oblique position, as determined by the separation of the left clavicle from the left border of the spine, the trachea remained in the midline (interspinous line) in 57%, was displaced toward the left in 39%, and was deviated to the right in 3%.

C. Visible right tracheal border (right paratracheal line)—800 cases

1. After discarding many films because of underpenetration of the tracheal region, the *outside* margin of the right border of the trachea below the clavicular level was examined in 500 cases (Figs. 11–25 and 11–30). It was visi-

ble for much of its intrathoracic extent in 63% and invisible in 37%. In about 20% of all individuals, the outside right tracheal border was also visible above the clavicles. How do you explain it? Simple—the posterior half of the trachea makes contact with the lungs.

2. The region of the azygos vein in the crotch between the right tracheal margin and RUL (Fig. 5–44) was scrutinized in 300 individuals after discarding many others because of inadequate visibility of the area due to rotation or underpenetration. In 76%, not even the slightest thickening of the tracheobronchial wall could be seen. 15% showed slight mural thickening; and only 8.6% demonstrated a round or oval azygos shadow in this angle, but never over 1 cm in transverse diameter.

V. THE DIAPHRAGM

A. Elevation—500 cases

As is well known, the right hemidiaphragm is normally slightly higher than the left. However, in 11% of the cases in this series one of the hemidiaphragms appeared abnormally elevated. In 9%, the left hemidiaphragm was at the same level or higher than the right. In half of these, there was obvious distention of the stomach or colon. The right hemidiaphragm was more than 3 cm higher than the left in the remaining 2%.

B. Scalloping—500 cases

A scalloped or polyarcuate diaphragm was seen in 5.5%. In nearly all the cases it was present on the right, although in one fifth it was bilateral. In only one instance was it confined to the left side. Scalloping was usually mild in degree.

C. Obliteration of a costophrenic angle—600 cases

In 1.2%, one or both costophrenic angles were obliterated, presumably by past pleural disease.

D. Visibility of the subcardiac segment of the left hemidiaphragm—800 cases

The silhouette of the left leaf as seen under the heart from the spine to the fat pad was examined (K in Fig. 15–2) on adequately penetrated films. In 90%, more than half of this segment could be discerned—it often was totally visible. In 8%, less than half was evident, and in 2% the entire inferior cardiophrenic border was obliterated.

E. Gastric bubble—700 cases

The gas bubble was visible in only about 500 of 700 individuals. Among the 200 in whom it could not be seen were many with films inadequately penetrated or positioned for the purpose. It is possible that in some the bubble was invisible because of a low position of the stomach. When seen, the top of the gas shadow lay within 1 cm of the dome of the hemidiaphragm in 88%, 1 to 2 cm from it in 11%, and more than 2 cm below it in 0.7%.

VI. THE LUNGS

A. Apical "cap" — 300 cases

7.3% showed apical pleural thickening, although in only 1% was this of more than slight degree. The left apex was much more commonly involved than the right. In about 1% both apices were affected.

B. Lung density — 800 cases

1. Comparison of right and left lung density was made in 500 cases. Only true PA films were utilized. If bullae were visible, the case was excluded. Radiolucency of the right and left lungs was compared area by area. The two lungs were equally lucent in 72%. One lung was *locally* slightly more radiolucent than the other in 25%; it was distinctly so in an additional 0.6%. The increased blackness was generally seen in the upper lung, more commonly on the left. A *diffuse* increase in radiolucency of one lung was found in 2%, mild in degree in two thirds, and moderate in one third; the finding was about equal in frequency on each side.

2. The effects of expiration were studied in 300 cases. Inspiration and expiration films were available in one group of individuals. Comparison of the lucency of the lung bases on the two films was made after first ascertaining that a change in level of the diaphragm had occurred. Alteration in apparent heart size with respiration was ignored. In 25%, little or no clouding of the lung bases occurred on expiration. Moderate clouding was seen in 46% and marked opacification, similar in degree to that of congestive failure, was found in 25%.

C. Hilar shadows — 5100 cases

1. The relative levels of the two hilar shadows were compared in 500 cases. These figures have already been recorded in Table 3–1 (page 105) and will not be repeated here.

2. The size of the hilar shadows was correlated with age in 1100 patients. No actual measurements were made but the sizes of the two hila were averaged and classified as small, medium, or large. It was found that a slight increase in size of the hilar shadows occurs with advancing years.

3. The size of the right hilum was compared to the left in 1000 cases. In 84%, the two sides were approximately equal. In the remaining 16% there was inequality, the larger hilum occurring on the right in 8% and on the left in 8%. Asymmetry was seldom striking in degree. No increase in the incidence of asymmetry with advancing years was noted.

4. The density of the two hila was compared in 1000 cases. It was equal in 88%, slightly greater on the right in 8%, and slightly greater on the left in 4%. In only one instance was the difference in density on the two sides moderate in degree.

5. The incidence of obliteration of the silhouette of the heart by the pulmonary vessels in the left hilum was studied in 500 cases (L in Fig. 15–2), after discarding many cases because of underpenetration or of overlapping of the descending aorta. This cardiac segment was obliterated in 71% and preserved in 29%.

6. The right hilum was studied for similar obliteration of the ascending aorta in 500 cases (M in Fig. 15–2). Again, many cases were discarded, mostly because the spine overlapped the area. In 24%, the ascending aorta was obliterated; in 76%, it was preserved.

7. The location of the bifurcation of the left pulmonary artery in relation to the middle segment of the left cardiac border was determined in 500 cases. In 91.5%, the first pulmonary bifurcation occurred lateral to the heart; in 8% it was seen slightly behind the left edge of the heart; and in 0.2% (one instance) it lay well over a centimeter medial to the left border.

D. Calcification — 2200 cases

1. In 37% of 1350 cases, no pulmonary or lymph node calcification was seen in the chest. In 35%, there were one or more small calcifications, all under 5 mm in diameter in the hilum or mediastinum and under 3 mm in diameter in the lung. In 24%, there were calcifications 5 to 10 mm in di-

ameter in the nodes and/or 3 to 5 mm in the parenchyma. In 3.2%, the calcifications were larger. In 5% of the 1350 cases, both the parenchymal and lymph node components of a primary complex were visible. There appeared to be no increase in the incidence or average size of the calcifications with advancing age.

2. The hila were studied in another 850 cases for the presence of calcification. In 61%, calcification was not apparent and in another 14% its presence was uncertain. Definite hilar calcification was noted in 25%.

E. Vascular patterns — 4550 cases

1. The vascular markings in the outer third of the lungs were studied in 800 cases. Only 5% of the cases showed many distinct branching vessels in this region. Two thirds of those showing these prominent vascular markings were in the age group over 40.

2. Visibility of the pulmonary veins was tested in 850 cases. The only criterion used was the demonstration of one or more individual vessels coursing toward the left atrium rather than toward the hilum. From the trial run, it quickly became apparent that I could not identify the veins in the upper lung fields; therefore, only the lower pulmonary vessels were studied and tabulated. On the right side, the pulmonary veins were clearly seen in 48% of 500 cases, questionably recognized in 40%, and not identified at all in 12%. Corresponding figures for the left lower lung in 350 cases were 15%, 36%, and 49%, respectively. The striking difference between the figures on the two sides was attributable to the much greater obscuration by the left side of the heart. Although the technical quality of the film and the body habitus of the subject had considerable bearing on the visibility of the veins, there were also wide variations from one individual to the next, unrelated to these factors.

3. In 900 subjects, the right cardiophrenic angle was studied. The difficulty in differentiating between normal confluent vascular markings and pulmonary infiltrate in this region is well known. In about half the cases, the right cardiophrenic angle showed a hazy increase in density, usually ill-defined but definitely more radiopaque than the lung elsewhere. In many, the vessels were indistinctly delineated within this haze. The type of body habitus bore no significant relationship to this appearance. It is apparent that the hazy increase in opacity in the right cardiophrenic angle in these normal individuals may occasionally be confused with pneumonic or other pulmonary infiltrate, especially since its counterpart on the left side cannot be used for comparison because of the overlying heart shadow.

4. The lateral costophrenic regions were examined in 1000 cases for evidence of transverse markings resembling the septal lines of Kerley (B lines). On the right side, 17% of 500 cases showed a few faint but definite transverse lines, probably representing small vessels. In 2%, the lines were more numerous and better shown, but relatively thin. In one case, typical septal lines indistinguishable from those described by Kerley were seen. The remaining 81% showed no transverse lines. On the left, 77% of 500 cases were normal, 19% showed a few faint transverse lines, 3% revealed well-defined but thin lines, and three cases showed typical septal lines.

5. The upper and lower pulmonary vessels were compared in size and number in 1000 cases. Covering the hila with the thumbs seemed to help in the comparisons. The upper vessels were smaller than the lower in 63%, the two were about equal in 34%, and the upper lung vessels were more prominent than the lower in 3%, similar in degree to that seen in patients with pulmonary venous hypertension.

F. Pulmonary septa — 1000 cases

1. The minor septum was completely invisible in 44% of 500 cases. In 32%, less than half the normal extent of the septum could be seen; in 23%, more than half was visible. The position of the outer end of the septum, seen in 280 of the 500 cases, was studied in relation to the topography of the thoracic cage. It was found to be at the level of the fourth anterior interspace in 67%, the fifth rib or interspace in 15%, and below this in 3%. It lay over the third rib or interspace in 13% and above this level in 2%. It was concluded that there is so much variation

in the level of the minor septum that abnormal displacement cannot be recognized unless it is striking or unless other considerations, such as alterations in shape and direction, are taken into account. The medial end of the minor septum nearly always terminated at the lateral margin of the right inferior pulmonary artery within about a centimeter of the origin of this vessel at the hilum.

2. A segment of the inferior accessory fissure was visible in 5% of 500 chests. In 2%, less than one fourth of its estimated length was seen; in 3%, from one fourth to three fourths. In no instance in the series was more than three fourths seen, although I have seen the full length of this accessory fissure on a number of other occasions (Fig. 3–8).

REFERENCES

Listed here in the left-hand column are references cited in the text and in the right-hand column the page(s) on which each reference appears.

1. Aaron, B. L.: Intradiaphragmatic cyst: a rare entity. J. Thorac. Cardiovasc. Surg. 49:531, 1965. — 426

2. Abeles, H., and Chaves, A. D.: The significance of calcification in pulmonary coin lesions. Radiology 58:199, 1952. — 479

3. Abrams, H. L.: Radiologic aspects of increased pulmonary artery pressure and flow: preliminary observations. Stanford Med. Bull. 14:97, 1956. — 217

4. Addington, E. A., and Kirklin, B. R.: The incidence and significance of apical lesions in pulmonary tuberculosis: a pathologic and roentgenologic study. Radiology 34:327, 1940. — 303

4a. Addington, W. W., Cugell, D. W., Westerhoff, T. R., Shapiro, B., and Smith, R. T.: The pulmonary edema of heroin toxicity—an example of the stiff lung syndrome. Chest 62:199, 1972. — 299, 345

5. Albo, R. J., and Grimes, O. F.: The middle lobe syndrome: a clinical study. Dis. Chest 50:509, 1966. — 95

6. Alexander, C.: Diaphragm movements and the diagnosis of diaphragmatic paralysis. Clin. Radiol. 17:79, 1966. — 435, 436

7. Alexander, S. C., Fiegiel, S. J., and Class, R. N.: Congenital absence of the left pulmonary artery. Amer. Heart J. 50:465, 1955. — 189, 290

8. Allen, R. P., Taylor, R. L., and Reiquam, C. W.: Congenital lobar emphysema with dilated septal lymphatics. Radiology 86:929, 1966. — 142, 246

8a. Alroy, G. G., Lichtig, C., and Kaftori, J. K.: Tracheobronchopathia osteoplastica: end stage of primary lung amyloidosis? Chest 61:465, 1972. — 489

9. Anderson, R. C., Adams, P., Jr., and Burke, B.: Anomalous inferior vena cava with azygos continuation (infrahepatic interruption of the inferior vena cava): report of 15 new cases. J. Pediat. 59:370, 1961. — 236

10. Andrews, N. C., Pratt, P. C., and Christoforidis, A. J.: Identification of active pulmonary cavitary disease by barium bronchogram technique. Dis. Chest 51:596, 1967. — 16

11. Anson, B. J., Siekert, R. G., Richmond, T. E., and Bishop, W. E.: Accessory pulmonary lobe of azygos vein: anatomical report, with record of incidence. Quart. Bull. Northwestern Univ. Med. School 24:285, 1950. — 74

12. Anton, H. C.: Multiple pleural plaques. Brit. J. Radiol. 40:685, 1967. — 377

13. Arendt, J., and Wolf, A.: The vallecular sign: its diagnosis and clinical significance. Amer. J. Roentgen. 57:435, 1947. — 267

14. Arnett, N. L., and Schulz, D. M.: Primary pulmo-   339
    nary eosinophilic granuloma. Radiology 69:224,
    1957.
15. Arnois, D., Silverman, F. N., and Turner, M. E.:   224
    The radiographic evaluation of pulmonary vascu-
    lature in children with congenital cardiovascular
    disease. Radiology 72:689, 1959.
16. Aronoff, A., Bywaters, E. G. L., and Fearnley, G.   340
    R.: Lung lesions in rheumatoid arthritis. Brit.
    Med. J. 2:228, 1955.
17. Aronstam, E. M., and Thomas, P. A., Jr.: In-   315
    trathoracic fibrocaseous granuloma of obscure ori-
    gin: a ten year survey. Dis. Chest 41:547, 1962.
18. Aschoff, L.: Lectures on Pathology: II. Pathogen-   296
    esis of Human Pulmonary Consumption. New
    York, Paul B. Hoeber, Inc., 1924.
19. Ashba, J. K., and Ghanem, M. H.: The lungs in   339
    systemic sclerosis. Dis. Chest 47:52, 1965.
20. Asp, K., Heikel, P.-E., Pasila, M., and Sulamaa,   160
    M.: Pulmonary sequestration in children. Ann.
    Paediat. Fenn. 9:270, 1963.
21. Austrian, C. R., and Brown, W. H.: Miliary dis-   289, 433
    eases of lung. Amer. Rev. Tuberc. 45:751, 1942.
22. Avery, E. E., Mörch, E. T., and Benson, D. W.:   433
    Critically crushed chests: a new method of treat-
    ment with continuous mechanical hyperventila-
    tion to produce alkalotic apnea and internal pneu-
    matic stabilization. J. Thoracic Surg. 32:291, 1956.
23. Avnet, N. L.: Roentgenologic features of congeni-   419, 426
    tal bilateral anterior diaphragmatic eventration.
    Amer. J. Roentgen. 88:743, 1962.
24. Baarsma, P. R., and Dirken, M. N. J.: Collateral   180
    ventilation. J. Thoracic Surg. 17:238, 1948.
25. Bachman, A. L., Hewitt, W. R., and Beekley, H.   96, 98, 143, 290
    C.: Bronchiectasis: a bronchographic study of
    sixty cases of pneumonia. Arch. Intern. Med.
    91:78, 1953.
26. Bachman, A. L., Sara, N. O., and Mantz, H. E.:   25, 97, 290
    Pleuritic involvement associated with primary
    atypical pneumonia: a roentgenographic and clin-
    ical study. Amer. J. Roentgen. 53:244, 1945.
27. Bachynski, J. E.: Absence of the air bronchogram   61
    sign: a reliable finding in pulmonary embolism
    with   infarction   or   hemorrhage.   Radiology
    100:547, 1971.
28. Bachynski, J. E.: Selective bronchography of soli-   269
    tary mass lesions in the lung. J. Canad. Assoc.
    Radiol. 22:65, 1971.
29. Badger, T. L., Gottlieb, L., and Gaensler, E. A.:   305, 479
    Pulmonary alveolar microlithiasis, or calcinosis of
    the lungs. New Eng. J. Med. 253:709, 1955.
30. Baghdassarian, O. M., Avery, M. E., and Neu-   344
    hauser, E. B. D.: A form of pulmonary insuf-
    ficiency in premature infants: pulmonary dysma-
    turity? Amer. J. Roentgen. 89:1020, 1963.
31. Baghdassarian, O. M., and Weiner, S.: Pneuma-   321
    tocele formation complicating hydrocarbon pneu-
    monitis. Amer. J. Roentgen. 95:104, 1965.
32. Bagshawe, K. D., and Garnett, E. S.: Radiological   315
    changes in the lungs of patients with trophoblas-
    tic tumours. Brit. J. Radiol. 36:673, 1963.
33. Bahl, O. P., Oliver, G. C., Rockoff, S. D., and   299
    Parker, B. M.: Localized unilateral pulmonary
    edema: an unusual presentation of left heart fail-
    ure. Chest 60:277, 1971.
34. Balestra, G.: Le calcificazioni a guscio d'uovo   467
    sono patognomoniche della silicosi? Radiol. Med.
    38:829, 1952.

35. Balikian, J. P., Fuleihan, F. J. D., and Nucho, C. N.: Pulmonary alveolar microlithiasis: report of five cases with special reference to roentgen manifestations. Amer. J. Roentgen. 103:509, 1968. — 479

36. Barden, R. P.: Pulmonary edema: correlation of roentgenologic appearance and abnormal physiology. Amer. J. Roentgen. 92:495, 1964. — 290, 299

37. Bariety, M., Coury, C., Monod, O., Gimbert, J. L., and Wargon, H.: Twelve years' experience with gas mediastinography (770 cases): results obtained in cancer of the lung. Dis. Chest 48:449, 1965. — 21

38. Barnett, T. B., and Herring, C. L.: Lung abscess: initial and late results of medical therapy. Arch. Intern. Med. 127:217, 1971. — 346

39. Baron, M. G., and Whitehouse, W. M.: Primary lymphosarcoma of the lung. Amer. J. Roentgen. 85:294, 1961. — 304

40. Bartley, T. D., and Arean, V. M.: Intrapulmonary neurogenic tumors. J. Thorac. Cardiovasc. Surg. 50:114, 1965. — 315

41. Barzó, P.: Bronchographic changes in chronic bronchitis. Fortschr. Roentgenstr. 105:679, 1966. — 288

42. Bateson, E. M.: The solitary circumscribed bronchogenic carcinoma: a radiological study of 100 cases. Brit. J. Radiol. 37:598, 1964. — 319

43. Baum, G. L., Bernstein, I. L., and Schwarz, J.: Broncholithiasis produced by histoplasmosis. Amer. Rev. Tuberc. 77:162, 1958. — 465

44. Baum, G. L., Racz, I., Bubis, J. J., Molho, M., and Shapiro, B. L.: Cystic disease of the lung: report of eighty-eight cases, with ethnologic relationship. Amer. J. Med. 40:578, 1966. — 313

45. Bayindir, S., Bikfalvi, A., and Sailer, F. X.: Zur Frage der Lungen-Hypoplasie. Fortschr. Roentgenstr. 107:423, 1967. — 81

46. Beatty, O. A., Saliba, A., and Levene, N.: A study of cavities and bronchi in pulmonary fungus diseases. Dis. Chest 47:409, 1965. — 346

47. Beber, B. A., Litt, R. E., and Altman, D. H.: A new radiographic finding in mongolism. Radiology 86:332, 1966. — 453

48. Behlke, F. M.: Hepatodiaphragmatic interposition in children. Amer. J. Roentgen. 91:669, 1964. — 425

49. Behrendt, D. M., and Scannell, J. G.: Pericardial fat necrosis: an unusual cause of severe chest pain and thoracic "tumor." New Eng. J. Med. 279:473, 1968. — 419, 463

50. Beigelman, P. M., Miller, L. V., and Martin, H. E.: Mediastinal and subcutaneous emphysema in diabetic coma with vomiting: report of four cases. J.A.M.A. 208:2315, 1969. — 392

51. Belcher, J. R.: Large air cysts of the lung. Brit. J. Clin. Pract. 12:87, 1958. — 321

52. Belcher, J. R., and Pattinson, J. N.: Hypoplasia of the lobar pulmonary arteries: a report of three cases. J. Thoracic Surg. 34:357, 1957. — 189

53. Belgrad, R.: Fungus ball—an unusual manifestation of coccidioidomycosis: a case report. Radiology 101:289, 1971. — 329

54. Belgrad, R., Good, C. A., and Woolner, L. B.: The alveolar-cell carcinoma (terminal bronchiolar carcinoma): a study of surgically excised tumors with special emphasis on localized lesions. Radiology 79:789, 1962. — 304, 305, 315

55. Bellini, F., and Ghislandi, E.: Calcificazioni "a guscio d'uovo" a sede extrailare in silicotubercolotico. Med. Lavoro 51:600, 1960. — 467

56. Benoit, H. W., Jr., and Ackerman, L. V.: Solitary pleural mesotheliomas. J. Thoracic Surg. 25:346, 1953.   382

57. Benton, C., and Gerard, P.: Thymolipoma in a patient with Graves' disease: case report and review of the literature. J. Thorac. Cardiovasc. Surg. 51:428, 1966.   41, 392, 419

58. Benton, C., and Silverman, F. N.: Some mediastinal lesions in children. Seminars in Roentgenology 4:91, 1969.   419

59. Berger, G.: Intralobuläre Lungensequestration. Z. Kinderchir. 5:458, 1968.   160, 163

60. Berger, H. W., and Seckler, S. G.: Pleural and pericardial effusions in rheumatoid disease. Ann. Intern. Med. 64:1291, 1966.   351

61. Berger, M., and Thompson, J. R.: Cavitary carcinomatosis of the lungs: report of a case. Dis. Chest 52:106, 1967.   319

62. Bergmann, M., Flance, I. J., and Blumenthal, H. T.: Thesaurosis following inhalation of hair spray: a clinical and experimental study. New Eng. J. Med. 258:471, 1958.   304

63. Berk, R. N.: Dilatation of the left superior intercostal vein in the plain-film diagnosis of chronic superior vena caval obstruction. Radiology 83:419, 1964.   236

64. Berkmen, Y. M.: The many facets of alveolar-cell carcinoma of the lung. Radiology 92:793, 1969.   304, 305

65. Berkmen, Y. M.: Bronchial obstruction in unresolved pneumonia. To be published.   272

66. Berlin, H. S., Stein, J., and Poppel, M. H.: Congenital superior ectopia of the kidney. Amer. J. Roentgen. 78:508, 1957.   446

67. Bernard, J., Sauvegrain, J., and Nahum, H.: Tomography of the lungs in infancy and childhood: techniques, indications and results. In Kaufmann, H. J. (Ed.): Progress in Pediatric Radiology, Vol. 1. Chicago, Year Book Medical Publishers, 1967.   15

68. Berne, A. S., Gerle, R. D., and Mitchell, G. E.: The mediastinum: normal roentgen anatomy and radiologic technics. Seminars in Roentgenology 4:3, 1969.   350, 409

69. Berne, A. S., and Heitzman, E. R.: The roentgenologic signs of pedunculated pleural tumors. Amer. J. Roentgen. 87:892, 1962.   377, 395

70. Berne, A. S., Ikins, P. M., Straehley, C. J., Jr., and Bugden, W. F.: Diagnostic carbon dioxide pneumomediastinography as an extension of scalene-lymph-node biopsy. New Eng. J. Med. 267:225, 1962.   21, 389

71. Berrigan, T. J., Jr., Carsky, E. W., and Heitzman, E. R.: Fat embolism: roentgenographic pathologic correlation in 3 cases. Amer. J. Roentgen. 96:967, 1966.   299

72. Berthelot, P., Walker, J. G., Sherlock, S., and Reid, L.: Arterial changes in the lungs in cirrhosis of the liver—lung spider nevi. New Eng. J. Med. 274:291, 1966.   213

73. Beskin, C. A., Colvin, S. H., Jr., and Beaver, P. C.: Pulmonary dirofilariasis: cause of pulmonary nodular disease. J.A.M.A. 198:665, 1966.   315

74. Bessolo, R. J., and Maddison, F. E.: Scimitar syndrome: report of a case with unusual variations. Amer. J. Roentgen. 103:572, 1968.   83, 87

75. Bidstrup, P., Nordentoft, J. M., and Petersen, B.: Hernia of the lung: brief survey and report of two cases. Acta Radiol. (Diagn) 4:490, 1966.   463

76. Birnbaum, G. L.: Anatomy of the Bronchovascular   161

System: Its Application to Surgery. Chicago, Year Book Medical Publishers, Inc., 1954.

77. Bischoff, M. E.: Noninfectious necrotizing granulomatosis: the pulmonary roentgen signs. Radiology 75:752, 1960.   347

78. Blades, B., and Dugan, D. J.: Pseudobronchiectasis. J. Thoracic Surg. 13:40, 1944.   284

79. Blades, B., and Paul, J. S.: Chest wall tumors. Ann. Surg. 131:976, 1950.   97, 385

80. Blajot, I.: Radiología Clínica del Tórax. Barcelona, Ediciones Toray, S.A., 1970.   453

81. Bland, E. F., and Castleman, B.: Pseudocoarctation of the aorta. New Eng. J. Med. 280:1466, 1969.   474

82. Blank, E., and Zuberbuhler, J. R.: Left to right shunt through a left atrial left superior vena cava. Amer. J. Roentgen. 103:87, 1968.   213

83. Blank, N., and Castellino, R. A.: Chest roentgen patterns of pleural reflections from the aortic arch to the left heart border and the diagnosis of lymphadenopathy. Presented at The Radiological Society of North America meeting, Chicago, 1970.   416

84. Blatt, E. S., Schneider, H. J., Wiot, J. F., and Felson, B.: Roentgen findings in obstructed diaphragmatic hernia. Radiology 79:648, 1962.   438, 442, 444

85. Bledsoe, F. H., and Seymour, E. Q.: Acute pulmonary edema associated with parathion poisoning. Radiology 103:53, 1972.   299

86. Blichert-Toft, M.: Fatigue fracture of the first rib. Acta Chir. Scand. 135:675, 1969.   457

87. Bliek, A. J., and Mulholland, D. J.: Extralobar lung sequestration associated with fatal neonatal respiratory distress. Thorax 26:125, 1971.   160

88. Blomquist, G., and Mahoney, P. S.: Non-collapsing air-filled esophagus in diseased and postoperative chests. Acta Radiol. 55:32, 1961.   392, 396

89. Bloomer, W. E., Liebow, A. A., and Hales, M. R.: Surgical Anatomy of the Bronchovascular Segments. Springfield, Ill., Charles C Thomas, Publisher, 1960.   156, 158

90. Blount, H. C., Jr.: Localized mesothelioma of the pleura: a review with six new cases. Radiology 67:822, 1956.   382

91. Blundell, J. E.: Pneumothorax complicating pulmonary infarction. Brit. J. Radiol. 40:226, 1967.   371

92. Bobrowitz, I. D.: Round densities within cavities: lung lesions simulating the pathognomonic roentgen sign of echinococcus cyst. Amer. Rev. Tuberc. 50:305, 1944.   327

93. Bogdonoff, M. L.: Comparative study of patients with pneumonia, atelectasis, and lung infarction following inhalation of various gas mixtures. Radiology 82:679, 1964.   305

94. Bogedain, W., and Carpathios, J.: Lesions of the azygos node area. Ohio Med. J. 59:596, 1963.   258

95. Bonte, F. J., and Schonfeld, M. D.: The axillary mass sign on lateral chest roentgenograms. Amer. J. Roentgen. 87:900, 1962.   461

96. Bookstein, J. J.: Pulmonary thromboembolism with emphasis on angiographic-pathologic correlation. Seminars in Roentgenology 5:29, 1970.   101

97. Boone, M. L., Swenson, B. E., and Felson, B.: Rib notching: its many causes. Amer. J. Roentgen. 91:1075, 1964.   454, 455, 456

98. Borman, C. N.: Broncho-pulmonary segmental anatomy and bronchography. Minn. Med. 41:820, 1958.   147

99. Botenga, A. S. J.: The role of bronchopulmonary anastomoses in chronic inflammatory processes of   231

the lung: selective arteriographic investigation. Amer. J. Roentgen. 104:829, 1968.

100. Bourassa, M. G.: The scimitar syndrome: report of two cases of anomalous venous return from a hypoplastic right lung to the inferior vena cava. Canad. Med. Assoc. J. 88:115, 1963. — 83, 87

101. Bovornkitti, S., Kangsadal, P., Sangvichien, S., and Chatikavanij, K.: Neurogenic muscular aplasia (eventration) of the diaphragm. Amer. Rev. Resp. Dis. 82:876, 1960. — 436

102. Bower, G. C.: So-called bronchiolar emphysema: its relationship to diffuse pulmonary fibrosis and pulmonary emphysema. Amer. Rev. Resp. Dis. 96:1049, 1967. — 341

103. Bowerman, D. L., and Towbin, M. N.: Bronchiolar emphysema: its significance in industrial medicine: report of a case. Dis. Chest 46:349, 1964. — 341

104. Boyd, J. F., Park, S. D. S., and Smith, G.: The correlation between various assessments of pulmonary arterial pressure in mitral stenosis. Brit. Heart J. 20:466, 1958. — 95

105. Boyden, E. A.: Cleft left upper lobes and the split anterior bronchus. Surgery 26:167, 1949. — 78

106. Boyden, E. A.: Segmental Anatomy of the Lungs. A Study of the Patterns of the Segmental Bronchi and Related Pulmonary Vessels. New York, Blakiston Division, McGraw-Hill Book Co., 1955. — 143, 147, 150, 155, 156, 158

107. Boyden, E. A.: Bronchogenic cysts and the theory of intralobar sequestration: new embryologic data. J. Thoracic Surg. 35:604, 1958. — 161

108. Boyden, E. A.: The pulmonary artery and its branches. *In* Luisada, A. (Ed.): Cardiology, Vol. I. New York, Blakiston Division, McGraw-Hill Book Co., 1959. — 187

109. Boyden, E. A.: The segmental anatomy of the lungs. *In* Myers, J. A. (Ed.): Diseases of the Chest—Including the Heart. Springfield, Ill., Charles C Thomas, Publisher, 1959. — 143

110. Boyden, E. A.: Personal communication, 1960. — 160

111. Boyden, E. A.: Respiratory system, anatomy of. Encyclopaedia Britannica, 1960. — 289

112. Boyden, E. A.: The nomenclature of the bronchopulmonary segments and their blood supply. Dis. Chest 39:1, 1961. — 147, 201, 205

113. Boyden, E. A.: The developing bronchial arteries in a fetus of the twelfth week. Amer. J. Anat. 129:357, 1970. — 230

114. Boyden, E. A.: Didactic-preclinical development of the pulmonary airways. Minn. Med. 54:894, 1971. — 289

115. Boyden, E. A.: The structure of the pulmonary acinus in a child of six years and eight months Amer. J. Anat. 132:275, 1971. — 289, 295

116. Boyden, E. A.: Development of the human lung. *In* Kelley, V. C. (Ed.): Brennemann's Practice of Pediatrics, Vol. IV. Hagerstown, Md., Harper & Row, 1972. — 289

117. Boyden, E. A., Bill, A. H., Jr., and Creighton, S. A.: Presumptive origin of a left lower accessory lung from an esophageal diverticulum. Surgery 52:323, 1962. — 160, 161

118. Boyden, E. A., and Tompsett, D. H.: Anomalous splitting of the upper lobe bronchus in right and left lungs: with a note on the incidence in the London area of left medial basal segments. J. Thoracic Surg. 37:460, 1959. — 147, 153, 157

119. Boyden, E. A., and Tompsett, D. H.: Congenital absence of the medial basal bronchus in a child: with preliminary observations on postnatal growth of the lungs. J. Thorac. Cardiovasc. Surg. 43:517, 1962. — 156

120. Boyer, R. C.: Bronchography in chronic lobar collapse. Amer. J. Roentgen. 69:28, 1953.   **16, 273**

121. Bradham, R. R., Sealy, W. C., and Young, W. G., Jr.: Chronic middle lobe infection: factors responsible for its development. Ann. Thorac. Surg. 2:612, 1966.   **327**

122. Brannan, H. M., Good, C. A., Divertie, M. B., and Baggenstoss, A. H.: Pulmonary disease associated with rheumatoid arthritis. J.A.M.A. 189:914, 1964.   **340**

123. Brauer, L.: Erfahrungen und Überlegungen zur Lungenkollapstherapie. Beitr. Klin. Tuberk. 12:49, 1909.   **433**

124. Brettner, A., Heitzman, E. R., and Woodin, W. G.: Pulmonary complications of drug therapy. Radiology 96:31, 1970.   **299, 344**

125. Bridges, R. A., Berendes, H., and Good, R. A.: A fatal granulomatous disease of childhood: the clinical, pathological, and laboratory features of a new syndrome. A.M.A. J. Dis. Child. 97:387, 1959.   **346**

126. Brijs, A.: Pneumomediastinum bei Neugeborenen. Fortschr. Roentgenstr. 110:687, 1969.   **392**

127. Broch, O. J., Moe, T., and Wehn, M.: Pulmonary fibrosis. Acta Med. Scand. 148:189, 1954.   **338, 340**

128. Brock, R. C.: The Anatomy of the Bronchial Tree (2nd ed.). London, Oxford University Press, 1954.   **71, 77, 143, 147, 150, 155**

129. Brody, J. S., and Levin, B.: Interlobular septa thickening in lipid pneumonia. Amer. J. Roentgen. 88:1061, 1962.   **245**

130. Brown, B. St. J., Dunbar, J. S., and MacEwan, D. W.: Foreign bodies in the tracheobronchial tree in childhood. J. Canad. Assoc. Radiol. 14:158, 1963.   **96**

131. Brown, O. L., Garvey, J. M., and Stern, C. A.: Diffuse intrapulmonary hemorrhage caused by Coumadin intoxication. Dis. Chest 48:525, 1965.   **302**

132. Brünner, S.: Lung Cysts. A Clinical Radiological Study. Copenhagen, Munksgaard, 1964.   **313, 321**

133. Brünner, S.: Tracheography and bronchography: techniques and indications during infancy and childhood. *In* Kaufmann, H. J. (Ed.): Progress in Pediatric Radiology. Vol. 1. Respiratory Tract. Chicago, Year Book Medical Publishers, Inc., 1967.   **16, 20, 163**

134. Bruwer, A. J.: Posteroanterior chest roentgenogram in two types of anomalous pulmonary venous connection. J. Thoracic Surg. 32:119, 1956.   **83**

135. Bruwer, A. J., and Brandenburg, R. O.: Pulmonic stenosis: posteroanterior roentgenographic appearance in 15 patients more than 34 years of age. Proc. Staff Meet. Mayo Clin. 32:567, 1957.   **192**

136. Bruwer, A. J., Clagett, O. T., and McDonald, J. R.: Intralobar bronchopulmonary sequestration. Amer. J. Roentgen. 71:751, 1954.   **160**

137. Bryant, L. R., Wiot, J. F., and Kloecker, R. J.: A study of the factors affecting the incidence and duration of postoperative pneumoperitoneum. Surg. Gynec. Obstet. 117:145, 1963.   **447**

138. Bryk, D.: Dilated right pulmonary veins in mitral insufficiency. Chest 58:24, 1970.   **138**

139. Buechner, H. A., and Ansari, A.: Acute silico-proteinosis: a new pathologic variant of acute silicosis in sandblasters, characterized by histologic features resembling alveolar proteinosis. Dis. Chest 55:274, 1969.   **304**

140. Buechner, H. A., Rabin, C. B., Schepers, G. W. H., Spain, D. M., and Ziskind, M. M.: Diffuse pulmonary lesions: the problems of differential diagnosis. Dis. Chest 43:155, 1963.   **289, 304, 305, 479**

141. Bunner, R.: Lateral intrathoracic meningocele.   389, 419
     Acta Radiol. 51:1, 1959.

142. Burchell, H. B., and Pugh, D. G.: Uncomplicated   104
     isolated dextrocardia ("dextroversio cordis" type).
     Amer. Heart J. 44:196, 1952.

143. Burke, J. F.: Early diagnosis of traumatic rupture   272
     of the bronchus. J.A.M.A. 181:682, 1962.

144. Burko, H.: Considerations in the roentgen diag-   70
     nosis of pneumonia in children. Amer. J.
     Roentgen. 88:555, 1962.

145. Burko, H., Carwell, G., and Newman, E.: Size,   201, 217
     location, and gravitational changes of normal
     upper lobe pulmonary veins. Amer. J. Roentgen.
     111:687, 1971.

146. Burman, S. O., and Kent, E. M.: Bronchiolar   341
     emphysema (cirrhosis of the lung). J. Thorac. Car-
     diovasc. Surg. 43:253, 1962.

147. Burrows, F. G. O.: Pulmonary nodules in rheuma-   315, 321
     toid disease: a report of two cases. Brit. J. Radiol.
     40:256, 1967.

148. Burton, J. F., Zawadski, E. S., Wetherell, H. R.,   299
     and Moy, T. W.: Mainliners and blue velvet. J.
     Forensic Sci. 10:466, 1965.

149. Bush, J. K., McLean, R. L., and Sieker, H. O.: Dif- 341
     fuse lung disease due to lymphangiomyoma.
     Amer. J. Med. 46:645, 1969.

150. Butt, W. P.: Mesothelioma of the pleura. J. Canad.   374
     Assoc. Radiol. 13:40, 1962.

151. Butterfield, J., Moscovici, C., Berry, C., and   321
     Kempe, C. H.: Cystic emphysema in premature
     infants: a report of an outbreak with the isolation
     of type 19 ECHO virus in one case. New Eng. J.
     Med. 268:18, 1963.

152. Caceres, J., and Felson, B.: Double primary car-   131, 315, 320
     cinoma of the lung. Radiology 102:45, 1972.

153. Caffey, J., and Silverman, F. N.: Pediatric X-Ray   403
     Diagnosis (5th ed.). Chicago, Year Book Medical
     Publishers, Inc., 1967.

154. Caffrey, P. R., and Altman, R. S.: Pulmonary al-   479
     veolar microlithiasis occurring in premature
     twins. J. Pediat. 66:758, 1965.

155. Campbell, A. H.: Spontaneous disappearance of   316
     tuberculomata of the lung. Med. J. Aust. 2:242,
     1955.

156. Campbell, D. C., Jr., Murney, J. A., and Dominy,   160, 207
     D. E.: Systemic arterial blood supply to a normal
     lung. J.A.M.A. 182:497, 1962.

157. Campbell, M.: Visible pulsation in relation to   216
     blood flow and pressure in the pulmonary artery.
     Brit. Heart J. 13:438, 1951.

158. Campbell, M. J., and Clayton, Y. M.: Bronchopul-   163, 328
     monary aspergillosis: a correlation of the clinical
     and laboratory findings in 272 patients inves-
     tigated for bronchopulmonary aspergillosis.
     Amer. Rev. Resp. Dis. 89:186, 1964.

158a. Campbell, R. E.: Intrapulmonary interstitial   392
     emphysema: a complication of hyaline membrane
     disease. Amer. J. Roentgen. 110:449, 1970.

159. Canfield, C. J., Davis, T. E., and Herman, R. H.:   302
     Hemorrhagic pulmonary-renal syndrome: report
     of three cases. New Eng. J. Med. 268:230, 1963.

160. Capitanio, M. A., and Kirkpatrick, J. A., Jr.: Pneu- 301
     mocystis carinii pneumonia. Amer. J. Roentgen.
     97:174, 1966.

161. Carabasi, R. J., Christian, J. J., and Brindley. H. 456
     H.: Costosternal chondrodynia: a variant of
     Tietze's syndrome? Dis. Chest 41:559, 1962.

162. Carlson, V., Martin, J. E., Keegan, J. M., and   164, 273

Dailey, J. E.: Roentgenographic features of mucoid impaction of the bronchi. Amer. J. Roentgen. 96:947, 1966.

163. Carmichael, J. H. E., Julian, D. G., Jones, G. P., and Wren, E. M.: Radiological signs in pulmonary hypertension: the significance of lines B of Kerley. Brit. J. Radiol. 27:393, 1954.   246

164. Carr, D. T., and Olsen, A. M.: Tracheopathia osteoplastica. J.A.M.A. 155:1563, 1954.   489

164a. Carrington, C. B.: Personal communication, 1972.   344

165. Carrington, C. B., Addington, W. W., Goff, A. M., Madoff, I. M., Marks, A., Schwaber, J. R., and Gaensler, E. A.: Chronic eosinophilic pneumonia. New Eng. J. Med. 280:787, 1969.   301

166. Carter, B. N., Giuseffi, J., and Felson, B.: Traumatic diaphragmatic hernia. Amer. J. Roentgen. 65:56, 1951.   437, 438, 440, 443

167. Castellino, R. A., and Blank, N.: Adenopathy of the cardiophrenic angle (diaphragmatic) lymph nodes. Amer. J. Roentgen. 114:509, 1972.   260

168. Castellino, R. A., Blank, N., and Adams, D. F.: Dilated azygos and hemiazygos veins presenting as paravertebral intrathoracic masses. New Eng. J. Med. 278:1087, 1968.   395

169. Cathcart, R. T., Theodos, P. A., and Fraimow, W.: Anthracosilicosis: selected aspects related to the evaluation of disability, cavitation, and the unusual X-ray. A.M.A. Arch. Intern. Med. 106:368, 1960.   345

170. Cauldwell, E. W., Siekert, R. G., Lininger, R. E., and Anson, B. J.: The bronchial arteries: an anatomic study of 150 human cadavers. Surg. Gynec. Obstet. 86:395, 1948.   230

171. Cha, E. M., and Khoury, G. H.: Persistent left superior vena cava: radiologic and clinical significance. Radiology 103:375, 1972.   213

172. Chait, A., and Zucker, M.: The superior vena cava in the evaluation of atrial septal defect. Amer. J. Roentgen. 103:104, 1968.   236

173. Chang, C. H.: The normal roentgenographic measurement of the right descending pulmonary artery in 1,085 cases. Amer. J. Roentgen. 87:929, 1962.   187

174. Chang, C. H.: The value of the lateral chest roentgenogram in the diagnosis of pulmonary venous hypertension. Radiology 92:117, 1969.   189

175. Chang, C. H., and Smith, C. A.: Postictal pulmonary edema. Radiology 89:1087, 1967.   299

176. Chang, L. W. M., Lee, F. A., and Gwinn, J. L.: Normal lateral deviation of the trachea in infants and children. Amer. J. Roentgen. 109:247, 1970.   269

177. Chapman, J. S.: Spontaneous irruption of air from the lung. I. Pneumomediastinum. Amer. J. Med. 18:547, 1955.   395

178. Charrette, E. E., Mariano, A. V., and Laforet, E. G.: Solitary mast cell "tumor" of lung: its place in the spectrum of mast cell disease. Arch. Intern. Med. 118:358, 1966.   315

179. Chasler, C. N.: Pneumothorax and pneumomediastinum in the newborn. Amer. J. Roentgen. 91:550, 1964.   370

180. Chavez, C. M., and Conn, J. H.: Thoracic duct laceration: closure under conservative management based on lymphangiography evaluation. J. Thorac. Cardiovasc. Surg. 51:724, 1966.   21, 250

181. Chen, J. T. T., Capp, M. P., Johnsrude, I. S., Goodrich, J. K., and Lester, R. G.: Roentgen appearance of pulmonary vascularity in the diag-   192

nosis of heart disease. Amer. J. Roentgen. 112:559, 1971.

182. Chen, J. T. T., Robinson, A. E., Goodrich, J. K., and Lester, R. G.: Uneven distribution of pulmonary blood flow between left and right lungs in isolated valvular pulmonary stenosis. Amer. J. Roentgen. 107:343, 1969. — 192

183. Chinachoti, N., and Tangchai, P.: Pulmonary alveolar microlithiasis associated with the inhalation of snuff in Thailand. Dis. Chest 32:687, 1957. — 305, 479

184. Chipman, C. D., Aikens, R. L., and Nonamaker, E. P.: Pericardial fat necrosis. Canad. Med. Assoc. J. 86:237, 1962. — 419, 463

185. Christie, A., and Peterson, J. C.: Pulmonary calcification in negative reactors to tuberculin. Amer. J. Public Health 35:1131, 1945. — 464

186. Christoforidis, A. J.: Radiological manifestations of endobronchial obstruction: experimental study of dogs. Doctoral thesis, Ohio State University, Columbus, 1957. — 97, 288

187. Christoforidis, A. J., Nelson, S. W., and Pratt, P. C.: Bronchiolar dilatation associated with muscular hyperplasia: polycystic lung. Emphasis on the roentgenologic findings. Amer. J. Roentgen. 92:513, 1964. — 341

188. Churchill, E. D., and Belsey, R.: Segmental pneumonectomy in bronchiectasis: lingula segment of left upper lobe. Ann. Surg. 109:481, 1939. — 143

189. Ciaglia, P.: Intrathoracic meningocele. J. Thoracic Surg. 23:283, 1942. — 419

190. Ciba Foundation Symposium: Terminology, definitions, and classification of chronic pulmonary emphysema and related conditions; a report. Thorax 14:286, 1959. — 307

191. Cicciarelli, F. E., Soule, E. H., and McGoon, D. C.: Lipoma and liposarcoma of the mediastinum: a report of 14 tumors including one of the thymus. J. Thorac. Cardiovasc. Surg. 47:411, 1964. — 419

192. Cimmino, C. V.: The esophageal-pleural stripe on chest teleroentgenograms. Radiology 67:754, 1956. — 409

193. Cimmino, C. V.: Modification (pharmacogenic?) of subphrenic abscess. Virginia Med. Monthly 84:444, 1957. — 423, 436

194. Cimmino, C. V.: The anterior mediastinal line on chest roentgenograms. Radiology 82:459, 1964. — 409

195. Clark, R. L., Goldenberg, D. B., and Blazek, J. V.: Abnormal vascular communications. Amer. J. Roentgen. 107:413, 1969. — 162, 213

196. Clark, R. L., Margulies, S. I., and Mulholland, J. H.: Histiocytosis X: a fatal case with unusual pulmonary manifestations. Radiology 95:631, 1970. — 321

197. Cody, P. H.: Pneumothorax of the newborn. J. Coll. Radiol. Aust. 5:18, 1961. — 366

198. Cohen, A. G.: Atelectasis of the right middle lobe resulting from perforation of tuberculous lymph nodes into bronchi in adults. Ann. Intern. Med. 35:821, 1951. — 465

199. Cohen, A. G., and Geffen, A.: Roentgenographic methods in pulmonary disease. Amer. J. Med. 10:375, 1951. — 11, 95

200. Cohen, A. S.: Amyloidosis. New Eng. J. Med. 277:628, 1967. — 341

201. Cohen, W. N., and McAlister, W. H.: Pneumocystis carinii pneumonia: report of four cases. Amer. J. Roentgen. 89:1032, 1963. — 301

201a. Collins, J. D., Furmanski, S., Steckel, R. J., and Snow, H. D.: Minimum calcification demonstra- — 479 ble in pulmonary nodules: a roentgen pathology model. Radiology 105:49, 1972.

202. Collins, V. P., Loeffler, R. K., and Tivey, H.: Observations on growth rates of human tumors. Amer. J. Roentgen. 76:988, 1956.   315

203. Condon, V. R., and Phillips, E. W.: Bronchial adenoma in children: a review of the literature and report of three cases. Amer. J. Roentgen. 88:543, 1962.   272

204. Conte, P., Heitzman, E. R., and Markarian, B.: Viral pneumonia: roentgen pathological correlations. Radiology 95:267, 1970.   301

205. Cooke, C. R., and Hyland, J. W.: Pathological calcification of the lungs following intravenous administration of calcium. Amer. J. Med. 29:363, 1960.   479

206. Cooley, J. C., and Gillespie, J. B.: Mediastinal emphysema: pathogenesis and management. Report of a case. Dis. Chest 49:104, 1966.   392

207. Cooley, R. N.: Pulmonary thromboembolism— the case for the pulmonary angiogram. Amer. J. Roentgen. 92:693, 1964.   21

208. Cosemans, J., and Gyselen, A.: Osteoplastic tracheopathy: report of a case. Dis. Chest 45:332, 1964.   489

209. Coventry, W. D., and LaBree, R. H.: Heterotopia of bone marrow simulating mediastinal tumor: a manifestation of chronic hemolytic anemia in adults. Ann. Intern. Med. 53:1042, 1960.   419

210. Craig, J. M., Kirkpatrick, J., and Neuhauser, E. B. D.: Congenital cystic adenomatoid malformation of the lung in infants. Amer. J. Roentgen. 76:516, 1956.   304, 343

211. Cranz, H. J., and Pribram, H. F. W.: The pulmonary vessels in the diagnosis of lobar collapse. Amer. J. Roentgen. 94:665, 1965.   107

211a. Cremin, B. J., and Movsowitz, H.: Lobar emphysema in infants. Brit. J. Radiol. 44:692, 1971.   135

212. Cross, C. E., Shaver, J. A., Wilson, R. J., and Robin, E. D.: Mitral stenosis and pulmonary fibrosis: special reference to pulmonary edema and lung lymphatic function. Arch. Intern. Med. 125:248, 1970.   241, 246

213. Crutcher, R., and Plott, C.: Mediastinal lipoma. J. Thoracic Surg. 27:261, 1954.   392, 419

214. Cubillo, E., and Rockoff, S. D.: Milk of calcium fluid in an intrapulmonary bronchogenic cyst. Chest 60:608, 1971.   180, 492

215. Cubillo-Herguera, E., and McAlister, W. H.: The pulmonary meniscus sign in a case of bronchogenic carcinoma. Radiology 92:1299, 1969.   327

216. Cudkowicz, L.: The Human Bronchial Circulation in Health and Disease. Baltimore, Williams & Wilkins Co., 1968.   230

217. Cueto, J. C., McFee, A. S., and Bernstein, E. F.: Intrathoracic pheochromocytoma. Dis. Chest 48:539, 1965.   419

218. Culiner, M. M.: Obliterative bronchitis and bronchiolitis with bronchiectasis. Dis. Chest 44:351, 1963.   313

219. Culiner, M. M.: Bronchial cysts and collateral ventilation. Dis. Chest 45:627, 1964.   180, 282

220. Culiner, M. M.: Collateral ventilation and the hyperlucent lung. Amer. J. Med. 36:395, 1964.   282

221. Culiner, M. M.: The hyperlucent lung, a problem in differential diagnosis. Dis. Chest 49:578, 1966.   223, 282

222. Culiner, M. M.: The right middle lobe syndrome, a non-obstructive complex. Dis. Chest 50:57, 1966.   95, 96, 282

223. Culiner, M. M., and Reich, S. B.: Collateral ventilation and localized emphysema. Amer. J. Roentgen. 85:246, 1961. — 180, 184, 273

224. Cumming, G.: Unilateral hyperlucent lung. J. Pediat. 78:250, 1971. — 223

225. Currarino, G., and Silverman, F. N.: Premature obliteration of the sternal sutures and pigeon-breast deformity. Radiology 70:532, 1958. — 459

226. Curry, T. S., III, and Curry, G. C.: Atresia of the bronchus to the apical posterior segment of the left upper lobe. Amer. J. Roentgen. 98:350, 1966. — 180

227. Dabbs, C. H., Berg, R., and Peirce, E. C.: Intrapericardial bronchogenic cysts: report of two cases and probable embryologic explanation. J. Thoracic Surg. 34:718, 1957. — 491

228. Dalith, F., and Neufeld, H.: Radiological diagnosis of anomalous pulmonary venous connection: a tomographic study. Radiology 74:1, 1960. — 83, 87

229. Dalton, C. J., and Schwartz, S. S.: Evaluation of the paraspinal line in roentgen examination of the thorax. Radiology 66:195, 1956. — 382, 409

230. D'Angio, G. J., and Iannaccone, G.: Spontaneous pneumothorax as a complication of pulmonary metastases in malignant tumors of childhood. Amer. J. Roentgen. 86:1092, 1961. — 371

231. Danner, P. K., McFarland, D. R., and Felson, B.: Massive pulmonary gangrene. Amer. J. Roentgen. 103:548, 1968. — 327

232. Darke, C. S., Chrispin, A. R., and Snowden, B. S.: Unilateral lung transradiancy: a physiological study. Thorax 15:74, 1960. — 223

233. Darke, C. S., and Middleton, R. S. W.: Calcification of the lungs after chicken pox. Brit. J. Dis. Chest 61:198, 1967. — 474

234. Daves, M. L.: Skiagraphing the mediastinal moguls. New Physician, p. 49, January, 1970. — 399, 497

235. Daves, M. L., and Walsh, J. A.: Minihemithorax. Amer. J. Roentgen. 109:528, 1970. — 83, 105

236. Davidson, J. W.: Pulmonary complications of lymphography. New Eng. J. Med. 285:237, 1971. — 245, 299

237. Davidson, S. W.: Some anomalies of the respiratory system. J. Fac. Radiol. 8:1, 1956. — 83, 153, 160

238. Davies, L. G., Goodwin, J. F., Steiner, R. E., and Van Leuven, B. D.: The clinical and radiological assessment of the pulmonary arterial pressure in mitral stenosis. Brit. Heart J. 15:393, 1953. — 216

239. Davila, J. C., Hamilton, G. B., and Charbonneau, A.: Systemic-pulmonary arterioarterial fistula: report of a case. A.M.A. Arch. Surg. 76:496, 1958. — 232, 456

240. Davis, J. G., and Simonton, J. H.: Mediastinal carinal bronchogenic cysts. Radiology 67:391, 1956. — 3, 4, 304

241. Davis, L. A.: The vertical fissure line. Amer. J. Roentgen. 84:451, 1960. — 72

242. Davis, S., Gardner, F., and Qvist, G.: The shape of a pleural effusion. Brit. Med. J. 1:436, 1963. — 351

243. Davis, W. S., and Allen, R. P.: Accessory diaphragm: duplication of the diaphragm. Radiol. Clin. N. Amer. 6:253, 1968. — 83, 92, 120, 386, 428

244. Davison, L. M.: Neurofibromatosis with diffuse interstitial pulmonary fibrosis and phaeochromocytoma. Brit. J. Radiol. 40:549, 1967. — 341

245. Dawson, J.: Pulmonary tuberous sclerosis and its relationship to other forms of the disease. Quart. J. Med. 23:113, 1954. — 341

246. D'Cruz, I. A., and Arcilla, R. A.: Anomalous venous drainage of the left lung into the inferior vena cava. Amer. Heart J. 67:549, 1964. — 81

247. DeMasi, C. J.: Allergic pulmonary infiltrates probably due to nitrofurantoin. Arch. Intern. Med. 120:631, 1967.   246

248. Demy, N. G., and Gewanter, A. P.: Correlation of upper lobe vascularization with certain congenital intracardiac shunts. Radiology 62:329, 1954.   220

249. Desai, M. G.: Widened and kinked descending part of the thoracic aorta simulating intra-thoracic tumour. Brit. J. Radiol. 30:391, 1957.   419

250. Dévé, F.: Le signe radiologique de la "calotte aérienne" n'est pas rigoureusement pathognomonique du kyste hydatique du poumon. Semana Méd. 1:1081, 1938.   327

251. Dietrich, D. E.: Intrathoracic herniation of the kidney. Dis. Chest 44:315, 1963.   437

252. Di Guglielmo, L., and Bonomo, B.: The significance of the lateral subsegments of the lung in pulmonary disease: a review of 500 cases. Acta Radiol. 44:217, 1955.   151

253. Dijkstra, C.: Technique and hazards of bronchography general classification of bronchial diseases. Medicamundi 3:101, 1957.   288

254. Dijkstra, C.: Bronchography. Springfield, Ill., Charles C Thomas, Publisher, 1958.   16

255. Diner, W. C., Kniker, W. T., and Heiner, D. C.: Roentgenologic manifestations in the lungs in milk allergy. Radiology 77:564, 1961.   302

256. Dines, D. E.: Diagnostic significance of pneumatocele of the lung. J.A.M.A. 204:1169, 1968.   321

257. Di Rienzo, S.: Radiologic Exploration of the Bronchus. Springfield, Ill., Charles C Thomas, Publisher, 1949.   16, 135, 147, 269, 285

258. Dixon, A. St. J., and Ball, J.: Honeycomb lung and chronic rheumatoid arthritis: a case report. Ann. Rheum. Dis. 16:241, 1957.   340

259. Dodd, G. D., and Boyle, J. J.: Excavating pulmonary metastases. Amer. J. Roentgen. 85:277, 1961.   321

260. Doig, A. T.: Atelectatic bronchiectasis of the right middle lobe. Tubercle 27:173, 1946.   13

261. Don, C., and Gray, D. G.: Cavitating secondary carcinoma of the lung. J. Canad. Assoc. Radiol. 19:310, 1967.   321

262. Donegan, C. K., and Nouse, D. C.: Diagnostic difficulties in evaluating pulsating mediastinal masses. J.A.M.A. 157:798, 1955.   1

263. Doniach, I., Morrison, B., and Steiner, R. E.: Lung changes during hexamethonium therapy for hypertension. Brit. Heart J. 16:101, 1954.   344

264. Doppman, J. L.: Infrahepatic interruption of the inferior vena cava with azygos continuation. Dis. Chest 53:349, 1968.   236

265. Doppman, J. L., and Lavender, J. P.: The hilum and the large left ventricle. Radiology 80:931, 1963.   185, 192, 201, 217

266. Dornhorst, A. C., and Pierce, J. W.: Pulmonary collapse and consolidation: the role of collapse in the production of lung field shadows and the significance of segments in inflammatory lung disease. J. Fac. Radiol. 5:276, 1954.   143, 180

267. Doub, H. P., and Jones, H. C.: Hernia of the mediastinum. Amer. J. Roentgen. 38:297, 1937.   105

268. Doyle, A. E., Goodwin, J. F., Harrison, C. V., and Steiner, R. E.: Pulmonary vascular patterns in pulmonary hypertension. Brit. Heart J. 19:353, 1957.   217

269. Doyle, F. H., Read, A. E., and Evans, K. T.: The mediastinum in portal hypertension. Clin. Radiol. 12:114, 1961.   395

270. Doyle, O. W.: Misleading shadows on chest films.   **461**
     Southern Med. J. 52:1516, 1959.
271. Dozois, R. R., Bernatz, P. E., Woolner, L. B., and   **419**
     Andersen, H. A.: Sclerosing mediastinitis involv-
     ing major bronchi. Mayo Clin. Proc. 43:557, 1968.
272. Dragsted, P. J., and Rodbro, P.: Pseudocysts of   **321**
     the lungs in kerosene poisoning: report of two
     cases. Dis. Chest 48:87, 1965.
273. Drake, E. H., and Lynch, J. P.: Bronchiectasis as-   **428**
     sociated with anomaly of right pulmonary vein
     and right diaphragm: report of a case. J. Thoracic
     Surg. 19:433, 1950.
274. Dressler, W., and Kleinfeld, M.: Tic of the respi-   **433**
     ratory muscles: report of three cases and review of
     literature. Amer. J. Med. 16:61, 1954.
275. Drevvatne, T., and Frimann-Dahl, J.: Peripheral   **314**
     bronchial carcinomas: a radiological and patho-
     logical study. Brit. J. Radiol. 34:180, 1961.
276. Dulfano, M. J., and Di Rienzo, A.: Laminagraphic   **223**
     observations of the lung vasculature in chronic
     pulmonary emphysema. Amer. J. Roentgen.
     88:1043, 1962.
277. Dulfano, M. J., and Hewetson, J.: Radiologic con-   **53, 288**
     tributions to the nosology of obstructive lung
     disease entities. Dis. Chest 50:270, 1966.
278. Dunbar, J. S.: Fractures and pseudoarthroses of   **457**
     the first rib. J. Canad. Assoc. Radiol. 7:14, 1956.
279. Dunbar, J. S., and Favreau, M.: Infrapulmonary   **351, 366**
     pleural effusion with particular reference to its oc-
     currence in nephrosis. J. Canad. Assoc. Radiol.
     10:24, 1959.
280. Dunham, H. K.: Personal communication.   **24**
281. Dunham, H. K.: The stereoscopic x-ray examina-   **14**
     tion of the chest with special reference to the
     diagnosis of pulmonary tuberculosis. Bull. Johns
     Hopkins Hosp. 22:229, 1911.
282. Dunphy, B.: Acute occupational cadmium poison-   **299, 344**
     ing: a critical review of the literature. J. Occupat.
     Med. 9:22, 1967.
283. Durnin, R. E., Lababidi, A., Butler, C., Selke, A.,   **161**
     and Flege, J. B.: Bronchopulmonary sequestra-
     tion. Chest 57:454, 1970.
284. Edge, J. R., Millard, F. J. C., Reid, L., and Simon,   **308**
     G.: The radiographic appearances of the chest in
     persons of advanced age. Brit. J. Radiol. 37:769,
     1964.
285. Edland, R. W., Levine, S., Serfas, L. S., and Flair,   **419**
     R. C.: Seminoma-like tumor in the hyperplastic
     thymus gland: a case report and literature review.
     Amer. J. Roentgen. 103:25, 1968.
286. Edling, N. P. G.: The radiologic appearances of   **459**
     the heart, oesophagus and lungs in funnel chest
     deformity. Acta Radiol. 39:273, 1953.
287. Eggenschwyler, H.: Schalenförmige Hilus-   **467**
     verkalkungen ohne Silikose. Radiol. Clin. 19:77,
     1950.
288. Eiken, M., Nielsen, R., and Baden, H.: Intra-os-   **21**
     seous costal venography: assessment of the
     method in studies on portal hypertension. Amer.
     J. Roentgen. 94:172, 1965.
289. Eklöf, O., and Gooding, C. A.: Paravertebral wi-   **405**
     dening in cases of neuroblastoma. Brit. J. Radiol.
     40:358, 1967.
290. Elliott, G. B., Belkin, A., and Donald, W. A. J.:   **133, 272**
     Cystic bronchial papillomatosis. Clin. Radiol.
     13:62, 1962.
291. Ellis, F. H., Jr., and Bruwer, A. J.: The roentgeno-   **258**
     graphic image of the azygos vein: a possible

source of diagnostic confusion. Proc. Staff Meet. Mayo Clin. 29:508, 1954.

292. Ellis, F. H., Jr., et al.: Surgical implications of the mediastinal shadow in the thoracic roentgenograms of infants and children. Surg. Gynec. Obstet. 100:532, 1955. 403

293. Ellis, K.: Lymphangiomyomatosis of the lung. To be published. 341

294. Ellis, K., and Gregg, H. G.: Thymomas—roentgen considerations. Amer. J. Roentgen. 91:105, 1964. 403

295. Ellis, K., Leeds, N. E., and Himmelstein, A.: Congenital deficiencies in the parietal pericardium. Amer. J. Roentgen. 82:125, 1959. 395

296. Ellis, K., Seaman, W. B., Griffiths, S. P., Berdon, W. E., and Baker, D. H.: Some congenital anomalies of the pulmonary arteries. Seminars in Roentgenology 2:325, 1967. 104, 160, 205, 207

297. Ellis, P. R., Jr., et al.: Massive pulmonary cavitary bleeding. Dis. Chest 40:18, 1961. 251, 327

298. Ellis, R. H.: Disease of the right middle lobe in pneumoconiosis. Brit. J. Dis. Chest 58:169, 1964. 272

299. Ellman, P.: Discussion on the lungs as an index of systemic disease. Proc. Roy. Soc. Med. 51:654, 1958. 340

300. Engel, S.: Handbuch der Röntgendiagnostik und -Therapie im Kindesalter. Leipzig, Georg Thieme Verlag, 1933. 251

300a. Ennis, J. T., et al.: Intralobar pulmonary sequestration in association with bilateral systemic arterialization of the lungs. Brit. J. Radiol. 45:949, 1972. 163

301. Epstein, B. S.: Diaphragmatic changes incident to hepatic neoplasms. Amer. J. Roentgen. 82:114, 1959. 436

302. Eraklis, A. J., Griscom, N. T., and McGovern, J. B.: Bronchogenic cysts of the mediastinum in infancy. New Eng. J. Med. 281:1150, 1969. 405

303. Ernst, S. M. P. G., and Bruschke, A. V. G.: An aberrant systemic artery to the right lung with normal pulmonary tissue. Chest 60:606, 1971. 207

304. Esser, C.: Topographische Ausdeutung der Bronchien im Röntgenbild unter besonderer Berücksichtigung des Raumfaktors. Stuttgart, Georg Thieme Verlag, 1957. 147, 150, 168

305. Esser, C.: Body-section radiography of the bronchial tree: with special reference to a modified lateral projection. Med. Radiogr. Photogr. 36:38, 1960. 15

306. Evander, L. C.: Pleural fat pads: a cause of thoracic shadows. Amer. Rev. Tuberc. 57:495, 1948. 377

307. Evans, B. H., and Haight, C.: Surgical removal of unsuspected mediastinal lymphoblastomas: report of four cases and a review of the literature. Arch. Surg. 57:307, 1948. 260

308. Evans, K. T., Cockshott, W. P., and Hendrickse, P. de V.: Pulmonary changes in malignant trophoblastic disease. Brit. J. Radiol. 38:161, 1965. 289

309. Eyler, W. R.: Pulmonary findings in the collagen diseases. Radiology 73:109, 1959. 340

310. Fagan, C. J.: Traumatic lung cyst. Amer. J. Roentgen. 97:186, 1966. 346

311. Fagan, C. J., and Swischuk, L. E.: The opaque lung in lobar emphysema. Amer. J. Roentgen. 114:300, 1972. 142

312. Falconer, B.: Calcification of hyaline cartilage in man. Arch. Path. 26:942, 1938. 452

313. Falkenbach, K. H., et al.: Pneumocystis carinii pneumonia. Amer. J. Roentgen. 85:706, 1961. 301

314. Falkenbach, K. H., Zheutlin, N., Dowdy, A. H., and O'Loughlin, B. J.: Pulmonary hypertension due to pulmonary arterial coarctation. Radiology 73:575, 1959.   205

315. Favez, G., and Soliman, O.: L'exploration radiologique du poumon et du médiastin à l'aide de la tomographie oblique posterieure à 55°. Basel, S. Karger, 1966.   15

316. Favour, C. B., and Sosman, M. C.: Erythema nodosum. Arch. Intern. Med. 80:435, 1947.   260

317. Feder, B. H., and Wilk, S. P.: Localized interlobar effusion in heart failure: phantom lung tumor. Dis. Chest 30:289, 1956.   360

318. Feinberg, S. B., Lester, R. G., and Burke, B. A.: The roentgen findings in pneumocystis carinii pneumonia. Radiology 76:594, 1961.   301

319. Feist, J. H.: Selective cinebronchography in obstructive and restrictive pulmonary disease. Amer. J. Roentgen. 99:544, 1967.   272

320. Feldman, D. J.: Localized interlobar effusion in heart failure. J.A.M.A. 146:1408, 1951.   360

321. Felman, A. H.: Neurogenic pulmonary edema: observations in 6 patients. Amer. J. Roentgen. 112:393, 1971.   299

322. Felman, A. H.: Lingular and upper lobe atelectasis and cardiomegaly: an unusual pattern simulating pleural effusion. Brit. J. Radiol. 45:299, 1972.   72

323. Felson, B.: Acute miliary diseases of the lung. Radiology 59:32, 1952.   289, 301

324. Felson, B.: Fluoroscopy of the chest. Dis. Chest 27:322, 1955.   2

325. Felson, B.: The lobes and interlobar pleura: fundamental roentgen considerations. Amer. J. Med. Sci. 230:572, 1955.   59, 71, 100, 101, 109, 133, 379

326. Felson, B.: Some special signs in chest roentgenology. *In* Rabin, C. B. (Ed.): Roentgenology of the Chest. Springfield, Ill., Charles C Thomas, Publisher, 1958.   58, 124, 131, 255, 256, 258, 316, 362, 380, 489

327. Felson, B.: Uncommon roentgen patterns of pulmonary sarcoidosis. Dis. Chest 34:357, 1958.   302, 337, 340

328. Felson, B.: Less familiar roentgen patterns of pulmonary granulomas: sarcoidosis, histoplasmosis and noninfectious necrotizing granulomatosis (Wegener's syndrome). Amer. J. Roentgen. 81:211, 1959.   341

329. Felson, B.: Some less familiar roentgen manifestations of intrathoracic histoplasmosis. Arch. Intern. Med. 103:54, 1959.   257, 263

330. Felson, B.: Fundamentals of Chest Roentgenology. Philadelphia, W. B. Saunders Co., 1960.   147, 428

331. Felson, B.: Disseminated interstitial diseases of the lung. Ann. Radiol. 9:325, 1966.   330, 332, 335, 336, 339, 342, 344

332. Felson, B.: Letter from the editor. Seminars in Roentgenology 2:221, 1967.   272, 467, 474

333. Felson, B.: The roentgen diagnosis of disseminated pulmonary alveolar diseases. Seminars in Roentgenology 2:3, 1967.   292, 293, 333, 479

334. Felson, B.: Abdominal gas: a roentgen approach. Ann. N.Y. Acad. Sci. 150:141, 1968.   449

335. Felson, B.: Letter from the editor. Seminars in Roentgenology 3:323, 1968.   213, 419

336. Felson, B.: More chest roentgen signs and how to teach them. Radiology 90:429, 1968.   41

337. Felson, B.: Letter from the editor. Seminars in Roentgenology 4:1, 1969.   28

338. Felson, B.: The mediastinum. Seminars in Roentgenology 4:41, 1969.   39, 382, 383, 397, 404, 419

339. Felson, B.: Thoracic calcifications. Dis. Chest 56:330, 1969. — 473

340. Felson, B.: Pulmonary agenesis and related anomalies. Seminars in Roentgenology 7:17, 1972. — 428

341. Felson, B.: The many faces of pulmonary sequestration. Seminars in Roentgenology 7:3, 1972. — 160

342. Felson, B., and Braunstein, H.: Noninfectious necrotizing granulomatosis: Wegener's syndrome, lethal granuloma, and allergic angiitis and granulomatosis. Radiology 70:326, 1958. — 272, 346, 347

343. Felson, B., and Felson, H.: Localization of intrathoracic lesions by means of the postero-anterior roentgenogram: the silhouette sign. Radiology 55:363, 1950. — 26, 29, 33, 34, 35, 37, 38, 78

344. Felson, B., and Felson, H.: Acute diffuse pneumonia of asthmatics. Amer. J. Roentgen. 74:235, 1955. — 301

345. Felson, B., Fleischner, F. G., McDonald, J. R., and Rabin, C. B.: Some basic principles in the diagnosis of chest diseases. Radiology 73:740, 1959. — 241, 300, 319, 323, 354, 355, 356

346. Felson, B., Jones, G. F., and Ulrich, R. P.: Roentgenologic aspects of diffuse miliary granulomatous pneumonitis of unknown etiology. Amer. J. Roentgen. 64:740, 1950. — 474

347. Felson, B., and Lessure, A. P.: "Downhill" varices of the esophagus. Dis. Chest 46:740, 1964. — 236, 465

348. Felson, B., and Palayew, M. J.: The two types of right aortic arch. Radiology 81:745, 1963. — 414, 419

349. Felson, B., Rosenberg, L. S., and Hamburger, M., Jr.: Roentgen findings in acute Friedländer's pneumonia. Radiology 53:559, 1949. — 133, 136, 183, 184

350. Felson, B., Weinstein, A. S., and Spitz, H. B.: Principles of Chest Roentgenology: A Programed Text. Philadelphia, W. B. Saunders Co., 1965. — 454

351. Felson, B., and Wiot, J. F.: Case of the Day. Springfield, Ill., Charles C Thomas, Publisher, 1967. — 395, 400, 467, 474, 493

352. Felson, H., and Heublein, G. W.: Some observations on diffuse pulmonary lesions. Amer. J. Roentgen. 59:59, 1948. — 29, 289

352a. Fennessy, J. J.: Bronchial brushing in the diagnosis of peripheral lung lesions: a preliminary report. Amer. J. Roentgen. 98:474, 1966. — 265

353. Ferencz, C., and Currarino, G.: Personal communication. — 83, 87

354. Ferencz, C., Johnson, A. L., and Goldbloom, A.: Problem of differential diagnosis in infants with large hearts and increased blood flow to the lungs. Pediatrics 13:30, 1954. — 216

355. Ferguson, T. B., and Burford, T. H.: The changing pattern of pulmonary suppuration: surgical implications. Dis. Chest. 53:396, 1968. — 327

356. Field, C. E.: Pulmonary agenesis and hypoplasia. Arch. Dis. Child. 21:61, 1946. — 83

357. Fifer, W. R., Woellner, R. C., and Gordon, S. S.: Mediastinal histoplasmosis: report of three cases with dysphagia as the presenting complaint. Dis. Chest 47:518, 1965. — 419

358. Figiel, S. J., Figiel, L. S., and Rush, D. K.: Changes in the linear thoracic paraspinal shadow due to para-aortic hemorrhage: a new sign of dissecting aortic aneurysm. Dis. Chest 49:379, 1966. — 419

359. Figley, M. M.: Mediastinal minutiae. Seminars in Roentgenology 4:22, 1969. — 409

360. Figley, M. M., Gerdes, A. J., and Ricketts, H. J.: Radiographic aspects of pulmonary embolism. Seminars in Roentgenology 2:389, 1967. — 21

361. Findlay, C. W., Jr., and Maier, H. C.: Anomalies — 81, 213

of the pulmonary vessels and their surgical significance: with a review of literature. Surgery 29:604, 1951.

362. Fischer, E.: Verkalkungsformen der Rippenknorpel. Fortschr. Roentgenstr. 82:474, 1955.   **452, 453**

363. Fischer, H. W., and Blaug, S. M.: Aerosol bronchography. Radiology 92:150, 1969.   **16, 267**

364. Fiser, F.: Branching of the bronchi with special reference to lung subsegments. Fortschr. Roentgenstr. 97:425, 1962.   **150**

365. Fishbone, G.: The azygos vein in right aortic arch. Radiology 96:45, 1970.   **236**

366. Fisher, A. M. H., Kendall, B., and Van Leuven, B. D.: Hodgkin's disease: a radiological survey. Clin. Radiol. 13:115, 1962.   **260, 489**

367. Fleischner, F. G.: Personal communication.   **49, 107**

368. Fleischner, F. G.: Das Röntgenbild der interlobaren Pleuritis und seine Differentialdiagnose. Ergeb. Med. Strahlforsch. 2:197, 1926.   **12, 360**

369. Fleischner, F. G.: Der sichtbare Bronchialbaum, ein differentialdiagnostisches Symptom im Röntgenbild der Pneumonia. Fortschr. Roentgenstr. 36:319, 1927.   **60**

370. Fleischner, F. G.: Über das Wesen der basalen horizontalen Schattenstreifen im Lungenfeld. Wien. Arch. Inn. Med. 28:461, 1936.   **436**

371. Fleischner, F. G.: The visible bronchial tree: a roentgen sign in pneumonic and other pulmonary consolidations. Radiology 50:184, 1948.   **60**

372. Fleischner, F. G.: The pathogenesis of bronchiectasis: a roentgen contribution. Radiology 53:818, 1949.   **96, 97, 98**

373. Fleischner, F. G.: The esophagus and mediastinal lymphadenopathy in bronchial carcinoma. Radiology 58:48, 1952.   **8**

374. Fleischner, F. G.: Unilateral pulmonary embolism with increased compensatory circulation through the unoccluded lung. Radiology 73:591, 1959.   **223, 299**

375. Fleischner, F. G.: Pulmonary embolism. Clin. Radiol. 13:169, 1962.   **224**

376. Fleischner, F. G.: Atypical arrangement of free pleural effusion. Radiol. Clin. N. Amer. 1:347, 1963.   **351, 352, 354, 366**

377. Fleischner, F. G.: Roentgenology of the pulmonary infarct. Seminars in Roentgenology 2:61, 1967.   **305**

378. Fleischner, F. G.: The butterfly pattern of acute pulmonary edema. Amer. J. Cardiol. 20:39, 1967.   **290**

379. Fleischner, F. G., Bernstein, C., and Levine, B. E.: Retrosternal infiltration in malignant lymphoma. Radiology 51:350, 1948.   **260, 463**

380. Fleischner, F. G., and Castleman, B.: Mesothelioma of pleura. New Eng. J. Med. 276:230, 1967.   **377, 489**

381. Fleischner, F. G., Hampton, A. O., and Castleman, B.: Linear shadows in the lungs (interlobar pleuritis, atelectasis and healed infarction). Amer. J. Roentgen. 46:610, 1941.   **436**

382. Fleischner, F. G., and Reiner, L.: Linear x-ray shadows in acquired pulmonary hemosiderosis and congestion. New Eng. J. Med. 250:900, 1954.   **241, 243**

383. Fleischner, F. G., and Sachsse, E.: Retrotracheal lymphadenopathy in bronchial carcinoma, revealed by the barium-filled esophagus. Amer. J. Roentgen. 90:792, 1963.   **255**

384. Fleischner, F. G., and Sagall, E. L.: Pulmonary arterial oligemia in mitral stenosis as revealed on the plain roentgenogram. Radiology 65:857, 1955.   **216**

385. Fleischner, F. G., and Udis, S. W.: Dilatation of the azygos vein: a roentgen sign of venous engorgement. Amer. J. Roentgen. 67:569, 1952. **258**

386. Fleming, P. R., and Simon, M.: The haemodynamic significance of intrapulmonary septal lymphatic lines (lines B of Kerley). J. Fac. Radiol. 9:33, 1958. **241**

387. Fleming, R. J., Medina, J., and Seaman, W. B.: Roentgenographic aspects of tracheal tumors. Radiology 79:628, 1962. **269**

388. Fletcher, B. C., Outerbridge, E. W., and Dunbar, J. S.: Pulmonary interstitial emphysema in the newborn. J. Canad. Assoc. Radiol. 21:273, 1970. **366, 392**

389. Fletcher, D. E.: Asbestos-related chest disease in joiners. Proc. Roy. Soc. Med 64:837, 1971. **377**

390. Fletcher, D. E., and Edge, J. R.: The early radiological changes in pulmonary and pleural asbestosis. Clin. Radiol. 21:355, 1970. **377**

391. Flynn, M. W., and Felson, B.: The roentgen manifestations of thoracic actinomycosis. Amer. J. Roentgen. 110:707, 1970. **272, 279, 345, 346, 379, 388, 457**

392. Forrest, J. V.: Radiographic findings in *Pneumocystis carinii* pneumonia. Radiology 103:539, 1972. **301**

393. Forsee, J. H., and Blake, H. A.: Pulmonary cystic changes in xanthomatosis. Ann. Surg. 139:76, 1954. **321**

394. Foster-Carter, A. F.: The anatomy of the bronchial tree. Brit. J. Tuberc. 36:19, 1942. **147**

395. Foster-Carter, A. F.: Broncho-pulmonary abnormalities. Brit. J. Tuberc. 40:111, 1946. **71, 77, 78, 143**

396. Foster-Carter, A. F., and Hoyle, C.: The segments of the lungs: a commentary on their investigation and morbid radiology. Dis. Chest 11:511, 1945. **143**

397. Frack, M. D., Simon, L., and Dawson, B. H.: The lymphangiomyomatosis syndrome. Cancer 22:428, 1968. **341**

398. Fraimow, W., and Cathcart, R. T.: Clinical and physiological considerations in pulmonary muscular hyperplasia. Ann. Intern. Med. 56:752, 1962. **341**

399. Franch, R. H., and Gay, B. B., Jr.: Congenital stenosis of the pulmonary artery branches: a classification, with postmortem findings in two cases. Amer. J. Med. 35:512, 1963. **205**

400. Fraser, R. G., and Bates, D. V.: Body section roentgenography in the evaluation and differentiation of chronic hypertrophic emphysema and asthma. Amer. J. Roentgen. 82:39, 1959. **223**

401. Fraser, R. G., Macklem, P. T., and Brown, W. G.: Airway dynamics in bronchiectasis: a combined cinefluorographic-manometric study. Amer. J. Roentgen. 93:821, 1965. **285**

402. Fraser, R. G., and Paré, J. A. P.: Diagnosis of Diseases of the Chest, Vol. I. Philadelphia, W. B. Saunders Co., 1970. **309, 311, 315, 321, 435, 457, 463**

403. Fraser, R. G., and Wortzman, G.: Acute pneumococcal lobar pneumonia: the significance of nonsegmental distribution. J. Canad. Assoc. Radiol. 10:37, 1959. **143**

404. Freed, T. A., Buja, L. M., Berman, M. A., and Roberts, W. C.: Pulmonary hemorrhage: radiographic and pathological correlation in patients with congenital cardiac disease dying following cardiac surgery. Radiology 94:555, 1970. **301**

405. Freedman, E., and Billings, J. H.: Active bronchopulmonary lithiasis. Radiology 53:203, 1949. **465**

406. Freundlich, I. M., Libshitz, H. I., Glassman, L. **327**

M., and Israel, H. L.: Sarcoidosis. Typical and atypical thoracic manifestations and complications. Clin. Radiol. 21:376, 1970.

407. Friedman, E.: Further observations on the vertical fissure line. Amer. J. Roentgen. 97:171, 1966.   72

408. Friedman, P. S., Solis-Cohen, L., and Levine, S.: Accessory lobe of the liver and its significance in roentgen diagnosis. Amer. J. Roentgen. 57:601, 1947.   426

409. Friedman, R. L.: Infrapulmonary pleural effusions. Amer. J. Roentgen. 71:613, 1954.   354

410. Frimann-Dahl, J.: Examination of the soft tissues of the chest. Acta Radiol. 37:246, 1952.   380

411. Frye, R. L., and Braunwald, E.: Bilateral diaphragmatic contraction synchronous with cardiac systole. New Eng. J. Med. 263:775, 1960.   435

412. Frye, R. L., Marshall, H. W., Kincaid, O. W., and Burchell, H. B.: Anomalous pulmonary venous drainage of the right lung into the inferior vena cava. Brit. Heart J. 24:696, 1962.   87

413. Fulton, H.: The roentgenologic significance of funnel chest. Amer. J. Roentgen. 71:524, 1954.   459

414. Gaensler, E. A., Goff, A. M., and Prowse, C. M.: Desquamative interstitial pneumonia. New Eng. J. Med. 274:113, 1966.   305, 341

415. Gaensler, E. A., and Strieder, J. W.: Progressive changes in pulmonary function after pneumonectomy: the influence of thoracoplasty, pneumothorax, oleothorax, and plastic sponge plombage on the side of pneumonectomy. J. Thoracic Surg. 22:1, 1951.   433

416. Gagliardi, R. A., Feigelson, H. H., and Shufro, A. S.: Transient paradoxical movement of the diaphragm. J. Thoracic Surg. 37:636, 1959.   421

417. Galassi, L.: Calcificazioni nel quadro della silicosi polmonare. Riv. Infort. Mal. Prof. 52:215, 1965.   467

418. Galatius-Jensen, F., and Halkier, E.: Radiological aspects of pleural hyalo-serositis. Brit. J. Radiol. 38:944, 1965.   377

419. Gale, G. L., and Delarue, N. C.: Leiomyosarcoma of the bronchus: report of a case. Dis. Chest 52:257, 1967.   272

420. Gallagher, P. G., Lynch, J. P., and Christian, H. J.: Intralobar bronchopulmonary sequestration of the lung: report of two cases and review of the literature. New Eng. J. Med. 257:643, 1957.   160

421. Galland, F., Serviansky, B., Bialostozky, D., Aceves, S., and Dorbecker, N.: Edema pulmonar agudo correlacion clinico radiologica estudio de diez casos comprobados en la necropsia. Arch. Inst. Cardiol. Mex. 29:517, 1959.   299

422. Galloway, R. W., Epstein, E. J., and Coulshed, N.: Pulmonary ossific nodules in mitral valve disease. Brit. Heart J. 23:297, 1951.   475

423. Garber, R. L.: Congenital aplasia of the lung. Amer. J. Roentgen. 53:129, 1945.   83

424. Garland, L. H., Beier, R. L., Coulson, W., Heald, J. H., and Stein, R. L.: The apparent sites of origin of carcinomas of the lung. Radiology 78:1, 1962.   319

425. Garrison, C. O., Dines, D. E., Harrison, E. G., Jr., Douglas, W. W., and Miller, W. E.: The alveolar pattern of pulmonary lymphoma. Mayo Clin. Proc. 44:260, 1969.   304

426. Gasul, B. M., Arcilla, R. A., and Lev, M.: Anomalous systemic venous connection. *In* Gasul, B. M., Arcilla, R. A., and Lev, M. (Eds.): Heart Disease in Children. Philadelphia, J. B. Lippincott Co., 1966.   213

427. Gay, B. B., Jr.: Normal pulsations in the pulmonary vascular tree as seen with roentgenoscopic image amplification. Amer. J. Roentgen. 81:801, 1959.   216

428. Gay, B. B., Jr., and Franch, R. H.: Pulsations in the pulmonary arteries as observed with roentgenoscopic image amplification: observations in patients with isolated pulmonary valvular stenosis. Amer. J. Roentgen. 83:335, 1960.   216

429. Gay, B. B., Jr., and Franch, R. H.: Pulsations in the pulmonary arteries as observed with roentgenoscopic image amplification: observations in patients having increased pulmonary blood flow. Amer. J. Roentgen. 85:1025, 1961.   216

430. Gayola, G., Janis, M., and Weil, P. H.: Intrathoracic nerve sheath tumor of the vagus. J. Thorac. Cardiovasc. Surg. 49:412, 1965.   419

431. Gefferth, K.: Über die hyaline Membrane-Erkrankung der Neugeborenen. Fortschr. Roentgenstr. 106:62, 1967.   301

432. Geffin, B., Grillo, H. C., Cooper, J. D., and Pontoppidan, H.: Stenosis following tracheostomy for respiratory care. J.A.M.A. 216:1984, 1971.   269

433. Gelfand, D. W., Goldman, A. S., Law, E. J., MacMillan, B. G., Larson, D. L., Abston, S., and Schreiber, J. T.: Thymic hyperplasia in children recovering from thermal burns. J. Trauma 12:813, 1972.   255, 403

434. Gelfand, M. L., Hammer, H., and Hevizy, T.: Asymptomatic pulmonary atelectasis in drug addicts. Dis. Chest 52:782, 1967.   96

435. Genereux, G. P.: Bronchial atresia: a rare cause of unilateral hypertranslucency. J. Canad. Assoc. Radiol. 22:71, 1971.   273

436. Gephart, T., and Castleman, B.: Partial obstruction of right-middle-lobe bronchus by metastasis from carcinoma of breast. New Eng. J. Med. 262:1238, 1960.   94

437. Gerle, R. D.: Personal communication, 1969.   453

438. Gerle, R. D., and Felson, B.: Metastatic endobronchial hypernephroma. Dis. Chest 44:225, 1963.   94, 272

439. Gerle, R. D., Jaretzki, A., III, Ashley, C. A., and Berne, A. S.: Congenital bronchopulmonary-foregut malformation: pulmonary sequestration communicating with the gastrointestinal tract. New Eng. J. Med. 278:1413, 1968.   160, 161

440. Gerson, C. E., and Rothstein, E.: An anomalous tracheal bronchus to the right upper lobe. Amer. Rev. Tuberc. 64:686, 1951.   153

441. Gianturco, C.: Intrathoracic pressure and position of the patient in the roentgen examination of the mediastinum. Amer. J. Roentgen. 71:870, 1954.   7

442. Ginés, A. R.: Calcificaciones pleuropulmonares. I. Bronquiolitiasis. II. Calcificaciones gangliopulmonares. III. Asociación de focos calcificados y carcinoma bronquial. IV. Calcificaciones pleurales. Hoja Tisiol. 19:18, 1959.   465, 474, 484, 489

443. Gladnikoff, H.: A roentgenographic study of the mediastinum in health and in primary pulmonary carcinoma. Acta Radiol. Suppl. 73:5, 1948.   188, 260, 350, 409

444. Gleason, D. C., and Steiner, R. E.: The lateral roentgenogram in pulmonary edema. Amer. J. Roentgen. 98:279, 1966.   246, 290, 300, 333

445. Glover, L. B., Barcia, A., and Reeves, T. J.: Congenital absence of the pericardium: a review of the literature with demonstration of a previously unreported fluoroscopic finding. Amer. J. Roentgen. 106:542, 1969.   395

446. Gold, R., Wilt, J. C., Adhikari, P. K., and Macpherson, R. I.: Adenoviral pneumonia and its complications in infancy and childhood. J. Canad. Assoc. Radiol. 20:218, 1969.   301

447. Goldberg, B.: Radiological appearances in pulmonary aspergillosis. Clin. Radiol. 13:106, 1962.   327

448. Golden, R.: The effect of bronchostenosis upon the roentgen-ray shadows in carcinoma of the bronchus. Amer. J. Roentgen. 13:21, 1925.   121

449. Golden, R.: cited by Sante, L. R.: Principles of Roentgenological Interpretation (3rd ed.). Ann Arbor, Mich., Edwards Brothers, Inc., 1940.   121

450. Goldenberg, D. B., and Brogdon, B. G.: Congenital anomalies of the pectoral girdle demonstrated by chest radiography. J. Canad. Assoc. Radiol. 18:472, 1967.   463

451. Goldfischer, J., and Rubin, E. H.: Dermatomyositis with pulmonary lesions. Ann. Intern. Med. 50:194, 1959.   339

452. Goldstein, M. J., Snider, G. L., Liberson, M., and Poske, R. M.: Bronchogenic carcinoma and giant bullous disease. Amer. Rev. Resp. Dis. 97:1062, 1968.   319

453. Gondos, B: The roentgen image of the subclavian artery in the pulmonary apex. Amer. J. Roentgen. 86:1058, 1961.   416

454. Gonzalez, E., Weill, H., Ziskind, M. M., and George, R. B.: The value of the single breath diffusing capacity in separating chronic bronchitis from pulmonary emphysema. Dis. Chest 53:229, 1968.   307

455. Good, C. A.: Roentgenologic findings in myasthenia gravis associated with thymic tumor. Amer. J. Roentgen. 57:305, 1947.   11

456. Good, C. A.: Certain vascular abnormalities of the lungs. Amer. J. Roentgen. 85:1009, 1961.   205

457. Goodman, N.: The "air bronchiologram" and the solitary pulmonary nodule: report of a case. Dis. Chest 51:104, 1967.   305

458. Goodpasture, E. W.: The significance of certain pulmonary lesions in relation to the etiology of influenza. Amer. J. Med. Sci. 158:863, 1919.   302

459. Goodwin, J. F.: Pulmonary hypertension: a symposium. I. The nature of pulmonary hypertension. Brit. J. Radiol. 31:174, 1958.   217

460. Gordon, J., and Zinn, W. B.: Pulmonary distention as seen in the lordotic roentgenogram. J. Thoracic Surg. 26:261, 1953.   105

461. Gorlin, R. J., and Goltz, R. W.: Multiple nevoid basal-cell epithelioma, jaw cysts and bifid rib: a syndrome. New Eng. J. Med. 262:908, 1960.   453

462. Gorske, K. J., and Fleming, R. J.: Mycetoma formation in cavitary pulmonary sarcoidosis. Radiology 95:279, 1970.   321, 328

463. Gottesman, L., and Weinstein, A.: Varicosities of the pulmonary veins: a case report and survey of the literature. Dis. Chest 35:322, 1959.   223

464. Gough, J.: Correlation of radiological and pathological changes in some diseases of the lungs. Lancet 1:161, 1955.   241

465. Gough, J.: Pulmonary fibrosis and collagen diseases of the lungs: a symposium. II. Generalised and primary fibrosis of the lungs. Brit. J. Radiol. 29:641, 1956.   340, 341

466. Gould, D. M., and Dalrymple, G. V.: A radiological analysis of disseminated lung disease. Amer. J. Med. Sci. 238:621, 1959.   289

467. Gould, D. M., and Torrance, D. J.: Pulmonary edema. Amer. J. Roentgen. 73:366, 1955.   299

468. Grainger, R. G.: Pulmonary hypertension: a sym-   241, 300
     posium. III. Interstitial pulmonary oedema and
     its radiological diagnosis. A sign of pulmonary
     and capillary hypertension. Brit. J. Radiol. 31:
     201, 1958.

469. Grainger, R. G., and Hearn, J. B.: Intrapulmonary   241, 246
     septal lymphatic lines (B lines of Kerley): their
     significance and their prognostic evaluation be-
     fore mitral valvotomy. J. Fac. Radiol. 7:66, 1955.

470. Gramiak, R., and Koerner, H. J.: A roentgen diag-   385
     nostic observation in subpleural lipoma. Amer. J.
     Roentgen. 98:465, 1966.

471. Gray, H.: The lymphatic system. *In* Goss, C. M.   460
     (Ed.): Gray's Anatomy of the Human Body (28th
     ed.). Philadelphia, Lea & Febiger, 1966.

472. Gray, J. M., and Hanson, G. C.: Mediastinal em-   392
     physema: aetiology, diagnosis, and treatment.
     Thorax 21:325, 1966.

473. Grayson, C. E., and Blumenfeld, H.: "Egg shell"   467
     calcifications in silicosis. Radiology 53:216, 1949.

474. Green, G. J.: The radiology of tuberose sclerosis.   341
     Clin. Radiol. 19:135, 1968.

475. Green, R. A.: Nodular aspirational pulmonary   302, 341
     hemosiderosis. Amer. J. Roentgen. 92:561, 1964.

476. Greenberg, H. B.: Benign subpleural lymph node   260, 315
     appearing as a pulmonary "coin" lesion. Radio-
     logy 77:97, 1961.

477. Greenfield, H., and Herman, P. G.: Papilloma-   133, 272
     tosis of the trachea and bronchi. Amer. J.
     Roentgen. 89:45, 1963.

478. Greenspan, R. H.: Chronic disseminated alveolar   299, 301, 303
     diseases of the lung. Seminars in Roentgenology
     2:77, 1967.

479. Greenspan, R. H., and Capps, J. H.: Pulmonary   222
     angiography: its use in diagnosis of the chest.
     Radiol. Clin. N. Amer. 1:315, 1963.

480. Greenspan, R. H., Scanlon, G. T., Harrington, G.   21
     J., and McAlister, W. H.: Magnification and mi-
     croangiography. Part A. Magnification tech-
     niques. *In* Felson, B. (Ed.): Roentgen Techniques
     in Laboratory Animals: Radiography of the Dog
     and Other Experimental Animals. Philadelphia,
     W. B. Saunders Co., 1968.

481. Greenspan, R. H., and Steiner, R. E.: The radio-   223
     logic diagnosis of pulmonary thromboembolism.
     In Simon, M., Potchen, E. J., and Le May, M.
     (Eds.): Frontiers of Pulmonary Radiology. New
     York, Grune & Stratton, Inc., 1969.

482. Grishman, A., and Kane, I. J.: Disseminated cal-   475
     cified and bony nodules in the lungs associated
     with mitral disease. Amer. J. Roentgen. 53:575,
     1945.

483. Gross, R. E., Neuhauser, E. B. D., and Longino,   405
     L. A.: Thoracic diverticula which originate from
     the intestine. Ann. Surg. 131:363, 1950.

484. Gross, R. J., Null, R., and Loeb, W.: Pseudocyst of   446
     the pancreas associated with hydrothorax. Amer.
     J. Roentgen. 67:585, 1952.

485. Groth, J. F., and Friedman, S.: The occurrence of   213
     cyanosis in chronic hepatic disease: report of a
     case in a child. Pediatrics 25:63, 1960.

486. Gruenfeld, G. E., and Gray, S. H.: Malformations   74, 153
     of the lung. Arch. Path. 31:392, 1941.

487. Gudbjerg, C. E.: Pulmonary hamartoma. Amer. J.   315
     Roentgen. 86:842, 1961.

488. Guenter, C. A., Welch, M. H., Russell, T. R.,   308
     Hyde, R. M., and Hammarsten, J. F.: The pattern
     of lung disease associated with alpha$_1$ antitrypsin
     deficiency. Arch. Intern. Med. 122:254, 1968.

489. Guillaudeu, R. L., and Stewart, D. B.: Diaphrag-   **446**
matic pneumocele complicating therapeutic
pneumoperitoneum: a review and report of four
cases. Amer. Rev. Tuberc. 69:745, 1954.

490. Gvozdanovič, V., and Oberhofer, B.: Mediastinal   **21, 255**
phlebography: a bilateral simultaneous injection
technique. Acta Radiol. 40:395, 1953.

491. Haber, J., Benkoe, G., and Barna, K.: Bronchial   **98**
changes in pneumonia. Fortschr. Roentgenstr.
91:576, 1959.

492. Haber, S.: Retroperitoneal and mediastinal che-   **419**
modectoma: report of a case and review of the literature. Amer. J. Roentgen. 92:1029, 1964.

493. Hagen, H., and Heinz, K.: Varices in the lingular   **222**
branch of the pulmonary vein. Fortschr.
Roentgenstr. 93:151, 1960.

494. Hair-sprays. Lancet 1:709, 1964.   **304**

495. Halasz, N. A., Halloran, K. H., and Liebow, A. A.:   **78**
Bronchial and arterial anomalies with drainage of
the right lung into the inferior vena cava. Circulation 14:826, 1956.

495a. Hall, R. M., and Margolin, F. R.: Oxygen al-   **299**
veolopathy in adults. Clin. Radiol. 23:11, 1972.

496. Hamilton, L. C.: Personal communication, 1967.   **21, 288**

497. Hamman, L.: Spontaneous mediastinal emphy-   **395**
sema. Bull. Johns Hopkins Hosp. 64:1, 1939.

498. Hamman, L., and Rich, A. R.: Acute diffuse inter-   **336**
stitial fibrosis of the lungs. Johns Hopkins Hosp.
Bull. 74:177, 1944.

499. Hampton, A. O., and Castleman, B.: Correlation   **372**
of postmortem chest teleroentgenograms with autopsy findings: with special reference to pulmonary embolism and infarction. Amer. J. Roentgen.
43:305, 1940.

500. Hampton, A. O., and King, D. S.: The middle lobe   **112, 170**
of the right lung: its roentgen appearance in
health and disease. Amer. J. Roentgen. 35:721,
1936.

501. Hanelin, J., and Eyler, W. R.: Pulmonary artery   **192, 224**
thrombosis: roentgen manifestations. Radiology
56:689, 1951.

502. Hanke, R.: Lymphknoten- oder Gefäbschatten am   **236**
Aortenbogen? Fortschr. Roentgenstr. 108:197,
1968.

503. Hanke, R.: Rundatelektasen (Kugel- und Wal-   **184**
zenatelektasen): Ein Beitrag zur Differentialdiagnose intrapulmonaler Rundherde. Fortschr.
Roentgenstr. 114:164, 1971.

504. Harden, K. A., and Barthakur, A.: "Cavitary" le-   **321**
sions in sarcoidosis. Dis. Chest 35:607, 1959.

505. Hardie-Neil, J., and Gilmour, W.: Broncho-pul-   **150**
monary segments of the lung and their terminology. Brit. Med. J. 2:309, 1949.

505a. Hargreave, F., Hinson, K. F., Reid, L., Simon,   **301**
G., and McCarthy, D. S.: The radiological appearances of allergic alveolitis due to bird sensitivity
(bird fancier's lung). Clin. Radiol. 23:1, 1972.

506. Harle, T. S., Kountoupis, J. T., Boone, M. L. M.,   **299**
and Fred, H. L.: Pulmonary edema without cardiomegaly. Amer. J. Roentgen. 103:555, 1968.

507. Harper, R. A. K., and Guyer, P. B.: The radiologi-   **419**
cal features of thymic tumours: a review of sixty-
five cases. Clin. Radiol. 16:97, 1965.

508. Harris, G. B. C.: The newborn with respiratory   **301**
distress: some roentgenographic features. Radiol.
Clin. N. Amer. 1:497, 1963.

509. Harris, G. B. C., and Scully, R. E.: Congenital   **142**
lobar emphysema, right upper lobe. New Eng. J.
Med. 271:100, 1964.

510. Harris, J. H., Jr.: The pulmonary arteries and veins: their radiographic identification. Med. Radiogr. Photogr. 39:52, 1963.   **201**

511. Harrison, B. B.: Influenzal pneumonia—recent experiences. Brit. J. Radiol. 24:392, 1951.   **301**

512. Harvey, R. A.: Mediastinal pleurisy in infants. Amer. J. Roentgen. 49:145, 1943.   **399**

513. Hasche, E.: Die intralobäre Sequestration. Thoraxchirurgie 10:15, 1962.   **160**

514. Haubrich, R.: Zur Klinik und Theorie der plattenförmigen Lungenatelektase. Fortschr. Roentgenstr. 79:32, 1953.   **437**

515. Hawley, C., and Felson, B.: Roentgen aspects of intrathoracic blastomycosis. Amer. J. Roentgen. 75:751, 1956.   **266, 345, 346, 379, 386**

516. Heard, B. E., Steiner, R. E., Herdan, A., and Gleason, D.: Oedema and fibrosis of the lungs in left ventricular failure. Brit. J. Radiol. 41:161, 1968.   **300, 333**

517. Heaton, T. G.: Cardiospasm with associated pulmonary disease. Dis. Chest 14:425, 1948.   **8**

518. Heidenblut, A.: Tracheal bronchus: contribution to its recognition. Fortschr. Roentgenstr. 95:77, 1961.   **153**

519. Heikel, P.-E., and Pasila, M.: Intralobar sequestration of the lung. *In* Kaufmann, H. J. (Ed.): Progress in Pediatric Radiology. Vol. 1. Respiratory Tract. Chicago, Year Book Medical Publishers, Inc., 1967.   **160, 161**

520. Heimburger, I., Battersby, J. S., and Vellios, F.: Primary neoplasms of the mediastinum: a fifteen-year experience. Arch. Surg. 86:978, 1963.   **419**

521. Heimburger, I., and Battersby, J. S.: Primary mediastinal tumors of childhood. J. Thorac. Cardiovasc. Surg. 50:92, 1965.   **419**

522. Heitzman, E. R.: Personal communication.   **243**

523. Heitzman, E. R.: Personal communication, 1972.   **333**

524. Heitzman, E. R., Markarian, B., Berger, I., and Dailey, E.: The secondary pulmonary lobule: a practical concept for interpretation of chest radiographs. I. Roentgen anatomy of the normal secondary pulmonary lobule. Radiology 93:507, 1969.   **289**

525. Heitzman, E. R., Markarian, B., and Dailey, E. T.: Pulmonary thromboemoblic disease: a lobular concept. Radiology 103:529, 1972.   **306**

526. Heitzman, E. R., Scrivani, J. V., Martino, J., and Moro, J.: The azygos vein and its pleural reflections. I. Normal roentgen anatomy. Radiology 101:249, 1971.   **409**

527. Heitzman, E. R., Scrivani, J. V., Martino, J., and Moro, J.: The azygos vein and its pleural reflections. II. Applications in the radiological diagnosis of mediastinal abnormality. Radiology 101:259, 1971.   **409**

528. Heitzman, E. R., and Ziter, F. M., Jr.: Acute interstitial pulmonary edema. Amer. J. Roentgen. 98:291, 1966.   **246**

529. Heitzman, E. R., Ziter, F. M., Jr., Markarian, B., McClennan, B. I., and Sherry, H. S.: Kerley's interlobular septal lines: roentgen pathologic correlation. Amer. J. Roentgen. 100:578, 1967.   **243**

530. Heller, R. M., Dorst, J. P., James, A. E., Jr., and Rowe, R. D.: A useful sign in the recognition of azygos continuation of the inferior vena cava. Radiology 101:519, 1971.   **236**

531. Hemmati, A.: Le déplacement normal et pathologique de la limite supérieure du poumon provoqué par la toux. Ann. Radiol. 10:708, 1967.   **463**

532. Heppleston, A. G.: The pathology of honeycomb lung. Thorax 11:77, 1956.   331, 341

533. Hering, N., Templeton, J. Y., III, Haupt, G. J., and Theodos, P. A.: Primary sarcoma of the lung. Dis. Chest 42:315, 1962.   315

534. Hermann, R. E., and Barber, D. H.: Congenital diaphragmatic hernia in the child beyond infancy. Cleveland Clin. Quart. 30:73, 1963.   440

535. Hermann, W. R., and Walther, H.: Pneumopathia osteoplastica racemosa. Fortschr. Roentgenstr. 95:73, 1961.   475

536. Herrnheiser, G.: An anatomico-roentgenological analysis of the normal hilar shadow. Amer. J. Roentgen. 48:595, 1942.   185

537. Herrnheiser, G., and Hinson, K. F. W.: An anatomical explanation of the formation of butterfly shadows. Thorax 9:198, 1954.   290

538. Hessén, I.: Roentgen examination of pleural fluid: a study of the localization of free effusions, the potentialities of diagnosing minimal quantities of fluid and its existence under physiological conditions. Acta Radiol. Suppl. 86:7, 1951.   351, 353

539. Hilding, A. C.: Production of negative pressure in the respiratory tract by ciliary action and its relation to postoperative atelectasis. Anesthesiology 5:225, 1944.   96

540. Hilgert, F.: Der Spalt zwischen Ober- und Mittellappen der Lunge. Fortschr. Roentgenstr. 78:291, 1953.   73

541. Hill, M. C., Muto, C. N., Mani, J. R., and Dozier, W. E.: The value of pneumoperitoneum in diagnosis of sequestered lung. Amer. J. Roentgen. 91:291, 1964.   161

542. Hinchcliffe, W. A., Zamel, N., Fishman, N. H., Dedo, H. H., Greenspan, R. H., and Nadel, J.: Roentgenographic study of the human trachea with powdered tantalum. Radiology 97:327, 1970.   267

543. Hindle, W., Posner, E., Sweetnam, M. T., and Tan, R. S. H.: Pleural effusion and fibrosis during treatment with methysergide. Brit. Med. J. 1:605, 1970.   351

544. Hinshaw, H. C.: Diseases of the diaphragm. Diseases of the Chest (3rd ed.). Philadelphia, W. B. Saunders Co., 1969.   435, 464

545. Hinshaw, R. J., and Guilfoil, P. H.: Intramural cystic lesion of the esophagus due to *Histoplasma capsulatum*. Dis. Chest 47:555, 1965.   465, 470, 484

546. Hirshfield, H. J., Krainer, L., and Coe, G. C.: Cystic pulmonary cirrhosis (bronchiolar emphysema) (muscular cirrhosis of the lungs). Dis. Chest 42:107, 1962.   341

547. Hislop, A., and Reid, L.: New pathological findings in emphysema of childhood: 1. Polyalveolar lobe with emphysema. Thorax 25:682, 1970.   142

548. Hladik, M.: Rontgenuntersuchung bei Pectus excavatum. Fortschr. Roentgenstr. 104:773, 1966.   16, 459

549. Hochholzer, L., Theros, E. G., and Rosen, S. H.: Some unusual lesions of the mediastinum: roentgenologic and pathologic features. Seminars in Roentgenology 4:74, 1969.   392, 395, 419

550. Hodes, P. J., Johnson, J., and Atkins, J. P.: Traumatic bronchial rupture with occlusion. Amer. J. Roentgen. 60:448, 1948.   92, 94

551. Hodgson, J. H., Good, C. A., and Hall, B. E.: The roentgenographic aspects of polycythemia vera. Proc. Staff Meet. Mayo Clin. 21:152, 1946.   220

552. Hodson, C. J.: Pulmonary oedema and the "batswing" shadow. J. Fac. Radiol. 1:176, 1950.   290

553. Hodson, C. J.: The localization of pulmonary collapse-consolidation. J. Fac. Radiol. 8:41, 1956.   **23**

554. Hodson, C. J., and Trickey, S. E.: Bronchial wall thickening in asthma. Clin. Radiol. 11:183, 1960.   **64**

555. Hoffbrand, B. I., and Beck, E. R.: "Unexplained" dyspnoea and shrinking lungs in systemic lupus erythematosus. Brit. Med. J. 1:1273, 1965.   **340**

556. Holden, W. S., and Ardran, G. M.: Observations on the movements of the trachea and main bronchi in man. J. Fac. Radiol. 8:267, 1957.   **267**

557. Holinger, P. H.: Clinical aspects of congenital anomalies of the larynx, trachea, bronchi and oesophagus. J. Laryng. 75:1, 1961.   **153, 157**

558. Holinger, P. H., and Johnston, K. C.: Clinical aspects of congenital anomalies of the trachea and bronchi. Dis. Chest 31:613, 1957.   **135**

559. Holinger, P. H., and Rigby, R. G.: Bronchial obstruction in infants and children. Med. Clin. N. Amer. 30:105, 1946.   **5, 142**

560. Hollinshead, W. H.: Anatomy for Surgeons: Vol. 2. The Thorax, Abdomen, and Pelvis. New York, Paul B. Hoeber, Inc., 1956.   **74**

561. Holman, E.: "On circumscribed dilatation of an artery immediately distal to a partially occluding band": poststenotic dilatation. Surgery 36:3, 1954.   **192**

562. Hood, R. M., and Sloan, H. E.: Injuries of the trachea and major bronchi. J. Thorac. Cardiovasc. Surg. 38:458, 1959.   **272**

563. Hope, J. W., and Koop, C. E.: Differential diagnosis of mediastinal masses. Pediat. Clin. N. Amer. 6:379, 1959.   **416**

564. Horner, J. L.: Premature calcification of the costal cartilages: its frequent association with symptoms of non-organic origin. Amer. J. Med. Sci. 218:186, 1949.   **453**

565. Howells, J. B.: Alveolar cell carcinoma of the lung. Clin. Radiol. 15:112, 1964.   **304**

566. Howland, W. J., Curry, J. L., and Dickinson, D. W.: Tracheobronchiectasis: report of a case with eight year interval studies. Dis. Chest 45:558, 1964.   **268**

567. Howland, W. J., Jr., and Good, C. A.: The radiographic features of tracheopathia osteoplastica. Radiology 71:847, 1958.   **489**

568. Huber, J. F.: Practical correlative anatomy of the bronchial tree and lungs. J. Nat. Med. Assoc. 41:49, 1949.   **147**

569. Hublitz, U. F., and Shapiro, J. H.: Atypical pulmonary patterns of congestive failure in chronic lung disease: the influence of pre-existing disease on the appearance and distribution of pulmonary edema. Radiology 93:995, 1969.   **295**

570. Hudson, H. L., and McAlister, W. H.: Obstructing tracheal hemangioma in infancy. Amer. J. Roentgen. 93:428, 1965.   **269**

571. Huff, R. W., and Fred, H. L.: Postictal pulmonary edema. Arch. Intern. Med. 117:824, 1966.   **299**

572. Hughes, V. P.: Bronchiectasis with pulmonary bony metaplasia. Dis. Chest 47:441, 1965.   **474**

573. Hughes, W. F.: Hypersensitivity pneumonitis. I. A discussion of farmer's lung. Ohio Med. J. 67:730, 1971.   **301**

574. Huizinga, E.: Bronchography in bronchial cancer and collateral ventilation. J. Thoracic Surg. 23:445, 1952.   **180**

575. Huizinga, E., and Smelt, G. J.: Bronchography. Assen, Netherlands, Van Gorcum & Co., Publishers, 1949.   **150, 153, 156**

576. Huizinga, E., and van Weering, I. F.: Broncho-   **83**
graphy in agenesia and hypoplasia of the lung.
Ann. Otol. 73:26, 1964.

577. Hunt, R. B., and Sahler, O. D.: Mediastinal em-   **392**
physema produced by air turbine dental drills.
J.A.M.A. 205:241, 1968.

578. Hurwich, J. J.: Lung hernia: a case report and   **463**
review of literature. J. Thoracic Surg. 18:261,
1949.

579. Hurwitz, M.: Roentgenologic aspects of asbes-   **489**
tosis. Amer. J. Roentgen. 85:256, 1961.

580. Hutchinson, W. B., and Friedenberg, M. J.: In-   **382**
trathoracic mesothelioma. Radiology 80:937,
1963.

581. Hutchinson, W. B., Friedenberg, M. J., and Saltz-   **304**
stein, S.: Primary pulmonary pseudolymphoma.
Radiology 82:48, 1964.

582. Hutchison, J. H.: Bronchoscopic studies in pri-   **143**
mary tuberculosis in childhood. Quart. J. Med.
18:21, 1949.

583. Huzly, A.: Middle-lobe syndrome. Fortschr.   **95**
Roentgenstr. 97:407, 1962.

584. Hyde, I.: Traumatic para-mediastinal air cysts.   **346**
Brit. J. Radiol. 44:380, 1971.

585. Hyde, L.: Spontaneous pneumothorax. Dis. Chest   **370**
43:476, 1963.

586. Ingegno, A. P., D'Albora, J. B., Edson, J. N., and   **301**
Gianquinto, P. J.: Pneumonia associated with
acute salmonellosis: report of a case of salmonella
bronchopneumonia and fourteen cases of interstitial pneumonia. Arch. Intern. Med. 81:476, 1948.

587. Irmscher, G.: Egg-shell calcification of hilar   **467**
lymph glands without silicosis. Jötton, K. W.,
Klosterkötter, W., and Pfefferkorn, C.: Die Staub-
lungen-Tagung des Staatsinstitutes für Staub-
lungenforschung und Gewerbehygiene beim
Hygiene-Institut der Westfälischen Wilhelms-
Universität, Münster/Westfälia, 1953. Abstracted
in Bull. Hyg. 30:387, 1955.

588. Irvin, J. M., and Snowden, P. W.: Idiopathic pul-   **302**
monary hemosiderosis: report of a case with ap-
parent remission from cortisone. A.M.A. J. Dis.
Child. 93:182, 1957.

589. Isley, J. K., Jr., Bacos, J., Hickam, J. B., and   **285**
Baylin, G. J.: Bronchiolar behavior in pulmonary
emphysema and in bronchiectasis. Amer. J.
Roentgen. 87:853, 1962.

590. Israel, H. L., and Diamond, P.: Recurrent pulmo-   **299**
nary infiltration and pleural effusion due to nitrofurantoin sensitivity. New Eng. J. Med.
266:1024, 1962.

591. Israel-Asselain, R., Chebat, J., Sors, Ch., Basset,   **341, 346**
F., and Le Rolland, A.: Diffuse interstitial pulmo-
nary fibrosis in a mother and son with von Recklinghausen's disease. Thorax 20:153, 1965.

592. Jackson, C. L., and Huber, J. F.: Correlated ap-   **143, 147, 150**
plied anatomy of the bronchial tree and lungs
with a system of nomenclature. Dis. Chest 9:319,
1943.

593. Jacob, G., and Bohlig, H.: Die röntgenologischen   **377**
Komplikationen der Lungenasbestose. Fortschr.
Roentgenstr. 83:515, 1955.

594. Jacobs, R. C., Gershengorn, K., and Chait, A.:   **205**
Dysphagia associated with a distended pulmo-
nary vein. Brit. J. Radiol. 45:225, 1972.

595. Jacobson, G., Felson, B., Pendergrass, E. P.,   **467**
Flinn, R. H., and Lainhart, W. S.: Eggshell cal-
cifications in coal and metal miners. Seminars in
Roentgenology 2:276, 1967.

596. Jacobson, G., and Sargent, E. N.: Apical roentgen-   13
ographic views of the chest. Amer. J. Roentgen.
104:822, 1968.

597. Jaffe, R. B., and Koschmann, E. B.: Septic pulmo-   349
nary emboli. Radiology 96:527, 1970.

598. Jakimow, I. L., and Sheehan, F. R.: Kyphotic   13
view. Dis. Chest 47:636, 1965.

599. James, A. E., Jr., MacMillan, A. S., Eaton, S. B.,   269
and Grillo, H. C.: Roentgenology of tracheal stenosis resulting from cuffed tracheostomy tubes.
Amer. J. Roentgen. 109:455, 1970.

600. James, D. G., and Carstairs, L. S.: Miliary dis-   333
eases of the lungs. Disease-a-Month, July, 1962.

601. James, U., Brimblecombe, F. S.W., and Wells, J.   97, 98
W.: The natural history of pulmonary collapse in
childhood. Quart. J. Med. 25:121, 1956.

602. Janower, M. L., and Blennerhassett, J. B.:   245
Lymphangitic spread of metastatic cancer to the
lung: a radiologic-pathologic classification. Radiology 101:267, 1971.

603. Janower, M. L., Grillo, H. C., MacMillan, A. S.,   416, 419
Jr., and James, A. E., Jr.: The radiological appearance of carcinoma of the trachea. Radiology 96:39,
1970.

604. Jeanneret, P., and Sommer, E.: Über kurz-   361
dauernde Atelektasen des Mittellappens. Radiol.
Clin. 21:332, 1952.

605. Jervey, L. P., Jr., and Hamburger, M.: The treat-   133
ment of acute Friedlaender's bacillus pneumonia:
a continuing problem. Arch. Intern. Med. 99:1,
1957.

606. Jimenez, J. P., and Lester, R. G.: Pulmonary   301
complications following furniture polish ingestion: a report of 21 cases. Amer. J. Roentgen.
98:323, 1966.

607. Joffe, N.: Cavitating primary pulmonary tubercu-   133
losis in infancy. Brit. J. Radiol. 33:430, 1960.

608. Johnson, R. J., and Boyden, E. A.: Congenital   153
hypoplasia of the middle lobe of the lung, with
displacement of the anterior basal bronchus to the
middle lobe stem. Dis. Chest 35:360, 1959.

609. Johnson, T. H., Jr., Gajaraj, A., and Feist, J. H.:   330
Patterns of pulmonary interstitial disease. Amer.
J. Roentgen. 109:516, 1970.

610. Johnson, T. H., Jr., and Howland, W. J.: Aerosol   16, 267
bronchography: a preliminary report. Amer. J.
Roentgen. 104:787, 1968.

611. Johnston, R. F., and Flegel, E. E.: Displaced   153
bronchus, lung abscess and retrograde perfusion.
Dis. Chest 55:69, 1969.

612. Johnston, R. F., and Loo, R. V.: Hepatic hydro-   446
thorax: studies to determine the source of the
fluid and report of thirteen cases. Ann. Intern.
Med. 61:385, 1964.

613. Jones, D. B.: Basal pleural fluid accumulations   354
resembling elevated diaphragm. Radiology
50:227, 1948.

614. Jönsson, G.: Book review. Acta Radiol. 52:95,   377
1959.

615. Joseph, W. L., Murray, J. F., and Mulder, D. G.:   419
Mediastinal tumors—problems in diagnosis and
treatment. Dis. Chest 50:150, 1966.

616. Kahn, B., and Amer, N. S.: Multiple bronchial   272
polyps. Chest 57:279, 1970.

617. Kale, M. K., Rafferty, R. E., and Carton, R. W.:   207
Aberrant left pulmonary artery presenting as a
mediastinal mass: report of a case in an adult.
Arch. Intern. Med. 125:121, 1970.

618. Kalter, J. E., Bubis, J. J., Wolman, M., and Pauzner, Y.: Diaphragmatic hernia associated with accessory lung. Dis. Chest 42:429, 1962.   160

619. Kaltreider, H. B., Baum, G. L., Bogaty, G., McCoy, M. D., and Tucker, M.: So-called "metastatic" calcification of the lung. Amer. J. Med. 46:188, 1969.   479

620. Kamberg, S., and Loitman, B. S.: Histiocytosis X. Dis. Chest 41:338, 1962.   321, 339

621. Kane, I. J.: Segmental localization of pulmonary disease on the postero-anterior roentgenogram. Radiology 59:229, 1952.   147, 169

622. Kane, I. J.: Sectional Radiography of the Chest. New York, Springer Publishing Co., Inc., 1953.   15

623. Kaplan, B. M., Schlichter, J. G., Graham, G., and Miller, G.: Idiopathic congenital dilatation of the pulmonary artery. J. Lab. Clin. Med. 41:697, 1953.   192

624. Kassay, D.: Clinical Applications of Bronchology. New York, Blakiston Division, McGraw Hill Book Co., 1960.   435, 436

625. Kassay, D.: Comments on some controversial questions of bronchial classification and nomenclature. Dis. Chest 40:364, 1961.   151, 155

626. Kattan, K. R.: High kilovoltage oblique roentgenography of the chest: its advantage in differential diagnosis in diseases of the lung and the pleura. Dis. Chest 50:605, 1966.   15

627. Kattan, K. R., Spitz, H. B., and Moskowitz, M.: Intercostal bulging of the lung without emphysema. Amer. J. Roentgen. 112:542, 1971.   461

628. Katz, H. L.: Traction diverticula of the esophagus in middle lobe syndrome. Amer. Rev. Tuberc. 65:455, 1952.   95

629. Katz, I., LeVine, M., and Herman, P.: Trancheobronchiomegaly: the Mounier-Kuhn syndrome. Amer. J. Roentgen. 88:1084, 1962.   268

630. Kaye, J., Cohen, G., Sandler, A., and Tabatznik, B.: Massive pulmonary embolism without infarction. Brit. J. Radiol. 31:326, 1958.   192, 224

631. Keating, D. R., Burkey, J. N., Hellerstein, H. K., and Feil, H.: Chronic massive thrombosis of pulmonary arteries: a report of seven cases with clinical and necropsy studies. Amer. J. Roentgen. 69:208, 1953.   192, 224

631a. Keats, T. E.: The aortic-pulmonary mediastinal stripe. Amer. J. Roentgen. 116:107, 1972.   416

632. Keats, T. E., and Crane, J. F.: Cystic changes of the lungs in histiocytosis. Amer. J. Dis. Child. 88:764, 1954.   339

633. Keats, T. E., Kreis, V. A., and Simpson, E.: The roentgen manifestations of pulmonary hypertension in congenital heart disease. Radiology 66:693, 1956.   216

634. Keats, T. E., Lipscomb, G. E., and Betts, C. S., III: Mensuration of the arch of the azygos vein and its application to the study of cardiopulmonary disease. Radiology 90:990, 1968.   236

635. Keers, R. Y., and Smith, F. A.: A case of multiple pulmonary "hamartomata" of unusual type. Brit. J. Dis. Chest. 54:349, 1960.   315

636. Kegel, R. F. C., and Fatemi, A.: The ruptured pulmonary hydatid cyst. Radiology 76:60, 1961.   327

637. Keil, P. G., and Schissel, D. J.: The differential diagnosis of unresolved pneumonia and bronchiogenic carcinoma by pulmonary angiography. J. Thoracic Surg. 20:62, 1950.   21, 255

638. Kemp, F. H., Morley, H. M. C., and Emrys-   399

Roberts, E.: A sail-like triangular projection from the mediastinum: a radiographic appearance of the thymus gland. Brit. J. Radiol. 21:618, 1948.

639. Kent, E. M., and Blades, B.: The anatomic approach to pulmonary congestion. Ann. Surg. 116:782, 1942.   **73**

640. Kent, G., Gilbert, E. S., and Meyer, H. H.: Pulmonary microlithiasis: microlithiasis alveolaris pulmonum. Arch. Path. 60:556, 1955.   **479**

641. Kergin, F. G.: Congenital cystic disease of lung associated with anomalous arteries. J. Thoracic Surg. 23:55, 1952.   **160**

642. Kergin, F. G.: Silicotic and tuberculosilicotic lesions simulating bronchiogenic carcinoma. J. Thoracic Surg. 24:545, 1952.   **272**

643. Kerley, P.: Personal communication.   **151, 475**

644. Kerley, P.: Radiology in heart disease. Brit. Med. J. 2:594, 1933.   **241**

645. Kerley, P.: Respiratory system. *In* Shanks, S. C., and Kerley, P. (Eds.): A Textbook of X-Ray Diagnosis (2nd ed.), Vol. II. Philadelphia, W. B. Saunders Co., 1951.   **241**

646. Kerley, P.: Lung changes in acquired heart disease. Amer. J. Roentgen. 80:256, 1958.   **290, 344**

647. Kerr, I. H., Simon, G., and Sutton, G. C.: The value of the plain radiograph in acute massive pulmonary embolism. Brit. J. Radiol. 44:751, 1971.   **224**

648. Kher, G. A., and Makhani, J. S.: A preliminary study of the lengths of the two main bronchi and angle at the carina. J. Indian Med. Assoc. 34:262, 1960.   **267**

649. Khomiakov, I. S., and Fedorova, R. G.: Effect of nature of the exudate and retractile capacity of the lung on the fluid level curve in pleural effusion. Vestn. Rentgen. Radiol. 37:8, 1962.   **351**

650. Kiely, J. M., and Holley, K. E.: Idiopathic pulmonary hemosiderosis. Mayo Clin. Proc. 43:592, 1968.   **301**

651. Kilburn, K. H., and Asmundsson, T.: Anteroposterior chest diameter in emphysema: from maxim to measurement. Arch. Intern. Med. 123:379, 1969.   **308**

652. Kinare, S. G., Parulkar, C. B., Panday, S. R., and Sen, P. K.: Extensive ossification in a pulmonary plasmacytoma. Thorax 20:206, 1965.   **484**

653. King, D. S.: Roentgenograms of diffuse pulmonary lesions. Amer. Rev. Tuberc. 60:536, 1949.   **289**

654. King, J. B.: Calcification of the costal cartilages. Brit. J. Radiol. 12:2, 1939.   **452**

655. Kirklin, B. R., and Hodgson, J. R.: Roentgenologic characteristics of diaphragmatic hernia. Amer. J. Roentgen. 58:77, 1947.   **440**

656. Kirkpatrick, J. A., Jr., and Di George, A. M.: Congenital absence of the thymus. Amer. J. Roentgen. 103:32, 1968.   **403**

657. Kittredge, R. D., and Finby, N.: Bilateral tuberculous mediastinal lymphadenopathy in the adult. Amer. J. Roentgen. 96:1022, 1966.   **251**

658. Kittredge, R. D., and Finby, N.: Pericardial cysts and diverticula. Amer. J. Roentgen. 99:668, 1967.   **405**

659. Kiviluoto, R.: Pleural calcification as a roentgenologic sign of non-occupational endemic anthophyllite-asbestosis. Acta Radiol. Suppl. 194, 1960.   **377, 489, 492**

660. Kiviluoto, R.: Radiological aspects of pleural hyalo-serositis. Brit. J. Radiol. 39:233, 1966.   **377, 489**

661. Kjellberg, S. R., and Olsson, S. E.: Roentgenological studies of experimental pulmonary embolism   **224**

without complicating infarction in dog. Acta Radiol. 33:507, 1950.

662. Klebanoff, S. J., and White, L. R.: Iodination defect in the leukocytes of a patient with chronic granulomatous disease of childhood. New Eng. J. Med. 280:460, 1969.   346

663. Kleinfeld, M.: Acute pulmonary edema of chemical origin. Arch. Environ. Health 10:942, 1965.   299

664. Klemperer, P., and Rabin, C. B.: Primary neoplasms of the pleura: a report of five cases. Arch. Path. 11:385, 1931.   374, 382

665. Knowles, J. H., and Castleman, B.: Pulmonary sarcoidosis. New Eng. J. Med. 273:1268, 1965.   479

666. Knyvett, A. F.: The pulmonary lesions of chickenpox. Quart. J. Med. 35:313, 1966.   474

667. Koerner, H. J., and Sun D. I-C.: Mediastinal lipomatosis secondary to steroid therapy. Amer. J. Roentgen. 98:461, 1966.   392

668. Kohn, H. N.: Zur Histologie der indurirenden fibrinösen Pneumonie. München. Med. Wschr. 40:42, 1893.   180

669. Korsten, J., Grossman, H., Winchester, P. H., and Canale, V. C.: Extramedullary hematopoiesis in patients with thalassemia anemia. Radiology 95:257, 1970.   457

670. Krabbenhoft, K. L., and Evans, W. A., Jr.: Some pulmonary changes associated with intracardiac septal defects in infancy. Radiology 63:498, 1954.   220

671. Krause, G. R., and Lubert, M.: The anatomy of the bronchopulmonary segments: clinical applications. Radiology 56:333, 1951.   147, 169

672. Krause, G. R., and Lubert, M.: Gross anatomicospatial changes occurring in lobar collapse: a demonstration by means of three-dimensional plastic models. Amer. J. Roentgen. 79:258, 1958.   107, 112

673. Krech, W. G., Storey, C. F., and Umiker, W. C.: Thymic cysts: a review of the literature and report of two cases. J. Thoracic Surg. 27:477, 1954.   2, 419

674. Kremens, V.: Demonstration of the pericardial shadow on the routine chest roentgenogram: a new roentgen finding. Preliminary report. Radiology 64:72, 1955.   28, 392

675. Kricun, M. E., and Pais, M. J.: The lateral sternum—the first clue to disease. Exhibit, The Radiological Society of North America, Chicago, 1970.   459, 463

676. Křivinka, R.: Über einem Fall von linksseitigem Vorkommen des Lobus Wrisbergi. Roentgenpraxis 11:234, 1939.   77

677. Kruse, R. L., and Lynn, H. B.: Lobar emphysema in infants. Mayo Clin. Proc. 44:525, 1969.   142

678. Kubik, St., and Müntener, M.: Bronchusanomalien: tracheale, eparterielle und präeparterielle Bronchi. Fortschr. Roentgenstr. 114:145, 1971.   153

679. Kuenast, W.: Über die intralobäre Sequestration der Lunge; Bericht eines Falles. Fortschr. Roentgenstr. 87:476, 1957.   160

680. Kuhn, J. P., Fletcher, B. D., and DeLemos, R. A.: Roentgen findings in transient tachypnea of the newborn. Radiology 92:751, 1969.   301

681. Kuisk, H., and Sanchez, J. S.: Diffuse bronchiolectasis with muscular hyperplasia ("muscular cirrhosis of the lung"): relationship to chronic form of Hamman-Rich syndrome. Amer. J. Roentgen. 96:979, 1966.   341, 344

682. Kuisk, H., and Sanchez, J. S.: Desquamative interstitial pneumonia and idiopathic diffuse pulmonary fibrosis with their advanced final stages as   331, 341

"muscular cirrhosis of the lung" (diffuse bronchiolectasis with muscular hyperplasia): fibrosing alveolitis. Amer. J. Roentgen. 107:258, 1969.

683. Kurlander, G. J., and Helmen, C H.: Subpulmonary pneumothorax. Amer. J. Roentgen. 96:1019, 1966.   370

684. Kyllonen, K. E. J., and Perasalo, O.: Acute pericardial fat necrosis. Acta Chir. Scand. 122:275, 1961.   419, 463

685. Lachman, E.: Visceral topography in the light of the roentgenologic approach. Amer. J. Roentgen. 70:832, 1953.   72

686. Lachman, E.: Comparison of posterior boundaries of lungs and pleura as demonstrated on cadaver and on roentgenogram of the living. Anat. Rec. 83:521, 1942.   350, 351, 409

687. Lacquet, L. K., Fornhoff, M. R., and Buyssens, N.: Bronchial atresia with corresponding segmental pulmonary emphysema. Thorax 26:68, 1971.   135

688. Laforet, E. G., and Laforet, M. T.: Nontuberculous cavitary disease of the lungs. Dis. Chest 31:665, 1957.   345

689. Lambert, M. W.: Accessory bronchiole-alveolar communications. J. Path. Bact. 70:311, 1955.   180

690. Lampe, W. T., II: Klebsiella pneumonia: a review of forty-five cases and re-evaluation of the incidence and antibiotic sensitivities. Dis. Chest 46:599, 1964.   133

690a. Landing, B. H., Lawrence, T-Y. K., Payne, V. C., Jr., and Wells, T. R.: Bronchial anatomy in syndromes with abnormal visceral situs, abnormal spleen and congenital heart disease. Amer. J. Cardiol. 28:456, 1971.   205

691. Lane, E. J., Jr., and Carsky, E. W.: Epicardial fat: lateral plain film analysis in normals and in pericardial effusion. Radiology 91:1, 1968.   463

692. Lane, E. L., Jr., and Whalen, J. P.: A new sign of left atrial enlargement: posterior displacement of the left bronchial tree. Radiology 93:279, 1969.   189

693. Lane, S. D., Burko, H., and Scott, H. W.: Congenital bronchopulmonary-foregut malformation. Radiology 101:291, 1971.   161

694. Lansden, F. T., and Falor, W. H.: Congenital esophagorespiratory fistula in the adult. J. Thorac. Cardiovasc. Surg. 39:246, 1960.   269

695. Lansing, A. M.: Radiological changes in pulmonary atelectasis. Arch. Surg. 90:52, 1965.   96

696. Lanuza, A.: The sign of the cane: a new radiological sign for the diagnosis of small Morgagni hernias. Radiology 101:293, 1971.   440

697. Larose, J. H.: Cavitation of missile tracks in the lung. Radiology 90:995, 1968.   346

698. Larson, N. E., Larson, R. H., and Dorsey, J. M.: Mechanism of obstruction and strangulation of the esophageal hiatus. Surg. Gynec. Obstet. 119:835, 1964.   442

699. Lasser, E. C.: Some aspects of pulmonary dynamics revealed by concurrent roentgen kymography of spirometric movements and diaphragmatic excursions. Radiology 77:434, 1961.   435

700. Latham, W. J.: Hydatid disease: Part I. J. Fac. Radiol. 5:65, 1953.   327

701. Lattanzio, E.: Un particolare aspetto die versamenti pleurici liberi; il segno del galleggiamento del polmone e l'espansibilità respiratoria. Radiol. Med. 37:917, 1951.   353

702. Laumonier, P., Lachapèle, A.-P., Couraud, L., Hugues, A., Lagarde, C., and Mage, J.: Une appli-   21, 250

cation de la lymphangiographie au diagnostic et au traitement du chylothorax. Presse Méd. 70:2630, 1962.

703. Lavender, J. P.: Letter to the editor. Brit. J. Radiol. 37:243, 1964.   185

704. Lavender, J. P., and Doppman, J.: The hilum in pulmonary venous hypertension. Brit. J. Radiol. 35:303, 1962.   217

705. Lavender, J. P., Doppman, J., Shawdon, H., and Steiner, R. E.: Pulmonary veins in left ventricular failure and mitral stenosis. Brit. J. Radiol. 35:293, 1962.   217

706. Laws, J. W.: Personal communication.   233

707. Laws, J. W., and Heard, B. E.: Emphysema and the chest film: a retrospective radiological and pathological study. Brit. J. Radiol. 35:750, 1962.   305, 308

708. Lawson, J. P.: Pleural calcification as a sign of asbestosis: a report of three cases. Clin. Radiol. 14:414, 1963.   489

709. Ledesma, J., and Girdany, B. R.: Congenital lobar emphysema: a case report with a thirty-two year follow-up. Ann. Radiol. 15:181, 1971.   142

710. Lees, A. W.: Atelectasis and bronchiectasis in pertussis. Brit. Med. J. 2:1138, 1950.   97

711. Lefebvre, J. E., and Plainfosse, M. C.: Pulmonary angiography in children: methods and indications. *In* Kaufmann, H. J. (Ed.): Progress in Pediatric Radiology. Vol. 1. Respiratory Tract. Chicago, Year Book Medical Publishers, 1967.   21, 201

712. Lehman, J. A., Jr., and Cross, F. S.: Bilateral multiple carcinoma of the lung. Cancer 19:1931, 1966.   315

713. Lehman, J. S., and Crellin, J. A.: The normal human bronchial tree. Med. Radiogr. Photogr. 31:81, 1955.   147

714. Leigh, T. F., Abbott, O. A., Rogers, J. V., Jr., and Gay, B. B., Jr.: Venous aneurysms of the mediastinum. Radiology 63:696, 1954.   258

715. Leigh, T. F., and Weens, H. S.: The Mediastinum. Springfield, Ill., Charles C Thomas, Publisher, 1959.   255, 392, 416, 419, 492

716. Leigh, T. F., and Weens, H. S.: Roentgen aspects of mediastinal lesions. Seminars in Roentgenology 4:59, 1969.   419

717. LeMay, M., and Piro, A. J.: Cavitary pulmonary metastases. Ann. Intern. Med. 62:59, 1965.   321

718. Lemire, P., Trepanier, A., and Hebert, G.: Bronchocele and blocked bronchiectasis. Amer. J. Roentgen. 110:687, 1970.   273

719. Lenczner, M., Spaulding, W. B., and Sanders, D. E.: Pulmonary manifestations of parasitic infestations. Canad. Med. Assoc. J. 91:421, 1964.   346

720. Lennon, E. A., and Simon, G.: The height of the diaphragm in the chest radiograph of normal adults. Brit. J. Radiol. 38:937, 1965.   421

721. Leopold, J. G., and Gough, J.: Post-mortem bronchography in the study of bronchitis and emphysema. Thorax 18:172, 1963.   288

722. Lerner, M. A., Rosbash, H., Frank, H. A., and Fleischner, F. G.: Radiologic localization and management of cytologically discovered bronchial carcinoma. New Eng. J. Med. 264:480, 1961.   15

723. LeRoux, B. T.: Pleuro-pulmonary amoebiasis. Thorax 24:91, 1969.   351

724. LeRoux, B. T.: Opacities of the middle and upper lobes in combination. Thorax 26:55, 1971.   128, 133

725. Lesser, M. B.: Left azygos lobe: report of a case. Dis. Chest 46:95, 1964.   77

726. Lessure, A. P.: Multiple hemangiomas of mediastinum. Dis. Chest 35:433, 1959.   383

727. Lester, R. G.: Radiological concepts in the evalua-   217
     tion of heart disease (I). Mod. Conc. Cardiovasc.
     Dis. 37:113, 1968.
728. Leszczynski, S., and Pawlicka, L.: Les signes   135
     radiologiques de l'hypoventilation pulmonaire
     causée par une sténose bronchique (à propos de
     15 observations). Ann. Radiol. 7:11, 1964.
729. Levin, B.: On the recognition and significance of   241
     pleural lymphatic dilatation. Amer. Heart J.
     49:521, 1955.
730. Levin, B.: Subpleural interlobular lymphectasia   245
     reflecting metastatic carcinoma. Radiology 72:
     682, 1959.
731. Levin, D. C.: Pulmonary abnormalities in the   347
     necrotizing vasculitides and their rapid response
     to steroids. Radiology 97:521, 1971.
732. Levin, E. J.: Pulmonary intracavity fungus ball.   **11, 327**
     Radiology 66:9, 1956.
733. Levin, L., Kernohan, J. W., and Moersch, H. J.:   346
     Pulmonary abscess secondary to bland infarction.
     Dis. Chest 14:218, 1948.
734. Levitin, J., and Brunn, H.: A study of the   71
     roentgenologic appearance of the lobes of the
     lung and the interlobar fissures. Radiology
     25:651, 1935.
735. Liberson, M.: Diagnostic significance of the me-   354
     diastinal profile in massive unilateral pleural ef-
     fusions. Amer. Rev. Resp. Dis. 88:176, 1963.
736. Lieber, A., Rosenbaum, H. D., Hanson, D. J., and   **217, 224**
     Kwaan, H. M.: Accuracy of predicting pulmonary
     blood flow, pulmonary arteriolar resistance and
     pulmonary venous pressure from chest roentgen-
     ograms. Amer. J. Roentgen. 103:577, 1968.
737. Lieberman, F. L., Hidemura, R., Peters, R. L., and   446
     Reynolds, T. B.: Pathogenesis and treatment of
     hydrothorax complicating cirrhosis with ascites.
     Ann. Intern. Med. 64:341, 1966.
738. Lieberman, F. L., and Peters, R. L.: Cirrhotic   446
     hydrothorax: further evidence that an acquired
     diaphragmatic defect is at fault. Arch. Intern.
     Med. 125:114, 1970.
739. Liebow, A. A.: Personal communication.   **96, 315, 341, 344**
740. Liebow, A. A.: Pathology of carcinoma of the lung   489
     as related to the roentgen shadow. Amer. J.
     Roentgen. 74:383, 1955.
741. Liebow, A. A., and Carrington, C. B.: The intersti-   **305, 341**
     tial pneumonias. *In* Simon, M., Potchen, E. J., and
     Le May, M. (Eds.): Frontiers of Pulmonary Radio-
     logy. New York, Grune & Stratton, Inc., 1969.
742. Liebow, A. A., Hales, M. R., and Lindskog, G. E.:   **163, 230**
     Enlargement of the bronchial arteries, and their
     anastomoses with the pulmonary arteries in bron-
     chiectasis. Amer. J. Path. 25:211, 1949.
743. Liebow, A. A., Steer, A., and Billingsley, J. G.:   **305, 341**
     Desquamative interstitial pneumonia. Amer. J.
     Med. 39:369, 1965.
744. Liess, G.: Ein beachtenswertes Zeichen für die   327
     Röntgendiagnose des chronischen Lungenabs-
     zesses. Fortschr. Roentgenstr. 79:613, 1953.
745. Lillard, R. L., and Allen, R. P.: The extrapleural   **392, 409**
     air sign in pneumomediastinum. Radiology
     85:1093, 1965.
746. Lillie, W. I., McDonald, J. R., and Clagett, O. T.:   419
     Pericardial celomic cysts and diverticula: a con-
     cept of etiology and report of cases. J. Thoracic
     Surg. 20:494, 1950.
747. Lindskog, G. E., and Liebow, A. A.: Thoracic   433
     Surgery and Related Pathology. New York, Ap-
     pleton-Century-Crofts, Inc., 1953.

748. Llamas, R., Ortiz, J., Perez, A. R., and Baum, G.   267
L.: Experimental bronchography by tantalum in-
sufflation. Dis. Chest 56:75, 1969.

749. Locke, G. B.: Carcinoma of the middle-lobe bron-   112
chus. J. Fac. Radiol. 5:1, 1953.

750. Locke, G. B.: Rheumatoid lung. Clin. Radiol.   340
14:43, 1963.

751. Lodge, T.: The anatomy of the blood vessels of   **71, 72, 203**
the human lung as applied to chest radiology.
Brit. J. Radiol. 19:1, 1946.

752. Lodge, T.: Recent Advances in Radiology (3rd   **231**
ed.). Boston, Little, Brown and Co., 1955.

753. Lodin, H. L.: The value of tomography in exami-   **15**
nation of the intrapulmonary bronchi. Acta Ra-
diol. Suppl. 101:7, 1953.

754. Lodin, H. L.: Tomography of the middle and   **15**
lingular bronchi. Acta Radiol. (Diagn) 6:26, 1967.

755. Loeschcke, H.: Die Morphologie des normalen   **295**
und emphysematosen Acinus der Lunge. Beitr.
Path. Anat. 68:213, 1921.

756. Löffler, W.: The transient infiltrate with eosino-   **301**
philia. Schweiz. Med. Wschr. 66:45, 1936.

757. Loftis, J. W., Susen, A. F., Marcy, J. H., and Sher-   **395**
man, F. E.: Pneumopericardium in infancy.
Amer. J. Dis. Child. 103:61, 1962.

758. Loftus, L. R., Rooney, P. A., and Webster, C. M.:   **302**
Idiopathic pulmonary hemosiderosis and glo-
merulonephritis: report of a case. Dis. Chest
45:93, 1964.

759. Logan, W. D., Jr., Rohde, F. C., Abbott, O. A., and   **315**
Meltzer, H. D.: Multiple pulmonary fibroleio-
myomatous hamartomas: report of a case and
review of the literature. Amer. Rev. Resp. Dis.
91:101, 1965.

760. Longin, F.: The recognition of shrinkage of the   **107**
lower lobe of the left lung on the plain chest film.
Fortschr. Roentgenstr. 90:665, 1959.

761. Longin, F., and Schehl, R.: Increased distance be-   **424**
tween the diaphragm and the gastric fundus on
the roentgen picture: cause and simulation.
Fortschr. Roentgenstr. 92:20, 1960.

762. Longmire, W. P., Goodwin, W. E., and Buckberg,   **419**
G. D.: Management of sclerosing fibrosis of the
mediastinal and retroperitoneal areas. Ann. Surg.
165:1013, 1967.

763. Longcope, W. T., and Freiman, D. G.: A study of   **303**
sarcoidosis: based on a combined investigation of
160 cases including 30 autopsies from The Johns
Hopkins Hospital and Massachusetts General
Hospital. Medicine 31:1, 1952.

764. Louria, D. B.: Rickettsial and parasitic infection   **346**
of the lungs and embolic lung infections. *In*
Baum, G. L. (Ed.): Textbook of Pulmonary Diseases. Boston, Little, Brown and Co., 1965.

765. Lowman, R. M., Bloor, C. M., and Newcomb, A.   **419**
W.: Roentgen manifestations of thoracic extramedullary hematopoiesis. Dis. Chest 44:154,
1963.

766. Lubert, M., and Krause, G. R.: Patterns of lobar   **107, 110, 112, 115, 120**
collapse as observed radiographically. Radiology
56:165, 1951.

767. Lubert, M., and Krause, G. R.: Total unilateral   **42, 95, 120**
pulmonary collapse: a study of the roentgen ap-
pearance in the lateral view. Radiology 67:175,
1956.

768. Lull, G. F., Jr.: Pericardial celomic cyst: a re-   **419**
evaluation. Radiology 71:534, 1958.

769. Lundin, P., Simonsson, B., and Winberg, T.:   **315, 486**

Pneumopleural amyloid tumour: report of a case. Acta Radiol. 55:139, 1961.

770. Lyon, J. A., Jr.: Pneumomediastinum in the new-born. Radiol. Clin. N. Amer. 1:51, 1963. 392

771. Lyons, H. A., Calvy, G. L., and Sammons, B. P.: The diagnosis and classification of mediastinal masses. I. A study of 782 cases. Ann. Intern. Med. 51:897, 1959. 419

772. Lyons, J. P., and Watson, A. J.: The significance of radiographic 'calcification' in the lungs of coal-workers. Tubercle 42:457, 1961. 475

773. MacEwan, D. W., Dunbar, J. S., Smith, R. D., and Brown, B. St. J.: Pneumothorax, its recognition and evaluation particularly in young infants. To be published. 366

774. Mack, J. F., Moss, A. J., Harper, W. M., and O'Loughlin, B. J.: The bronchial arteries in cys-tic fibrosis. Brit. J. Radiol. 38:422, 1965. 231

775. Mack, R. M., Stevenson, J. K., and Graham, C. B.: Gigantic solitary congenital cyst of the lung in a nine-year-old boy: case report. Amer. Surg. 32:549, 1966. 321

776. Mackay, J. B., and Cairney, P.: Pulmonary cal-cification following varicella. New Zeal. Med. J. 59:453, 1960. 474

777. Mackenzie, F. A. F.: The radiological investiga-tion of the early manifestations of exposure to as-bestos dust. Proc. Roy. Soc. Med. 64:834, 1971. 377

778. Macklin, M. T., and Macklin, C. C.: Malignant in-terstitial emphysema of the lungs and medias-tinum as an important occult complication in many respiratory diseases and other conditions: an interpretation of the clinical literature in the light of laboratory experiment. Medicine 23:281, 1944. 370, 395

779. Macpherson, R. I.: Respiratory therapy in the newborn: the role of the radiologist. Exhibit, The Radiological Society of North America, Chicago, 1971. 344

780. Macpherson, R. I., Cumming, G. R., and Cher-nick, V.: Unilateral hyperlucent lung: a complica-tion of viral pneumonia. J. Canad. Assoc. Radiol. 20:225, 1969. 223

781. Maddison, F. E., Lim, R. C., Jr., Blaisdell, F. W., and Amberg, J. R.: Pulmonary microembo-lism—radiologic findings. Radiology 90:1176, 1968. 217

782. Madoff, I. M., Gaensler, E. A., and Strieder, J. W.: Congenital absence of the right pulmonary artery: diagnosis by angiocardiography, with car-diorespiratory studies. New Eng. J. Med. 247:149, 1952. 189

783. Madsen, E.: Dysphagia in bulbar and pseudobul-bar lesions simulating oesophageal carcinoma. Acta Radiol. 41:517, 1954. 95, 267

784. Magalhães, J. P.: Plate atelectasis and Kerley's lines. Rev. Brasil Radiol. 4:151, 1961. 436

785. Magbitang, M. H., Hayford, F. C., and Blake, J. M.: Dilated azygos vein simulating a mediastinal tumor: report of a case. New Eng. J. Med. 263:598, 1960. 236

786. Maier, H. C.: Bronchiogenic cysts of the medias-tinum. Ann. Surg. 127:476, 1948. 3, 4, 95

787. Maier, H. C.: Absence or hypoplasia of a pulmo-nary artery with anomalous systemic arteries to the lung. J. Thoracic Surg. 28:145, 1954. 189

788. Maier, H. C.: Lymphatic cysts of the medias-tinum. Amer. J. Roentgen. 73:15, 1955. 419

789. Maloney, J. V., Jr., Schmutzer, K. J., and Raschke, E.: Paradoxical respiration and "pendelluft." J. Thorac. Cardiovasc. Surg. 41:291, 1961. 433

790. Mangiulea, V. G., and Stinghe, R. V.: The accessory cardiac bronchus: bronchologic aspect and review of the literature. Dis. Chest 54:35, 1968. 156

791. Marchal, M., and Marchal, M. T.: La mesure rapide de la croissance des tumeurs par une nouvelle méthode: La microdensitométrie pulmonaire. C. R. Acad. Sci. 266:2032, 1968. 21

792. Margolin, H. N., Rosenberg, L. S., Felson, B., and Baum, G. L.: Idiopathic unilateral hyperlucent lung: a roentgenologic syndrome. Amer. J. Roentgen. 82:63, 1959. 135, 223, 228

793. Margolis, J.: Chronic interstitial pneumonitis of the azygos lobe. Dis. Chest 40:661, 1961. 77

794. Marks, C.: The ectopic tracheal bronchus: management of a child by excision and segmental pulmonary resection. Dis. Chest 50:652, 1966. 153

795. Marks, C., Wiener, S. N., and Reydman, M.: Pulmonary sequestration. Chest 61:253, 1972. 160

796. Marks, J. L., and Nathan, A.: The linear atelectatic sign in intra-abdominal lesions. Radiology 52:363, 1949. 437

797. Martel, W., Abell, M. R., Mikkelsen, W. M., and Whitehouse, W. M.: Pulmonary and pleural lesions in rheumatoid disease. Radiology 90:641, 1968. 340

798. Martin, E. J.: Incidence of bifidity and related rib abnormalities in Samoans. Amer. J. Phys. Anthrop. 18:179, 1960. 453

799. Maruyama, Y., Wilkins, E. W., Jr., and Wyman, S. M.: An evaluation of angiocardiography in pulmonary carcinoma with particular emphasis on prognosis. Radiology 79:617, 1962. 21

800. Mason, W. E., and Templeton, A. W.: Bronchographic signs useful in the diagnosis of lung cancer. Dis. Chest 49:284, 1966. 269, 272

801. Massaro, D., and Katz, S.: Fibrosing alveolitis; its occurrence, roentgenographic and pathologic features in von Recklinghausen's neurofibromatosis. Amer. Rev. Resp. Dis. 93:934, 1966. 341

802. Maurer, E. R.: Successful removal of tumor of the heart. J. Thoracic Surg. 23:479, 1952. 392, 419

803. Maurer, E. R., Mendez, F. L., Jr., and Alexander, J. W.: Modern methods of managing traumatic rupture and amputation of the bronchus. Dis. Chest 48:587, 1965. 272

804. McAdams, A. J.: Pulmonary hemorrhage in the newborn. Amer. J. Dis. Child. 113:255, 1967. 301

805. McAdams, A. J., Jr.: Bronchiolitis obliterans. Amer. J. Med. 19:314, 1955. 299

806. McAlister, W. H., and Blatt, E.: Calcified pulmonary artery thrombus. Amer. J. Roentgen. 87:908, 1962. 474

807. McAlister, W. H., and Gleason, D. C.: Alveolar diseases in children. Seminars in Roentgenology 2:98, 1967. 299, 301

808. McCarthy, D. S., Simon, G., and Hargreave, F. E.: The radiological appearances in allergic bronchopulmonary aspergillosis. Clin. Radiol. 21:366, 1970. 273

809. McCort, J. J.: Radiographic identification of lymph node metastases from carcinoma of the esophagus. Radiology 59:694, 1952. 255

810. McCort, J. J., and Robbins, L. L.: Roentgen diagnosis of intrathoracic lymph-node metastases in carcinoma of the lung. Radiology 57:339, 1951. 254

811. McGuire, J., and Bean, W. B.: Spontaneous inter-   395
     stitial emphysema of the lungs. Amer. J. Med. Sci.
     197:502, 1939.

812. McKusick, V. A., and Cooley, R. N.: Drainage of   87
     right pulmonary vein into inferior vena cava:
     report of case, with a radiologic analysis of the
     principal types of anomalous venous return from
     the lung. New Eng. J. Med. 252:291, 1955.

813. McLachlan, M. S. F., Wallace, M., and Sene-   479
     viratne, C.: Pulmonary calcification in renal fail-
     ure: report of three cases. Brit. J. Radiol. 41:99,
     1968.

814. McLetchie, N. G. B., and Reynolds, D. P.: His-   339
     tiocytic reticulosis and honeycomb lungs. Canad.
     Med. Assoc. J. 71:44, 1954.

815. McLoughlin, M. J.: Obstruction of the right ven-   223
     tricular outflow tract due to metastasis. Brit. J.
     Radiol. 43:573, 1970.

816. McPeak, E. M., and Levine, S. A.: The prepon-   359
     derance of right hydrothorax in congestive heart
     failure. Ann. Intern. Med. 25:916, 1946.

817. McPhail, J. L., and Arora, T. S.: Intrathoracic   315, 321
     hydatid disease. Dis. Chest 52:772, 1967.

818. Medlar, E. M.: Variations in interlobar fissures.   71
     Amer. J. Roentgen. 57:723, 1947.

819. Melamed, M. R., Koss, L. G., and Cliffton, E. E.:   15
     Roentgenologically occult lung cancer diagnosed
     by cytology: report of 12 cases. Cancer 16:1537,
     1963.

820. Melhem, R. E., Dunbar, J. D., and Booth, R. W.:   246
     The "B" lines of Kerley and left atrial size in mi-
     tral valve disease: their correlation with the mean
     left atrial pressure as measured by left atrial punc-
     ture. Radiology 76:65, 1961.

821. Melhem, R. E., Habbal, A. M., and Imad, A. P.:   57
     The "silhouette" sign in urinary tract calculi. Ex-
     perimental demonstration. Clin. Radiol. 21:313,
     1970.

822. Mendelson, E.: Abdominal wall masses: the use-   60
     fulness of the incomplete border sign. Radiol.
     Clin. N. Amer. 2:161, 1964.

823. Meriel, P., Galinier, F., and Desandre, M.:   360
     Formes atypiques des épanchements in-
     terlobaires chez les cardiaques. J. Radiol. Électr.
     35:545, 1954.

824. Meschan, I.: Roentgen Signs in Clinical Practice,   187
     Vol. II. Philadelphia, W. B. Saunders Co., 1966.

825. Meszaros, W. T.: Lung changes in left heart fail-   217
     ure. Presented at The American Roentgen Ray
     Society meeting, Miami Beach, 1970.

826. Métras, H., and Thomas, P.: "L'image en grelot"   327
     en radiologie pulmonaire. Presse Méd. 54:644,
     1946.

827. Meyer, E. C., and Liebow, A. A.: Relationship of   331, 344
     interstitial pneumonia honeycombing and atypi-
     cal epithelial proliferation to cancer of the lung.
     Cancer 18:322, 1965.

828. Michelson, E., and Salik, J. O.: The vascular pat-   201
     tern of the lung as seen on routine and tomogra-
     phic studies. Radiology 73:511, 1959.

829. Middlemass, I. B. D.: Deformity of the oeso-   8, 257
     phagus in bronchogenic carcinoma. J. Fac. Ra-
     diol. 5:121, 1953.

830. Middlemiss, H.: Tropical Radiology. New York,   474
     Intercontinental Medical Book Corp., 1961.

831. Millard, D. G.: Displacement of the linear thora-   409
     cic paraspinal shadow of Brailsford: an early sign
     in osteomyelitis of the thoracic spine. Amer. J.
     Roentgen. 90:1231, 1963.

832. Milledge, R. D., Gerald, B. E., and Carter, W. J.: 341
Pulmonary manifestations of tuberous sclerosis.
Amer. J. Roentgen. 98:734, 1966.

833. Miller, R. D., Fowler, W. S., and Helmholz, F. M., 339
Jr.: Scleroderma of the lungs. Staff Meet. Mayo
Clin. 34:66, 1959.

834. Miller, R. E., and Nelson, S. W.: The roentgeno- 447
logic demonstration of tiny amounts of free intraperitoneal gas: experimental and clinical studies. Amer. J. Roentgen. 112:574, 1971.

835. Miller, W. S.: The Lung. Springfield, Ill., Charles **241, 288**
C Thomas, Publisher, 1937.

836. Mills, N. L.: Pericardial cyst in the superior me- **419**
diastinum. Brit. J. Radiol. 32:554, 1959.

837. Milne, E. N. C.: Physiological interpretation of **217, 220**
the plain radiograph in mitral stenosis, including
a review of criteria for the radiological estimation
of pulmonary arterial and venous pressures. Brit.
J. Radiol. 36:902, 1963.

838. Milne, E. N. C.: Personal communication, 1971. **217**

839. Milne, E. N. C., and Bass, H.: The roentgenologic **307**
diagnosis of early chronic obstructive pulmonary
disease. J. Canad. Assoc. Radiol. 20:3, 1969.

840. Mindell, H. J.: Roentgen findings in farmer's **301**
lung. Radiology 97:341, 1970.

841. Mitchell, R. S.: Diffuse pulmonary emphysema **311**
and occupation. J.A.M.A. 181:71, 1962.

842. Molnar, W., and Riebel, F. A.: Bronchography: an **269**
aid in the diagnosis of peripheral pulmonary carcinoma. Radiol. Clin. N. Amer. 1:303, 1963.

843. Monod, O., Dieudonné, P., and Tardieu, P.: Post- **327, 329**
operative pulmonary aspergillosis. J. Franc. Med.
Chir. Thorac. 18:579, 1964.

844. Moore, R. L., and Lattes, R.: Papillomatosis of **133**
larynx and bronchi: case report with 34-year
follow-up. Cancer 12:117, 1959.

845. Morgan, W. K. C., and Wolfel, D. A.: The lungs **340**
and pleura in rheumatoid arthritis. Amer. J.
Roentgen. 98:334, 1966.

846. Mori, P. A., Anderson, A. E., Jr., and Eckert, P.: **307, 308**
The radiological spectrum of aging and emphyse-
matous lungs. Radiology 83:48, 1964.

847. Mornet, J., and Renard, J.: Le syndrome granu- **299**
lique des cardiopathies fébriles. Arch. Mal. Coeur
39:75, 1946.

848. Mortensson, W., and Lundström, N. -R.: Broncho- **87**
pulmonary vascular malformation syndrome causing left heart failure during infancy. Acta Radiol.
11:449, 1971.

848a. Moskowitz, H., Platt, R. T., Schacher, R., and **352**
Mellins, H. Z.: Roentgen visualization of minute
pleural effusion. Presented at The Radiological
Society of North America meeting, Chicago, 1972.

849. Moskowitz, M. M.: To brush or not to brush: is **265, 301**
there really a question? Brush biopsy of the lung.
Chest 59:648, 1971.

850. Mullard, K. S.: Congenital tracheoesophageal fis- **269**
tula without atresia of the esophagus. J. Thoracic
Surg. 28:39, 1954.

851. Müller, R., and Löfstedt, S.: The reaction of the **352**
pleura in primary tuberculosis of the lungs. Acta
Med. Scand. 122:105, 1945.

852. Müller, W., and Musshoff, K.: Ampullary bron- **285**
chiectasis, a rare malformation of the bronchi.
Fortschr. Roentgenstr. 91:701, 1959.

853. Mulvey, R. B.: The thymic "wave" sign. Radio- **403**
logy 81:834, 1963.

853a. Mulvey, R. B.: Peripheral bone metastases. **47**
Amer. J. Roentgen. 91:155, 1964.

854. Mulvey, R. B.: The effect of pleural fluid on the diaphragm. Radiology 84:1080, 1965. **428**

855. Munk, J., and Lederer, K. T.: Inspiratory widening of the heart shadow: a fluoroscopic sign in acute obstructive laryngo-tracheitis. Brit. J. Radiol. 27:294, 1954. **7**

856. Munsell, W. P.: Pneumomediastinum: a report of 28 cases and review of the literature. J.A.M.A. 202:689, 1967. **392**

857. Murray, G. F.: Congenital lobar emphysema. Surg. Gynec. Obstet. 124:611, 1967. **142**

858. Murray, M. J., and Kronenberg, R.: Pulmonary reactions simulating cardiac pulmonary edema caused by nitrofurantoin. New Eng. J. Med. 273:1185, 1965. **299**

859. Mustard, W. T., Trimble, A. W., and Trusler, G. A.: Mediastinal vascular anomalies causing tracheal and esophageal compression and obstruction in childhood. Canad. Med. Assoc. J. 87:1301, 1962. **419**

860. Naclerio, E. A.: The "V sign" in the diagnosis of spontaneous rupture of the esophagus (an early roentgen clue). Amer. J. Surg. 93:291, 1957. **370, 392**

861. Nadeau, P. J., Ellis, F. H., Jr., Harrison, E. G., Jr., and Fontana, R. S.: Primary pulmonary histiocytosis X. Dis. Chest 37:325, 1960. **338**

862. Nadel, J. A., Wolfe, W. G., and Graf, P. D.: Powdered tantalum as a medium for bronchography in canine and human lungs. Invest. Radiol. 3:229, 1968. **16, 267**

863. Nadelhaft, J., and Ellis, K.: Roentgen appearances of the lungs in 1,000 apparently normal full term newborn infants. Amer. J. Roentgen. 78:440, 1957. **201**

864. Nash, B., Friedenberg, R. M., and Goetz, R.: Aberrant insertion of a pulmonary vein into the left atrium simulating an intrinsic lesion of the esophagus. Amer. J. Roentgen. 86:888, 1961. **205**

865. Nash, G., Blennerhassett, J. B., and Pontoppidan, H.: Pulmonary lesions associated with oxygen therapy and artificial ventilation. New Eng. J. Med. 276:368, 1967. **343**

866. Nathan, M. H., Collins, V. P., and Adams, R. A.: Differentiation of benign and malignant pulmonary nodules by growth rate. Radiology 79:221, 1962. **315**

867. Nathan, M. T.: Cysts and duplications of neurenteric origin. Pediatrics 23:476, 1959. **405, 419**

868. National Tuberculosis Association. Chronic Obstructive Emphysema. A Manual for Physicians. New York, The National Tuberculosis Assoc., 1963. **288, 307**

869. Navani, S., Shah, J. R., and Levy, P. S.: Determination of sex by costal cartilage calcification. Amer. J. Roentgen. 108:771, 1970. **452**

870. Neaman, M. P.: Peripheral pulmonary embolism: a distinctive clinical-radiologic entity. J. Canad. Assoc. Radiol. 18:464, 1967. **217**

871. Nelson, S. W., Christoforidis, A. J., and Pratt, P. C.: Further experience with barium sulfate as a bronchographic contrast medium. Amer. J. Roentgen. 92:595, 1964. **16**

872. Nelson, T. G., Shefts, L. M., and Bowers, W. F.: Mediastinal tumors: an analysis of 141 cases. Dis. Chest 32:123, 1957. **419**

873. Nelson, W. P., Hall, R. J., and Garcia, E.: Varicosities of the pulmonary veins simulating arteriovenous fistulas. J.A.M.A. 195:13, 1966. **222**

874. Nemec, S. S.: Differential diagnosis of retrocardiac shadows. Radiology 50:174, 1948.   23

875. Nessa, C. B., and Rigler, L. G.: The roentgenological manifestations of pulmonary edema. Radiology 37:35, 1941.   290, 299

876. Ngan, H., Millard, R. J., Lant, A. F., and Trapnell, D. H.: Nitrofurantoin lung. Brit. J. Radiol. 44:21, 1971.   246

877. Nice, C. M., Jr., and Ostrolenk, D. G.: Asbestosis and nodular lesions of the lung: a radiologic study. Dis. Chest 54:226, 1968.   340

878. Nicholson, D. P.: Pulmonary collapse and pertussis. Arch. Dis. Child. 24:29, 1949.   97

879. Nicklaus, T. M., Stowell, D. W., Christiansen, W. R., and Renzetti, A. D., Jr.: The accuracy of the roentgenologic diagnosis of chronic pulmonary emphysema. Amer. Rev. Resp. Dis. 93:889, 1966.   309

880. Nicklaus, T. M., and Sutton, R. B.: Personal communication.   77

881. Nigogosyan, G., and Ozarda, A.: Accessory diaphragm: a case report. Amer. J. Roentgen. 85:309, 1961.   428

882. Nofsinger, C. D., and Vinson, P. P.: Intrabronchial metastasis of hypernephroma simulating primary bronchial carcinoma. J.A.M.A. 119:944, 1942.   94

883. Noguera, O. F., and Noguera, O. M.: Las lineas A y B de Kerley. Corroboracion de su substructum anatomo-patologico. Rev. Interamer. Radiol. 5:36, 1969.   245

884. Nohl, H. C.: An investigation into lymphatic and vascular spread of carcinoma of the bronchus. Thorax 11:172, 1956.   245

885. Nohl, H. C.: The Spread of Carcinoma of the Bronchus. London, Lloyd-Luke Ltd., 1962.   245, 254

886. Nordenström, B.: Transjugular approach to the mediastinum for mediastinal needle biopsy: a preliminary report. Invest. Radiol. 2:134, 1967.   254

887. Nordenström, B.: Personal communication, 1972.   308

888. Norlin, U. A. T.: Traumatic rupture of the main bronchi. Acta Radiol. 43:305, 1955.   92, 94

889. North, L. B.: Cavitary pulmonary infarction. Amer. Rev. Resp. Dis. 96:1056, 1967.   346

890. Northway, W. H., Jr., Rosan, R. C., and Porter, D. Y.: Pulmonary disease following respirator therapy of hyaline-membrane disease: bronchopulmonary dysplasia. New Eng. J. Med. 276:357, 1967.   343

891. Nowell, S.: Value of tomography in lesions of the main bronchi and their larger sub-divisions. Proc. Roy. Soc. Med. 40:399, 1947.   15, 269

892. Nusbaum, M., Baum, S., Hedges, R. C., and Blakemore, W. S.: Roentgenographic and direct visualization of thoracic duct. Arch. Surg. 88:105, 1964.   250

893. Odegaard, H.: The roentgenological picture in chronic, non-specific fibrosis of the middle lobe, with special regard to the value of planigraphy. Acta Radiol. 37:17, 1952.   95

894. Oderr, C.: Radiologic assessment of pulmonary insufficiency and cough effectiveness. Dis. Chest 49:46, 1966.   21

895. Oechsli, W. R., Jacobson, G., and Brodeur, A. E.: Diatomite pneumoconiosis: roentgen characteristics and classification. Amer. J. Roentgen. 85:263, 1961.   272

896. O'Gorman, L. D., Cottingham, R. A., Sargent, E. N., and O'Loughlin, B. J.: Mediastinal emphy-   392

sema in the newborn: a review and description of the new extrapleural gas sign. Dis. Chest 53:301, 1968.

897. Oh, K. S., Fleischner, F. G., and Wyman, S. M.: Characteristic pulmonary finding in traumatic complete transection of a main-stem bronchus. Radiology 92:371, 1969.   94, 272, 366

898. Ohba, S., Takashima, T., Hamada, S., and Kitagawa, M.: Multiple cystic cavitary alveolar-cell carcinoma. Radiology 104:65, 1972.   315

899. O'Keefe, M. E., Jr., Good, C. A., and McDonald, J. R.: Calcification in solitary nodules of the lung. Amer. J. Roentgen. 77:1023, 1957.   15, 484

900. Oliner, H., Schwartz, R., Rubio, F., Jr., and Dameshek, W.: Interstitial pulmonary fibrosis following busulfan therapy. Amer. J. Med. 31:134, 1961.   344

901. Ongley, P. A., Titus, J. L., Khoury, G. H., Rahimtoola, S. H., Marshall, H. J., and Edwards, J. E.: Anomalous connection of pulmonary veins to right atrium associated with anomalous inferior vena cava, situs inversus and multiple spleens: a developmental complex. Mayo Clin. Proc. 40:609, 1965.   236

902. Oosthuizen, S. F., and Fainsinger, M. H.: Pulmonary actinomycosis. Brit. J. Radiol. 22:152, 1949.   386

903. Ormond, R. S., Drake, E. H., and Hildner, F. J.: Pulmonary hypertension: an angiographic study. Radiology 88:680, 1967.   217

904. Ormond, R. S., and Eyler, W. R.: Roentgen diagnosis of cardiac competence. Radiology 79:378, 1962.   217, 220

905. Ormond, R. S., Jaconette, J. R., and Templeton, A. W.: The pleural esophageal reflection: an aid in the evaluation of esophageal disease. Radiology 80:738, 1963.   409

906. Ormond, R. S., Poznanski, A. K., and Templeton, A. W.: Pulmonary veins in congenital heart disease in the adult. Radiology 67:885, 1961.   220

907. Ovenfors, C-O.: Pulmonary interstitial emphysema: an experimental roentgen-diagnostic study. Acta Radiol. (Suppl.) 224:1964.   366, 392

908. Overholt, R. H.: Extrapleural pneumothorax: a report of experiences and present day indications. Dis. Chest 7:80, 1941.   217, 386

909. Owen, W. R., Thomas, W. A., Castleman, B., and Bland, E. F.: Unrecognized emboli to lungs with subsequent cor pulmonale. New Eng. J. Med. 249:919, 1953.   205

910. Pachter, M. R., and Lattes, R.: Mediastinal cysts: a clinicopathologic study of twenty cases. Dis. Chest 44:416, 1963.   419

911. Pachter, M. R., and Lattes, R.: Mesenchymal tumors of the mediastinum. I. Tumors of fibrous tissue, adipose tissue, smooth muscle, and striated muscle. Cancer 16:74, 1963.   419

912. Pachter, M. R., and Lattes, R.: Uncommon mediastinal tumors: report of two parathyroid adenomas, one nonfunctional parathyroid carcinoma and one "bronchial-type-adenoma." Dis. Chest 43:519, 1963.   419

913. Pachter, M. R., and Lattes, R.: "Germinal" tumors of the mediastinum: a clinicopathologic study of adult teratomas, teratocarcinomas, choriocarcinomas and seminomas. Dis. Chest 45:301, 1964.   419

914. Pais, M. J.: To be published.   346

915. Pajewski, M.: The diagnostic value of the laterooblique tomogram of the lungs. Brit. J. Radiol. 38:430, 1965.   15

915a. Palayew, M. J.: Progressive multinodular pulmonary histoplasmosis. Presented at The Radiological Society of North America meeting, Chicago, 1972. 486

916. Palazzo, W. L., and Garrett, T. A.: Cervical hernia of the lung. Radiology 56:575, 1951. 463

917. Papaioannou, A. N., and Watson, W. L.: Primary lymphoma of the lung: an appraisal of its natural history and a comparison with other localized lymphomas. J. Thorac. Cardiovasc. Surg. 49:373, 1965. 305

918. Parker, G. W, Sturtevant, H. N., Reed, J. E., and Flaherty, R. A.: Segmental localization of pulmonary disease. Amer. J. Roentgen. 83:217, 1960. 143

919. Parsonett, A. E., Klosk, E., and Bernstein, A.: Pleural transudates: unusual roentgenological configuration associated with congestive failure. Amer. Rev. Tuberc. 53:599, 1946. 360

920. Patel, C. V., and Anand, A. L.: A fatal case of pneumopericardium: probably due to a patent pleuropericardial defect. Radiology 74:626, 1960. 395

921. Patel, S., and Maso, C. J.: Ossification in metastases from carcinoma of the breast. J.A.M.A. 198:1309, 1966. 489

922. Patterson, C. D., Harville, W. E., and Pierce, J. A.: Rheumatoid lung disease. Ann. Intern. Med. 62:685, 1965. 339

923. Paul, L. W.: Neurogenic tumors at the pulmonary apex. Dis. Chest 11:648, 1945. 380, 385

924. Paul, L. W.: Basal mass shadows in chest roentgenograms. Texas J. Med. 52:132, 1956. 426, 440

925. Paul, L. W., and Richter, M. R.: Funnel chest deformity and its recognition in posteroanterior roentgenograms of the thorax. Amer. J. Roentgen. 46:619, 1941. 53

926. Paulson, D. L., and Shaw, R. R.: Chronic atelectasis and pneumonitis of the middle lobe. J. Thoracic Surg. 18:747, 1949. 95

927. Paunier, J.-P., and Candardjis, G.: Les opacités thoraciques sous-pariétales dans les lymphomes. Ann. Radiol. 8:547, 1965. 385

928. Peabody, J. W., Jr., Rupnik, E. J., and Hanner, J. M.: Bronchial carcinoma masquerading as a thin-walled cyst. Amer. J. Roentgen. 77:1051, 1957. 319

929. Pear, B. L.: Idiopathic disseminated pulmonary ossification. Radiology 91:746, 1968. 475

930. Peck, W. A., Jr.: Right-sided diaphragmatic liver hernia following trauma. Amer. J. Roentgen. 78:99, 1957. 424

931. Peirce, C. B., and Stocking, B. W.: The oblique projection of the thorax: an anatomic and roentgenologic study. Amer. J. Roentgen. 38:245, 1937. 11

932. Peleg, H., and Pauzner, Y.: Benign tumors of the lung. Dis. Chest 47:179, 1965. 315

933. Pendergrass, R. C., and Allbritten, F. F., Jr.: Pulmonary complications of dorsal sympathectomy. Amer. J. Roentgen. 57:205, 1947. 386

933a. Pernice, N., Renner, R. R., Markarian, B., and Heitzman, E. R.: The apical pleural cap. Presented at The Radiological Society of North America meeting, Chicago, 1972. 372

934. Petersen, J. A.: Recognition of infrapulmonary pleural effusion. Radiology 74:34, 1960. 352

935. Petersen, R. W.: Infrahepatic interruption of the inferior vena cava with azygos continuation (persistent right cardinal vein). Radiology 84:304, 1965. 42

936. Peterson, H. G., Jr., and Pendleton, M. E.: Contrasting roentgenographic pulmonary patterns of the hyaline membrane and fetal aspiration syndromes. Amer. J. Roentgen. 74:800, 1955. — 61

937. Petty, T. L., and Wilkins, M.: The five manifestations of rheumatoid lung. Dis. Chest 49:75, 1966. — 340

938. Pfister, R. C., Oh, K. S., and Ferrucci, J. T., Jr.: Retrosternal density: a radiological evaluation of the retrosternal-premediastinal space. Radiology 96:317, 1970. — 405, 463

939. Phillips, L. A.: Mediastinal chemodectoma and thoracic aortography: a case report. Clin. Radiol. 14:129, 1963. — 419

940. Pierce, J.: Allergic diseases of the lung. Unpublished data. — 143, 301

941. Pimentel, J. C.: Tridimensional photographic reconstruction in a study of the pathogenesis of honeycomb lung. Thorax 22:444, 1967. — 313, 331

942. Pirnar, T., and Neuhauser, E. B. D.: Asphyxiating thoracic dystrophy of the newborn. Amer. J. Roentgen. 98:358, 1966. — 457

943. Pitman, R. G., Steiner, R. E., and Szur, L.: The radiological appearances of the chest in polycythaemia vera. Clin. Radiol. 12:276, 1961. — 220

944. Plessinger, V. A., and Jolly, P. N.: Rasmussen's aneurysm and fatal hemorrhage in pulmonary tuberculosis. Amer. Rev. Tuberc. 60:589, 1949. — 327

945. Plum, G. E., Hayles, A. B., Bruwer, A. J., and Clagett, O. T.: Supernumerary intrathoracic rib: a case report. J. Thoracic Surg. 34:800, 1957. — 493

946. Poirier, T. J., and Van Ordstrand, H. S.: Pulmonary chondromatous hamartomas: report of seventeen cases and review of the literature. Chest 59:50, 1971. — 315

947. Polachek, A. A., and Pijanowski, W. J.: Extrathoracic egg-shell calcifications in silicosis. Amer. Rev. Resp. Dis. 82:714, 1960. — 467

948. Poppe, J. K.: Transient paradoxic motion of diaphragm with pneumonia. Dis. Chest 45:187, 1964. — 421

949. Portes, Y., Lopez, F., and Celis, A.: Roentgenologic representation of the exacerbation of chronic bronchitis with obstructive pulmonary emphysema. Electromedica 3:61, 1969. — 288

950. Pratt, P. C.: Pulmonary capillary proliferation induced by oxygen inhalation. Amer. J. Path. 34:1033, 1958. — 343

951. Preger, L.: Pulmonary alveolar proteinosis. Radiology 92:1291, 1969. — 304

952. Prowse, C. M., Fuchs, J. E., Kaufman, S. A., and Gaensler, E. A.: Chronic obstructive pseudoemphysema: a rare cause of unilateral hyperlucent lung. New Eng. J. Med. 271:127, 1964. — 223

953. Pump, K. K.: The bronchial arteries and their anastomoses in the human lung. Dis. Chest 43:245, 1963. — 230, 288

954. Pump, K. K.: Morphology of the acinus of the human lung. Dis. Chest 56:126, 1969. — 289

955. Rabin, C. B.: Radiology of the chest. *In* Golden's Diagnostic Roentgenology. Baltimore, Williams & Wilkins Co., 1952. — 1, 11, 290

956. Rabin, C. B.: Radiology of the chest. *In* Robbins, L. L. (Ed.): Golden's Diagnostic Roentgenology, Vol. II. Baltimore, Williams & Wilkins Co., 1964. — 492

957. Rabinowitz, J. G., and Wolf, B. S.: Roentgen significance of the pulmonary ligament. Radiology 87:1013, 1966. — 366

958. Race, G. A., Scheifley, C. H., and Edwards, J. E.: — 359

Hydrothorax in congestive heart failure. Amer. J. Med. 22:83, 1957.

959. Raffensperger, J. G., Diffenbaugh, W. G., and Strohl, E. L.: Postoperative massive collapse of the lungs. J.A.M.A. 174:1386, 1960.   96

960. Ramirez-R., J.: Pulmonary alveolar proteinosis: a roentgenologic analysis. Amer. J. Roentgen. 92:571, 1964.   304

961. Ramirez-R., J., and Campbell, G. D.: Rheumatoid disease of the lung with cavitation: report of two cases. Dis. Chest 50:544, 1966.   315, 321

962. Ramirez-R., J., and Levy, D. A.: Pseudocavitary histoplasmosis: infection of emphysematous bullae by *Histoplasma capsulatum.* Dis. Chest 48:442, 1965.   349

963. Ransome-Kuti, O., Veiga-Pires, A., and Audu, I. S.: Mediastinal emphysema in infants. Clin. Radiol. 19:47, 1968.   392

964. Raphael, M. J.: Mediastinal haematoma: a description of some radiological appearances. Brit. J. Radiol. 36:921, 1963.   395, 419

965. Rasmussen, V.: "On hemoptysis, especially when fatal, in its anatomical and clinical aspects," translated from Hospitals-Tidende, 11th year Nos. 9–13, Copenhagen, February and March, 1868, by Moore, W. D.: Edinburgh Med. J. 14:385, 1868.   327

966. Rawlings, M. S.: The "straight back" syndrome: a new cause of pseudoheart disease. Amer. J. Cardiol. 5:333, 1960.   461

967. Rayl, J. E., Peasley, E. D., and Joyner, J. T.: Differential diagnosis of bronchiectasis and bronchitis. Dis. Chest 39:591, 1961.   288

968. Rayl, J. E., and Smith, D. E.: Recent advances in bronchography. Dis. Chest 33:235, 1958.   20, 288

969. Read, J.: Diffuse lung disease: clinical and radiological features. Med. J. Aust. 2:241, 1961.   330, 331

970. Recavarren, S., Benton, C., and Gall, E. A.: The pathology of acute alveolar diseases of the lung. Seminars in Roentgenology 2:22, 1967.   289, 291, 296, 297

970a. Reeder, M. M., and Felson, B.: Gamuts in Radiology—Comprehensive Lists of Roentgen Differential Diagnosis. To be published by Audiovisual Radiology of Cincinnati.   vi

971. Rees, D. O., and Ruttley, M. S. T.: The bronchocele in bronchial neoplasm. Clin. Radiol. 21:62, 1970.   180

972. Reich, S. B.: Personal communication.   96

973. Reich, S. B., and Abouav, J.: Interalveolar air drift. Radiology 85:80, 1965.   180, 319

974. Reid, L.: The secondary lobule in the adult human lung, with special reference to its appearance in bronchograms. Thorax 13:110, 1958.   289

975. Reid, L.: The Pathology of Emphysema. London, Lloyd-Luke Ltd., 1967.   308

976. Reid, L., and Millard, F. J. C.: Correlation between radiological diagnosis and structural changes in emphysema. Clin. Radiol. 15:307, 1964.   307

977. Reid, L., and Simon, G.: The peripheral pattern in the normal bronchogram and its relation to peripheral pulmonary anatomy. Thorax 13:103, 1958.   288, 289, 296

978. Reid, L., and Simon, G.: III. Pathological findings and radiological changes in chronic bronchitis and emphysema. Brit. J. Radiol. 32:291, 1959.   64

979. Reid, L., Simon, G., Zorab, P. A., and Seidelin, R.: The development of unilateral hypertransradiancy of the lung. Brit. J. Dis. Chest 61:190, 1967.   223

980. Reid, L. M.: Correlation of certain bronchographic abnormalities seen in chronic bronchitis with the pathological changes. Thorax 10:199, 1955.　288

981. Reingold, I. M., and Amromin, G. D.: Extraosseous osteosarcoma of the lung. Cancer 28:491, 1971.　475, 489

982. Reingold, I. M., and Mizunoue, G. S.: Idiopathic disseminated pulmonary ossification. Dis. Chest 40:543, 1961.　484

983. Reinhardt, K.: Atélectasie pulmonaire gauche totale après bronchographie. J. Radiol. Électr. 32:470, 1951.　94, 97

984. Reisner, H., and Huzly, A.: Pleurogene Tumoren und Pseudotumoren der Pleura. Die Mesotheliome und ihre Einordnung. I. Fortschr. Roentgenstr. 106:775, 1967.　374

985. Reisner, H., and Huzly, A.: Pleurogene Tumoren und Pseudotumoren der Pleura. Die Mesotheliome und ihre Einordung. II. Fortschr. Roentgenstr. 107:68, 1967.　374

986. Rémy, J.: Le Signe de la Silhouette et le Bronchogramme Aérien. Presse Méd. 77:543, 1969.　28

987. Rendich, R. A., Levy, A. H., and Cove, A. M.: Pulmonary manifestations of azotemia. Amer. J. Roentgen. 46:802, 1941.　290

987a. Renner, R. R., Coccaro, A. P., Heitzman, E. R., Dailey, E. T., and Markarian, B.: *Pseudomonas* pneumonia: a prototype of hospital-based infection. Radiology 105:555, 1972.　301

988. Reynolds, J., and Davis, J. T.: Injuries of the chest wall, pleura, pericardium, lungs, bronchi and esophagus. Radiol. Clin. N. Amer. 4:383, 1966.　351, 392

989. Richards, G. E.: The interpretation of the triangular basal shadows in roentgenograms of the chest. Amer. J. Roentgen. 30:289, 1933.　23

990. Richards, P.: Pulmonary oedema and intracranial lesions. Brit. Med. J. 2:83, 1963.　299

991. Richman, S. R., and Harris, R. D.: Acute pulmonary edema associated with Librium abuse: a case report. Radiology 103:57, 1972.　299

992. Richter, K.: Pulmonale Gefässveränderungen bei Polycythaemia vera. Fortschr. Roentgenstr. 90:179, 1959.　220

993. Richter, K., et al.: The anomaly of the epibronchial right pulmonary artery as guiding symptom of a pulmo-cardiovascular syndrome. Fortschr. Roentgenstr. 107:31, 1967.　87, 205

994. Rigler, L. G.: Roentgen diagnosis of small pleural effusions: new roentgenographic position. J.A.M.A. 96:104, 1931.　352

995. Rigler, L. G.: Roentgenologic observations on the movement of pleural effusions. Amer. J. Roentgen. 25:220, 1931.　351, 354

996. Rigler, L. G.: A roentgen study of the mode of development of encapsulated interlobar effusions. J. Thoracic Surg. 5:295, 1936.　360

997. Rigler, L. G.: The density of the central shadow in the diagnosis of intrathoracic lesions. Radiology 32:316, 1939.　23

998. Rigler, L. G.: Bronchial obstruction: roentgenologic observations. Modern Med. 12:55, 1944.　97, 143

999. Rigler, L. G.: Roentgen examination of the chest: its limitations in the diagnosis of disease. J.A.M.A. 142:773, 1950.　297, 329, 333

1000. Rigler, L. G.: The Chest. A Handbook of Roentgen Diagnosis (2nd ed.). Chicago, Year Book Medical Publishers, Inc., 1954.　7, 11

1001. Rigler, L. G.: The roentgen signs of carcinoma of the lung. Amer. J. Roentgen. 74:415, 1955. — 479

1002. Rigler, L. G.: A new roentgen sign of malignancy in the solitary pulmonary nodule. J.A.M.A. 157:907, 1955. — 314

1003. Rigler, L. G.: A roentgen study of the evolution of carcinoma of the lung. J. Thoracic Surg. 34:283, 1957. — 316, 319

1004. Rigler, L. G.: Functional roentgen diagnosis: anatomical image – physiological interpretation. Amer. J. Roentgen. 82:1, 1959. — 7, 220

1005. Rigler, L. G., and Ericksen, L. G.: Inferior accessory lobe of the lung. Amer. J. Roentgen. 29:384, 1933. — 78

1006. Rigler, L. G., and Heitzman, E. R.: Planigraphy in the differential diagnosis of the pulmonary nodule: with particular reference to the notch sign of malignancy. Radiology 65:692, 1955. — 15, 314

1007. Rigler, L. G., and Kelby, G. M.: Emphysema: an early roentgen sign of bronchogenic carcinoma. Radiology 49:578, 1947. — 4

1008. Rigler, L. G., and Merner, T. B.: Planigraphy in the diagnosis of bronchogenic carcinoma. Amer. J. Roentgen. 58:267, 1947. — 15, 269

1009. Rigler, L. G., O'Loughlin, B. J., and Tucker, R. C.: Significance of unilateral enlargement of the hilus shadow in the early diagnosis of carcinoma of the lung: with observations on a method of mensuration. Radiology 59:683, 1952. — 187

1010. Rigler, L. G., and Surprenant, E. L.: Pulmonary edema. Seminars in Roentgenology 2:33, 1967. — 299

1011. Rigos, F. J.: A roentgenographic study of pleural effusion. Radiology 36:568, 1941. — 354

1012. Riley, E. A., and Tennenbaum, J.: Pulmonary aspergilloma or intracavitary fungus ball: report of five cases. Ann. Intern. Med. 56:896, 1962. — 327

1013. Ringel, L.: Personal communication. — 453

1014. Rinker, C. T., Garrotto, L. J., Lee, K. R., and Templeton, A. W.: Bronchography: diagnostic signs and accuracy in pulmonary carcinoma. Amer. J. Roentgen. 104:802, 1968. — 269

1015. Rinker, C. T., and McGraw, J. P.: Cytomegalic inclusion disease in childhood leukemia. Cancer 20:36, 1967. — 301

1016. Ritvo, M., and Nikolaidis, D.: Roentgen diagnosis of air embolism due to criminal abortion. Amer. J. Roentgen. 88:119, 1962. — 395

1017. Rivkin, L. M., Read, R. C., Lillehei, C. W., and Varco, R. L.: Massive atelectasis of the left lung in children with congenital heart disease. J. Thoracic Surg. 34:116, 1957. — 94

1018. Robbins, L. L.: The roentgenological appearance of parenchymal involvement of the lung by malignant lymphoma. Cancer 6:80, 1953. — 304

1019. Robbins, L. L., and Hale, C. H.: The roentgen appearance of lobar and segmental collapse of the lung. Radiology 44:107, 1945; 45:120, 260, 347, 1945. — 24, 105, 107, 169

1020. Robbins, L. L., Hale, C. H., and Merrill, O. E.: The roentgen appearance of lobar and segmental collapse of the lung. I. Technic of examination. Radiology 44:471, 1945. — 11, 24, 38, 107

1021. Robertson, C. L., Schackelford, G. D., and Armstrong, J. D.: Chronic eosinophilic pneumonia. Radiology 101:57, 1971. — 301

1022. Robillard, G., Bertrand, R., Gregoire, H., Berdnikoff, G., and Favreau-Ethier, M.: Plasma cell pneumonia in infants: review of 51 cases. J. Canad. Assoc. Radiol. 16:161, 1965. — 301

1023. Robin, E. D., and Thomas, E. D.: Some relations between pulmonary edema and pulmonary inflammation (pneumonia). Arch. Intern. Med. 93:713, 1954.   301

1024. Rodman, T., Hurwitz, J. K., Pastor, B. H., and Close, H. P.: Cyanosis, clubbing and arterial oxygen unsaturation associated with Laennec's cirrhosis. Amer. J. Med. Sci. 238:534, 1959.   213

1025. Rogers, J. V., Jr., and Leigh, T. F.: Differential diagnosis of right cardiophrenic angle masses. Radiology 61:871, 1953.   419, 440

1026. Rogers, L. F., and Osmer, J. C.: Bronchogenic cyst: a review of 46 cases. Amer. J. Roentgen. 91:273, 1964.   419

1027. Roland, A. S., Merdinger, W. F., and Froeb, H. F.: Recurrent spontaneous pneumothorax: a clue to the diagnosis of histiocytosis X. New Eng. J. Med. 270:73, 1964.   339

1028. Ropes, M. W., and Castleman, B.: Talc pneumoconiosis. New Eng. J. Med. 276:972, 1967.   489

1028a. Rose, R. W., and Ward, B. H.: Spherical pneumonias in children simulating pulmonary and mediastinal masses. Radiology 106:179, 1973.   64

1029. Rosen, A., Vaudagna, J., and Jamplis, R. W.: Spontaneous pneumopericardium. Amer. Rev. Resp. Dis. 87:764, 1963.   395

1030. Rosen, S. H., Castleman, B., and Liebow, A. A.: Pulmonary alveolar proteinosis. New Eng. J. Med. 258:1123, 1958.   304

1031. Rosenbaum, H. D., Alavi, S. M., and Bryant, L. R.: Pulmonary parenchymal spread of juvenile laryngeal papillomatosis. Radiology 90:654, 1968.   133, 272

1032. Rosenbaum, H. D., Lieber, A., Hanson, D. J., and Bernard, J. D.: Roentgen findings in ventricular septal defect. Seminars in Roentgenology 1:47, 1966.   217

1033. Rosenow, E. C., III, DeRemee, R. A., and Dines, D. E.: Chronic nitrofurantoin pulmonary reaction: report of five cases. New Eng. J. Med. 279:1258, 1968.   344

1034. Rosenthal, D. S., and Weg, J. G.: Intrapulmonary lymph node presenting as a solitary pulmonary nodule: report of a case. Dis. Chest 51:336, 1967.   315

1035. Roshe, J.: Bronchovascular anomalies of the right upper lobe: an unusual case report and review of the literature. J. Thorac. Cardiovasc. Surg. 50:86, 1965.   153

1036. Rothstein, E.: Infected emphysematous bullae: report of 5 cases. Amer. Rev. Tuberc. 69:287, 1954.   349

1037. Rothstein, E., and Landis, F. B.: Infrapulmonary pleural effusion simulating elevation of the diaphragm. Amer. J. Med. 8:46, 1950.   354

1038. Rottenberg, L. A., and Golden, R.: Spontaneous pneumothorax: a study of 105 cases. Radiology 53:157, 1949.   392

1039. Rouvière, H.: Anatomie des lymphatiques de l'homme. Paris, Masson et Cie, 1932.   251, 254

1040. Rovida, F.: Degli ascessi extrapleurici. Radiol. Med. 27:768, 1940.   380

1041. Rowlands, D. T., Jr.: Fibroepithelial polyps of the bronchus: a case report and review of the literature. Dis. Chest 37:199, 1960.   133, 272

1042. Roy, P. H., Carr, D. T., and Payne, W. S.: The problem of chylothorax. Mayo Clin. Proc. 42:457, 1967.   21, 250

1043. Rubenstein, L., Gutstein, W. H., and Lepow, H.:   341

Pulmonary muscular hyperplasia (muscular cirrhosis of the lungs). Ann. Intern. Med. 42:36, 1955.

1044. Rubin, E. H.: Pulmonary lesions in "rheumatoid disease" with remarks on diffuse interstitial pulmonary fibrosis. Amer. J. Med. 19:569, 1955.   340

1045. Rubin, E. H.: The Lung as a Mirror of Systemic Disease. Springfield, Ill., Charles C Thomas, Publisher, 1956.   220

1046. Rubin, E. H., and Rubin, M.: The shrunken right middle lobe with reference to the so-called "middle lobe syndrome." Dis. Chest 18:127, 1950.   112

1047. Rubin, M., and Mishkin, S.: The relationship between mediastinal lipomas and the thymus. J. Thoracic Surg. 27:494, 1954.   395

1048. Rudhe, U., and Ozonoff, M. B.: Pneumomediastinum and pneumothorax in the newborn. Acta Radiol. (Diagn) 4:193, 1966.   370

1049. Rudhe, U., Whitley, J. E., and Herzenberg, H.: Mild pulmonary valvular stenosis studied functionally and anatomically. Acta Radiol. 57:161, 1962.   192

1050. Ruttley, M., and Mills, R. A.: Subcutaneous emphysema and pneumomediastinum in diabetic keto-acidosis. Brit. J. Radiol. 44:672, 1971.   392

1051. Salinger, H.: The roentgen examination of the mediastinal lung hernia with reference to tomography. Acta Radiol. 29:130, 1948.   105

1052. Salzman, E.: Lung Calcifications in X-Ray Diagnosis. Springfield, Ill., Charles C Thomas, Publisher, 1968.   474, 479, 486, 492

1053. Samet, P., and Anderson, W.: Pendular motion of the mediastinum. Amer. J. Med. 20:860, 1956.   5

1054. Samson, P. C., and Childress, M. E.: Primary neurofibrosarcoma of the diaphragm: report of two cases. J. Thoracic Surg. 20:901, 1950.   426

1055. Samuel, E.: Pneumomediastinography. Unpublished data.   21

1056. Samuels, M. L., Howe, C. D., Dodd, G. D., Jr., Fuller, L. M., Shullenberger, C. C., and Leary, W. L.: Endobronchial malignant lymphoma: report of five cases in adults. Amer. J. Roentgen. 85:87, 1961.   272

1057. Sanders, C. F.: Sexing by costal cartilage calcification. Brit. J. Radiol. 39:233, 1966.   452

1058. Sanders, D. E., Delarue, N. C., and Lau, G.: Angiography as a means of determining resectability of primary lung cancer. Amer. J. Roentgen. 87:884, 1962.   21

1059. Sanders, R. C.: Post-operative pleural effusion and subphrenic abscess. Clin. Radiol. 21:308, 1970.   351, 423

1060. Sanger, P. W., Taylor, F. H., and Robicsek, F. F.: Deformities of the anterior wall of the chest. Surg. Gynec. Obstet. 116:515, 1963.   453, 459

1061. Sappington, T. B., Jr., and Daniel, R. A., Jr.: Accessory diaphragm: a case report. J. Thoracic Surg. 21:212, 1951.   428

1062. Sargent, E. N.: Personal communication.   302

1063. Sargent, E. N., Balchum, E., Freed, A. L., and Jacobson, G.: Multiple pulmonary calcifications due to coccidioidomycosis. Amer. J. Roentgen. 109:500, 1970.   464, 484

1064. Sargent, E. N., Barnes, R. A., and Schwinn, C. P.: Multiple pulmonary fibroleiomyomatous hamartomas: report of a case and review of the literature. Amer. J. Roentgen. 110:694, 1970.   315

1065. Sargent, E. N., Carson, M. J., and Reilly, E. D.: 301
Roentgenographic manifestations of varicella
pneumonia with postmortem correlation. Amer.
J. Roentgen. 98:305, 1966.

1066. Sargent, E. N., and Sherwin, R.: Selective 289
wedge bronchography: pilot study in animals for
development of a proper technique. Amer. J.
Roentgen. 113:660, 1971.

1067. Sauer, R., Eugenidis, N., and Endrei, E.: Die 319
zystische Erscheinungsform maligner Tumoren
in der Lunge. Fortschr. Roentgenstr. 114:190,
1971.

1068. Scadding, J. G.: Pulmonary fibrosis and collagen 340
diseases of the lungs: a symposium. I. Clinical
problems of diffuse pulmonary fibrosis. Brit. J.
Radiol. 29:633, 1956.

1069. Scadding, J. G.: Calcification in sarcoidosis. 479
Proc. Tuberc. Res. Council 48:30, 1962.

1070. Scadding, J. G., and Wood, P.: Systolic clicks 395
due to left-sided pneumothorax. Lancet 2:1208,
1939.

1071. Scharf, J.: Aseptic cavitation in pulmonary in- 346
farction. Chest 59:456, 1971.

1072. Scheff, S., Bednarz, W. W., and Levene, G.: 386
Roentgenologic aspects of retropleural hema-
tomas following sympathectomy. Radiology
68:224, 1957.

1073. Scheff, S., and Laforet, E. G.: The internal thora- 463
cic muscle and the lateral chest roentgenogram.
Radiology 86:27, 1966.

1074. Scheibel, R. L., Dedeker, K. L., Gleason, D. F., 245
Pliego, M., and Kieffer, S. A.: Radiographic and
angiographic characteristics of pulmonary veno-
occlusive disease. Radiology 103:47, 1972.

1075. Schepers, G. W. H.: Lung disease caused by 340
inorganic and organic dust. Dis. Chest 44:133,
1963.

1076. Schinz, H. R., Baensch, W. E., Friedl, E., and 475
Uehlinger, E.: Roentgen-Diagnostics, Vol. III
(1st ed.). New York, Grune & Stratton, Inc.,
1953.

1077. Schinz, H. R., Baensch, W. E., Frommhold, W., 27
Glauner, R., Uehlinger, E., and Wellauer, J.
(Eds.): Roentgen Diagnosis, Vol. I. (2nd ed.).
New York, Grune & Stratton, Inc., 1968.

1078. Schissel, D. J., and Keil, P. G.: Further observa- 21, 255
tions on the diagnostic value of pulmonary
angiography in bronchiogenic carcinoma. Amer.
J. Roentgen. 67:51, 1952.

1079. Schlanger, P. M., and Schlanger, H.: Hydatid 327
disease and its roentgen picture. Amer. J.
Roentgen. 60:331, 1948.

1080. Schmidt, W. R.: Dilatation of major azygos vein 258
simulating a mediastinal tumor: a case report. J.
Thoracic Surg. 27:251, 1954.

1081. Schneider, H. J., and Felson, B.: Buckling of the 419
innominate artery simulating aneurysm and
tumor. Amer. J. Roentgen. 85:1106, 1961.

1082. Schneider, L.: Bronchopulmonary hypogenesis: 81
clinical and roentgenologic features in the adult,
with long follow up observations. Amer. J. Med.
Sci. 215:665, 1948.

1083. Schneider, L., and Wimpfheimer, F.: Multiple 489
progressive calcific pleural plaque formation: a
sign of silicosis. J.A.M.A. 189:328, 1964.

1084. Schnietz-Cliever, E.: Über das Vorkommen des 77
Lobus venae azygos des lenken Lungenseite.
Fortschr. Roentgenstr. 72:728, 1950.

1085. Schoch, G.: Das Silhouettezeichen. Fortschr.   **39**
Roentgenstr. 88:503, 1958.

1086. Schoenbaum, S. W.: Subepithelial endobron-   **272**
chial metastases. Presented at The Radiological
Society of North America meeting, Chicago,
1970.

1087. Schoenmackers, J., and Vieten, H.: Das postmor-   **21**
tale Angiogram der Lunge bei Tuberkulose, Sili-
kose und Bronchialkarzinom. Fortschr. Roentgenstr. 77:14, 1952.

1088. Scholtze, H., and St. Stender, H.: Roentgeno-   **143**
logical segmental diagnosis of localized pulmonary tuberculosis. Fortschr. Roentgenstr. 93:44,
1960.

1089. Schüller, H., Bolin, H., Linder, E., and Stenram,   **315**
U.: Tumor-forming amyloidosis of the lower respiratory system: report of a case in the lung and a
short review of the literature. Dis. Chest 42:58,
1962.

1090. Schwab, R. S., and Viets, H. R.: Roentgenoscopy   **267**
of the pharynx in myasthenia gravis before and
after prostigmine injection. Amer. J. Roentgen.
45:357, 1941.

1091. Schwartz, H.: Roentgen diagnosis of pleural me-   **374**
sothelioma (endothelioma): case report. Amer. J.
Roentgen. 63:530, 1950.

1092. Schwarz, J.: Histoplasmosis. *In* Lubarsch, O.,   **474, 484**
and Henke, F. (Eds.): Handbuch der Speziellen
Pathologischen Anatomie und Histologie. Berlin, Springer-Verlag, 1970.

1093. Schwarz, J., Baum, G. L., and Straub, M.: Cavi-   **328**
tary histoplasmosis complicated by fungus ball.
Amer. J. Med. 31:692, 1961.

1094. Scott, J. T.: Mediastinal emphysema and left   **392, 395**
pneumothorax. Dis. Chest 32:421, 1957.

1095. Scott, S. M., Peasley, E. D., and Crymes, T. P.:   **346**
Pulmonary sporotrichosis: report of two cases
with cavitation. New Eng. J. Med. 265:453,
1961.

1096. Selikoff, I. J., Churg, J., and Hammond, E. C.:   **374**
Asbestos exposure and neoplasia. J.A.M.A.
188:22, 1964.

1097. Seltzer, R. A.: Subpleural lipoma. Lancet 84:100,   **385, 386**
1964.

1098. Seltzer, R. A., Mills, D. S., Baddock, S. S., and   **419, 492**
Felson, B.: Mediastinal thymic cyst. Dis. Chest
53:186, 1968.

1099. Semple, T., and Lancaster, W. M.: Noisy pneu-   **395**
mothorax: observations based on 24 cases. Brit.
Med. J. 1:1342, 1961.

1100. Servelle, M., Bastin, R., Tricot, R., Andrieux, J.,   **20, 250**
Demangel, C., Poncey, J.-P.: Reflux du chyle
dans les lymphatiques pulmonaires. Gaz. Med.
France 75:6349, 1968.

1101. Servelle, M., Soulie, J., Andrieux, J., Cornu, C.,   **250**
Poncey, J.-P., Deloche, A., and Nussaume, O.:
Les lymphatiques du poumon cardiaque. Gaz.
Med. France 75:6365, 1968.

1102. Seybold, W. D., McDonald, J. R., Clagett, O. T.,   **419**
and Good, C. A.: Tumors of the thymus. J. Thora-
cic Surg. 20:195, 1950.

1103. Seybold, W. D., McDonald, J. R., Clagett, O. T.,   **383**
and Harrington, S. W.: Mediastinal tumors of
blood vascular origin. J. Thoracic Surg. 18:503,
1949.

1104. Shanks, S. C., and Kerley, P. (Eds.): A Textbook   **453**
of X-Ray Diagnosis, Vol. II (2nd ed.) Philadel-
phia, W. B. Saunders Co., 1951.

1105. Shapiro, J., et al.: Atypical pulmonary patterns of congestive failure in chronic lung disease. Presented at The Radiological Society of North America meeting, Chicago, 1969.   295

1106. Shapiro, R., Wilson, G., and Gabriele, O. F.: The roentgen-ray diagnosis of intrapulmonary lymph nodes. Dis. Chest. 51:621, 1967.   260

1107. Shapiro, W., Wilson, G. L., Yesner, R., and Shuman, H.: A useful roentgen sign in the diagnosis of localized bronchioloalveolar carcinoma. Amer. J. Roentgen. 114:516, 1972.   314

1108. Sharp, M. E., and Danino, E. A.: An unusual form of pulmonary calcification: "microlithiasis alveolaris pulmonum." J. Path. Bact. 65:389, 1953.   479

1109. Sheft, D. J., and Moskowitz, H.: Pulmonary muscular hyperplasia. Amer. J. Roentgen. 93:836, 1965.   341

1110. Sherrick, D. W., Kincaid, O. W., and DuShane, J. W.: Agenesis of a main branch of the pulmonary artery. Amer. J. Roentgen. 87:917, 1962.   189, 205

1111. Shields, D. O., Meador, R. S., DuBose, H. M., and Richburg, P. L.: Differential diagnosis of bronchogenic carcinoma and pneumonia in patients more than forty years old. Amer. Rev. Tuberc. 76:47, 1957.   97

1112. Shook, C. D., and Felson, B.: Inhalation bronchography. Chest 58:333, 1970.   16, 19, 267

1113. Shopfner, C. E., Jansen, C., and O'Kell, R. T.: Roentgen significance of the transverse thoracis muscle. Amer. J. Roentgen. 103:140, 1968.   463

1114. Short, D. S.: Radiology of the lung in severe mitral stenosis. Brit. Heart J. 17:33, 1955.   243, 246

1115. Siegal, W., Smith, A. R., and Greenburg, L.: The dust hazard in tremolite talc mining, including roentgenological findings in talc workers. Amer. J. Roentgen. 49:11, 1943.   377, 489

1116. Siegelman, S. S., Shanser, J. D., and Attai, L. A.: Cervical herniation of the lung associated with transient venous occlusion: report of a case. Dis. Chest 53:785, 1968.   463

1117. Sieniewicz, D. J., Martin, J. R., Moore, S., and Miller, A.: Rheumatoid nodules in the lung. J. Canad. Assoc. Radiol. 13:73, 1962.   315, 321

1118. Silverman, N. R., Borns, P. F., Goldstein, A. H., Greening, R. R., and Hope, J. W.: Thrombus calcification in the inferior vena cava: a specific roentgenologic entity. Amer. J. Roentgen. 106:97, 1969.   474

1119. Silverstein, C. M.: Pulmonary manifestations of leptospirosis. Radiology 61:327, 1953.   301

1120. Silverstein, C. M., and Mitchell, G. L., Jr.: Tuberous sclerosis: report of a case with unusual pulmonary manifestations. Amer. J. Med. 16:764, 1954.   341

1121. Simon, G.: Personal communication.   97, 143, 223

1122. Simon, G.: The x-ray appearances of acquired atelectasis of the upper lobes. J. Fac. Radiol. 1:223, 1950.   99, 112

1123. Simon, G.: Radiology and emphysema. Clin. Radiol. 15:293, 1964.   105, 169, 192, 309

1124. Simon, G.: The value of radiology in critical mitral stenosis. Clin. Radiol. 15:99, 1964.   76, 217

1125. Simon, G.: The cause and significance of some long line shadows in the chest radiograph. Proc. Roy. Soc. Med. 58:861, 1965.   78

1126. Simon, G.: Further observations on the long line shadow across a lower zone of the lung. Brit. J. Radiol. 43:327, 1970.   437

1127. Simon, G.: Principles of Chest X-Ray Diagnosis   **7, 107, 112, 344, 492**
      (3rd ed.). New York, Appleton-Century-Crofts,
      Inc., 1971.

1128. Simon, G., Bonnell, J., Kazantzis, G., and Waller,   **435**
      R. E.: Some radiological observations on the
      range of movement of the diaphragm. Clin. Ra-
      diol. 20:231, 1969.

1129. Simon, M.: The pulmonary veins in mitral sten-   **220**
      osis. J. Fac. Radiol. 9:25, 1958.

1130. Simon, M.: The radiologic assessment of pulmo-   **185, 216, 217**
      nary hemodynamics. *In* Simon, M., Potchen, E.
      J., and Le May, M. (Eds.): Frontiers of Pulmo-
      nary Radiology. New York, Grune & Stratton,
      Inc., 1969.

1131. Singleton, E. B., and Wagner, M. L.: Radiologic   **133, 142, 269, 272, 392**
      Atlas of Pulmonary Abnormalities in Children.
      Philadelphia, W. B. Saunders Co., 1971.

1132. Sisk, P. B.: Pulmonary thromboembolism: atypi-   **223**
      cal clinical and roentgen manifestations. Dis.
      Chest 47:539, 1965.

1133. Skarby, H. G.: Über die Diagnostik ex-   **386**
      trapleuraler Abszesse. Acta Radiol. 19:259, 1938.

1134. Skinner, D. B., Dreyfuss, J. R., and Nardi, G. L.:   **21**
      Azygography in the evaluation of operability of
      pulmonary carcinoma. New Eng. J. Med.
      267:232, 1962.

1135. Skorneck, A. B.: Roentgen aspects of Tietze's   **456**
      syndrome: painful hypertrophy of costal carti-
      lage and bone—osteochondritis? Amer. J.
      Roentgen 83:748, 1960.

1136. Smedal, M. I., and Lippincott, S. W.: Ex-   **386**
      trapleural fluid complicating thoracic and thora-
      columbar sympathectomy. Surg. Clin. N. Amer.
      30:829, 1950.

1137. Smith, A. R.: Pleural calcification resulting from   **377, 489**
      exposure to certain dusts. Amer. J. Roentgen.
      67:375, 1952.

1138. Smith, K. R., and Morris, J. F.: Reversible bron-   **98**
      chial dilatation: report of a case. Dis. Chest
      42:652, 1962.

1139. Smith, M. J.: Roentgenographic aspects of com-   **437**
      plete and incomplete pulmonary infarction. Dis.
      Chest 23:532, 1953.

1140. Smith, P. L., and Gerald, B.: Empyema in child-   **351**
      hood followed roentgenographically: decortica-
      tion seldom needed. Amer. J. Roentgen.
      106:114, 1969.

1141. Smith, R. A.: Some controversial aspects of intra-   **160**
      lobar sequestration of the lung. Surg. Gynec.
      Obstet. 114:57, 1962.

1142. Smith, W. W., and Rothermich, N. O.: Diffuse in-   **340**
      terstitial fibrosis complicating rheumatoid arthri-
      tis: report of a case. Ohio Med. J. 53:773, 1957.

1143. Sobin, S. S., Carson, M. J., Johnson, J. L., and   **192**
      Baker, C. R.: Pulmonary valvular stenosis with
      intact ventricular septum: isolated valvular sten-
      osis and valvular stenosis associated with inter-
      atrial shunt. Amer. Heart J. 48:416, 1954.

1144. Soila, P.: Geometric enlargement in radiopho-   **21**
      tography of schoolchildren. Acta Radiol. 1:1053,
      1963.

1145. Soll, E. L., and Bergeron, R. B.: Pulmonary cryp-   **379**
      tococcosis—a case diagnostically confirmed by
      transbronchial brush biopsy. Chest 59:454, 1971.

1146. Sorsdahl, O. A., and Powell, J. W.: Cavitary pul-   **21, 346**
      monary lesions following non-penetrating chest
      trauma in children. Amer. J. Roentgen. 95:118,
      1965.

1147. Sosman, M. C., Dodd, G. D., Jones, W. D., and Pillmore, G. U.: The familial occurrence of pulmonary alveolar microlithiasis. Amer. J. Roentgen. 77:947, 1957.   **305, 479**

1148. Soter, C.: The azygos vein as a cause of mediastinal widening and a diagnostic roentgenologic sign. Northwest Community Hosp. Bull., 1965.   **236**

1149. Soter, C., Berkmen, Y., Gür, H., Hadzidakis, A. A., and Gilmore, J. H.: Ossifying pneumonitis and calcinosis: report of a case. Acta Radiol. 54:195, 1960.   **475**

1150. Southard, M. E.: Roentgen findings in chickenpox pneumonia. Amer. J. Roentgen. 76:533, 1956.   **301**

1151. Spain, D. M.: Acute non-aeration of lung: pulmonary edema versus atelectasis. Dis. Chest 25:550, 1954.   **93**

1152. Spillane, J. D.: Four cases of diabetes insipidus and pulmonary disease. Thorax 7:134, 1952.   **339**

1153. Spitz, H. B.: Eisenmenger's syndrome. Seminars in Roentgenology 3:373, 1968.   **459**

1154. Spitz, H. B., and Felson, B.: Unpublished data.   **101**

1155. Sprunt, W. H., Peters, R. M., and Holder, D. L.: The significance of alterations in the lung arterial pattern. Radiology 73:1, 1959.   **230**

1156. Sreenivasan, B. R.: Broncho-pulmonary segments. Proc. Alum. Assoc. King Edward VII Coll. Med. 4:181, 1951. Abstracted in Amer. J. Roentgen. 68:994, 1952.   **97**

1157. Stankey, R. M.: Pulmonary agenesis and hypoplasia: a case report. Ohio Med. J. 64:449, 1968.   **81**

1158. Stankey, R. M., Roshe, J., and Sogocio, R. M.: Carcinoma of the lung and dysphagia. Dis. Chest 55:13, 1969.   **254**

1159. Stauffer, H. M., LaBree, J., and Adams, F. H.: The normally situated arch of the azygos vein: its roentgenologic identification and catheterization. Amer. J. Roentgen. 66:353, 1951.   **236**

1160. Stead, E. A., and Castleman, B.: Sarcoidosis with calcified nodes. New Eng. J. Med. 281:375, 1969.   **467**

1161. Stead, W. W., Kerby, G. R., Schlueter, D. P., and Jordahl, C. W.: The clinical spectrum of primary tuberculosis in adults: confusion with reinfection in pathogenesis of chronic tuberculosis. Ann. Intern. Med. 68:731, 1968.   **257**

1162. Stead, W. W., and Soucheray, P. H.: Physiologic studies following thoracic surgery. I. Immediate effects of thoracoplasty. J. Thorac. Surg. 23:453, 1952.   **433**

1163. Steel, S. J.: Hodgkin's disease of the lung with cavitation. Amer. Rev. Resp. Dis. 89:736, 1964.   **321, 346**

1164. Steele, R. W., and Copeland, G. A.: Delayed resorption of pulmonary alveolar fluid in the neonate. Radiology 103:637, 1972.   **301**

1165. Stein, G. H.: Pneumonic densities obscured by the cardiac shadow. Radiology 41:576, 1943.   **23**

1166. Stein, H. L.: Roentgen diagnosis of congenital absence of pectoralis muscles. Radiology 83:63, 1964.   **223, 463**

1167. Stein, I. F., and Elson, R.: Meigs' syndrome. Dis. Chest 14:722, 1948.   **446**

1168. Steinbach, H. L., and Johnstone, H. G.: The roentgen diagnosis of Armillifer infection (porocephalosis) in man. Radiology 68:234, 1957.   **474, 493**

1169. Steinbach, H. L., Keats, T. E., and Sheline, G. E.: The roentgen appearance of the pulmonary veins in heart disease. Radiology 65:157, 1955.   **201**

1170. Steinberg, I.: Anomalous pulmonary venous   87
drainage of right lung into inferior vena cava
with malrotation of the heart: report of three
cases. Ann. Intern. Med. 47:227, 1957.

1171. Steinberg, I.: Congenital absence of a main   189
branch of the pulmonary artery: report of three
new cases associated respectively with bronchiectasis, atrial septal defect and Eisenmenger's complex. Amer. J. Med. 24:559, 1958.

1172. Steinberg, I.: Roentgen diagnosis of anomalous   87
pulmonary venous drainage of right lung into inferior vena cava: report of three new cases.
Amer. J. Roentgen. 81:280, 1959.

1173. Steinberg, I.: Dilatation of the hemiazygos veins 236
in superior vena caval occlusion simulating mediastinal tumor. Amer. J. Roentgen. 87:248,
1962.

1174. Steinberg, I., Bluth, I., and Steger, B.: Idiopathic 421
diaphragmatic paralysis. Amer. J. Roentgen.
104:590, 1968.

1175. Steinberg, I., and Robb, G. P.: Mediastinal and   255
hilar angiography in pulmonary disease. Amer.
Rev. Tuberc. 38:557, 1938.

1176. Steinberg, I., and Stein, H. L.: Angiocar-   87
diography in diagnosis of agenesis of a lung.
Amer. J. Roentgen 96:991, 1966.

1177. Steinberg, I., and Watson, R. C.: Lymphangio-   460
graphic and angiographic diagnosis of persistent
jugular lymph sac: report of a case. New Eng. J.
Med. 275:1471, 1966.

1178. Steiner, R. E.: II. Radiological appearances of   216
the pulmonary vessels in pulmonary hyper-
tension. Brit. J. Radiol. 31:188, 1958.

1179. Steiner, R. E.: Radiology of pulmonary circula- 185, 217
tion. Amer. J. Roentgen. 91:249, 1964.

1180. Stengel, B. F., Watson, R. R., and Darling, R. J.: 315, 321
Pulmonary rheumatoid nodule with cavitation
and chronic lipid effusion. J.A.M.A. 198:1263,
1966.

1181. Stern, W. Z., and Bloomberg, A. E.: Idiopathic   236
azygos phlebectasis simulating mediastinal
tumor. Radiology 77:622, 1961.

1182. Stivelman, B. P., and Malev, M.: Rassmussen   327
aneurysm: its roentgen appearance: report of
case with necropsy. J.A.M.A. 110:1829, 1938.

1183. Storch, C. B.: Fundamentals of Clinical Fluoros-   1, 2
copy: With Essentials of Roentgen Interpreta-
tion. New York, Grune & Stratton, Inc., 1951.

1184. Storch, C. B.: Fundamental Aids in Roentgen   3
Diagnosis. New York, Grune & Stratton, Inc.,
1964.

1185. Storey, C. F.: Encapsulated pleural effusion sim- 360
ulating mediastinal tumor: report of two cases.
Radiology 58:408, 1952.

1186. Stout, A. P., and Himadi, G. M.: Solitary (local- 374
ized) mesothelioma of the pleura. Ann. Surg.
133:50, 1951.

1187. Straub, M., and Schwarz, J.: The healed primary 464, 475
complex in histoplasmosis. Amer. J. Clin. Path.
25:727, 1955.

1187a. Strieder, D. J., and Nash, G.: Dyspnea and bi-   301
lateral pulmonary infiltrates: pigeon breeder's
pneumonia. New Eng. J. Med. 287:92, 1972.

1188. Suwanik, R., and Harinsuta, C.: Pulmonary   474
paragonimiasis: an evaluation of roentgen findings in 38 positive sputum patients in an endemic area in Thailand. Amer. J. Roentgen.
81:236, 1959.

1189. Swaye, P., Van Ordstrand, H. S., McCormack, L. J., and Wolpaw, S. E.: Familial Hamman-Rich syndrome: report of eight cases. Dis. Chest 55:7, 1969.   338

1190. Sweany, H. C., Porsche, J. D., and Douglass, J. R.: Chemical and pathologic study of pneumonoconiosis, with special emphasis on silicosis and silicotuberculosis. Arch. Path. 22:593, 1936.   467

1191. Swingle, J. D., Logan, R., and Juhl, J. H.: Inversion of the left hemidiaphragm. J.A.M.A. 208:863, 1969.   433

1192. Swischuk, L. E.: Transient respiratory distress of the newborn (TRDN): a temporary disturbance of a normal phenomenon. Amer. J. Roentgen. 108:557, 1970.   301

1193. Sybers, R. G., Sybers, J. L., Dickie, H. A., and Paul, L. W.: Roentgenographic aspects of hemorrhagic pulmonary-renal disease (Goodpasture's syndrome). Amer. J. Roentgen. 94:674, 1965.   302

1194. Szelei, B., and Benedict, J.: Roentgenomorphological studies on Fleischner's plate-like atelectasis. Fortschr. Roentgenstr. 91:709, 1959.   436

1195. Szücs, S., Miskovits, G., and Gaál, J.: The presence of azygos lobes, proven by azygography. Radiol. Diag. 1:119, 1960.   77

1196. Tager, S. N.: Use of over-penetrated film technic in diagnosis of cavities. Radiology 39:389, 1942.   14

1197. Taguchi, J. T.: Obstructing calcified thrombus of the aortic isthmus: a diagnostic roentgenological appearance. Amer. J. Cardiol. 12:567, 1963.   474, 475

1198. Talner, L. B., Gmelich, J. T., Liebow, A. A., and Greenspan, R. H.: The syndrome of bronchial mucocele and regional hyperinflation of the lung. Amer. J. Roentgen. 110:675, 1970.   273

1199. Taybi, H.: Congenital malformations of the larynx, trachea, bronchi and lungs. *In* Kaufmann, H. J. (Ed.): Progress In Pediatric Radiology. Vol. 1. Respiratory Tract. Chicago, Year Book Medical Publishers, Inc., 1967.   81, 87, 135, 269

1200. Taybi, H., Kurlander, G. J., Lurie, P. R., and Campbell, J. A.: Anomalous systemic venous connection to the left atrium or to a pulmonary vein. Amer. J. Roentgen. 94:62, 1965.   213

1201. Taylor, D. A., and Jacobson, H. G.: Post-traumatic herniation of the lung. Amer. J. Roentgen. 87:896, 1962.   463

1202. Tchertkoff, V., Lee, B. Y., and Wagner, B. M.: Plasma cell granuloma of lung: case report and review of literature. Dis. Chest 44:440, 1963.   315

1203. Temple, H. L., and Evans, J. A.: The bronchopulmonary segments. Amer. J. Roentgen. 63:26, 1950.   147, 169

1204. Templeton, A. W., and Garrotto, L. J.: Acquired extracardiac causes of pulmonary ischemia. Dis. Chest 51:166, 1967.   223

1205. Templeton, A. W., Moffat, R., and Nelson, D.: Bronchography and bronchial adenomas. Chest 59:59, 1971.   272

1206. Teplick, J. G., Haskin, M. E., and Steinberg, S. B.: Changes in the main pulmonary artery segment following pulmonary embolism. Amer. J. Roentgen. 92:557, 1964.   192

1207. Theander, G.: Motility of diaphragm in children with bronchial foreign bodies. Acta Radiol. (Diagn) 10:113, 1970.   435

1208. Theros, E. G.: An exercise in radiologic-pathologic correlation. Radiology 91:807, 1968.   479

1209. Thomas, M. P., Storer, J., Goodsit, E., and   341
      Snearly, R.: Pulmonary muscular hyperplasia: a
      report of functional data in three cases with a
      brief review of the literature. Dis. Chest 51:1,
      1967.

1210. Thomas, T. V.: Nonparalytic eventration of the   421
      diaphragm. J. Thorac. Cardiovasc. Surg. 55:586,
      1968.

1211. Thomson, W. N.: Pulmonary changes in collagen   339
      diseases. Clin. Radiol. 14:451, 1963.

1212. Thurn, P., and Schaede, A.: Zur röntgenologis-   192
      chen Diagnose der angeborenen Herzfehler mit
      vorspringendem Pulmonalisbogen (Pseudofor-
      men). Fortschr. Roentgenstr. 79:476, 1953.

1213. Tillotson, J. R., and Lerner, A. M.: Character-   301
      istics of nonbacteremic pseudomonas pneumo-
      nia. Ann. Intern. Med. 68:295, 1968.

1214. Ting, Y. M.: Pulmonary parenchymal findings in   346
      blunt trauma to the chest. Amer. J. Roentgen.
      98:343, 1966.

1215. Titus, J. L., Harrison, E. G., Clagett, O. T., An- 315
      derson, M. W., and Knaff, L. J.: Xanthomatous
      and inflammatory pseudotumors of the lung.
      Cancer 15:522, 1962.

1216. Torelli, G.: Studio stratigraficodelle iper-   117
      chiarezze para-aortiche. Ann. Radiol. Diag.
      23:274, 1951.

1217. Tori, G., and Garusi, G. F.: The azygos vein arch 236
      and its valvular apparatus: angiographic obser-
      vations. Amer. J. Roentgen. 87:235, 1962.

1218. Torrance, D. J., Jr.: The Chest Film in Massive   223
      Pulmonary Embolism. Springfield, Ill., Charles
      C Thomas, Publisher, 1963.

1219. Tourniaire, A., Blum, J., Tartulier, M., and   339
      Dayrieux, F.: Coeur pulmonaire chronique sclér-
      odermique. Presse Méd. 72:2269, 1964.

1220. Townsend, J. B.: Lipid pneumonia (paraffinoma)   25
      of right middle lobe. New Eng. J. Med. 241:579,
      1949.

1221. Toye, D. K. M.: The thoracic cage. In Kaufmann,   459
      H. J. (Ed.): Progress in Pediatric Radiology. Vol.
      1. Respiratory Tract. Chicago, Year Book Medi-
      cal Publishers, Inc., 1967.

1222. Trackler, R. T., and Brinker, R. A.: Widening of   354
      the left paravertebral pleural line on supine
      chest roentgenograms in free pleural effusions.
      Amer. J. Roentgen. 96:1027, 1966.

1223. Trapnell, D. H.: The peripheral lymphatics of   243
      the lung. Brit. J. Radiol. 36:660, 1963.

1224. Trapnell, D. H.: Recognition and incidence of   260
      intrapulmonary lymph nodes. Thorax 19:44,
      1964.

1225. Trapnell, D. H.: Radiological appearance of   245
      lymphangitis carcinomatosa of the lung. Thorax
      19:251, 1964.

1226. Trapnell, D. H.: Septal lines in pneumoconiosis.   245
      Brit. J. Radiol. 37:805, 1964.

1227. Trapnell, D. H.: Septal lines in sarcoidosis. Brit. 245
      J. Radiol. 37:811, 1964.

1228. Trapnell, D. H.: Personal communication, 1971.

1229. Trapnell, D. H., and Thurston, J. G. B.: Unilat-   299
      eral pulmonary oedema after pleural aspiration.
      Lancet 1:1367, 1970.

1230. Troupin, R. H.: Ossifying bronchial carcinoid: a   484
      case report. Amer. J. Roentgen. 104:808, 1968.

1231. Tuazon, R. A., Firestone, F., and Blaustein, A.   315
      U.: Human pulmonary dirofilariasis manifesting
      as a "coin" lesion: a case report. J.A.M.A. 199:45,
      1967.

1232. Tucker, R. M., and Brown, A. L., Jr.: Goodpasture's syndrome: résumé of case. Mayo Clin. Proc. 43:449, 1968.   302

1233. Tuddenham, W. J.: Visual physiology of roentgen diagnosis: A. Basic concepts. Amer. J. Roentgen 78:116, 1957.   22, 42, 120

1234. Tuddenham, W. J.: Problems of perception in chest roentgenology: facts and fallacies. Radiol. Clin. N. Amer. 1:277, 1963.   22, 28

1235. Tuddenham, W. J., Hale, J., and Pendergrass, E. P.: Supervoltage diagnostic roentgenography: a preliminary report. Amer. J. Roentgen. 70:759, 1953.   255

1236. Tuffanelli, D. L., and Winkelmann, R. K.: Systemic scleroderma: a clinical study of 727 cases. Arch. Derm. 84:359, 1961.   339

1237. Twigg, H. L., de Leon, A. C., Perloff, J. K., and Majd, M.: The straight-back syndrome: radiographic manifestations. Radiology 88:274, 1967.   461

1238. UICC/Cincinnati classification of the radiographic appearances of pneumoconioses: a cooperative study by the UICC committee. Chest 58:57, 1970.   331, 474

1239. Unger, J. B., Fink, J. N., and Unger, G. F.: Pigeon breeder's disease: a review of the roentgenographic pulmonary findings. Radiology 90:683, 1968.   345

1240. Van Allen, C. M., and Lindskog, G. E.: Collateral respiration in the lung: rôle in bronchial obstruction to prevent atelectasis and to restore patency. Surg. Gynec. Obstet. 53:16, 1931.   180

1241. van Mierop, L. H. S.: Anatomy of the heart. Ciba Clin. Symposia 17:67, 1965.   39

1242. Vastine, J. H., II, Vastine, M. F., and Arango, O.: Genetic influence on osseous development with particular reference to the deposition of calcium in the costal cartilages. Amer. J. Roentgen. 59:213, 1948.   452

1243. Veeneklaas, G. M. H.: Pathogenesis of intrathoracic gastrogenic cysts. Amer. J. Dis. Child. 83:500, 1952.   330, 405

1244. Věšína, S.: Roentgenologic symptomatology of diaphragmatic tumors. Acta Radiol. Cancerol. Bohemoslov. 6:109, 1952.   426

1245. Viamonte, M., Jr.: Selective bronchial arteriography in man: preliminary report. Radiology 83:830, 1964.   231

1246. Viamonte, M., Jr.: Intrathoracic extracardiac shunts. Seminars in Roentgenology 2:342, 1967.   213, 230, 231, 232

1247. Viamonte, M., Jr., Parks, R. E., and Barrera, F.: Roentgenographic prediction of pulmonary hypertension in mitral stenosis. Amer. J. Roentgen. 87:936, 1962.   220

1248. Villar, T. G., Pimentel, J. C., and Avila, R.: Some aspects of pulmonary aspergilloma in Portugal. Dis. Chest 51:402, 1967.   327

1249. Villar, T. G., Pimentel, J. C., and E Costa, M. F.: The tumour-like forms of aspergillosis of the lung (pulmonary aspergilloma): a report of five new cases and a review of the Portuguese literature. Thorax 17:22, 1962.   492

1250. Viswanathan, R.: Pathogenesis of pulmonary atelectasis. Dis. Chest 15:460, 1949.   96, 97

1251. Vix, V. A., and Klatte, E. C.: The lateral chest radiograph in the diagnosis of hilar and mediastinal masses. Radiology 96:307, 1970.   189, 419

1252. Waddell, J. A., Simon, G., and Reid, L.: Bronchial atresia of the left upper lobe. Thorax 20:214, 1965.   273

1253. Walker, J. H.: Significance and demonstration of   25
      lobar and segmental pulmonary collapse. North-
      west Med. 48:241, 1949.

1254. Walls, W. L.: Lobe of the azygos vein occurring   76, 77
      on the left. Lancet 79:308, 1959.

1255. Walther, R., and Blaschke, B.: Differential diag-   223, 463
      nosis in unilaterally increased transparency of
      the lungs, caused by congenital defects of the
      major pectoral muscle. Fortschr. Roentgenstr.
      91:488, 1959.

1256. Walton, T. T., Jr.: Tietze's syndrome: a benign   456
      cause of chest pain. Med. Times 96:166, 1968.

1257. Wang, C. C., and Robbins, L. L.: Amyloid dis-   341
      ease: its roentgen manifestations. Radiology
      66:489, 1956.

1258. Ward, H. N., Lipscomb, T. S., and Cawley, L. P.:   299
      Pulmonary hypersensitivity reaction after blood
      transfusion. Arch. Intern. Med. 122:362, 1968.

1259. Ward, R., and Stalker, R.: Sheep cell agglutina-   340
      tion test in chronic interstitial pulmonary fi-
      brosis. Ann. Rheum. Dis. 24:246, 1965.

1260. Warner, W. P., and Graham, D.: Lobar atelec-   23, 107
      tasis as a cause of triangular roentgen shadows in
      bronchiectasis. Arch. Intern. Med. 52:888, 1933.

1260a. Warren, W. P.: Hypersensitivity pneumonitis   301
      due to exposure to budgerigars. Chest 62:170,
      1972.

1261. Watson, W. L., and Farpour, A.: Terminal bron-   304
      chiolar or "alveolar cell" cancer of the lung: two
      hundred sixty-five cases. Cancer 19:776, 1966.

1262. Weaver, E. J. M.: Acquired communication be-   366
      tween the pleural cavities: report of a case. Brit.
      J. Dis. Chest 54:353, 1960.

1263. Webb, W. A., and Thoroughman, J. C.: Solitary   315
      pulmonary nodule due to Brucella suis: report of
      a case. Dis. Chest 49:222, 1966.

1264. Webber, M. M., and O'Loughlin, B. J.: Varia-   72
      tions of the pleural vertical fissure line. Radio-
      logy 82:461, 1964.

1265. Weber, W. N., Margolin, F. R., and Nielsen, S.   305
      L.: Pulmonary histiocytosis X: a review of 18 pa-
      tients with reports of 6 cases. Amer. J. Roentgen.
      107:280, 1969.

1266. Weed, L. A., and Andersen, H. A.: Etiology of   465
      broncholithiasis. Dis. Chest 37:270, 1960.

1267. Weens, H. S., and Thompson, E. A.: The pulmo-   327
      nary air meniscus. Radiology 54:700, 1950.

1268. Weidman, W. H., and Kieffer, J.: Laminagraphy   15
      in chest conditions. Amer. Rev. Tuberc. 43:202,
      1941.

1269. Weill, H., Ferrans, V. J., Gay, R. M., and Ziskind, 305
      M. M.: Early lipoid pneumonia: roentgenologic,
      anatomic and physiologic characteristics. Amer.
      J. Med. 36:370, 1964.

1270. Weiner, M. A.: Chronic infiltrates of lung as-   304
      sociated with dyspnea. J.A.M.A. 205:581, 1968.

1271. Weinstein, A. S., and Mueller, C. F.: In-   492, 493
      trathoracic rib. Amer. J. Roentgen. 94:587, 1965.

1272. Weiss, W., Boucot, K. R., and Gefter, W. I.:   360
      Localized interlobar effusion in congestive heart
      failure. Ann. Intern. Med. 38:1177, 1953.

1273. Wells, J. A. T.: A left eparterial bronchus and a   81
      tri-lobed left lung: a case report. Dis. Chest
      37:129, 1960.

1274. Welsh, R. A., and Felson, B.: Uncomplicated   104
      dextroversion of the heart. Radiology 66:24,
      1956.

1275. Wenger, M. E., Dines, D. E., Ahmann, D. L.,   419 and Good, C. A.: Primary mediastinal choriocarcinoma. Mayo Clin. Proc. 43:570, 1968.

1276. Wesenberg, R. L., Graven, S. N., and McCabe, E. B.: Radiological findings in wet-lung disease. Radiology 98:69, 1971. 301

1277. Wesselhoeft, C. W., Jr., and Keshishian, J. M.: Acquired nonmalignant esophagotracheal and esophagobronchial fistulas. Ann. Thorac. Surg. 6:187, 1968. 269

1278. Westermark, N.: Importance of intra-alveolar pressure in the diagnosis of pulmonary diseases. Radiology 50:610, 1948. 7

1279. Westermark, N.: Roentgen Studies of the Lungs and Heart. Minneapolis, The University of Minnesota Press, 1948. 224

1280. Westfall, R. E.: Obliteration of segmental pulmonary artery borders: a method of localizing right lower lobe infiltrates. Dis. Chest 56:305, 1969. 39, 173

1281. Westgaard, T., and Keats, T. E.: Diffuse spasm and muscular hypertrophy of the lower esophagus. Radiology 90:1001, 1968. 409

1282. Westing, S. W.: Roentgenologic examination of the pharynx. Amer. J. Roentgen. 49:587, 1943. 267

1283. Westling, P., Sundberg, K., and Söderberg, G.: Systemic reticuloendothelial granuloma. Acta Radiol. Suppl. 149, 1957. 338

1284. Weston, W. J.: Left-sided lobe of the azygos vein. J. Fac. Radiol. 5:286, 1954. 77

1285. Westwood, L. A., and Levin, S.: The eosinophilic lung. Tubercle 32:98, 1951. 301

1286. Whalen, J. P., and Lane, E. J., Jr.: Bronchial rearrangements in pulmonary collapse as seen on the lateral radiograph. Radiology 93:285, 1969. 189

1287. Whalen, J. P., Meyers, M. A., Oliphant, M., Caragol, W., and Evans, J. A.: The retrosternal line: a new sign of an anterior mediastinal mass. In press. 463

1288. Whalen, J. P., and Shaheen, G. A.: Visualization of the subdiaphragmatic fat: an aid in the localization of the diaphragm. Brit. J. Radiol. 44:224, 1971. 447

1289. Whitaker, W., and Lodge, T.: The radiological manifestations of pulmonary hypertension in patients with mitral stenosis. J. Fac. Radiol. 5:182, 1954. 220

1290. Whitcomb, M. E., and Schwarz, M. I.: Pleural effusion complicating intensive mediastinal radiation therapy. Amer. Rev. Resp. Dis. 103:100, 1971. 351

1291. White, P. D., August, S., and Michie, C. R.: Hydrothorax in congestive heart failure. Amer. J. Med. Sci. 214:243, 1947. 359

1292. White, W. F., Saxton, H. M., and Dawson, I. M. P.: Pneumocystis pneumonia: report of three cases in adults and one in a child with a discussion of the radiological appearances and predisposing factors. Brit. Med. J. 2:1327, 1961. 301

1293. White, W. F., and Urquhart, W.: The demonstration of pulmonary lymphatics by lymphography in a patient with chylothorax. Clin. Radiol. 17:92, 1966. 21, 250

1294. Whitley, J. E., Rudhe, U., and Herzenberg, H.: Decreased left lung vascularity in congenital left to right shunts. Acta Radiol. 1:1125, 1963. 223

1295. Whittaker, L. D., Jr., Lynn, H. B., Dawson, B., and Chaves, E.: Hernias of the foramen of Bochdalek in children. Mayo Clin. Proc. 43:580, 1968. 440

1296. Wier, J. A.: Congenital anomalies of the lung.   **160**
Ann. Intern. Med. 52:330, 1960.

1297. Wigh, R., and Gilmore, F. R.: Solitary pulmonary   **379**
necrosis: a comparison of neoplastic and inflammatory conditions. Radiology 56:708, 1951.

1298. Wigh, R., and Montague, E. D.: Evaluation of in-   **260**
trapulmonic adenopathy in sarcoidosis. Radio-
logy 64:810, 1955.

1299. Wilder, C. E., and Lindgren, I.: Catheterization   **236**
and roentgen visualization of the azygos vein
and its tributaries in Laennec's cirrhosis: a new
technic. Radiology 79:953, 1962.

1300. Williams, A. W., Dunnington, W. G., and Berte,   **338, 339**
S. J.: Pulmonary eosinophilic granuloma: a clini-
cal and pathologic discussion. Ann. Intern. Med.
54:30, 1961.

1301. Williams, J. R., and Bonte, F. J.: Pulmonary dam-   **301**
age in nonpenetrating chest injuries. Radiol.
Clin. N. Amer. 1:439, 1963.

1302. Williams, J. R., and Stembridge, V. A.: Pulmo-   **302**
nary contusion secondary to nonpenetrating
chest trauma. Amer. J. Roentgen. 91:284, 1964.

1303. Williams, T. N., and Schreiber, M. H.: A schema   **299**
for roentgenographic diagnosis of disseminated
alveolar disease. Texas Med. 66:56, 1970.

1304. Willman, K. H.: Das Röntgenbild des "Mit-   **95**
tellappensyndroms." Fortschr. Roentgenstr.
76:346, 1952.

1305. Wilson, E. S., Jr., and McCarty, R. J.: Nitrofuran-   **246**
toin pneumonia. Amer. J. Roentgen. 103:540,
1968.

1306. Wilson, M. G., and Mikity, V. G.: A new form of   **313**
respiratory disease in premature infants. J. Dis.
Child. 99:489, 1960.

1307. Wilson, W.: Mucoid impaction of the bronchi.   **184, 273, 315**
Brit. J. Radiol. 37:590, 1964.

1308. Wilson, W. J., and Amplatz, K.: Unequal vascu-   **223**
larity in tetralogy of Fallot. Amer. J. Roentgen.
100:318, 1967.

1309. Wilt, K. E., Andrews, N. C., Meckstroth, C. V.,   **16, 269, 288**
Molnar, W., and Klassen, K. P.: The role of
bronchography in the diagnosis of bronchogenic
carcinoma. Dis. Chest 35:517, 1959.

1310. Winter, F. S.: Persistent left superior vena cava: **213**
survey of world literature and report of thirty
additional cases. Angiology 5:90, 1954.

1311. Wiot, J. F., Benton, C., and McAlister, W. H.:   **447**
Postoperative pneumoperitoneum in children.
Radiology 89:285, 1967.

1312. Wishart, D. L.: Normal azygos vein width in   **236**
children. Radiology 104:115, 1972.

1312a. Wisoff, C. P., and Felson, B.: Bronchography   **325**
with oily Dionosil. J. Thoracic Surg. 29:435,
1955.

1313. Witt, R. L., and Wiot, J. F.: Cinebronchography.   **16, 269**
In Tice-Harvey Practice of Medicine, Vol. II.
Hagerstown, Md., W. F. Prior Co., Inc., 1965.

1314. Witten, R. M., Fayos, J. V., and Lampe, I.: The   **409**
dorsal paraspinal mass in Hodgkin's disease.
Amer. J. Roentgen. 94:947, 1965.

1315. Wittenborg, M. H., and Aviad, I.: Organ influ-   **421**
ence on the normal posture of the diaphragm: a
radiological study of inversions and hetero-
taxies. Brit. J. Radiol. 36:280, 1963.

1316. Wittenborg, M. H., Gyepes, M. T., and Crocker,   **269**
D.: Tracheal dynamics in infants with respira-
tory distress, stridor, and collapsing trachea. Radiology 88:653, 1967.

1317. Woesner, M. E., Sanders, I., and White, G. W.:   306
The melting sign in resolving transient pulmonary infarction. Amer. J. Roentgen. 111:782,
1971.

1318. Wohl, G. T., and Shore, L.: Lesions of the car-   424
diac end of the stomach simulating carcinoma.
Amer. J. Roentgen. 82:1048, 1959.

1319. Wójtowicz, J.: Some tomographic criteria for an   205
evaluation of the pulmonary circulation. Acta
Radiol. (Diagn) 2:215, 1964.

1320. Wolfel, D. A., and Dennis, J. M.: Multiple mye-   457
loma of the chest wall. Amer. J. Roentgen.
89:1241, 1963.

1321. Wong, R. K. L.: Postoperative pulmonary atelec-   96
tasis. Dis. Chest 40:302, 1961.

1322. Wood, P.: Pulmonary hypertension. Mod. Conc.   215
Cardiovasc. Dis. 28:513, 1959.

1323. Woods, F. M., and Buente, L.: Extraperiosteal   433
Lucite ball plombage. Amer. Rev. Tuberc.
68:902, 1953.

1324. Wooldridge, W. E., and Hagemann, P. O.: Be-   446
nign pelvic tumors with ascites and hydrothorax:
Meigs' syndrome. Amer. J. Med. 5:237, 1948.

1325. Wright, J. T.: The radiological sign of "clicking"   395
pneumothorax. Clin. Radiol. 16:292, 1965.

1326. Wyatt, J. P., Fischer, V. W., and Sweet, H. C.:   288
The pathomorphology of the emphysema com-
plex. Amer. Rev. Resp. Dis. 89:533, 1964.

1327. Wychulis, A. R.: Acquired non-malignant eso-   269
phagotracheobronchial fistula. J.A.M.A. 196:117,
1966.

1328. Wyman, S. M.: Congenital absence of a pulmo-   189
nary artery: its demonstration by roentgenography. Radiology 62:321, 1954.

1329. Wyman, S. M., and Eyler, W. R.: Anomalous pul-   160
monary artery from the aorta associated with intrapulmonary cysts (intralobar sequestration of
lung): its roentgenologic recognition and clinical
significance. Radiology 59:658, 1952.

1330. Wyman, S. M., and Wilkins, E. W., Jr.: Angiocar-   255
diography as an aid to identification of nonresectable pulmonary carcinomas. J. Thoracic Surg.
35:452, 1958.

1331. Xalabarder, C.: What is atelectasis? Tubercle   97
30:266, 1949.

1332. Yamada, S.: Über die seröse Flüssigkeit in der   352
Pleurahöhle der gesunden Menschen. Z. Ges.
Exp. Med. 90:342, 1933.

1333. Yamamoto, K., and Sasaki, T.: Cinefluorographic   267, 285
observation of the tracheobronchial movements.
Dis. Chest 41:79, 1962.

1334. Young, B. R.: The value of body section   15
roentgenography (planigraphy) for the demonstration of tumors, non-neoplastic disease and
foreign bodies in the neck and chest. Amer. J.
Roentgen. 47:83, 1942.

1334a. Young, D. A., and Simon, G.: Certain move-   421, 435
ments measured on inspiration-expiration chest
radiographs correlated with pulmonary function
studies. Clin. Radiol. 23:37, 1972.

1335. Young, R. C., Bennett, J. E., Vogel, C. L., Car-   273, 328
bone, P. P., and DeVita, V. T.: Aspergillosis: the
spectrum of the disease in 98 patients. Medicine
49:147, 1970.

1336. Zawadowski, W.: Über die Schattenbildungen   453
an der Lungen-Weichteilgrenze. Fortschr.
Roentgenstr. 53:306, 1936.

1337. Zelefsky, M. N., Janis, M., Bernstein, R., Blatt,   163

C., Lin, A., and Meng, C-H.: Intralobar bronchopulmonary sequestration with bronchial communication. Chest 59:266, 1971.

1338. Zheutlin, N., Lasser, E. C., and Rigler, L. G.: Bronchographic abnormalities in alveolar cell carcinoma of the lung: a new diagnostic sign. Dis. Chest 25:542, 1954. 126

1339. Zil'berman, S. N.: Differential diagnosis of sequestral forms of pulmonary tuberculoma. Vestn. Rentgen. Radiol. 6:16, 1971. 327

1340. Zimmer, E. A.: Technique and Results of Fluoroscopy of the Chest. Springfield, Ill., Charles C Thomas, Publisher, 1954. 1

1341. Zinn, B., and Monroe, J.: The lordotic position in fluoroscopy and roentgenography of the chest. Amer. J. Roentgen. 75:682, 1956. 12

1342. Zintheo, C. J., Jr.: Auxiliary techniques in chest roentgenography. Amer. Rev. Tuberc. 37:14, 1938. 11

1343. Ziskind, M. M., George, R. B., and Weill, H.: Acute localized and diffuse alveolar pneumonias. Seminars in Roentgenology 2:49, 1967. 295, 301, 305, 336, 349

1344. Ziskind, M. M., Schwarz, M. I., George, R. B., Weill, H., Shames, J. M., Herbert, S. J., and Ichinose, H.: Incomplete consolidation in pneumococcal lobar pneumonia complicating pulmonary emphysema. Ann. Intern. Med. 72:835, 1970. 336, 349

1345. Ziskind, M. M., Weill, H., and Payzant, A. R.: The recognition and significance of acinus-filling processes of the lungs. Amer. Rev. Resp. Dis. 87:551, 1963. 295, 296, 301

1346. Zsebök, Z., Géher, F., Nagy, É. J., Török, I., and Wachtl, I.: Technic of Roentgenologic Investigations. New York, IMB Intercontinental Medical Book Corp., 1969. 7, 147, 435, 436

1347. Zylak, C. J.: Acute respiratory distress in adults. To be published. 344

INDEX